OXFORD MEDICAL PUBLICATIONS

Oxford Handbook of
**Expedition and
Wilderness Medicine**

Published and forthcoming Oxford Handbooks

Oxford Handbook for the Foundation Programme 4e
Oxford Handbook of Acute Medicine 3e
Oxford Handbook of Anaesthesia 3e
Oxford Handbook of Applied Dental Sciences
Oxford Handbook of Cardiology 2e
Oxford Handbook of Clinical and Laboratory Investigation 3e
Oxford Handbook of Clinical Dentistry 6e
Oxford Handbook of Clinical Diagnosis 3e
Oxford Handbook of Clinical Examination and Practical Skills 2e
Oxford Handbook of Clinical Haematology 3e
Oxford Handbook of Clinical Immunology and Allergy 3e
Oxford Handbook of Clinical Medicine – Mini Edition 8e
Oxford Handbook of Clinical Medicine 9e
Oxford Handbook of Clinical Pathology
Oxford Handbook of Clinical Pharmacy 2e
Oxford Handbook of Clinical Rehabilitation 2e
Oxford Handbook of Clinical Specialties 9e
Oxford Handbook of Clinical Surgery 4e
Oxford Handbook of Complementary Medicine
Oxford Handbook of Critical Care 3e
Oxford Handbook of Dental Patient Care
Oxford Handbook of Dialysis 3e
Oxford Handbook of Emergency Medicine 4e
Oxford Handbook of Endocrinology and Diabetes 3e
Oxford Handbook of ENT and Head and Neck Surgery 2e
Oxford Handbook of Epidemiology for Clinicians
Oxford Handbook of Expedition and Wilderness Medicine 2e
Oxford Handbook of Forensic Medicine
Oxford Handbook of Gastroenterology & Hepatology 2e
Oxford Handbook of General Practice 4e

Oxford Handbook of Genetics
Oxford Handbook of Genitourinary Medicine, HIV and AIDS 2e
Oxford Handbook of Geriatric Medicine 2e
Oxford Handbook of Infectious Diseases and Microbiology
Oxford Handbook of Key Clinical Evidence
Oxford Handbook of Medical Dermatology
Oxford Handbook of Medical Imaging
Oxford Handbook of Medical Sciences 2e
Oxford Handbook of Medical Statistics
Oxford Handbook of Neonatology
Oxford Handbook of Nephrology and Hypertension 2e
Oxford Handbook of Neurology 2e
Oxford Handbook of Nutrition and Dietetics 2e
Oxford Handbook of Obstetrics and Gynaecology 3e
Oxford Handbook of Occupational Health 2e
Oxford Handbook of Oncology 3e
Oxford Handbook of Ophthalmology 3e
Oxford Handbook of Oral and Maxillofacial Surgery
Oxford Handbook of Orthopaedics and Trauma
Oxford Handbook of Paediatrics 2e
Oxford Handbook of Pain Management
Oxford Handbook of Palliative Care 2e
Oxford Handbook of Practical Drug Therapy 2e
Oxford Handbook of Pre-Hospital Care
Oxford Handbook of Psychiatry 3e
Oxford Handbook of Public Health Practice 3e
Oxford Handbook of Reproductive Medicine & Family Planning 2e
Oxford Handbook of Respiratory Medicine 3e
Oxford Handbook of Rheumatology 3e
Oxford Handbook of Sport and Exercise Medicine 2e
Handbook of Surgical Consent
Oxford Handbook of Tropical Medicine 4e
Oxford Handbook of Urology 3e

Oxford Handbook of
Expedition and
Wilderness Medicine

2nd edition

Dr Chris Johnson

Consultant Anaesthetist, North Bristol NHS Trust, Westbury-on-Trym, Bristol, UK

Dr Sarah R. Anderson

Consultant in Health Protection, Public Health England, London, UK

Dr Jon Dallimore

GP and Specialty Doctor, Emergency Medicine, Bristol Royal Infirmary, Bristol, UK

Professor Chris Imray

Consultant Vascular and Renal Transplant Surgeon, Warwick Medical School and University Hospital Coventry and Warwickshire NHS Trust, UK

Shane Winser

Geography Outdoors: the centre supporting field research, exploration and outdoor learning, Royal Geographical Society (with IBG), London, UK

Mr James Moore

Director and Nurse Specialist, Travel Health Consultancy, Exeter, UK

Professor David A. Warrell

International Director, Royal College of Physicians; Emeritus Professor of Tropical Medicine, University of Oxford, UK

OXFORD
UNIVERSITY PRESS

OXFORD
UNIVERSITY PRESS

Great Clarendon Street, Oxford, OX2 6DP,
United Kingdom

Oxford University Press is a department of the University of Oxford.
It furthers the University's objective of excellence in research, scholarship,
and education by publishing worldwide. Oxford is a registered trade mark of
Oxford University Press in the UK and in certain other countries

© Oxford University Press 2015

The moral rights of the authors have been asserted

First Edition published 2008
Second Edition published 2015

Published in the United States of America by Oxford University Press
198 Madison Avenue, New York, NY 10016, United States of America

British Library Cataloguing in Publication Data
Data available

Library of Congress Control Number: 2015934834

ISBN 978-0-19-968841-8

Printed and bound in China by
C&C Offset Printing Co., Ltd.

Oxford University Press makes no representation, express or implied, that the
drug dosages in this book are correct. Readers must therefore always check
the product information and clinical procedures with the most up-to-date
published product information and data sheets provided by the manufacturers
and the most recent codes of conduct and safety regulations. The authors and
the publishers do not accept responsibility or legal liability for any errors in the
text or for the misuse or misapplication of material in this work. Except where
otherwise stated, drug dosages and recommendations are for the non-pregnant
adult who is not breast-feeding

Links to third party websites are provided by Oxford in good faith and
for information only. Oxford disclaims any responsibility for the materials
contained in any third party website referenced in this work.

Preface

Wilderness: 'a tract of solitude and savageness'
(*A Dictionary of the English Language*, Samuel Johnson, 1755)

Should the urge to explore, enjoy, and carry out research in wilderness environments be constrained in any way by issues of health, safety, the environment, and the well-being of the local inhabitants? We think it should, but please read on.

Expedition medicine (known in North America as 'wilderness medicine') is concerned with maintaining physical and psychological health under the stresses and challenges of expeditions to remote and challenging places. Its aim is to encourage adventure but, at the same time, to attempt to minimize the risk of trauma and disease by proper planning, preventive measures such as vaccinations, the acquisition of relevant medical skills and sensible behaviour. Responsible attitudes towards the environment and the welfare of indigenous peoples and other local helpers in the area of travel are also of great importance.

This book is a product of the Royal Geographical Society (with IBG) Expedition Medicine Cell, which was formed to provide medical advice to RGS-IBG expeditions and those seeking advice from the Society. In it, we have collected and summarized the experience and skills accumulated by explorers, expeditioners, researchers, and remote area travellers from all around the world.

The first edition, published in 2008, was designed to be a practical and portable guide to the prevention and treatment of those medical problems most likely to be encountered in extreme and remote environments. We are delighted that it proved so popular and has been used during the course of expeditions by doctors, nurses, paramedics, and first-aiders, as well as by non-medical expedition members.

The second edition builds upon this foundation, but includes additional topics. Since prevention of disease and accident is fundamental to working in remote and potentially hazardous areas, the sections on risk management have been expanded. To help decision-making, we include more treatment algorithms. We recognize that travel in remote areas is no longer limited to the young, fit, and experienced traveller.

Historically, exploration and wilderness travel have proved distinctly dangerous. Admiral Anson circumnavigated the globe in 1741–1742, losing five of his six ships and 626 of his 961 crew, a disaster eventually mitigated by the capture of a Spanish treasure ship which left him and his surviving sailors wealthy men. All 124 members of Sir John Franklin's ill-fated voyage to the North-West passage died. During Stanley's great trans-Africa expedition from Zanzibar to the Congo (1874–1847), 114 of his original 228 expedition members died from battle, murder, smallpox, dysentery, drowning, crocodile attack, fever, execution, insanity, getting lost, or falling victim to cannibalism, opium, or starvation. This level of expedition mortality was unacceptable even in those days, and led to Stanley being branded a ruthless and irresponsible leader. The twentieth century saw safety improve and mortality fall, but until the 1980s 1% of Antarctic base members died of accident or disease, while for every ten climbers who summited Everest, one person died on the mountain.

The twenty-first century has seen a vast increase in numbers of people visiting remote areas for research, education, and recreation. In 2010, over 400,000[1] UK nationals booked an 'adventure' holiday; during the 2012–2013 season, more than 25,000 tourists landed on Antarctica,[2] while on one day, 19 May 2012, 234 climbers summited Everest. With few un-trodden places remaining, the predominant aim of expeditions has shifted from discovery and sovereign possession in the nineteenth century to geographical and scientific investigation in the twentieth century, and has now added pleasure, personal development, and cultural exchange in the twenty-first. Travellers still find novel ways to fuel their desire for adventure; participation in extreme sporting and endurance challenges is increasing rapidly. Gap-year adventure is acquainting school leavers and their anxious parents with some of the realities of wilderness travel. The commercial opportunities have resulted in the marketing of adventurous journeys by numerous companies, blurring the distinction between an expedition and a leisure activity, and exposing people to physical and psychological hazards for which they may be unprepared. Explicit standards such as British Standard 8848: a specification for the provision of visits, fieldwork, expeditions, and adventurous activities, outside the United Kingdom set out good practice for organizing ventures and seek to optimize planning and risk management.

Many of the hazards encountered by previous generations of explorers still challenge expeditions in the twenty-first century, but we are now in a radically stronger position to minimize risk through careful planning based on a vast fund of physiological research, medical knowledge, and the development of drugs, vaccines, technology, and skills. Since our last edition was written, the advent of the smart phone, tablet, and e-reader have altered the way we access knowledge, while cellular and satellite networks link us to the Internet from previously isolated locations. Video communication with remote research stations in space or the heart of Antarctica may be only two mouse clicks away from a computer anywhere in the world. We expect a significant proportion of our future sales to be in electronic format.

Increasingly, doctors and other clinicians expect to receive appropriate training to equip themselves for new challenges. A number of organizations have produced competency-based syllabuses for expedition or wilderness medicine. We have tried to structure the book so that it covers most of the topics included in these courses.

1 http://www.apassporttoadventure.com/assets/pdf/adventure_050110.pdf

2 http://www.iaato.org/documents/10157/346545/touristsbynationality_landed.pdf/bd1e0d3c-ccb8-4b24-a552-b45c09d26a00

We hope that this handbook will encourage many people to experience and enjoy expeditions and wilderness travel in a responsible way, and to identify and minimize avoidable risks without allowing these concerns to detract from the essential excitement and sense of achievement.

Chris Johnson
Sarah R. Anderson
Jon Dallimore
Chris Imray
Shane Winser
James Moore
David A. Warrell

April 2015

Foreword

If an expedition team in a remote region includes a key member who is prone to cardiac trouble, common sense would suggest that they take a portable defibrillator with them. But there are those who would scoff at this . . . 'Why not take an X-ray machine and portable Intensive Care Unit, too?' This cynical point of view being that too much medical cover detracts from the very nature of a true wilderness expedition.

I once found myself, by myself, hauling a sledge towards the South Pole some 400 miles from the nearest human when the extreme pain of a kidney stone attack hit me without warning. Twenty years earlier, I would have been in terminal panic for, in those days, I usually spurned any medical cover beyond a very basic first-aid pack. But Doctor Mike Stroud had, on this occasion, furnished me with an extensive array of painkillers, antibiotics, and a mini handbook of instructions to cope with all likely and various less-likely ailments. So I was able to keep the agony of the stones at bay for the time it took to contact a ski-plane, and I was more than a little grateful for Mike's handbook and carefully thought out medical supplies.

Some years later, at 28,000 feet up the Tibetan side of Everest, the wire stitches that had held my chest-cage in position since a recent by-pass operation, suddenly felt as though they were tearing into and tightening my chest and lungs. Another heart attack, I realized, was imminent, and I grabbed for the glyceryl trinitrate (GTN) tablets which my wife had made me carry at all times on the climb. Thanks to their immediate 'dilating' effect, I survived the ensuing hasty midnight retreat back down to Base Camp, but a Scottish climber died of a heart attack at the same altitude the following night. He carried no GTN tablets, for he had no cardiac history.

If you can travel with a doctor, so much the better, but not everyone has that luxury. Full insurance cover is vital, and for Antarctica these days the Foreign Office Polar Department will, upfront, need to see proof that you have such cover.

The authors of this Handbook have all experienced travel in wild, remote parts of the world and have learnt the hard way exactly what level of medical knowledge and supplies should be available to anyone or any group heading beyond the response reach of a 999 call.

Ranulph Fiennes
Expedition Leader
Exmoor, Somerset

2015

Dedication

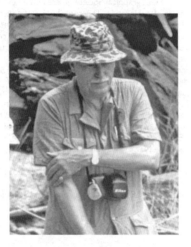

Dr Bent Einer Juel-Jensen (1922–2006)

MA, DM (Cand. Med. Copenhagen) FRCP,
MRCGP, HonFRGS

This book is dedicated to the memory of our late very dear friend Bent Juel-Jensen who stimulated, encouraged, and supported us together with generations of other young explorers and expeditioners at the Royal Geographical Society and the University of Oxford. He was the archetypal and model expedition medical officer.

Born in Odense, Denmark, Bent qualified in medicine in Copenhagen in 1949 but spent the rest of his life based in Oxford with his devoted wife Mary. At New College he studied physiology and Elizabethan literature and later became a loyal Fellow of St Cross College. His medical career began at the Radcliffe Infirmary with Dr Fred Hobson and Professor George Pickering, working on hypertension. In 1960, he became hospital Medical Officer and, from 1977 to 1990, University Medical Officer. Bent took charge of infectious diseases in Oxford and pioneered the treatment of herpes zoster with antiviral drugs. Many of his protégés became consultants or professors of infectious diseases.

Bent's greatest enthusiasm was exploration and expeditions. He was passionately committed to the Oxford University Exploration Club, eventually becoming its Honorary President. Bent greatly improved the medical preparedness and training of its largely undergraduate members and was the inspiration, advisor, and friend to many budding young explorers, including the editors of this Handbook. Pharmaceutical companies were pressurized into donating essential drugs for their medical kits. As founding medical advisor to the Royal Geographical Society he created a new awareness of the medical aspects of exploration. This contribution was recognized by his election to an Honorary Fellowship. The RGS-NMK Kora Research Project (Tana River, Kenya) in 1983 had Bent as its energetic medical officer. He was friend and advisor to many famous explorers and travellers, the likes of Sir Wilfred Thesiger, Sir Vivian Fuchs, and Bruce Chatwin.

After England and Denmark, Bent's favourite country was Ethiopia. Oxford expeditions to explore the rock-hewn churches of Tigre in 1973 and 1974 resulted in his forming a close friendship with the local ruler, Prince Ras Mangashia. Bent's enthusiasm for Ethiopia stimulated him to learn Amharic and the priests' language Ge'ez, to embrace its history, literature, culture, and food. He always carried his own supply of fiery berbera to ignite tame European dishes. His great physical courage, early displayed in his resistance to the Nazis in wartime Copenhagen, was again very much to the fore as he gave medical support across the Sudanese border to the Ethiopian Democratic Union's army battling the evil despot Mengistu Haile Mariam.

Bent Juel-Jensen, what an incredible man and a marvellous friend for all seasons!

Contents

Contributors *xiii*

Contributors to the first edition *xvii*

Symbols and abbreviations *xix*

1	Expedition medicine	1
2	Preparations	15
3	Caring for people in the field	81
4	Ethics and responsibilities	111
5	Crisis management	133
6	Emergencies: diagnosis	169
7	Emergencies: trauma	179
8	Emergencies: collapse and serious illness	211
9	Treatment: skin	265
10	Treatment: head and neck	299
11	Treatment: dental	337
12	Treatment: chest	369
13	Treatment: abdomen	383
14	Treatment: limbs and back	415
15	Treatment: infectious diseases	455
16	Psychological and psychiatric problems	515
17	Risks from animals	541
18	Plants and fungi	577
19	Anaesthesia in remote locations	585
20	Cold climates	607
21	Mountains and high altitude	637
22	Inland and coastal waters	675
23	Offshore	701

24 Underwater 72!

25 Hot, dry environments: deserts 74!

26 Hot, humid environments: tropical forest 76

27 Caving 78

28 Medical kits 79

Index *813*

Contributors

Dr Edi Albert
Senior lecturer in Remote
and Polar Medicine, and Rural
Generalist in Emergency Medicine,
University of Tasmania, Hobart,
Tasmania, Australia; Director,
Wilderness Education Group

Sarah R. Anderson
Consultant in Health Protection,
Public Health England, London, UK

Dr Kristina Birch
Consultant in Anaesthetics &
Intensive Care Medicine, North
Bristol NHS Trust UK

Dr Jules Blackham
Consultant Emergency Physician
& HEMS consultant, North Bristol
NHS Trust & Great Western Air
Ambulance, UK

Dr Jim Bond
Specialist in Travel & Expedition
Medicine, TrExMed Travel Clinic,
Edinburgh, UK

Dr Spike Briggs
Consultant in Intensive Care &
Anaesthesia, Poole Hospital NHS
Foundation Trust; Director of
Medical Support Offshore Ltd, UK

Tim Campbell-Smith
Consultant General & Colorectal
Surgeon, Surrey & Sussex NHS
Healthcare Trust UK

Mr Alistair R. M. Cobb
Consultant Oral & Maxillofacial
Surgeon, Southwest Regional Cleft
Service, Bristol, UK

Dr Robert Conway
Anaesthetist and Expedition Doctor,
Wild Medic Ltd, Brighton, UK

Dr Paul Cooper
Consultant Neurologist, Greater
Manchester Neuroscience Centre,
Salford Royal Foundation Trust,
UK

Dr Rachael Craven,
Consultant Anaesthetist, University
Hospitals, Bristol, UK

Jon Dallimore
GP, and Specialty Doctor in
Emergency Medicine, Bristol Royal
Infirmary, UK

Dr Claire Davies
Travel health doctor/GP,
InterHealth Worldwide, London,
UK

Dr Ian Davis
GP & Polar Explorer, UK

Dr Richard Dawood
Medical Director, Fleet Street
Clinic, London, UK

Dr Sundeep Dhillon
Honorary Research Fellow, Centre
for Altitude, Space & Extreme
Medicine (CASE), Institute of
Sport, Exercise & Health, London,
UK

Dr Rose Drew
Registrar in Anaesthesia &
Intensive Care Medicine, Sheffield
School of Anaesthesia, UK

Dr Matthew Dryden
Director of Infection, Rare &
Imported Pathogens Department,
Public Health England, Porton,
Hampshire Hospitals NHS
Foundation Trust & Southampton
School of Medicine, UK

Dr Linda Dykes
Consultant in Emergency Medicine, Ysbyty Gwynedd, Bangor, Wales, UK

Jonathan Ferguson
Consultant Cardiothoracic Surgeon, The James Cook University Hospital, Middlesbrough, UK

Prof Karen Forbes
Professorial Teaching Fellow & Consultant in Palliative Medicine, University of Bristol, UK

Prof Larry Goodyer
Head of the Leicester School of Pharmacy, De Montfort University, Leicester, UK

Paul F. Goodyer
CEO and Founder of Nomad Travel Stores and Travel Clinics, Enfield, UK

Penelope B. Granger
General dental practitioner, BASMU, Derriford Hospital, Plymouth, UK; Norrbottens Läns Landsting, Sweden

Rebecca Harris
Freelance TV Producer, London, UK

Peter Harvey
Risk Management Specialist, Hampshire, UK

Dr Debbie Hawker
Clinical Psychologist, InterHealth Worldwide, London, UK

Dr Amy Hughes
Clinical Lecturer in Emergency Response, Humanitarian & Conflict Response Institute, University of Manchester, UK

Prof Chris Imray
Consultant Vascular and Renal Transplant Surgeon, Warwick Medical School and University Hospital Coventry and Warwickshire NHS Trust, UK

Chris Johnson
Consultant Anaesthetist, North Bristol NHS Trust, Westbury-on-Trym, Bristol, UK

Clive Johnson
Polarsphere, Polar Logistics, Buxton, UK

Stephen Jones
Operations Manager, Antarctic Logistics & Expeditions LLC, UK

Burjor K. Langdana
General & Expedition Dental Practitioner, General Dental Practitioner Leeds, Dentist to British Antarctic Survey Medical Unit, UK

Dr Jonathan Leach
General Practitioner, Bromsgrove, UK

Dr Campbell MacKenzie
Specialist in remote and offshore medicine, Bristol, UK

Dr Carey M. McLellan
Extended Scope Physiotherapist in Emergency Care, University Hospitals, Bristol, UK

Iain McIntosh
Travel Health Consultant, St Ninians Travel Health Research Centre, Stirling, UK

Dr Alastair Miller
Consultant Physician (Infectious diseases), Royal Liverpool University Hospital & University of Liverpool, UK

James Moore
Director and Nurse Specialist, Travel Health Consultancy, Exeter, UK

Clare Morgan
Sexual Health Adviser, University Hospitals, Bristol, UK

Dr Paddy Morgan
Consultant Anaesthetist, North Bristol NHS Trust, Westbury-on-Trym, Bristol, UK

Mr Daniel S. Morris
Consultant Ophthalmologist, Cardiff Eye Unit, University of Wales, UK

Annabel H. Nickol
Clinical Lecturer in Respiratory and General Medicine, Oxford Centre for Respiratory Medicine, UK

Dr Howard Oakley
Associate Specialist in Environmental Medicine, Institute of Naval Medicine, Alverstoke, UK

Prof Andrew J. Pollard
Professor of Paediatric Infection & Immunity, Dept. of Paediatrics, University of Oxford, UK

Lt Col Harvey Pynn
Consultant in Emergency Medicine & Pre-hospital care, University Hospitals, Bristol; Medical Director, Wilderness Medical Training, UK

Paul Richards
General Practitioner & Travel Medicine Specialist. Honorary Lecturer, Centre for Altitude, Space & Extreme Medicine (CASE), UCL, London, UK

Barry Roberts
Director, Wilderness Medical Training, UK

George W. Rodway
Assistant Professor, Division of Health Sciences, University of Nevada, Reno, NV, USA

Prof Marc Shaw
Travel and Geographical Medicine Consultant; Professor, School of Public Health, James Cook University, Townsville, Medical Director, Worldwise Travellers Health Centres, New Zealand

Julian Thompson
Specialist Registrar in Anaesthesia & Intensive Care, Oxford University Hospitals, UK

Dr Lesley F. Thomson
Consultant Anaesthetist, Derriford Hospital, Plymouth, UK

Andrew Thurgood
Consultant Nurse—Prehospital Emergency Medicine, Mercia Accident Rescue Service & West Midlands CARE Team, UK

Prof David A. Warrell
International Director, Royal College of Physicians; Emeritus Professor of Tropical Medicine, University of Oxford, UK

Dr Andy Watt
Consultant Physician, Ayrshire and Arran NHS, UK

Dr Jane Wilson-Howarth
GP, and Medical Director, Travel Clinic Ltd., Cambridge & Ipswich, UK

Dr Jeremy Windsor
Consultant in Anaesthesia & Intensive Care, Chesterfield Royal Hospital, Derbyshire, UK

Shane Winser
Geography Outdoors: the centre supporting field research, exploration and outdoor learning, Royal Geographical Society (with IBG), London, UK

Contributors to the first edition

Mr James Calder
Trauma and Orthopaedic Consultant, North Hampshire Hospital, and Clinical Senior Lecturer, Imperial College, London, UK

Dr Charles Clarke
Honorary Consultant Neurologist, National Hospital for Neurology & Neurosurgery, Queen Square, London, UK and President of the British Mountaineering Council, UK

David Geddes
Dental Surgeon

Dr Mike Grocott
Senior Lecturer in Intensive Care Medicine, Centre for Altitude Space and Extreme Environment Medicine, UCL Institute of Human Health and Performance, London, UK

Dr Stephen Hearns
Consultant in Emergency Medicine, Lead Consultant Emergency Medical Retrieval Service, Royal Alexandra Hospital Paisley, UK

Dr Michael E. Jones
Consultant Physician, Regional Infectious Diseases Unit, Western General Hospital, Edinburgh, UK & HealthLink360 Edinburgh International Health Centre Carberry, Musselburgh, UK

Akbar Lalani

Christina Lalani

Nick Lewis

Prof David Lockey
Prof of Trauma and pre-hospital Emergency Medicine, North Bristol NHS Trust, UK

Prof Hugh Montgomery
Director, Institute for Human Health & Performance, University College London, UK

Dr Christopher Moxon
Research Associate, Malawi-Liverpool-Wellcome Clinical Research Programme, Honorary Paediatric Registrar, College of Medicine, Malawi

Prof Ian Palmer
Professor of Military Psychiatry, Head of Medical Assessment Programme, MoDUK, St Thomas' Hospital, London, UK

Dr Andy Pitkin
Department of Anesthesiology, University of Florida, Gainesville, Florida, USA

Dr Tariq Qureshi
Department of Emergency Medicine, John Radcliffe Hospital, Oxford Radcliffe Hospitals, NHS Trust, UK

Dr Charlie Siderfin
General Practitioner, Heilendi Family Medical Practice, Kirkwall, Orkney, UK

Dr Joe Silsby
Consultant in Anaesthesia and
ICM Taunton and Somerset NHS
Foundation Trust, UK

James Watson
Physiotherapy Officer, Medical
Support Unit, Headquarters,
Hereford Garrison, UK

Symbols and abbreviations

➔	cross-reference
>	greater than
<	less than
~	approximately
ABC	airway, breathing, circulation
ACE	angiotensin-converting enzyme
ACL	anterior cruciate ligament (knee)
ADL	activities of daily living (disability)
AED	automated external defibrillator
AIDS	acquired immune deficiency syndrome
AMS	acute mountain sickness
AMTS	Abbreviated Mental Test Score
ARDS	acute respiratory distress syndrome
ARI	acute lower respiratory infection
ART	atraumatic restorative technique (dental)
ASAP	as soon as possible!
ATLS	advanced trauma life support
AVPU	Scale to evaluate conscious level (awake/verbal/pain/unresponsive)
BAS	broad arm sling
BCG	bacillus Calmette–Guérin
BLS	basic life support
BM	blood glucose measurement
BMI	body mass index
BNF	British National Formulary
BP	blood pressure
BS	British Standard
BTS	British Thoracic Society
CAGE	cerebral arterial gas embolism
CMV	cytomegalovirus
CNS	central nervous system
CO	carbon monoxide
CO_2	carbon dioxide
COPD	chronic obstructive pulmonary disease
CPP	cerebral perfusion pressure
CPR	cardiopulmonary resuscitation

CRT	capillary refill time
CSF	cerebrospinal fluid
CVA	cerebral vascular accident (stroke)
DCI	decompression illness
DCS	decompression sickness
DEET	diethyl toluamide
DIPJ	distal interphalangeal joint
DKA	diabetic ketoacidosis
DSH	deliberate self-harm
DTI	Department of Trade & Industry
DVT	deep venous thrombosis
EAV	expired air ventilation
EBV	Epstein–Barr virus
ECG	electrocardiogram
EHS	exertional heat stroke
ELISA	enzyme-linked immunosorbent assay
ELT	emergency locator transmitters (aircraft)
ENT	ear, nose, throat
EPA	Environmental Protection Agency (US)
EPIRB	emergency position-indicating radio beacon
ERP	emergency response plan
ETEC	enterotoxigenic *Escherichia coli*
ETT	endotracheal tube
EU	European Union
FCO	Foreign and Commonwealth Office (UK)
FG	French gauge
g	gram
G	gauge
GCS	Glasgow Coma Scale
GI	gastrointestinal
GMC	General Medical Council (UK)
GORD	gastro-oesophageal reflux disease
GP	general practitioner
GPS	global positioning system
GSM	global system for mobile communications
GTN	glyceryl trinitrate
HAART	highly active anti-retroviral therapy
HACE	high-altitude cerebral oedema
HAH	high-altitude headache
HAPE	high-altitude pulmonary oedema

HAR	high-altitude retinopathy
HAS	high arm sling
HELP	heat escape lessening position
HiB	*Haemophilus influenzae* b
HIV	human immunodeficiency virus
HPV	human papilloma virus
HPVR	hypoxic pulmonary vasoconstrictive response
HR	heart rate
HRI	heat-related illness
HRT	hormone replacement therapy
HSV	herpes simplex virus
HVR	hypoxic ventilatory response
IBG	Institute of British Geographers
IBRD	International Beacon Registration Database
ICP	intracranial pressure
ID	intradermal
IHD	ischaemic heart disease
IM	intramuscular (drug administration)
IPJ	inter phalangeal joint (digits)
IRM	intermediate restorative material (dental)
IUCD	intrauterine contraceptive device
IV	intravenous
JME	juvenile myoclonic epilepsy
LA	local anaesthesia/anaesthetic (e.g. lidocaine)
LCL	lateral collateral ligament
LIF	left iliac fossa of abdomen
LMA	laryngeal mask airway
LUQ/RUQ	left/right upper quadrant of abdomen
LZ	landing zone (aircraft)
MAP	mean arterial pressure
MCA	Marine & Coastguard Agency
MCL	medial collateral ligament (knee)
MCPJ	metacarpophalangeal joint (digits)
mg	milligram
MI	myocardial infarction
mL	millilitre
MMR	mumps, measles, rubella
MO	medical officer
MRI	magnetic resonance imaging
NFCI	non-freezing cold injury

NGO	non-governmental organization
NHS	National Health Service (UK)
NICE	National Institute for Health and Care Excellence (UK)
NPA	nasopharyngeal airway
NSAID	non-steroidal anti-inflammatory drug (e.g. ibuprofen)
O_2	oxygen
OCP	oral contraceptive pill
OPA	oropharyngeal airway
ORS	oral rehydration solution
P	pulse
PASP	pulmonary artery systolic pressure
PCL	posterior cruciate ligament (knee)
PCR	polymerase chain reaction
PE	pulmonary embolism
PEFR	peak expiratory flow rate
PEPSE	post-exposure prophylaxis following sexual exposure
PF	peak flow (asthma)
pH	acid/base scale
P-I	pressure immobilization
PID	pelvic inflammatory disease
PIPJ	proximal interphalangeal joint
PLB	personal locator beacon (ground personnel)
PO	oral (drug administration)
PPE	personal protective equipment
PPI	proton-pump inhibitor
PR	rectal (drug administration)
PTRs	Package Travel Regulations 1992
PTSD	post-traumatic stress disorder
RGS	Royal Geographical Society
RICE	rest, ice, compression. elevation
RIF	right iliac fossa of abdomen
RIG	rabies immune globulin
RR	respiratory rate
RSI	repetitive strain injury
RSV	respiratory syncytial virus
RTC	road traffic collision
RUQ	right upper quadrant
SAR	search and rescue
SARS	severe acute respiratory syndrome

SC	subcutaneous (drug administration)
SCUBA	self-contained underwater breathing apparatus
SPC	Summary of Product Characteristics
SPF	sun protection factor (sunscreen)
STI	sexually transmitted infection
T	temperature
TB	tuberculosis
TDS	three times daily (drug administration)
TMJ	temporomandibular joint
TPR	temperature, pulse, respiration (chart)
UC	ulcerative colitis
UK	United Kingdom
URTI	upper respiratory tract infection
USA	United States of America
UTI	urinary tract infection
UV	ultraviolet
UVA, UVB, UVR	ultraviolet radiation
VEGF	vascular endothelial growth factor
VHF	very high frequency (radio waveband)
WBGT	wet bulb globe temperature
WHO	World Health Organization

Chapter 1

Expedition medicine

Section editor
Chris Johnson

Contributors
Sarah R. Anderson
Chris Johnson
Linda Dykes
David A. Warrell
Shane Winser

Wilderness travel 2
Scope of expedition medicine 4
Risk of death 6
Illness on expeditions 10
Conditions requiring hospital evacuation 12
Meeting the challenge 14

Wilderness travel

'Because it is there.'

George Mallory (1923)

This book is about the healthcare of travellers to remote areas. Remote areas are defined as places where access to sophisticated medical services is difficult or impossible, and the responsibility for dealing with medical problems falls on expedition members. In Europe this branch of medicine is usually called 'expedition medicine', while in North America it is called 'wilderness medicine'.

An expedition is an organized journey with a purpose. Early expeditions sought new lands to claim, develop, and exploit. In the twentieth century, as gaps on maps shrank, geologists, naturalists, and ecologists added detail to the knowledge, while physiologists explored human responses to extreme environments. Today, new scientific knowledge often requires a highly technological approach and considerable funding, so personal development, cultural exchange, and fund-raising have become increasingly important justifications for travel.

Adventure travel organizations send tens of thousands of people overseas each year to areas that 20 years ago could only be reached by a well-equipped expedition. Given a (very) thick wallet, trips to both Poles, the summit of Everest, and even outer space can be purchased. Age is no longer considered a bar to travel, with both healthy and less fit elderly clients expecting to reach remote and often physically demanding destinations—an octogenarian has reached the top of Everest. Attitudes to physical and mental disabilities have also changed enormously. A blind climber has summited Everest and limbless military veterans walked to the South Pole. The distinction between an expedition and a recreational journey is no longer obvious, but the challenges of caring for people far from a base hospital remain.

Technology has shrunk the world, potentially making even the remotest locations accessible from any Internet link. Superjeeps, helicopters, and satellite communications enable ready access to previously isolated parts of the globe. Increasingly, the wilderness is used as a playground for sporting endeavours that push the limits of human physiology.

Groups travelling to remote areas now include:
- Well-organized and funded expeditions.
- Small groups of independent travellers.
- Commercial trips to remote destinations.
- Charity fundraising treks to exotic destinations.
- Participants in 'adventure' holidays.
- Competitors in extreme sporting events.
- Gap-year travellers.

Despite the improvements in communications and technology, the physical, environmental, and health risks of remote areas remain. This book is about helping travellers understand and prepare for the hazards of remote environments. It is designed to assist doctors, nurses and paramedics who support groups far from formal medical facilities.

Increasingly during the past decade, military and disaster-relief organizations have developed the capability to provide portable but remarkably sophisticated healthcare in remote locations. This has been a response both to war in difficult environments such as the Middle East, and to better assist countries following major natural disasters such as tsunami and earthquakes. These capabilities rely on skilled manpower and costly logistic support, and this book does not deal with this type of healthcare.

Scope of expedition medicine

Expedition medicine is about:
- Preparing for an expedition—to minimize ill health and maximize expedition achievements.
- Working during the expedition—in a professional capacity to diagnose, treat, and manage health problems.
- Managing expedition emergencies and potential evacuations.
- Finally, advising on health issues once the expedition has returned home.

Organizing the medical care of an expedition takes time and includes tasks such as:
- The assessment and reduction of risk and therefore injury.
- Team selection.
- First-aid training.
- Preventive medicine both before departure and in the field.
- Organization of a suitable medical kit.
- Knowing about particular health problems in the area of the visit.
- Provision of medical skills in the field.
- Arrangements for medical back-up and evacuation.
- Organization of medical insurance.

Each of these aspects will be covered later in this book.

Expedition medicine is not just about the treatment of disease or coping with injuries; it should permeate all facets of the expedition. Health criteria must be considered when the location of the base camp is decided and the activities of the trip planned. Food, sanitation, and psychology are part of the expedition medic's work. The medic will fulfil many roles and will certainly be expected to be nurse as well as doctor. Sometimes the work will involve listening to and encouraging those who are finding the expedition stressful. The obligation to care for the sick or accompany a casualty during evacuation may mean that certain personal goals are not attained.

Not all expeditions will have a trained doctor, nurse, or paramedic attached to them, but all expeditions must consider how they can prevent disease, and cope with illness or trauma should it develop. Correctly practised, expedition medicine should not constrain the enthusiasms and ambitions of an expedition but, by anticipating preventable medical problems, facilitate the achievements and enjoyment of all participants.

Expedition destinations

When planning an adventure, people often seek novel experiences. Expedition medicine requires an understanding of how humans can physiologically acclimatize and technologically adapt to extreme environments. Contemporary travel is able to take someone within a few hours from a relatively benign to a potentially life-threatening environment. Newcomers may have no idea of the hazards they face and inadvertently place themselves in danger. Within an organized group it is the role of the leader, local guides, and medic to ensure that participants know how to behave to maintain safety, and that expedition plans match the physical and physiological capabilities of the weakest member of the group.

Between 1995 and 1997 the Royal Geographical Society and Institute of British Geographers (RGS-IBG) surveyed a large number of expeditions and at that time mountain ranges and tropical jungles were the most popular expedition destinations (Fig. 1.1).

Other destinations have increased in popularity and accessibility. During the 1970s, only a handful of tourists visited Antarctica. In the 1980s, numbers increased to around 2000 a year, and this expansion has continued to the current level (2013/14) of around 40,000 visitors a year. Iceland has become a very popular adventure destination and in 2013 attracted over 700,000 visitors, of which 90,000 came from the UK, more than half during the winter months. Mountain trekking in the great ranges has seen similar increases in popularity. In 2013, about 400,000 'adventure holiday' packages were sold in the UK, so it is increasingly likely that a family practitioner will be consulted about the preparations required for travel in remote areas. Chapters 20–27 of this book provide information about human health and physiology in extreme environments.

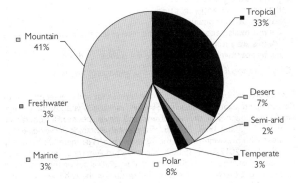

Fig. 1.1   Expedition destinations. Source: Royal Geographical Society Medical Database.

Risk of death

The explorer's worst nightmare may be to catch a dreadful tropical disease or to be attacked by a ferocious wild animal, but for most expeditions the reality is more mundane. Stomach upsets, sprains, bruises, and insomnia are the common problems. The risks of catching insect-borne diseases such as malaria or dengue, or being involved in a vehicle collision on the way to the expedition area are usually far greater than the more exotic risks of the wilderness.

Death during an expedition is rare and tragic but should be kept in perspective (Tables 1.1 and 1.2). The media love dramatic stories but ignore the hazards of daily life. With the exception of extreme sporting activities, the risk for participants in a well-planned expedition is not that different from the risks faced during an active life at home.[1] Fatal road accidents, drowning, or falls can occur anywhere; effective advanced planning can reduce their incidence. Proper briefing of travellers, together with good risk management, can reduce harm. Sadly, the risk of violent death overseas from crime or terrorism has climbed from a low point in the mid twentieth century.

Expeditions are getting safer . . .
  But society is less tolerant of risk.
Deaths occur on expeditions . . .
  But deaths also occur in the UK and receive less publicity.
All deaths are a tragedy . . .
  But by not travelling do you reduce the number of deaths?

Only join a trip if you know, understand, and accept the risks.

Expeditions are becoming safer. In the eighteenth and nineteenth centuries, complete expeditions such as Sir John Franklin's ill-fated Arctic Voyage, would disappear into the wilderness and never be heard from again. Between 1943 and 1983, 26 staff of the British Antarctic Survey died (1% of those who overwintered); in the 30 years since 1983 there has been only one death. In 2012, over 35,000 tourists visited Antarctica, most of them on cruise ships. The rate of those dying of natural causes on the ships is not recorded, but there were five recorded deaths on the continent, two as a result of a base fire, and three associated with a shipwreck.

In the twentieth century, the ratio of successful summit attempts to deaths on Mount Everest was 1:7; by 2007 the ratio had improved to six deaths for 500 successful summits[2] (Table 1.3). However, this reduction in relative risk has been associated with much greater numbers of people tackling the challenge, not a reduction in the absolute numbers of deaths—with nine climbers dying on the mountain in 2012 and ten in 2013. Overall around 6000 UK Nationals die abroad each year, but most of these are expatriate residents. The Foreign and Commonwealth office produces an annual report[3] summarizing the needs for consulate assistance overseas.

1 Anderson SR, Johnson CJH. Expedition health and safety—a risk assessment. *Journal of the Royal Society of Medicine* (2000); **93**: 557–62.
2 🔎 http://www.everestnews.com/history/everestsummits/summitsbyyear.htm
3 🔎 https://www.gov.uk/government/uploads/system/uploads/attachment_data/file/230013/British_Behaviour_Abroad_Report_2012-13_UPDATED_15_08_13.pdf

Table 1.1 Deaths abroad in UK travellers (2002)

Deaths from natural causes	1111
Non-natural causes	316
Total deaths	1427
Journeys made:	59,200,000
One death per 41,500 journeys	

Typically between one and three deaths a year are linked to expedition travel.

Table 1.2 Non-natural deaths abroad in UK travellers (2002)

Road accident	158
Suicide	57
Drowned	21
Air accident	14
Murder (non-terrorist)	10
Terrorism (Bali bombs 26)	29
Balcony accidents	14
Skiing and mountaineering	12
Rail death	1
Total deaths	316

Table 1.3 Relative risk of death in remote areas

Everest summit ratio (to 1999)	1 in 7
Himalayan mountaineering	1 in 34
Everest summit ratio (2007)	1 in 83
Antarctica over-wintering (1943–1983)	1 in 100
All-cause risk of death after major surgery	1 in 250
Royal Geographical Society Survey (1995–2000)	1 in 1500
Himalayan trekking	1 in 7000
Gap-year travel	1 in 7500
Low-altitude jogging	1 in 7700

Judged by the numbers of people dying, the much lower Kilimanjaro[4] is more hazardous than Everest with estimates of fatalities of between 10 and 30 deaths per year. But this reflects the ease of access—over 30,000 people attempt to climb the mountain each year, and the wide age profile of trekkers, some of whom may have a high underlying risk of cardiovascular problems before departure. But over 50% of the trekkers turn back below the summit due to cold, dehydration, and altitude sickness and this reflects the common use of inappropriate ascent profiles.

Fatalities amongst young people are always tragic and the dramatic circumstances in which they occur means that they are often highly publicized, giving the impression that such travel is more hazardous than it really is. Recent well-publicized deaths of UK nationals during youth expeditions include cases of hyperthermia, wild animal attack, electrocution, and inappropriate fluid ingestion.

Better weather forecasting, equipment, communications, training, and rescue services have all contributed to reducing the risk of travel in remote areas, but safety should not be taken for granted, and travellers to remote areas must strive to minimize risk and be self-sufficient.

Illness on expeditions

Gathering and collating information about health on expeditions is very difficult owing to concerns about confidentiality and data protection. The RGS study,[5] published in 2000, analysed health issues from 246 expeditions. Fig. 1.2 shows a summary of the key findings.

Gastrointestinal upsets (30%)

Diarrhoea and vomiting are an inevitable hazard of travel and are usually self-limiting. However, serious cases lead to dehydration and hospitalization. Dysentery, cholera, and giardiasis can infect the unwary. Simple hygiene measures can reduce the incidence of problems, but all travellers need to carry basic remedies for days when travel is unavoidable, and larger expeditions ought to have the facilities to rehydrate a seriously affected member.

Medical problems (21%)

Simple medical problems such as respiratory infections and headache are very common, and are usually easily treated. Insect-borne diseases such as malaria and dengue fever can be incapacitating and sometimes fatal. Appropriate precautions should be taken.

Orthopaedic problems (19%)

Sprains and back strain are common; rest and simple painkillers help. Fractures and serious trauma will require evacuation.

Environmental problems (14%)

Environmental extremes may cause problems for the unprepared. Altitude sickness affects many travellers ascending rapidly to altitude; heat exhaustion and heatstroke can be a serious problem, while at the other extreme frostbite and non-freezing cold injury can cause long-term disability. When environmental problems occur they can be serious, and require urgent treatment and evacuation, often in difficult circumstances.

Fauna (8%)

Unfamiliarity with local animal life can lead to injury. Scorpions and sea urchins commonly cause problems. Wherever rabies is endemic, dogs should be treated with caution. Although attacks are rare, large animals throughout the world present a hazard both directly and as a cause of road collision

Feet (4%)

Good foot care is always essential. Blisters cause misery and can become infected on a long expedition. Regular cleansing and use of foot powder reduces fungal infections and sores.

5 Anderson SR, Johnson CJH (2000). Expedition health and safety: a risk assessment. *J R Soc Med*, 93, 557–62.

Surgical problems (1%)

Acute abdominal crises, severe gynaecological pain, and renal stones are very alarming and often require evacuation of the patient, but fortunately are rare.

Evacuation and repatriation

In this study of 250 expeditions, 25 participants required temporary or permanent evacuation, and eight had to be repatriated. Eleven of these evacuations were caused by acute mountain sickness and were taken to a lower altitude, while 13 participants had to be admitted to hospital for malaria, dysentery, appendicitis, or renal stones.

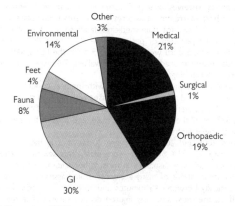

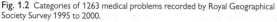

Fig. 1.2 Categories of 1263 medical problems recorded by Royal Geographical Society Survey 1995 to 2000.

Conditions requiring hospital evacuation

Fortunately, death and serious injury are nowadays very rare on expeditions, so epidemiological studies must study large numbers of people. Few results of these have been published, but data from the UK gives an idea of the type of issues arising in a frequently visited mountainous area. The Ysbyty Gwynedd hospital in Bangor, North Wales receives almost all the casualties from the mountains of the nearby Snowdonia National Park. The Park is a very popular destination for walkers, climbers, and tourists with 4.25 million visitors spending around 10.4 million days in the area during 2012. Military and civilian mountain rescue teams and helicopters provide search and rescue (SAR) cover to evacuate casualties beyond the reach of conventional ambulances.

The hospital receives over 100 casualties a year who require rescue and urgent hospital treatment as a result of events taking place within the mountains, and their mountain medicine database[4] has logged over 1000 incidents. Eleven per cent of patients were children, a third were in the 18–28 age group, a third were aged 29–49, with the remainder over 50. Two-thirds became injured or ill while hill-walking, 7% were scrambling, and 11% were rock climbing.

Only 19% of the patients presented with medical conditions although the incidence of medical problems increases with age—in those aged >60 medical problems were the cause of more than a third of the admissions. Overall, 63% of all the casualties were male, and 55% of the patients presented with lower limb injuries.

Between 2004 and 2011 there were 70 fatalities in the mountains of the National Park, 93% of whom were male. This sex ratio reflects the predominance of male casualties in most other trauma registries. Owing to the remote locations of many accidents, skilled assistance takes time to arrive—typically between 45 minutes and an hour—and this delay has a triage effect: the most seriously injured do not survive. The majority of trauma victims who die within this initial period have non-survivable head or spinal cord injuries. Of those with serious spinal fractures, 73% had spinal cord disruption at post-mortem.

The pattern of survivors is quite different. Half of Snowdonia mountain trauma casualties complain of back pain, or have a mechanism of injury that would mandate 'spinal packaging' in conventional pre-hospital practice. However, in the mountains providing such care may delay evacuation and create additional hazard to both rescuers and casualty. Analysis suggests that while 14% of this group of casualties prove to have some form of spinal fracture, most are stable transverse process fractures that are painful, but clinically insignificant. Less than 2% of mountain casualties found alive after a serious accident have an unstable spinal fracture—a comparable rate to most major trauma series in urban populations.

4 The Bangor Mountain Medicine database (unpublished) is maintained by Linda Dykes, Ben Hall, and Rhiannon Talbot and is quoted with their permission.

Pelvic fractures also cause concern to rescuers, because pelvic splints are difficult to apply in precarious locations. However, only 2% of the mountain trauma casualties had a pelvic fracture and severe pelvic disruption was only seen in those who died before help arrived.

Meeting the challenge

People enjoy the excitement and challenges of the great outdoors. Travels in remote areas will always carry risk, and if things go wrong help may be far away. Expedition medicine involves many aspects of care unfamiliar to clinicians used to working in conventional hospital or family practice. Good planning and logistics, effective risk management, communications, hygiene, and sanitation, together with an understanding of human health and physiology in extreme environmental conditions, form the core of the specialist knowledge necessary to work effectively.

Many people attracted to remote areas are risk-takers. Effective planning and risk management is about ensuring that the risks encountered are controlled and mitigated to the greatest possible degree. This is especially important when young or naïve clients join a group travelling to a remote area. Those with greater skills and knowledge have a 'duty of care' to the novices.

Many doctors, nurses, and paramedics seek to participate in expeditions, and the authors hope that this Handbook will provide a useful guide to the knowledge and skills that these clinicians will require as they head to distant parts.

Chapter 2

Preparations

Section editors
Sarah R. Anderson and James Moore

Contributors
Sarah R. Anderson
Jon Dallimore
Claire Davies
Richard Dawood
Peter Harvey
Iain McIntosh
James Moore
Barry Roberts
David A. Warrell
Jane Wilson-Howarth
Shane Winser
Tariq Qureshi (1st edition)

Joining an expedition *16*
Role of the expedition medical officer *20*
Creating expedition teams *26*
Immunization *28*
Medical kits and supplies *42*
Medical and first-aid training *44*
Medical screening *46*
Advising those with common pre-existing conditions *50*
The older traveller *58*
Child health in remote areas *62*
Risk management *68*
Medical insurance *74*
Legal liabilities and professional insurance *76*

Joining an expedition

The Royal Geographical Society (with IBG) estimates that >2500 overseas expeditions leave the UK annually. These will range from solo travellers or teams of two up to expeditions involving 100 or more participants. Expeditions typically last for as little as 1–2 weeks to many months, if not years in the case of continuing research programmes. The sheer volume of expedition traffic represents great scope for joining an expedition, assuming one is not inclined to organize a journey independently. Expeditions occur throughout the year but are usually timed for a variety of reasons; e.g. to coincide with a certain event (summer holidays, animal migration patterns), climatic conditions (avoiding monsoons or other 'rains'), and the seasons (avoiding the Himalayan or north polar areas in the northern hemisphere winter).

Potentially there is a huge choice of where to go and what to do. Think first about your motivation:
● Science.
● Adventure.
● Personal challenge.
● Community involvement.

Think second about your personal circumstances:
● Relevant skills and experience.
● The level of responsibility you desire.
● Time available.
● Financial commitments/resources.
● Personal interests.

Unless you fully appreciate the demands of expedition travel, as opposed to independent travel, it is worth initially considering joining a short expedition before committing yourself to a prolonged and arduous journey in a very remote area, with little chance of repatriation if you find you cannot cope or hate the experience.

Expeditions are costly enterprises and normally each participant has to pay their way. At best you might get your costs covered by the expedition but it is unrealistic to expect a wage, unless you have a special skill and/or are vastly experienced. There is also the opportunity cost to consider while on an expedition when mortgages, pensions, and other bills have to be paid, and there is no corresponding income. In addition there are 'hidden' costs which might include upgrading clothing, camera equipment, special insurance, etc. It all adds up.

Types of expedition

Institutional expeditions

Universities, research groups, and public institutions (such as the Natural History Museum, Royal Botanic Gardens, Kew and Edinburgh, the Zoological Society of London, and the British Antarctic Survey) are examples in this class.

Commercial expeditions

Commercial operators charge a fee to join their expeditions and aim to make a profit. They range from 'one-off' projects to 'adventure travel' companies who offer land-based expeditions and ocean sailing opportunities. Such businesses may be run by sole traders, as partnerships, or as limited companies and are subject to 'Package Travel Regulations 1992' (PTRs). Under these regulations a travel package is offered when at least two of the following three components are included: transport, accommodation, or other tourist service accounting for a significant proportion of the package. Anyone offering a 'travel package' is legally required to be 'bonded' so that any fees paid are protected if the organization folds prior to travel. Responsibility for implementation of the PTRs lies with the Department for Business, Innovation & Skills (BIS).

Charity organizations

The Charity Commission is the regulator and registrar of charities in England and Wales. There is great variety in the expedition activities of such bodies. For example, they range from medical research expeditions, aid and relief work, youth expeditions, conservation and science projects to expeditions for medically disadvantaged people and 'charity challenges' (such as treks, cycle rides, and climbs) in aid of a specific cause. See $\mathcal{R}$ http://www.charity-commission.gov.uk for the register of organizations. Remember that companies that run 'charity treks' on behalf of registered charities are not charities and may be profit-driven businesses.

Private expeditions

Anyone can set up an expedition and recruit team members to join it. This is not regulated and no qualifications are necessary to do so. A one-off expedition is outside the scope of the PTRs.

Film/TV projects

There is great public interest in the adventures and human dramas associated with expeditions. These adventures are made more accessible by low-cost filming and production techniques, and are another route by which aspiring medics might get an opportunity, sometimes paid, to join an expedition. The producers' aim to capture the 'drama'—both physical and emotional—of people in extreme circumstances may clash with a MO's ethical and moral obligations to promote safe practices, so the nature of a film project and its participants should be considered wisely. See ➔ Working with the media, p. 126.

Extreme challenges

Polar races, jungle and desert marathons, ocean sailing races, and multi-sport adventure races are some examples of extreme challenges set in remote environments that are becoming popular. Whilst not necessarily true 'expeditions', these events do represent opportunities for medics. Managing the health of competitive athletes under extreme environmental conditions in remote environments can be a high-pressure, stressful responsibility.

Assessing an expedition opportunity

While you may be grateful to any expedition that accepts you, you are about to invest a considerable amount of time, effort, and possibly money in the enterprise, so research the organization to satisfy yourself that it is likely to achieve its goals, and that the plans match your expectations.

- How long has the company/organization been trading and what is its financial structure and bonding system?
- Are they aligned to a standard, e.g. BS8848 (see Box 2.1) or screened via an external organization such as the RGS-IBG, or internally, e.g. by the Oxford University Expeditions Council?
- What are the credentials of the expedition leader(s)?
- How much do you have to pay and what does it include/exclude?
- How are participants selected and medically screened?
- What pre-expedition meeting/training plan is in place?
- What medical kit is provided?
- What insurance, risk assessment, and emergency back-up arrangements are in place?
- Will your medical defence organization cover you if there are Americans/Canadians or other internationals on the team?
- Will you be expected to treat locals and therefore be required to register with the local government as a medical practitioner?
- Don't ignore your instinct or 'gut feeling'; sloppy administration might be a tell-tale sign of poor field organization.

Information sources on expedition opportunities

- The Internet.
- Word of mouth.
- Contacts through companies that offer expedition medical training.
- The Royal Geographical Society maintains a:
  - Register of personnel available for expeditions, which is used to help expeditions to recruit medical personnel (🖰 http://www.rgs.org/expeditionmedicine).
  - Bulletin of expedition vacancies.
  - List of organizations that recruit expedition members (🖰 http://www.rgs.org/je).

Box 2.1 BS 8848

BS 8848 is the British Standard for organizing and managing visits, fieldwork, expeditions, and adventurous activities outside the UK.

BS 8848 aims to reduce the risk of injury or illness on overseas ventures by specifying the safety requirements that have to be met by providers of these activities.

BS 8848 documents establish good practice and specify the processes needed to manage overseas ventures, from gap-year activities to adventure holidays and charity treks. Providers, leaders, and participants need to know the risks involved, that they've been planned for, and that action has been taken to minimize them.

BS 8848 provides those that comply with the requirements of the standard with a way of being able to demonstrate to participants, leaders, and other interested parties that their venture provider is following good practice to manage safety on the venture. BS 8848 can also be used to identify areas for improvement in existing safety management procedures.

Following BS 8848 will help ensure that providers of adventure activities:
- Assign clear roles and responsibilities to those involved.
- Plan a venture to help ensure that key elements are not missed.
- Provide clear and accurate information to participants on the safety issues and on the nature of the activities.
- Appoint competent staff with the right skills, training, and know-how.
- Prepare risk management plans and make staff aware of the risks associated with specific activities and locations.

See ✆ http://www.bsigroup.com/BS8848 for further details.

Role of the expedition medical officer

The expedition MO is key to the success of an expedition. Success is achieved by preventing expedition members becoming ill and treating quickly and appropriately. This does not mean that, as MO, you must treat everything that is presented to you, but rather you must use your knowledge to advise on the best course of action. As MO you are unlikely to be busy with medical problems but, if someone is ill or injured, you may be the only person who can deal with the situation. These can be stressful times, with no advice available from seniors and no one to relieve you for a break. Good communication between you, your patient, and other expedition members is essential, as is strong decision-making, based on the knowledge and facilities available to you.

To prepare for the role of expedition MO
- Carefully research the area you will travel to.
- Improve your knowledge of local medical problems.
- Attend relevant courses in expedition medicine, first aid, advanced life support, basic dental skills and, if relevant, consider a Diploma in Tropical Medicine and Hygiene.
- Prepare physically.

Pre-expedition roles
- Advise and brief the team on medical issues (general and specific to the expedition environment).
- Undertake medical screening of all expedition members (➜ Medical screening, p. 46).
- Encourage all participants to have a pre-expedition dental check-up.
- Document the blood group of each expedition member (obtained free by donating blood at a local blood donor centre).
- Consider subscribing to the Blood Care Foundation to ensure access to safe blood abroad (℘ http://www.bloodcare.org.uk).
- Provide advice on immunizations and malaria prophylaxis (if medically qualified to do so); otherwise have an awareness of appropriate immunizations and antimalarials (➜ Immunization, p. 28; ➜ Antimalarials, p. 62; ➜ Prevention of malaria, p. 483).
- Organize appropriate first-aid training for all expedition members (➜ Medical and first-aid training, p. 44).
- Educate the team on health and hygiene issues (➜ Camp health and hygiene, p. 22).
- Obtain, pack, and transport medical supplies and kits (Chapter 28).
- Undertake a risk assessment and prepare associated documents (➜ Risk management, p. 68).
- Review local health services and medical facilities.
- Anticipate and plan evacuation of a severely ill or injured person.
- Prepare a communication network to support your medical diagnosis and decision-making in case of evacuation (➜ Telemedicine and communications, p. 160).
- Prepare an emergency response plan (ERP; ➜ Emergency response plan, p. 136).

- Organize medical insurance with full emergency evacuation cover
  (➲ Medical insurance, p. 74; ➲ Evacuation, p. 146).
- Confirm that your professional indemnity insurance will cover the role
  of an expedition medical officer.

Medical screening of expedition members is essential to ensure tailored
pre-travel advice and to expand the expedition first-aid kit. Ask each member to complete a personal medical questionnaire and emphasize the need
for full disclosure to enable proper preparation and appropriate insurance
cover. Make three copies of the questionnaire: leave one in the UK with a
nominated contact and take two on the expedition, in case an emergency
evacuation is needed.

Pre-Expedition Medical Questionnaire
Name:

Date of birth:

Address:

Next of kin:
  Name
  Address
  Tel./contact details
  Relationship

GP details:

Current medical problems:

Past medical history (including past psychiatric history):

Current medications:

Allergies:

Last dental check-up:

Immunizations:
Childhood vaccinations: did you receive all of your childhood vaccinations
including MMR (Mumps, Measles, Rubella)   Yes/No

Expedition-related vaccinations   *Date received*
  Tetanus/diphtheria/polio (within the last 10 years)
  Hepatitis A
  Typhoid
  Yellow fever (if certification required)
  Hepatitis B
  Rabies
  Meningococcal meningitis ACWY
  BCG
  Cholera
  Japanese B encephalitis
  Tick-borne encephalitis

Blood group:

Roles during the expedition

- Reiterate rules of camp and personal hygiene (➲ Camp health and hygiene, p. 22).
- Reinforce these at regular intervals during the expedition.
- Ensure a safe, copious water supply.
- Undertake brief medical review of expedition members on arrival.
- Revise basic first aid and management of minor injuries with all expedition members.
- Place expedition medical kits in a designated place and inform all expedition members.
- Organize a routine for patient consultations.
- Oversee the safety of expedition members.
- Reassess the risks posed by the natural environment, instruct the team on prevention and early suspicion (e.g. heat illness, altitude sickness), and alter emergency plans as appropriate.
- Review evacuation plans.
- Consider visiting the local hospital early to introduce yourself.
- Practise a mock evacuation.
- Write up accident reports as necessary.
- Enjoy being part of the expedition.

Camp health and hygiene

As MO you are responsible for base camp health and hygiene—see 'Caring for people in the field' for full details (Chapter 3). Contribute to the design of the camp layout to ensure water supplies and waste disposal are correct. Undertake regular checks of latrine and kitchen hygiene, food storage, and rubbish disposal. If anything is substandard bring it to the attention of all expedition members and rectify. Strict adherence to the rules of camp and personal hygiene is essential to minimize gastroenteritis, the most common complaint on all expeditions.

Consultations

A consultation service for non-urgent problems is one of the main roles of an MO; how you do this will depend on the size and structure of your expedition. Allocate a regular time each day when you are exclusively available for consultation; consider before or after meals. It is important to try to ensure complete privacy (not always easy). Briefly record consultations and any treatment given (➲ Documentation, p. 89).

Treatment

Size, weight, and cost considerations mean that most expedition medical kits are fairly basic, and the number of diagnostic aids limited. MOs should ensure that they have medical supplies sufficient for treating minor illnesses and are able to provide emergency care for more serious conditions until a patient can be evacuated.

Most problems are straightforward and can be dealt with on the spot. The role of the MO is therefore uncomplicated: to make a diagnosis and treat. In urban settings, help is available to confirm intuitive feelings or doubts; however, in the field it is not, and as expedition MO you therefore have to assume the worst-case scenario. This may mean causing a lot of inconvenience and concern, e.g. by sending someone with stomach ache to hospital with possible appendicitis, or making someone with a headache descend 1000 m. You will provoke grumbling and hostility if the person recovers without intervention, but you really have no choice other than to take the safest course of action.

MOs are also there to offer reassurance. People come with genuine symptoms, whether major or minor, and the significance may not always be apparent to the sufferer. You will not know what the situation is until you have made a serious attempt at a diagnosis, so *never fail to take this step*. If you think nothing is wrong, friendly reassurance is very important. Remember that psychological or psychiatric problems, fears, and tensions may manifest themselves as physical symptoms. Expeditioners tend to be self-sufficient people, and the circumstances of an expedition often reinforce this. There is a tendency for MOs to overdo the self-sufficiency; this can lead them to try and solve all problems single-handedly. Always ask yourself whether extra advice is available and if it would be useful.

Confidentiality

All patients rightly expect that medical information will be confidential. People also have a right to refuse treatment, even if, in the MO's view, this will not be in their best interest. However, the General Medical Council (GMC) has made it clear that doctors also have a duty to the public at large. On expeditions circumstances can arise where confidentiality may need to be broken so that the health and safety of other expedition members is not jeopardized. The expedition leader may need to be informed that an individual is concealing an illness or refusing treatment.

Consent

Without consent, treatment is assault. Consent to emergency life-saving treatment is usually presumed by the law if the patient is unconscious or too ill to consent. The law presumes that a reasonable person would wish his/her life to be saved. In the case of a healthcare professional acting within his/her sphere of clinical competence, consent is usually implied, i.e. the patient does not resist the treatment and therefore is presumed to consent. In other situations where treatment carries considerable risk, or is controversial, informed expressed consent should be obtained. For consent to be informed the individual must understand the proposed treatment and the risks involved in accepting or refusing that treatment. This means that the patient should be made aware of material risks and common or serious side effects, as well as the likely consequences should treatment be withheld. Verbal consent, especially in an expedition setting, is usually adequate.

For an individual over 16 years of age, only that individual is able to give consent. Remember, patients have the right to refuse treatment. Children under 16 can consent to medical treatment themselves if, in the opinion of the doctor, they are capable of understanding the nature and consequences of that treatment (Gillick competence). The child should, however, be given information that is relevant to his/her age and understanding. When taking under-16s on an expedition it is wise to gain written permission from the parent or guardian that medical care can be given if it is thought to be in the child's best interest.

Incident reports

Incidents may happen. One of the roles of the expedition MO is to write up an incident report if necessary. It is important that information collected is purely factual, and should include:

- The site and time of the incident/accident.
- The people involved.
- Who else was present (witnesses).
- What happened.
- What action was taken.
- The outcome.

Assessing health risk

Medical health risk management should form part of overall risk assessment (➔ Risk management, p. 68). People who commonly encounter specific hazards, such as experienced climbers, cavers, or divers, should also contribute. In these activities, field leaders are usually well informed and often trained to advise less experienced individuals. Risks can be minimized by the use of sensible and simple precautions such as avoiding travelling at night, selecting appropriate equipment, wearing seat belts in vehicles and helmets while climbing. An emergency response plan should be prepared (➔ Emergency response plan, p. 136).

Once in the field, it is important to *reassess* the situation, particularly the hazards of local flora and fauna, the climate (e.g. both heat and humidity), and the physical environment. Situations may arise in the field where the MO will either have to give an opinion about a proposed activity, or give unsolicited warnings once activities have begun.

Evacuation

An essential role of the MO is the ability to make a decision on evacuation. Consider the following:

- The need to choose the safest option when diagnosis cannot be confirmed by colleagues or tests.
- The often conflicting needs of the other expedition members.
- Lack of privacy and confidentiality, all part of expedition life.

Plans should be prepared on communication and transportation methods in case an emergency or evacuation occurs (see ➔ Evacuation, p. 146 for further details on evacuation). If the evacuation is to be funded by an insurance company it will be critical to liaise with the insurance company's medical assistance agent. This individual will hold the approval for financing evacuations. Failure to do this may result in the insurance company not paying for evacuation costs.

Dealing with local communities

Expeditions may employ local workers and will encounter local communities. MOs may be asked to assist with the medical care of someone who is sick or injured. Chapter 4 discusses the ethical dilemmas associated with such situations.

At the end of expedition

- When appropriate, repeat advice that participants should continue malaria prophylaxis for the full prescribed period.
- Warn team members about non-healing skin lesions (leishmaniasis) and the vital importance of seeking medical help early if a fever develops within the first few weeks after return. Malaria can develop and kill rapidly.
- Provide continuing medical advice and support as necessary.

If participants are fit and healthy at the end of an expedition, they probably don't require any follow-up. For participants with symptoms, the MO should recommend urgent review by a doctor, to examine, investigate, and treat as appropriate. The most helpful post-expedition tests are:

- Full blood count with white cell differential to detect an increase in eosinophils (an eosinophilia is seen with parasitic disease).
- Urine dipstick for blood, protein, or sugar.
- Stool specimen for microscopy, culture & antibiotic sensitivities (M,C & S) plus ova, cysts, and parasites.
- Urine specimen and serology for schistosomiasis (>6 weeks after expedition) if they were exposed to fresh water in an endemic area (➔ Schistosomiasis (bilharzia), p. 498).

Do not forget that tropical diseases such as malaria and schistosomiasis may present weeks, months, or even years after the expedition has ended. A single case in your expedition team should alert you to recommend the screening of other members, since they are likely to have shared the same risk of exposure. Usually the role of the expedition MO post-expedition will be to direct individuals to their best local health provider to investigate and treat the problem.

Creating expedition teams

Expeditions create their own unique social atmosphere. There can be enormous strain on individuals and the team, brought about by the intensity of living in a group, which is amplified by physical hardship, deprivation of normal Western comforts, climatic and cultural demands, and the stress of striving to achieve the expedition's objectives. This is one of the great attractions of expedition life: to put oneself to the test and willingly forego the relative safety and security of home in exchange for the deep satisfaction, elevated self-esteem, and close human bonds that can be one of the greatest benefits of the expedition experience.

To optimize the expedition experience for all participants, particular attention must be paid to appropriate team selection, team building, effective leadership, and an understanding of the dynamics of groups in the field.

Team building

Time is well-invested prior to the expedition in building the expedition members into an effective team so that the team is ready to handle the demands of the expedition. The time devoted to this should be proportional to the size of the team and the complexity and longevity of the expedition. For large multi-national expeditions it is impracticable to get the team together before the expedition; in these circumstances a period of time should be devoted in-country to team building, skill development, and briefings, before the party is deployed to the field.

Immunization

Introduction

Vaccines offer safe, reliable protection against an increasing range of important disease hazards abroad, but it is important to note that medical preparation for going abroad is not just about immunization: careful attention to the other health precautions covered in this book are also of paramount importance, before, during, and after every successful expedition. An important benefit of going to be vaccinated is the opportunity to discuss a wider range of health concerns and precautions that may be even more beneficial than the vaccines themselves, an opportunity that should always be used to the full. It is important for those with an incomplete or absent vaccination history to understand that vaccinations are not only there to protect the individual, but also the indigenous population from imported disease.

Timing

Ideally, immunization should commence at least 6 weeks before departure, to allow time for vaccines requiring more than one dose and sufficient time for the vaccines to become effective (Table 2.1). Vaccine supply problems do occur from time to time, and this can be a further reason for seeking protection well in advance.

Background

Everyone attending for immunization should bring with them any available records of previous vaccines received, to avoid unnecessary repeated doses.

Immunization schedules are becoming more complicated and especially where groups of young people are concerned, 'catch-up' protection may be necessary for any missed doses, notably MMR and diphtheria, tetanus, and polio (of note: significant outbreaks of mumps and measles have recently occurred in young people in whom MMR vaccine has been omitted).

Travel provides an important opportunity to ensure that the routine vaccination schedule is up to date. The UK childhood immunization schedule can be found at: ℛ http://www.nhs.uk/Conditions/vaccinations/Pages/vaccination-schedule-age-checklist.aspx.

Where expedition participants are drawn from more than one country, it may be important to be aware of differences between national schedules.

HIV-positive and other immunosuppressed people require special advice about immunizations, for further details see: ℛ http://wwwnc.cdc.gov/travel/yellowbook/2012/chapter-8-advising-travelers-with-specific-needs/immunocompromised-travelers.

Certificates and regulations

Yellow fever is the only disease for which international, WHO-approved vaccination certificates still apply as a condition of entry to some countries. Travellers to Saudi Arabia during the Haj or Umrah pilgrimage may be required to show proof of vaccination against meningitis ACWY.

Choosing which vaccines to have

Most travel vaccines are not required formally as a condition of entry, but are 'optional'—the choice is based on an assessment of the likely health risks such as locally prevalent diseases, the precise details of a trip or expedition, including its duration, conditions of accommodation, the likely level of contact with local people, and the environment.

In England, Wales, and Northern Ireland general guidelines are published by the National Travel Health Network and Centre (NaTHNaC) ($\wp$ http://www.nathnac.org); in Scotland by Health Protection Scotland; the WHO also issues information, and it may also be helpful to consult resources from other countries, such as the United States. Many medical practices, travel clinics, companies and other organizations also formulate their own policies.

On an expedition, participants inevitably compare the vaccines and medication they have received; inconsistencies tend to be the rule rather than the exception, which can lead to unnecessary anxiety and can undermine confidence in the advice that has been given.

The best option is therefore for an expedition's MO to draw up some general guidelines or a formal policy, seeking specialist advice if this is needed. The best care comes when one clinic or practice takes responsibility for the entire group. If this is not possible, the MO should circulate guidelines to all expedition members to give to the individual clinics or practices that will carry out immunization.

In the UK, only a small number of travel vaccines can be provided free of charge on the NHS, and escalating development costs mean that newer travel vaccines are costly—a factor that needs to be considered in the context of an expedition's overall budget.

Previous vaccinations or interrupted schedules

Individuals may have received either a full or partial vaccine courses in the past. It is important to note that vaccine courses rarely require restarting, irrespective of the time between doses. For example, if someone has received two hepatitis B vaccinations 3 years ago, they will only require a single hepatitis B vaccination to complete the primary course.

Table 2.1 Travel vaccine guide

Vaccine	No. of doses	Initial course — Primary course schedule	Notes	Duration of protection	Minimum age
Killed vaccines					
Cholera (Dukoral)	2	Adults & children 6–18 years: Day 0, 1–6 weeks		2 years	2 years
	3	Children 2–6 years: Day 0, 1–6 weeks, 1–6 weeks apart		6 months	
Diphtheria/tetanus/polio		Initial course usually completed in childhood. Unvaccinated adults: 3 doses one month apart		10 years	n/a
Hepatitis A	2	Day 0, then 6–12 months		25+ years	1 year
Hepatitis B—rapid schedule	4	Days 0, 7, 21, and 12 months	A single Hep B booster at 5 years for those at continuing risk	Life	18 years
Hepatitis B—standard schedule	3	Months 0, 1, and 2 or 6		Life	Birth
Hepatitis A & B—combined	3	Months 0, 1, and 2 or 6		25+ years	1 year
Influenza	1	Children need a 2nd dose 4 weeks later if first ever flu vaccine course		1 year	6 months
Japanese encephalitis (Ixiaro)	2	Days 0 and 28	Booster at 1year	Unknown	2 months
Meningitis ACWY (conjugated)	1	Single dose		Unknown	1 year
Meningitis B	2	Age 6 months to adults: Months 0 and 2	Booster between 12 & 24 months	Unknown	
	3	Age 2–5 months: Months 0, 1, and 2			
Pneumonia (Prevenar, Pneumovax)	1	Single dose		5+ years	

Vaccine	No. of doses	Schedule	Duration of protection	Minimum age
Rabies (im or intradermal)	3	Days 0, 7, and 21 or 28	Life in most cases	Birth
Tickborne encephalitis	2 or 3	Days 0, and 28–42	3+ years	1 year
Typhoid/ Hepatitis A (combined)	1	Hepatitis A booster at 6–12 months Typhoid booster at 3 years	Hep A 1year, then 25+ Typhoid 3 years	16 years
Typhoid injected (Typhim Vi)	1	Single dose	3 years	2 years
Live vaccines				
MMR (measles/mumps/rubella) adults	2	Day 0 and 28	Life	
TB: BCG (mantoux first if aged 6+ years)	1	Single dose		Birth
Typhoid oral (Vivotif)	3	Day 0, 2, and 4	3 years	6 years
Varicella (chickenpox)	2	Months 0, and 1–2	Unknown	1 year
Yellow fever	1	Single dose	Life	9 months
			Certificate lasts for 10 years	

Single dose vaccines require 10–14 days to become effective. Do NOT give live vaccines to immunosuppressed patients, and consider implications carefully during pregnancy. Vaccine schedules, indications, and booster recommendations are prone to change in the light of new evidence. For the most up-to-date information, including scheduling of live vaccines visit: ⅋ http://nathnac.org/pro/index.htm

Adapted from Table 13.2.1 in Travellers' Health: how to stay healthy abroad (OUP).

Individual vaccines for travel

Meningococcal meningitis

Most travel clinics are able to provide up-to-date information about areas of risk. Travellers who have had their spleen removed may be more vulnerable to this condition.

A new generation of 'conjugated' vaccines now offers robust protection against the A, C, W, and Y strains of the disease, lasting at least 5 years. A vaccine against the problematic B strain has now also been licensed, and hopefully a combination vaccine may soon be developed.

Vaccination is important for travellers at high risk (e.g. those who have had a splenectomy), and for travellers to high-risk destinations (see Fig. 2.1), especially if they will be in close contact with local populations (e.g. in schools, hospitals, or refugee camps). See also ➔ Meningitis, p. 473.

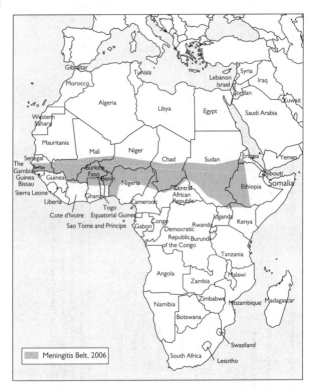

Fig. 2.1 Distribution of annual epidemics of meningococcal meningitis in Africa: the 'meningitis belt'.

intramuscular route but state that suitably qualified and experienced healthcare professionals may give the vaccine via the intradermal route. This method is known to be effective, is supported by the WHO, and is used routinely in many countries.)

- It is also acceptable to provide post-exposure prophylaxis by this method.

Tick-borne encephalitis

A safe vaccine is available, and medical experts in the affected regions strongly advise visitors to be vaccinated if they will be exposed to possible risk (Fig. 2.6). (In Austria, the entire population is vaccinated as a matter of routine!) The vaccine requires two, or preferably three, doses for protection, starting at least 4 weeks prior to travel and given on months 0, 1–3, with the final vaccine given 5 months after the second. The first two doses can be given 2 weeks apart.

Vaccination is strongly advised for people at risk, particularly those visiting forested areas in late spring, or those likely to drink unpasteurized milk from infected animals (e.g. Tibetan yaks). For short-term travellers, many advise tick avoidance measures only. See also ➲ Ticks, p. 288.

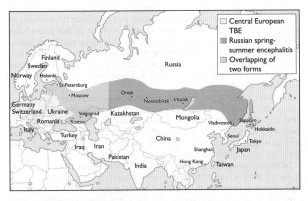

Fig. 2.6 Geographical distribution of tick-borne encephalitis.

Tuberculosis

Immunization with bacillus Calmette–Guérin (BCG) is not routinely offered to children in the UK, though it is offered at birth to targeted risk groups. Expeditions involving travel to parts of the world that are highly endemic for tuberculosis (TB)—especially if there will also be a close degree of contact with local people—should consider the need for BCG protection or TB testing with a skin test or blood test. See also ➲ Tuberculosis, p. 475.

Typhoid

Typhoid remains common in all low-income countries, and in most hot countries with poor hygiene conditions (➲ Typhoid and paratyphoid (enteric fevers), p. 477). Vaccination is advisable for travel to Africa, Asia (especially the Indian subcontinent), and Latin America, and should also be considered for travel to Mexico and the Caribbean.

Two vaccines are available: an oral vaccine (Ty 21a), consisting of three capsules to be swallowed on alternate days, that provide full protection for up to 5 years; and an (Vi antigen) injected vaccine, that provides 3-year protection after a single dose.

- The oral vaccine contains live, modified bacteria, so should not be taken at the same time as antibiotics (e.g. doxycycline used for bacterial infections and for malaria chemoprophylaxis).
- Previous generations of typhoid vaccines caused unpleasant reactions (local pain, fever, illness), so travellers may be concerned about side effects—current oral and injected vaccines are extremely safe and do not cause these effects.
- Vaccine protection is ~70–80% effective.

Yellow fever

Vaccination against yellow fever is necessary for travel to many parts of Africa and South America (Fig. 2.7), either as a certificate requirement or for personal protection (➲ Yellow fever, p. 464). It is also a certificate requirement in many countries outside the yellow fever endemic zones—notably in Asia, for travellers arriving from affected regions of Africa and South America. (Although yellow fever does not occur in Asia, it has the potential to cause serious outbreaks if inadvertently introduced by an infected traveller.)

The WHO now advise that a single yellow fever vaccine induces lifelong protection. However, yellow fever vaccination certificates are currently valid only for 10 years. Changes in the International Health Regulations can take many years to be introduced and fully implemented. In the meantime, seek up-to-date advice on requirements and recommendations, since these are likely to change in the near future.

Increasing awareness of vaccine side effects has coincided with efforts to define and map yellow fever risk more accurately, and to make sure that only people at genuine risk of exposure receive the vaccine. On the other hand, we now know that the vaccine offers long-lasting protection—both from yellow fever, and from vaccine risks in later life, and that many serious travellers do not know in advance where their travels will take them. There is an attractive case for vaccinating such people when they are younger, healthy, and immune-competent, regardless of their exact destination.

- Don't leave vaccination to the last minute—the vaccination certificate does not become valid until 10 days after vaccination.
- Be aware that international regulations are aimed at protecting countries from importation of the virus rather than at protecting travellers, and that some countries apply these public health rules very vigorously.
- The vaccine is only given at designated yellow fever vaccination centres.
- The vaccine is live, so should be avoided where possible in pregnancy and is contraindicated in those who are immunocompromised.

(a)

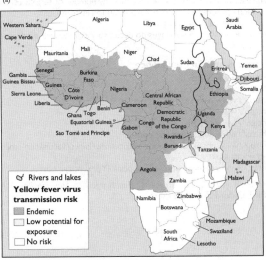

(b)

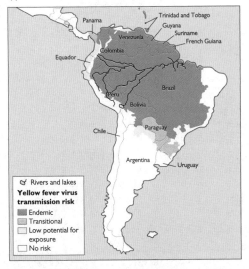

Fig. 2.7 Geographical distribution of yellow fever. Vaccination is strongly recommended for all travellers to both endemic and transitional areas.

- The vaccine is extremely safe, though a tiny number of serious reactions in elderly people has led to increased caution in its use.
- Only a single dose is necessary.
- Yellow fever vaccine shortages do occur, so vaccinate well in advance of needing it.

Resources and further advice

🖰 http://www.dh.gov.uk
🖰 http://www.travax.nhs.uk
🖰 http://www.nathnac.org
🖰 http://www.who.int/ith
🖰 http://www.cdc.gov
🖰 http://www.fleetstreetclinic.com
🖰 http://www.nhs.uk/Conditions/vaccinations/Pages/vaccination-schedule-age-checklist.aspx
🖰 http://www.nathnac.org/yellow_book/YBmainpage.htm

Dawood R (ed) (2012). *Travellers' Health: How to Stay Healthy Abroad.* Oxford: Oxford University Press.

Medical kits and supplies

Chapter 28 contains information about the type of supplies and drugs that need to be included in an expedition medical kit. The exact requirements will depend upon:

• The size of the party, the duration of the trip, and its remoteness.
• The environments visited.
• Access to local medical assistance and its quality.
• The number of outlying camps.
• The likelihood of having to treat local staff and villagers.
• The medical knowledge of the team members/medic.
• Communications with other camps and remote medical help.
• Ease and speed of evacuation in event of a serious incident.
• Transportability.
• Cost.
• All equipment must be packed in suitably protective containers and clearly labelled. Security is important to minimize the risk of theft—especially of drugs that could be used for recreational purposes or re-sold in developing countries.

Obtaining supplies

Buying medical supplies from a retailer can be costly, and acquiring, packing, and labelling a medical kit can be time-consuming. UK drug companies may provide samples or donate medication, particularly if there is some formal recognition of the company's sponsorship. Local pharmacists and NHS hospital trusts may be able to help by providing drugs at cost. Technically, GPs should not give NHS prescriptions for illnesses which may be acquired outside the UK, but many do.

In some parts of the world, prescription drugs are available over the counter but they may be counterfeit and the quality cannot be guaranteed.

Drug export

Expeditions carrying reasonable quantities of drugs are unlikely to encounter problems at customs when entering a country. However, it may be useful to have a doctor's letter stating that the drugs are for the personal use of the expedition team members and are not the subject of any commercial transaction.

Controlled drugs

Wherever possible, avoid taking 'controlled' drugs. A Home Office licence is required and must be returned within 28 days of return to the UK. For more details see: ℞ http://www.gov.uk/controlled-drugs-licences-fees-and-returns. Any controlled drugs dispensed should be recorded in a controlled drugs register. Local controls over drugs, especially painkillers and sedatives, vary and it is important not to be found to be carrying inappropriate medications for that part of the world. The International Narcotics Control Board (℞ http://www.INCB.org) provides information on country regulations regarding the transfer of drugs across borders.

Sometimes acceptance on a trip is provisional, pending performance on training exercises or a full medical examination and review.

Occasionally, significant pre-existing illness is not declared until the expedition is in the field. This can be a very risky situation where there is inadequate information about the condition, additional medication is not available, and the expedition is very remote from expert medical help. If the applicant is uninsured because the insurers will not cover this particular condition, it may be necessary to repatriate that person before an incident occurs.

Box 2.3 A health questionnaire for pre-existing conditions

1. Do you suffer from asthma, epilepsy, or diabetes?
2. Have you ever had any heart problems?
3. Do you suffer from recurring back or joint problems?
4. Do you have any condition that impairs your immune system?
5. Have you ever suffered from chronic fatigue syndrome or any other condition affecting your energy levels?
6. Do you have or have you ever had any significant infectious disease e.g. hepatitis B, HIV, or TB?
7. Have you ever had a psychological or psychiatric illness, including an eating disorder, deliberate self-harm, overdoses, depression, anxiety or panic attacks, psychotic episodes, schizophrenia, or bipolar disorder?
8. Do you have any other current medical problems or are you on treatment for any condition?
9. Are you currently undergoing any medical investigations?
10. What medication are you taking, if any?
11. Are you allergic to anything?
12. Have you ever used recreational drugs or had a problem controlling your alcohol intake?
13. Do you have any objections to any form of treatment, including blood transfusions or immunizations?
14. How many days off sick have you had over the last year?
15. Please record your height and weight.

Generic pre-expedition advice

- Staff and other team members should have a working knowledge of any disability or illness and immediate treatment that may be necessary, such as management of hypoglycaemia, anaphylaxis, or convulsions in fellow expeditioners.
- Review the group medical kit—will any extra items be required?
- Make contingency plans. Are there escape routes so that a journey can be curtailed if necessary?
- Ensure that the expedition's insurers are fully informed—some pre-existing medical conditions attract a higher insurance premium, and insurers are not required to meet a claim if they have not been informed of all material facts.

Pre-expedition advice for the participants
- The individual should be able to demonstrate a good level of fitness appropriate to expedition activities to be undertaken. Short, low-intensity trips to a similar environment with different activity levels will be particularly useful for people with conditions such as diabetes where the individual needs to learn to manage their illness in varied conditions.
- Optimize the illness and monitor with a diary of blood sugars, blood pressure, peak flow rates, etc.
- Each individual with a pre-existing medical condition should have a self-management plan after discussion with their GP, specialist nurse, or consultant. This can be summarized in a letter from the treating doctor together with any significant past illnesses and medications. Consider whether standby medications may be needed, e.g. prednisolone for acute asthma, antibiotics for those with immune suppression.
- Individuals need to carry their own medication with some in reserve.
- Discuss the risks openly, and ensure participants are prepared to accept them.

During the journey
- Flying west results in a long day, flying east a short day.
- Most people who take regular medication should stay on home time and then adjust timings on arrival. Those on anti-epileptics or with type 1 diabetes should seek advice from their specialist about how to adjust their medication.
- All travellers need to keep hydrated and mobile, particularly while flying.
- Pro-thrombotic conditions may benefit from compression stockings, even low-molecular-weight heparin injections on the advice of a haematologist. There is insufficient evidence at present to support the use of aspirin as prevention against flight-related deep venous thrombosis.

During the expedition
- Advice and support should be available—from group leaders/medical team or local medical staff.
- Where good communications exist it may be possible to obtain advice from the home country and treating doctors.
- Encourage the 'buddy system', particularly for younger groups, so that all individuals are looking out for any problems.

After the expedition
- Encourage reassessment of any medical condition with the expeditioner's GP/specialist.
- Send a report of any significant problems to the GP.
- Consider reporting back to the RGS-IBG Expedition Medicine Group any significant medical problems and 'near misses' using the forms available at: ℘ http://www.rgs.org/medicalcell

Advising those with common pre-existing conditions

Asthma

One in 12 adults has asthma (see ⟩ Asthma, p. 380):

- Optimize control before departure to enable a good level of fitness.
- Consider carrying a peak flow meter and spacer (probably not a nebulizer as this is bulky and heavy, but consider if on-board ship or on a larger expedition).
- Carry a supply of oral and injectable steroids.
- Consider standby antibiotics if an individual is prone to infections.
- Follow the British Thoracic Society (BTS) guidelines for management. See: ℘ http://www.brit-thoracic.org.uk/guidelines/asthma-guidelines. aspx
- Each individual should discuss a treatment plan with their GP, asthma nurse, or respiratory specialist before departure.
- May need to exclude those with severe or brittle asthma. Those with numerous or recent exacerbations will also need to consider carefully the risks of travelling remote from healthcare.
- High-altitude travel is not a provoking factor for asthma, but an asthma exacerbation at high altitude will be more serious because of the hypoxic environment and lack of access to medical care.
- Cold may trigger asthma attacks in some individuals.

The management of acute asthma is discussed on ⟩ Prevention of acute asthma attacks, p. 380.

Diabetes

Diabetes need not be a contraindication to travel; however, a person with type 1 diabetes needs to be confident monitoring their blood sugars and adjusting their diabetes control (⟩ Diabetic emergencies, p. 256). Those who have recently been diagnosed with diabetes should consider deferring a trip to a very remote area until they are completely confident that they can manage the disease safely without outside support.

The main concerns regarding travel with diabetes are:

- The risk of hypoglycaemia because of changes in time zones, food intake, and energy output. Some blood sugar monitors are less reliable in extreme conditions such as sub-zero temperatures.
- Infections are more likely and may be more serious, especially gastro-enteritis.
- In those who have had diabetes for many years there is an increased risk of heart attack or stroke. Reduced kidney function, disturbances in skin sensation (particularly the feet), and ulceration should also be considered.

Diabetics: before the expedition

Antimalarials and immunizations should be advised as for other travellers. Consider how insulin will be stored on the expedition (see Box 2.4).

It is useful to have the following information from the GP, diabetes nurse, or specialist:

- Date of diagnosis.
- How well controlled is the patient's diabetes (HbA1c level)?
- Do they follow medical advice?
- Insulin type, dosage, frequency?
- Have there been episodes of hypoglycaemia/hyperglycaemia?
- Any complications—neuropathy, ulceration, eye problems or insulin resistance?
- Has treatment varied over last year?

This information can be written in a letter and given to the patient. If appropriate, it can also usefully mention the need for carrying needles and syringes. Even if not eating, people with diabetes continue to need regular insulin, and frequent blood sugar testing becomes even more important. Intravenous fluids and injectable antiemetics may be needed if vomiting occurs, and the use of these items may need special training or the presence of a suitably qualified healthcare professional.

Other group members should be trained in recognizing the symptoms of hypoglycaemia and the treatment needed—GlucoGel®, glucagon, or, rarely, intravenous glucose 10%.

Diabetics: during the expedition
It is important to consider:

- Will there be medical/nursing staff available to supervise/advise treatment?
- The expedition organizers need to consider the dietary needs of those with diabetes. Snacks should be readily available in case of delays or low blood sugar levels.
- 'Ideal' blood sugar levels may not be possible because of varying diet and activity levels. The main concern is preventing hypoglycaemia, so a little latitude is reasonable for a few weeks during the trip.
- People with diabetes are more susceptible to infections and should report any symptoms at an early stage before blood sugar levels become erratic. Foot infections may be particularly serious in those who do not have normal sensation. Particular importance should be paid to keeping feet clean, dry, and inspecting for problems. Wounds and fungal infections must be treated promptly to prevent ulceration and other complications.

Checklist for the individual diabetic
- Ensure adequate supplies of insulin, lancets, sugar testing sticks, syringes/pens, needles, sharps disposal, glucometer, GlucoGel®, and glucagon and plans for correct insulin storage as appropriate (see Box 2.4).
- A talisman such as a MedicAlert® bracelet should be worn.
- Are the insurers aware, as diabetes is a significant pre-existing condition?
- If the individual suffers from travel sickness, consider an antiemetic to prevent vomiting/dehydration.
- Oral rehydration solutions should be available.

Box 2.4 Insulin storage

Ideally insulin should be stored at 4–8°C. At these temperatures it will remain active for up to 2 years. Insulin that has been opened can be kept at room temperature; viability is usually 28 days but individuals should check with the manufacturer of their insulin.

Frio® insulin storage pouches keep insulin vials cool in hot climates for up to 28 days (℠ http://www.friouk.com).

Insulin should be carried in hand luggage, although a medical letter of authorization should be obtained from the patient's GP. X-rays do not affect insulin.

Vacuum flasks can be used to protect insulin from climatic extremes. If insulin is 'clumped' or turbid it should not be used.

Other resources

℠ http://www.diabetes.org.uk

℠ http://www.diabetes-exercise.org

Hypertension

Isolated, well-controlled hypertension is not a problem for most people travelling to remote areas. However, if there is evidence of secondary organ damage due to hypertension (heart failure, renal failure) the risks of stroke or heart attack will be much higher (→ Hypertension, p. 52). Consider:

- Blood pressure should be stable before travel.
- Whether there are other significant cardiovascular risk factors and whether they have been addressed.
- Check renal function before travel.
- Ensure that there is a good level of fitness and that individuals can cope with activity levels similar to those likely on the trip.
- Blood pressure may improve with weight loss and increased exercise during an expedition. Consider whether measuring blood pressure during the trip will be feasible or even sensible.
- Antihypertensive medication:
  - May affect exercise tolerance.
  - Beta-blockers can cause lethargy and limit maximum heart rate response. They also reduce the blood flow to the extremities, which may become important when travelling to cold areas. They can also pre-dispose to heat illness.
  - Diuretics increase urine output, contribute to heat illness, and can lead to hypotension if an individual is already dehydrated.
  - Angiotensin-converting enzyme (ACE) inhibitors can also cause hypotension after exercising.
  - Calcium channel blockers affect heart rate during exercise and side effects include ankle swelling and flushing which may be worse in hot climates.
  - Consider carrying aspirin 300 mg for angina or heart attacks, glyceryl trinitrate (GTN) spray for angina, and blood pressure monitoring equipment.
- After return, people with hypertension should be medically reassessed to check blood pressure and renal function.

Cardiovascular disease

A history of angina, previous MI, or claudication will be worrying. Similarly those with multiple risk factors for cardiovascular disease (hypertension, hypercholesterolaemia, smokers, and/or a strong family history of cardio-vascular disease) need to consider carefully the risks of being remote from health care. Stresses of expedition life may provoke symptoms of chest pain (➜ Chest pain, p. 242) or breathlessness on exertion.

Six months after successful coronary artery bypass graft/angioplasty or stenting it is possible to undertake remote foreign travel provided there are no symptoms of chest pain or breathlessness while exercising to the level required on the expedition. The individual should be able to complete a full exercise electrocardiogram (ECG) without symptoms or ECG changes.

There always remains the risk of recurrence and this must be accepted by the individual and team members. Ask the question: can the individual undertake vigorous activity at the same level as expected on the expedition (i.e. can they spend long days walking in the British hills)?

Epilepsy

The consequences of a seizure during an expedition activity could be very serious; for instance, falling from the back of an open vehicle, being tossed overboard during white-water rafting, or collapsing on steep ground. Dehydration, alcohol, stress, and lack of sleep may all provoke convulsions. Gastroenteritis may affect antiepileptic levels and result in fitting.

Before the trip more information will be required regarding the frequency, severity, preventive medication, and treatment of convulsions. Other team members need to be aware and know what to do in the event of a fit (➜ Urgent treatment, p. 254). Those whose epilepsy is poorly controlled may not be suitable for expeditions. Antiepileptic medication may interact with other drugs, particularly antimalarials and quinolones such as cipro-floxacin. Chloroquine and mefloquine may provoke seizures and should not be used in those with epilepsy.

Treatment of status epilepticus (a seizure lasting longer than 30 min) is very difficult in a remote environment and the condition can be life-threatening. Those with epilepsy should follow guidance regarding swimming, driving, operating machinery, and dangerous activities such as diving and rock climb-ing as they would at home. Epilepsy is a significant pre-existing health prob-lem and insurers must be aware of the diagnosis in the event of a claim. Consider taking rectal and IV diazepam or buccal midazolam together with an oropharyngeal airway and a hand-held suction device.

People with epilepsy are definitely travelling at increased risk but this can be minimized with preparation—some activities such as scuba diving may be unacceptably risky and this should be understood before departure.

Allergy and anaphylaxis

Anaphylaxis is a severe form of allergic reaction (➲ Anaphylaxis and ana-phylactic shock, p. 236; Fig. 8.8). It may be provoked by food, drugs, insect bites, or stings. Knowledge of the allergy is essential for cooks, expedition staff, and other group members.

All expedition members need to be aware of the symptoms and signs of severe allergic reactions and should know how to give adrenaline (epi-nephrine), if required. A MedicAlert®/MediTag bracelet or similar should be worn at all times.

Adrenaline (epinephrine) auto-injectors in the form of an EpiPen® or Jext®, if recommended by the GP or specialist, needs to be carried at all times and must be kept in hand luggage during air travel. It is important that the person at risk knows how to use it in an emergency. Consider taking extra drugs for anaphylaxis—adrenaline (epinephrine), prednisolone, chlor-phenamine, hydrocortisone, and a salbutamol inhaler.

In those with severe allergies, consider oral antihistamine for the duration of the trip. This should be discussed with the GP or specialist. Remember that severe allergy can be induced by aspirin in some people, and that aspi-rin and widely used non-steroidal anti-inflammatory agents, such as ibupro-fen and diclofenac, can cause or aggravate urticaria and angioedema.

Useful resources for allergies
✍ http://allergyuk.org
✍ http://resus.org.uk

> *Suggested questions for those with allergies*
> 1. What are you allergic to?
> 2. How do you react to this substance and how often?
> 3. When did you last have an allergic reaction?
> 4. What treatment is needed when you have an allergic reaction?
> 5. When, if ever, have you required hospital treatment for an allergic reaction?

Inflammatory bowel disease

Inflammatory bowel disease such as Crohn's disease or ulcerative colitis (UC) may predispose individuals to severe, possibly life-threatening diar-rhoea and gastrointestinal (GI) haemorrhage. Other complications such as anaemia, dehydration, and generalized infection may also occur. The drugs used to treat inflammatory bowel disease may have an effect on the immune system so that infections may be easier to acquire. Some drugs, e.g. azathioprine, require periodic monitoring of blood tests. Infectious diar-rhoea may trigger a flare up of the underlying condition. On expedition, it may be very difficult to differentiate between the two.

Individuals with inflammatory bowel disease should be fully aware of the potential risks. Severe, bloody diarrhoea, particularly if associated with a fever or abdominal pain, require prompt medical attention.

For those with inflammatory bowel disease:
- Avoid traveller's diarrhoea if at all possible.
- Inform the MO immediately if there is any flare-up of disease—particularly bloody stools, abdominal pain, and fever.

- The group should carry oral rehydration solutions, IV fluids, antibiotics, and steroids.
- A casualty evacuation plan should be in place.

Further information may be found at ℰ http://www.crohns.org.uk and ℰ http://www.crohnsandcolitis.org.uk/information-and-support

Psychiatric illness

(See also Chapter 16.) Depression, anxiety, panic attacks, deliberate self-harm, and eating disorders are all common. Non-disclosure happens occasionally and will affect insurance cover. There is a wide variety in severity and risk of each illness. Those with a single episode of depression and subsequent recovery in response to a significant life event pose a lower level of risk than those with recurrent or chronic problems.

A carefully worded pre-expedition questionnaire is needed to ensure that psychiatric and psychological illness is not overlooked. Anyone with a history of psychiatric illness should be followed up with a more detailed discussion of the problem.

Some expedition companies will not accept those still taking antidepressant medication because of the difficulty of managing an exacerbation and for arranging regular supervision.

Dehydration predisposes to lithium toxicity which may be fatal.

Low body mass index (BMI) may mean that the individual has little physical reserve in the event of other illness. Binge eating or vomiting can be very disruptive for other group members to cope with.

Involve the GP and/or psychiatrist in making the decision regarding fitness to travel—an expedition is not the place to convalesce from a serious mental health problem.

If there is a history of psychotic illness most psychiatrists recommend that the individual should have been stable for 2 years, is off medication, and can show evidence of coping with stressful situations, including foreign travel.

Disabilities

Remarkable achievements on expeditions have been made by those with significant disabilities. Appropriate challenges can be identified which help to maintain independence and dignity by the use of special adaptations. A multidisciplinary team (occupational therapists, physiotherapists, nurses, rehabilitation physicians, and prosthetists) can all contribute to identifying these challenges and advising on safe travel.

The needs of those with disabilities may be considered under the following headings:
- Mobility (prostheses, wheelchair, ability to transfer).
- Seating (are specialized cushions required?).
- Activities of daily living (ADLs)—what help is needed for activities of daily living—washing, feeding, shaving, toileting?
- Communication—consider the safety aspects for those with hearing or visual impairment.
- Bladder/bowel control—self-catheterization, use of suppositories, changing ileostomy bags are all possible issues which will need sensitive management.

- Skin—prolonged walking, immersion in sea water, and the effects of heat may affect the skin under a prosthetic limb or the prosthesis itself. Those with paraplegia may quickly develop pressure sores or blisters without realizing, so skin care in this group is very important.
- Cognitive and behavioural—are there any difficulties with thinking, understanding, behaviour, or psychological issues?

HIV and immunosuppression

Expedition members who are HIV positive or immunosuppressed for other reasons need specialist advice about immunizations well in advance. Those who are immunosuppressed should be educated about the potential risks of infectious disease and there should be a low threshold for treatment as well as medical evacuation if needed (➲ Repatriation, p. 158). The individual risks of infectious disease in the location of the expedition need to be taken into account when deciding whether to accept a potential participant. Most of the immunosuppressed are unable to receive 'live' vaccines including yellow fever.

Those with HIV may need prophylaxis against opportunistic infections on the advice of their specialist. Those with a good CD4 count (>500) are considered to be without significant immune compromise. Consider whether any antiretroviral medication may need blood monitoring while away. Participants on immunosuppressive medications such as azathioprine may also require blood monitoring depending on the length of the expedition.

Splenectomized patients are at increased risk of bacterial infections caused by pneumococcus and meningococcus, as well as being more vulnerable to malaria. They should seek specialist pre-travel advice.

Those on prolonged courses of high-dose steroids (>20 mg prednisolone/day for >2 weeks) are at particularly high risk of infection.

Chronic fatigue syndrome

Participants with a history of chronic or post-viral fatigue should be able to demonstrate full recovery and ability to participate in normal daily activities for a significant period of time prior to the expedition. Infectious diseases or overexertion may contribute towards relapse.

Obesity

23% of adults in the UK are obese; some morbidly so (BMI >40). Obese travellers are at increased risk of heat acclimatization problems, dehydration, deep venous thrombosis (DVT), and musculoskeletal problems. In addition, there may be undiagnosed associated conditions such as hypertension and diabetes. Serious consideration should be given as to whether those with severe obesity are able to cope with the physical demands of an expedition. Encourage weight loss beforehand and consider assessment of physical capacity pre-expedition on training exercises.

The older traveller

Increasing numbers of older people are visiting remote and exotic places, or taking part in adventurous activities. Most travel without mishap. Advancing age, however, brings declining health and physical disability, which can increase health risk for the adventurous traveller. Pre-existing, chronic illness and medication increase overall health risk and older people are more likely to experience travel-related illness while abroad. The 65+ years age group differs from the young with potential adverse effects on global travel due to:

- Age-related physiological changes.
- Increased incidence of co-morbidity.
- Atypical disease presentations.
- Increased incidence of iatrogenic illness.
- Functional disability.

Effects of the ageing process

Adverse changes occur in:

- Renal function, water, and sodium regulation.
- Temperature regulation.
- Cardiopulmonary and GI function.
- Cell-mediated immune response.
- Neurological function.
- Metabolic response.

Health risks affected by ageing

- Reduced cardiac reserve decreases ability to cope with dehydration, high altitude, or physical exertion.
- Reduced lung capacity means less reserve to deal with reduced oxygen at altitude or from infections.
- Weakened immune system makes infection more likely.
- Deteriorating kidney function increases likelihood that dehydration will lead to kidney failure.
- Poor renal function diminishes ability for kidneys to cope with salt loss when diarrhoea occurs.
- Deteriorating brain function may result in confusion in stressful situations.
- Poor brain function causes difficulty in coping with new situations and can lead to serious anxiety.
- Poor vision and hearing can lead to accidents, or failure to see or hear public announcements.
- Poorer circulation and healing results in slower healing of injuries, wounds, and bites.
- Thinning bones from osteoporosis increase the risk of fractures with falls.
- Thinning skin increases the risk of nasty lacerations—especially over the shins.
- Reduced stomach acid increases risk from food poisoning and contaminated food and water.

Pre-expedition considerations for older travellers

A personalized pre-travel health review can identify potential problems and, with anticipation and precaution, overall risks to health can be reduced. In terms of health risk, the potential older traveller can be grouped in one of the following:

- *Group 1—low risk*—the 'young' old includes:
  - Those travelling to low-risk destinations.
  - Those on short-haul journeys.
  - Those free from any pre-disposing illness.
- *Group 2—medium risk*—where travel involves:
  - Environmental extremes.
  - Travel to tropical countries.
  - The 'frail old'—those with pre-existing illness, e.g. diabetes.
- *Group 3—high risk:*
  - The terminally ill.
  - Those with pre-existing illness *and* travelling to high-risk countries.
  - Pre-existing illness and visiting tropical countries or environmental extremes.

In addition to the regular pre-travel management plan, consider the following in relation to age, ability, and co-morbidities:
- Identify and analyse health hazards of expedition (actual and potential).
- Minimize impact of potential health hazards.
- Identify appropriate chemoprophylaxis/vaccination (include influenza and pneumococcal vaccination).
- Consider potential changes in routine drug medication.
- Assess effects of pre-existing disease in foreign environment.
- Clinical evaluation at specialist travel health clinic/GP for groups 2 and 3.
- Ensure adequate travel health insurance including repatriation cover.
- Ask 'what if . . . ?'

Expedition considerations for older travellers

Whilst on expedition it is vitally important that both the individual traveller and expedition medic have a heightened awareness as to the age-related problems that might occur. Ensure:
- Expedition activities can be adjusted to match the physical capabilities of all the participants.
- Medications for those with co-morbidities are stored appropriately.
- Changes to plans fall within acceptable and manageable risks for the whole team.
- Older individuals feel comfortable in voicing health concerns without feeling burdensome.
- A lower threshold for seeking medical advice when faced with illness in the older traveller.

Post-expedition considerations for older travellers

As with any expeditioner, health problems can arise in the months following an expedition. Age-related physiological changes put the older traveller at greater potential risk for developing travel-related illness on return, the complications of which can be severe. Expedition members should be encouraged to seek medical advice on return if there are:

- Changes in bowel habits.
- An onset of fevers or flu-like symptoms.
- Changes in co-morbidities, e.g. unstable blood glucose levels.
- Unusual rashes or dermatological changes.

Awareness of risk, sensible pre-travel preparation, and a rapid response to problems whilst away will help ensure elderly travellers journey in good health.

Resources for the older traveller

For further information see: ✆ http://www.interhealth.org.uk/home/around-the-world/health-information-a-z

McIntosh I (2013). *Travel and Health: Management and Care of the Older Traveller*. Exeter: Short Run Press.

Child health in remote areas

Exploring with children and adolescents broadens everyone's horizons and facilitates introductions to people who might otherwise have been passed by. It does, however, often mean adapting the style and pace of travel. Goal-driven trips where the targets have been set by adults without consulting younger members can be disastrous. Involve everyone in the planning and allow time for everyone to indulge their interests. The trip will be most successful if the adults are performing well within their levels of competence. Children are often more adaptable and resourceful than the adults with whom they travel.

Diagnosing illness in children, especially in the under-3s, is difficult—even for paediatricians—and so any adult travelling to remote places with small children must be well prepared, well read, and have a good back-out plan. The commonest causes of problems in travelling children are accidents, scrapes and bumps, swallowing things they shouldn't have, traveller's diarrhoea, skin sepsis, and common infections as at home: tonsillitis, ear, and chest infections. The responsible adult should either be carrying the wherewithal to treat these problems or should know someone who can.

Immunization

Parents will need to ensure their child is up to date with the routine childhood vaccines (Table 2.1) because, in less well-resourced regions, levels of local immunization will be low and thus 'herd' immunity is poor. Travellers are therefore at increased risk of measles, pertussis, diphtheria, etc. For other immunizations the family should consult a travel health expert. Intrepid children are more likely to get bitten by dogs and monkeys; rabies immunization is therefore especially relevant for any mobile child.

Yellow fever immunization is not given to infants under the age of 9 months so this might preclude family travel to regions where yellow fever is common.

Parenteral typhoid immunization has poor efficacy in children under the age of 18 months and gives no cover at all against paratyphoid. Oral typhoid immunization offers some cover against paratyphoid but is only licensed for children over the age of 6. Parents must therefore be especially aware of the means of reducing the risk of these and other faecal-oral infections (➔ Diarrhoea and vomiting, p. 398).

Antimalarials

Both mefloquine (Lariam®) and atovaquone + proguanil (Malarone®) can be given to small children. Mefloquine does not seem to cause the problems with mood that adults sometimes experience; the tablets crack easily into quarters for children's doses. It should be noted, however, that travel into highly malarious regions with small children or when pregnant may be unwise, and expert advice should be sought before travel.

Unfamiliar environments

Odd and unexpected things can faze children and adolescents, including weird food, unfamiliar lavatory arrangements (toddlers can't squat over long drops), and issues surrounding personal space. Small children prefer to be down at a level where they too can explore; they get bored if carried all day, and it is sobering to realize that every year in the Alps children die from hypothermia while being carried in backpacks by skiing or mountaineering parents. A thermometer is not necessary to assess if a baby or toddler is chilling dangerously. Compare his skin temperature on the limbs with trunk temperature; if the limbs feel colder then the child needs to be warmed in a place of shelter.

Sunshine

Sunburn in childhood is associated with an increased risk of skin cancer in adulthood. It also makes the whole family miserable. Severe sunburn can lead to hypothermia, disastrous loss of fluids, and secondary infection. It is crucial, therefore, that children are protected with long clothes, hats, sun-protective swimsuits, umbrellas (if carried in a backpack), sunscreens, and avoidance of exposure at the very hottest times of the day. So-called sun-blocks reduce exposure to the wavelengths that cause sunburn without necessarily giving adequate protection to cancer-causing wavelengths. SPFs of 15–30 are therefore recommended; sunscreens need to be reapplied frequently (see also ➔ Solar skin damage, p. 266). Sunscreens need replacing each year.

A fine pimply, very itchy rash is probably *prickly heat*. Unlike many of the other causes of itching in children, this is not a histamine-mediated response and so it doesn't respond to antihistamines. The treatment is getting the child cool—either by immersing or splashing with cold water, dabbing (not rubbing) with a damp cloth, and/or retreating to a room with a fan or air conditioning. Calamine lotion is soothing. Dressing the child in loose fitting, 100% cotton clothes will help avoid the problem, and so will a rest during the hottest part of the day.

Bite prevention for children

It is wise to embrace precautions that avoid insect and tick bites, not least because an itching bitten child is miserable but, in hot climates, scratched bites often lead to skin infections. Hydrocortisone 1% or betametasone diproprionate 0.025% ointments are the best treatment for bites and stings, although could promote sepsis if the skin is broken. Skin infections (➔ Wound infections, p. 278) cause spreading redness, oozing, sometimes red tracking on the affected limb, and, later, fever.

Choosing the right clothes and footwear helps keep biters away, as does spraying these clothes with permethrin. At dusk, any remaining exposed skin can be covered in a repellent based on up to 30% DEET, or Merck 3535. Repellents that are based on citronella or lemon eucalyptus are less effective alternatives. If the child is small then he can be protected under a cot net (preferably also proofed with permethrin), and older children are partially protected by the fact that malaria mosquitoes tend to hunt at ankle level; thus applying repellent to the clothes usually discourages mosquitoes from searching up and biting the face. Further information on bite avoidance, bed nets, etc., is on ➔ Prevention of malaria, p. 483.

The fretful small child—ill or bored?

When children become unwell, they can become precipitously ill within hours, and diagnosis can very difficult, especially if the patient isn't yet capable of explaining where it hurts. A toddler with tonsillitis, for example, will often point to his tummy when asked where the pain is. Many cautious paediatricians advise against intrepid travel with children who cannot yet talk because:

- It is difficult to distinguish boredom from disease.
- Small children are fearless and fall off things, or drown.
- Children explore and swallow things they shouldn't.
- Bacillary dysentery can make them dangerously ill rapidly.
- Dehydration becomes an issue sooner and can be difficult to manage.
- Malaria is a huge risk and bite precautions are difficult to enforce.
- Small children taken to altitude are at risk of hypothermia and mountain sickness (see ➲ Children at altitude, p. 670.)

Once a child has reached the age of 4 years they become fun to travel with, they'll enjoy sharing your adventures and are better able to communicate symptoms of illness. Illness with fever can initially be treated with both paracetamol and ibuprofen. In a non-malarial region it is probably safe to delay consulting a doctor if the child perks up, although meningitis or typhoid are always possible. In areas where malaria is a risk, a child with a fever over 38°C should be evacuated to a clinic or hospital.

Diagnostic aids for an ill child

Diagnosis in an ill child is challenging whoever you are and travel makes this task even more difficult. The designated adult responsible for children would be well advised to travel with *urine dipsticks*, a *thermometer* and a *child health book*. The *Baby Check* scoring system is invaluable for grading the severity of illness in babies under 6 months (see ➲ Resources: children's health abroad, p. 67). The responsible adult should also know the location of the nearest competent medical facility.

Common causes of high fever in children

- Tonsillitis (toddlers usually refuse food).
- Middle ear infection (with ear ache on one side only).
- Pneumonia/lung infection (>40 breaths/min).
- Bacillary dysentery (fever can start before the diarrhoea; blood is sometimes visible in the stools).
- Sepsis arising from wound infections.
- Malaria (has the child been in a malarious region for >1 week?).
- Meningitis and meningococcal septicaemia.
- Dengue fever (children raised in temperate zones often avoid the severe 'breakbone' illness of adults).

Common causes of drowsiness in children

- Fatigue.
- Dehydration, especially secondary to diarrhoea.
- Malaria.
- Significant infection, including typhoid, meningitis, UTI, etc.
- The child has swallowed something noxious (e.g. someone's sleeping pills or paraffin in a cola bottle).

Diarrhoea in children

In diarrhoea, fluids are lost through increased bowel actions and from sweating (especially if there is also fever), yet the appetite will be wanting and often it is difficult to get the child to drink. Standard oral rehydration salts and even fruit-flavoured oral rehydration solutions taste unpleasant because of the potassium content, and many children—even if somewhat dehydrated—will refuse them. In most situations all that the child needs is water with some kind of solute in it. Sugars and/or salts enhance fluid transport into the body, so that water is absorbed more efficiently than if pure water is drunk.

Examples of rehydration solutions include:

• Young coconut.
• Crackers and water.
• Thin soups.
• Colas (but not Diet Coke®); add a pinch of salt.
• Banana and water.
• Toast, jam, and fluids.
• Water or dilute squashes with honey or sugar added.
• Weak herb teas with sugar added.
• Blackcurrant juice.
• Sweet drinks that you can see through.
• Drinks made with Bovril®, Marmite®, or Oxo®.
• Plain carbohydrate foods such as boiled rice and noodles also enhance fluid absorption.

Dehydration in children

Paediatricians make meticulous calculations of what is required to rehydrate an ill child, but a child who is controlling fluid intake through drinking is most unlikely to overhydrate. An early sign of dehydration is to look at the lips and inside the mouth; if these areas look dry then the child needs more fluids. A child who is continuing to pass urine is not significantly dehydrated. Comparing the child's current weight with a recent reliable weight is a useful method of assessing whether there is dehydration. If the child becomes too drowsy to drink then IV or nasogastric fluids will be required.

Some causes of abdominal pain in children

• Diarrhoea/gastroenteritis (pain often relieved by passing wind or stool).
• Constipation (give more to drink, and lots of fruit; increasing pain often heralds stool passage).
• Tonsillitis (in the under-3s, antibiotics are recommended).
• Urinary tract ('bladder') infection (serious in the under-5s—treat with antibiotics and arrange further investigation on return).
• Fatigue (equivalent to a grown-up's migraine).
• Appendicitis (usually in children >5 years; pain starts around navel and moves to right lower abdomen; a child with an appetite does not have appendicitis, nor does one who can jump around, or sit up from lying without pain). Suspected appendicitis needs evacuation to a hospital.
• Meningitis, see ➜ Meningitis, p. 473 (an emergency—evacuate).
• Malaria, see ➜ Malaria, p. 480 (an emergency—evacuate).
• Pneumonia (respiratory rate is usually increased >40/min); antibiotics by mouth may cure. Hospital assessment is recommended.

- Typhoid or paratyphoid (note that paratyphoid is not covered by current injectable vaccines); this is a serious condition that needs expert treatment.
- Hepatitis A or E (often mild in small children) and some other viral infections.
- Intussusception (in child 3 months to 2 years; needs surgery).
- Threadworm (there will also be anal itching); treat with oral mebendazole and repeat after 1 week.
- Twisted testicle (some children are too shy to mention where it hurts); needs urgent surgery.

Generally the further away the pain is from the navel the more likely it is to have a significant or serious cause. Pain that wakes a child at night suggests real illness and is seldom benign.

Breathing problems in children

Respiratory problems are common in travelling children. Perhaps a fifth will have asthmatic tendencies yet they may not have an inhaler with them. Chest infections are common too. Noisy breathing (grunting or wheezing) is a sign of illness, and the breathing rate will give some indication of the severity. Flaring of the nostrils on inspiration suggests that the child is struggling to get enough air into the lungs. Whistling or high-pitched musical noises, mostly on breathing out, suggest asthma, while deeper sounds, mostly on breathing in, are most likely to be due to croup or obstruction above the level of the lungs. Remember that asthma and croup can kill so, if in doubt, or if the child is small, evacuate to a hospital.

Normal breathing rates

Newborn baby:	30–40 breaths/min (>60 suggests difficulties).
Child >2 months:	<30/min (>40 suggests significant problem).
Big kids and adults:	<20 breaths/min.

First-aid supplies for children

Those new to family travel tend to take too much. Probably the most important item is a knowledge base or book. Colourful dressings seem to have remarkable analgesic properties and so does chocolate: these are important items to have immediately to hand. Wound infections begin readily in hot climates and so an appropriate means of cleaning and dressing wounds is essential. Savlon® Dry spray is convenient, as are antiseptic wipes. For long periods in remote regions, potassium permanganate crystals are light, cheap, and portable; they are often available at the destination (make up to a rosé wine-coloured solution in water and use this to bathe wounds). Do not use antiseptic creams since these promote infection. Other medication will depend upon the level of knowledge of the carers or medic.

Suggested medical kit for children

- Insect repellent (up to 30% DEET can be used, with care, on children).
- Sunscreen 15–30 SPF, broad-brimmed hat and sun-protective clothes.
- Paracetamol and/or ibuprofen syrup. (NB If bought locally may not be so palatable.)
- Digital thermometer.
- Steri-Strips™.
- Colourful sticking plasters.
- 'Savlon® Dry iodine spray or other drying antiseptic.
- Hydrocortisone or betametasone diproprionate 0.025% ointment (for itchy bites and eczema).
- Amoxicillin syrup (if confident in use of antibiotics).
- Motion sickness preparation if child troubled by this (hyoscine is best for rapid onset one-dose situations or an antihistamine like cinnarizine if multi-dosing is likely).

Resources: children's health abroad

Baby Check: ℘ http://nicutools.org

KidsTravelDoc: ℘ http://www.kidstraveldoc.com. A website founded by a paediatrician dedicated to the health of children when travelling.

Wilson-Howarth J (2009). *The Essential Guide to Travel Health: Don't Let Bugs Bites & Bowels Spoil Your Trip.* London: Cadogan.

Wilson-Howarth J, Ellis M (2014). *Your Child Abroad: A Travel Health Guide* (3rd ed). Chalfont St Peter: Bradt Travel Guides. ℘ http://www.bradt-guides.com/your-child-abroad-ebook.html

Risk management

The concept of managing risk is to identify potential hazards and use control measures to reduce significant risks. This process is only effective if all members of the expedition understand the necessity for these control measures to be in place and are willing to behave accordingly.

Risk can never be completely eliminated, and different people have different thresholds of 'acceptable risk'. Therefore, it is essential to include all expedition members in risk management planning. This ensures that members are fully aware of the risks the expedition is likely to encounter and are able to make an informed decision as to whether to take part in the expedition.

Risk assessments

At the heart of planning a safe and responsible expedition is the process of compiling the risk assessment. The concept is simple; hazards need to be identified and assessed for the severity of risk they represent to the people associated with the expedition (Tables 2.2, 2.3, 2.4).

Risks that are identified are ranked on the basis of the relationship between severity of impact and likelihood of occurrence; the significant risks are then accepted or reduced using appropriate precautions (control measures) such as those identified in Table 2.5.

Definitions (source UK Health and Safety Executive (2006))

Five steps to risk assessment. Health and Safety Executive publication ref: INDG 163 (rev 2) 06/06.

- A *hazard* is anything that may cause harm, such as chemicals, electricity, working from ladders, an open drawer, etc.
- The *risk* is the chance, high or low, that somebody could be harmed by these and other hazards, together with an indication of how serious the harm could be.

Areas to cover in a risk assessment

- The group.
- The environment.
- The activities, e.g. glacier survey, white-water rafting.
- Travel and accommodation.
- Local people.
- Health.

The UK Health and Safety Executive refers to the process as *5 Steps to Risk Assessment* (2006). These are as follows:

1. Identify the hazards and associated risks.
2. Identify who is potentially at risk and how.
3. Identify the precautions or control measures to minimize the risk, including any further action required to reduce the risk to an acceptable level.
4. Record findings.
5. Review the risk assessment periodically.

Table 2.2 Relationship between likelihood and severity of risk

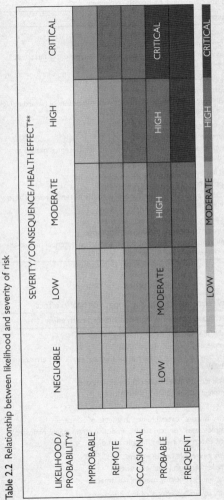

LIKELIHOOD/ PROBABILITY*	SEVERITY/CONSEQUENCE/HEALTH EFFECT**				
	NEGLIGIBLE	LOW	MODERATE	HIGH	CRITICAL
IMPROBABLE					
REMOTE					
OCCASIONAL					CRITICAL
PROBABLE	LOW	MODERATE	HIGH	HIGH	
FREQUENT					

LOW   MODERATE   HIGH   CRITICAL

* Definition see Table 2.3.
** Definition, see Table 2.4.

Table 2.3 Probability of impact of health exposure

Descriptor	Description of probability or health exposure
Frequent	Possibility of repeated incidents Approximately once or more per week *Health exposure*: frequent contact with the potential hazard at very high concentrations
Probable	Possibility of isolated incidents Approximately once per month *Health exposure*: frequent contact with the potential hazard at high concentrations
Occasional	Possibility of occurring some time Approximately once per year *Health exposure*: frequent contact with the potential hazard at moderate concentrations
Remote	Not likely to occur Approximately once in 10 years or less *Health exposure*: frequent contact with the potential hazard at low concentrations
Improbable	Practically impossible Approximately once in 100 years or more *Health exposure*: infrequent contact with the potential hazard at low concentrations

Table 2.4 Severity/consequence of the impact or health effect

Descriptor	Description of severity/consequence or health effect
Critical	*Health*: life-threatening or disabling illness Examples: HIV/AIDS, hepatitis B *Safety*: any fatality or potential for multiple fatalities. Permanent disability
High	*Health*: irreversible health effects of concern Examples: noise-induced hearing loss *Safety*: serious injuries with potential for a fatality
Moderate	*Health*: severe, reversible health effects of concern Examples: back/muscle strain, repetitive strain injury, heat stroke *Safety*: extensive injuries, hospitalization
Low	*Health*: reversible health effects Examples: sunburn, heat exhaustion *Safety*: injury requiring medical treatment
Negligible	*Health*: reversible effects of low concern Examples: minor muscular discomfort, skin rash *Safety*: minor injury requiring first-aid treatment

Focus on the serious risks

To ensure risk assessments are effective, it is important to focus on hazards that present a serious risk to the group. Many models exist but simply by considering the severity of probable illness or injuries, it is then possible to judge the likelihood of a risk occurring (see Table 2.4)

The five locations where injuries are most likely to occur are:
- Roads.
- Beach.
- Hotels (including balconies).
- Remote locations.
- Ski slopes.

Source: Foreign and Commonwealth Office, 2005.

The UK Foreign and Commonwealth Office (FCO) produces an annual report, *British Behaviour Abroad*, which includes information on the countries in which Britons are most likely to require assistance (⌖https://www.gov.uk/government/publications/british-behaviour-abroad-report-2013).

Research

The best tool for compiling risk assessments is the experience of similar groups/expeditions to the same specific destination involving similar and proposed activities. Reports from past expeditions and networking with individuals who have relevant experience will be useful.

Sources of expedition reports include:

Royal Geographical Society (with IBG)	⌖ http://www.rgs.org/expeditionreports
British Mountaineering Council	⌖ https://www.thebmc.co.uk/expedition-reports
Conservation Leadership Programme	⌖ http://www.conservationleadershipprogramme.org/Projects.asp
Royal Scottish Geographical Society	⌖ http://www.rsgs.org/expeditions

A record of incidents and accidents on expeditions, and near misses has been compiled by the Royal Geographical Society's Medical Cell ⌖ http://www.rgs.org/medicalcell and is summarized on ➧ Illness on expeditions, p. 10.

Expedition participants

Participants themselves create risk, e.g. through pre-existing medical conditions and inappropriate behaviour. People travel to remote places for various reasons, often involved with the wish to escape the confines and constraints of life at home and to take more risks. The data on increased levels of unprotected sexual contact by individuals on overseas visits reinforces this; however, extra risk-taking extends to all activities whilst on an expedition. It is the experience of many large expedition organizations that accidents tend to occur more often on days when expeditioners are relaxing (R-and-R 'off-duty' days), after hard work, and after drinking alcohol.

Assess the wider threats

Assessment of threat (including insurrection, political turmoil, anarchy, and lawlessness) can be completed via consultation with specialists or those who know the destination well. There are a number of risk consultancies that can be used, such as Control Risks Group, Kroll Security International, and Salamanca Risk.

Travel-related risks can also be researched using information sources provided by government representatives:

UK—Foreign and Commonwealth Office	℘ http://www.gov.uk/ foreign-travel-advice
Australia—Dept of Foreign Affairs and Trade	℘ http://www.dfat.gov.au
US—State Department	℘ http://www.travel.state.gov
Canada—Dept of Foreign Affairs and Trade	℘ http://www.voyage.gc.ca
World Health Organization (WHO)	℘ http://www.who.int
Centre for Disease Control	℘ http://www.cdc.gov/travel
MASTA—Medical advice site	℘ http://www.masta.org
BBC website	℘ http://www.bbc.co.uk
In-country contacts and agents	
Special interest clubs	
Local tourist board website	
Guidebooks	

Control measures

Once the serious risks have been identified, each one must be reduced to an acceptable level using a control measure (Table 2.5).

As Table 2.5 outlines, personal protective equipment (PPE; e.g. helmets) is one of the least effective methods of preventing risk and should not be used in isolation. A behavioural solution, such as avoiding areas of loose rock, should be used in combination with PPE.

Many control measures can be put in place by an expedition, e.g.:

- Providing first-aid training for all members.
- Getting immunized before exposure to disease.
- Preventing bites by disease-transmitting insects.

During the expedition more control measures may need to be implemented that were not identified in the planning process. Reactive plans should aim to reduce the consequence of the incident via effective incident management and good crisis management.

Table 2.5 Proactive and reactive risk-reduction measures

	Method	Description
Most effective	Elimination	Do not do the activity
	Substitution	Do it in a different way; consider a 'Plan B'
	Engineering	Implement mechanical solution to reduce risk
	Behaviour	Change behaviour to minimize risk
	PPE	Reduce the severity and likelihood of injury using PPE
Least effective	Reactive plans	First aid and emergency response plans to reduce severity of incident

Educate the group

It is important to share the outcomes of the risk assessment with the participants. This also provides the background for participants to understand why control measures are in place.

Therefore, the pre-expedition information should include the risk assessment or, as a minimum, the key risks and control measures in place to reduce them. Continual enforcement of control measures and frequent briefing of risks is considered good practice.

Employ sensible flexible control measures

The key to effective control measures is to be flexible. Unnecessary overuse of control measures will produce a negative response from expedition members.

The level of controls used must reflect the seriousness of the risk. For example, drowning is more serious than new boots causing blisters. However, both these hazards can be highlighted in different ways. For example, a note about new boots in the pre-trip information coupled with group observation would be an effective way of reducing the likelihood of blisters.

The severity of drowning would require a different approach. This would include gathering data on whether participants can swim, providing appropriate life jackets, ensuring competent supervision and, finally, having an ERP in case of capsize.

See also ➔ Emergency response plan, p. 136 and Chapter 5 for further information.

Medical insurance

Making sure that there is adequate and appropriate insurance cover in place for all participants is an essential part of pre-expedition planning and integral to the ERP (◆ Emergency response plan, p. 136).

Eligible travellers from the UK are entitled to receive free or reduced-cost medical care in many European countries on production of a completed EHIC form (available from local Post Offices or Department of Health website). The EHIC is valid in all European Community countries plus Iceland, Liechtenstein, and Norway. However, few European Union (EU) countries pay the full cost of medical treatment, and travellers visiting other parts of Europe even for a few days should take out insurance.

Most overseas visits will require insurance for the following elements:
• Medical treatment and additional expenses.
• Repatriation.
• Personal accident.
• Search and rescue.
• Replacement/rearrangement.
• Public/personal liability.

You might also want to consider insurance for:
• Cancellation and curtailment.
• Loss of baggage and equipment.

When buying insurance
• Do not under-insure; the costs of in-country medical expenses and repatriation can be high.
• Disclose all activities and risks to the insurer—including pre-existing medical conditions. Failure to do so will invalidate your policy.
• Check the small print and make sure cover is in place for all aspects of the visit and what exclusions apply.
• Ensure that specific risks are mentioned which concern your trip, e.g. death from hypothermia.
• If local staff are hired, make enquiries as to your responsibilities to them. Many countries have requirements for workers' compensation in the event of an accident or injury.
• Ensure that your policy will not expire if your expedition over-runs.
• For a group policy, be certain that the insurer has not limited the number of individuals covered in a single incident.
• The insurer should provide a 24-h phone number which can be called when an incident occurs.
• Report all claims as soon as possible; late claim notices may be affected by a time bar on the policy.

Types of insurance

Medical and additional expenses

Medical insurance should pay for treatment and travel expenses incurred for individuals following accidental injury or illness. The insurance should have a 24-h contact number available for the insurer to guarantee payment to treatment centres or emergency services should their help be required. The level of medical cover for each member should be at least £1 million for Europe and £2 million for the rest of the world (source: FCO). Medical expenses in the USA can be particularly high, especially if surgery or intensive care is involved, and some policies now offer £5–10 million for travel in North America. Any pre-existing medical conditions must be disclosed to the insurer.

Personal accident

This covers death and disablement due to an accident whilst on an expedition. An amount is paid to the injured party in the event of loss of use of limbs, eyes, disablement, or death.

Search and rescue considerations

Insurance may be found to fund a SAR, but SAR is very expensive, particular if it involves aircraft, and the price of insurance will reflect this. Pre-training and good communication will reduce the chance of individuals becoming detached from the group. The majority of search and rescues around the world are carried out via a mixture of police, army, and volunteers. The ERP should have links to these organizations. Emergency funds may be required to initiate this process.

Replacement and rearrangement

Insurance is available to cover the cost of replacing a key team member in the event of an expedition member being disabled or killed. It should also be possible to cover the costs of returning the injured person to the expedition when they have recovered.

Public/personal liability

Insurance against any legal liability incurred on the group or an individual or to a group or individual in the event of an incident is advisable. Leaders and medical professionals and expedition organizers have greater responsibilities than other members of the expedition.

Professional indemnity insurance

Doctors and other medical professionals should confirm that their professional indemnity insurance company will cover them to work with members of the expedition and/or host country nationals (see ➔ Legal Liabilities and professional insurance, p. 76).

Legal liabilities and professional insurance

An introduction to legal liability in UK

This section is based on UK law; please be aware that the laws of the country in which the expedition takes place may apply. When reading this section please note the legal principles but seek further specialist advice.

To date, there have been no reported cases where an expedition doctor has been successfully sued in a UK court. In this increasingly litigious climate however, no practitioner can afford to be complacent.

In 1997, a UK court held that a mountain guide's breach of duty of care resulted in the death of a client, and awarded damages to the client's infant son. In December 2005, *The Times* reported that a private prosecution for unlawful killing had been launched by the father of the youngest Briton to reach the summit of Mount Everest—the judge ruled that there was no negligence and stated in his ruling that high-altitude mountaineering is a hazardous sport where the risks are well recognized.

Relevant medical law is more likely to be found in case law (where judgments provide precedents) than in statute (enacted through parliament).

Negligence

Negligence for clinical practitioners under UK law requires a claimant to demonstrate the following (known as the 'Bolam test'):
- The plaintiff owed a duty of care.
- There was an accepted standard of care.
- The duty of care was breached.
- The claimant suffered harm.
- Causation (that is, that the breach of the duty of care led to, or materially contributed to, the harm that the claimant suffered).

This has subsequently been slightly modified by the Bolitho ruling in which the judge ruled that any standard of care would have to withstand logical analysis in a courtroom and that, exceptionally, a court may decide that expert medical opinion was flawed.

Courts have also extended these tests for negligence by a doctor to other cases where a defendant owes a duty of care to a claimant: e.g. in the case of the mountain guide discussed earlier in this section and in the case of the standard of care expected from a volunteer first-aider.

Duty of care

In the UK, an individual has no legal duty to assist members of the public when acting privately. The situation may differ in other countries. In France, for example, there is a legal obligation on every person to give emergency assistance at the scene of an accident, and failure to do so has resulted in prosecutions, most notably in the case of the paparazzi who abandoned the scene of the car crash involving Diana, Princess of Wales.

There may, however, be a professional obligation to render medical assistance. Even when off-duty, the GMC expects doctors to provide emergency assistance.

'In an emergency, wherever it arises, you must offer assistance, taking account of your own safety, your competence, and the availability of other options for care.'

GMC, *Good Medical Practice* guide.

The Nursing and Midwifery Council has indicated in its professional Code of Conduct that it requires similar actions of its registrants.

These professional obligations do not carry the full force of law, but penalties for failing to comply may be serious (e.g. recently the GMC issued a formal reprimand to a doctor who failed to render assistance to an injured person at the scene of a road accident) and, in the absence of legal precedent, this may be taken as instructive by courts.

Any person treating a patient, advising a patient, or advising an expedition company has, in law, a clear duty of care.

Standard of care

Where a duty of care is owed, the obligation is to exercise reasonable care and skill in the circumstances. The case of *Bolam* v *Friern Hospital Management Committee* (1957) produced the following definition of what is reasonable:

'The test is the standard of the ordinary skilled man exercising and professing to have that special skill. A man need not possess the highest expert skill at the risk of being found negligent . . . it is sufficient if he exercises the skill of an ordinary man exercising that particular art.'

This definition is supported and clarified by the case of *Bolitho* v *City and Hackney Health Authority* (1993).

Courts have indicated that they will not allow inexperience as a defence in actions of professional negligence: if a doctor is unable to exercise reasonable care in carrying out a particular task then he should not undertake this. Should a practitioner hold himself out to be an expedition doctor (and as such having a 'specialist' skill), therefore, his actions would be judged against what might reasonably be expected of a competent expedition doctor even if this were the first time the individual had ever taken on such a role.

At present, there are no established standards of care for expeditions, but a court may accept the expert advice of other practitioners who provide similar services to members of expeditions in defining what would currently be considered 'reasonable'. In the future, qualifications such as the recently established Diploma in Mountain Medicine may be cited as evidence of a standard to be expected of a doctor accompanying a mountaineering expedition (http://medex.org.uk/diploma/about_diploma.php).

Causation

A claimant must prove that the breach of duty caused the harm suffered. What has to be proved is illustrated by the case of *Barnett* v *Chelsea and Kensington Hospital Management Committee* (1969). A man was sent home from a hospital accident and emergency department after complaining of acute stomach pains and sickness. He died later that same day, of what later proved to be arsenic poisoning. The hospital admitted a breach of duty but the widow failed to recover damages because the patient would have died whatever the doctor had done, i.e. causation could not be demonstrated.

In the context of an expedition, the requirement to demonstrate causation may prove to be the main obstacle to a claimant trying to sue a doctor for negligence. For example, in the case of a patient who suffered an intracranial bleed secondary to a head injury, it would be a challenge to show that it was a doctor's failure to site burr holes that led to long-term disability rather than the injury caused by a falling rock.

Emergency situations

In an emergency, courts take into account the specific circumstances, such as the need to act with speed in a hazardous situation, and determine whether a practitioner had acted with reasonable care. A court will recognize the fact that medicine was being practised in a remote area and that medical resources would be limited. As one judge ruled:

'I accept that full allowance must be made for the fact that certain aspects of treatment may have to be carried out in what one witness [. . .] called "battle conditions". An emergency may overburden the available resources, and, if an individual is forced by circumstances to do too many things at once, the fact that he does one of them incorrectly should not lightly be taken as negligence.'

Wilsher v Essex Area Health Authority.

However, expedition members, as potential patients, must be informed of the skills and limitations of the expedition medic (such as equipment carried, distance to definitive care, evacuation times, etc.). Similarly, the risks that expedition members will be taking need to be clearly spelt out.

Liability on commercial expeditions

Most of the medical indemnity organizations will provide 'Good Samaritan' cover for doctors acting in any part of the world. However, this would apply only where a team member just happens to be a doctor. It would certainly not cover a doctor receiving any form of inducement (e.g. a 10% discount on the trip fee) that may imply the doctor has an official medical role on the expedition.

Particular caution is required where citizens of the USA or Canada are participating in the expedition. Indeed, it may be impossible for a UK-registered doctor to obtain professional indemnity insurance other than on a 'Good Samaritan' basis for treating or advising people who are ordinarily residents of North America. English courts have jurisdiction over the deaths of Britons wherever they occur and there is no formal time limit for criminal prosecutions for unlawful killing. There is little doubt that an American court would claim an analogous jurisdiction over the death of an American citizen.

Expedition companies have a responsibility in common law to ensure that any medic that they choose to employ is suitably experienced. In the event of a claim for negligence, any claim would normally be made against the expedition company but this would not cover the professional negligence of a doctor.

Expeditions departing without a doctor

Many smaller expeditions may not have the resources to be able to take a doctor into the field. However, the team will still require medical advice and the supply of a suitable medical kit. In these cases, doctors may be approached to perform various services:

- Provide advice on vaccinations or antimalarial chemoprophylaxis.
- Advise on contents of a suitable medical kit.
- Supply private prescriptions for an expedition (NB drugs may be used for the treatment of trip members previously unknown to the doctor).
- Medical advice by phone to expedition medics.
- Delegate the responsibility for initiating treatment to a trip leader.

In these situations, the administration of medication should be via a written protocol or verbal consultation with a doctor (e.g. by telephone, satellite phone, or email). All prescription medication should be accompanied by a letter from the prescribing doctor. It would also be prudent for the doctor to seek a written understanding from the person to whom prescriptions are supplied that the medication prescribed will only be used for the immediate treatment of expedition members while some distance from a hospital or clinic and not as a substitute for seeking professional medical advice where this is readily available.

Professional indemnity insurance

Most of the principal medical insurance bodies in the UK will extend the scope of their cover to include the practice of expedition medicine. However, this needs to be specifically requested (even if, depending on the grade and specialty of the practitioner, it were then provided at no extra cost) and, as mentioned earlier, may not extend to the care of North Americans.

Other factors to discuss with insurers would include:

- The scope of the treatment you propose to provide (especially if this were to fall well outside your normal full-time specialty).
- Whether you intend to extend this beyond your expedition members (such as to local workers employed by your team, other members of the local population, and perhaps other travellers not involved with your own trip).

Be aware of the differing organizational structures of the principal medical insurance bodies: the scope of their services may differ.

Summary

- Expedition medicine is an interesting and challenging vocation which needs to be practised with care.
- A clear written understanding of one's responsibilities as an MO is very important, but particularly so where charity or commercial expeditions are concerned.
- Drugs supplied to an expedition for administration or dispensing by non-medical personnel need to be prescribed via a written protocol or via a tele-medicine consultation.
- Finally, good specialist insurance cover needs to be actively sought, including professional indemnity insurance.

Chapter 3

Caring for people in the field

Section editors
James Moore and Shane Winser

Contributors
Larry Goodyer
Paul Goodyer
James Moore
Shane Winser
Akbar Lalani (1st edition)
Christina Lalani (1st edition)

Organization of a healthy base camp 82
Expedition health clinics 84
Field nursing care 88
Giving drugs 92
Kitchens and food preparation 96
Diet 98
Water purification 102
Sanitation and latrines 108

Organization of a healthy base camp

Clean water, good food, and a comfortable place to sleep are essential for a happy and healthy expedition. Tired and hungry people are significantly more prone to accidents and illness and caring for people in a well-organized, safe environment is much easier as 'any fool can be uncomfortable'. Expeditions can base themselves anywhere from luxury hotels to bivouacs under the stars. Whichever type of accommodation is used it should offer:

- Refuge from the elements.
- Security from personal attack or theft.
- Protection from the local fauna and flora.
- An acceptable level of comfort and privacy.

Camp location

When choosing the site for an expedition camp, consider:

- Weather and prevailing wind.
- Providing shelter from stormy weather.
- Avoiding areas prone to snow accumulation.
- Use of available shade and breeze in hot climates.
- Avoiding areas at risk of lightning strike.
- Floods:
  - Avoiding tidal regions and flood plains.
  - Dry river beds that may be liable to flash flooding.
  - Narrow valleys in areas of high rainfall.
- Dangers from falling rocks and mud slides, avalanche (snow/ice), dead trees and branches, or animal attacks.
- Animal hazards:
  - Not placing camp between animals and their watering holes.
  - Avoiding large animal mating and breeding areas.
  - Avoiding areas of insect infestation.
  - Avoiding routes of migration/travel.

Animal attacks are more likely during camp construction or new occupation, as humans initially invade the animals' environment. As the local fauna gets used to human presence, they may move closer to the camp to take advantage of food scraps etc. During camp deconstruction the animals may again be disturbed, making a hostile response more likely.

Local permissions and environmental impact

Permissions may need to be obtained from the landowner.

Avoid placing a campsite in an area that has religious or spiritual significance for the local people (see ➲ Interacting with local communities, p. 120).

Many cultures will readily offer supplies and hospitality even when this leaves them with shortages. Ensure that your presence does not deplete scarce local resources such as water, firewood, food, or fuel when these are in short supply.

Ensure that your campsites create no long-term ecological damage (see ➲ Environmental impact, p. 124).

Re-supply and casualty evacuation

Investigate the logistics of:
- Evacuating an injured casualty (➜ Evacuation, p. 146).
- Access to re-supplies of food, water, and fuel.
- Reliable communications with local agencies and emergency services, or others upon whom you may rely.

Campsite identification

In unfamiliar surroundings or poor weather conditions, it is easy to become disorientated, even within the vicinity of base camp. To reduce the risk of members getting lost, clearly identify key areas such as:
- Camp entrances, exits, and boundaries.
- Latrines.
- Washing areas.
- Refuse areas.
- Communication facilities.
- Medical and first aid facilities.
- Fire extinguishing equipment and fire exits.

When constructing a camp, consider the layout in relation to those with an illness or injury. Once sign-posted, ask the following question: 'Could I find who or what I need, in an emergency, in the dark or in poor visibility?'

Expedition health clinics

The majority of health problems experienced on expedition are not emergencies and can be dealt with at set times during the day. Outside clinic times, emergency healthcare can be provided using a basic first-aid kit (commonly known as a 'grab-bag').

Individuals should have a personal first-aid kit to enable self-care (see ◗ Personal medical kit, p. 800), although it is important for the medic to be aware of any self-administered medication.

Expedition health clinics described in this chapter are primarily concerned with providing healthcare for expedition team members and associates. The provision of healthcare dedicated to the indigenous population is more complex and largely outside the remit of this book (see ◗ Care of local staff, p. 118).

Clinic times

Expedition health clinics can be structured to suit both mobile and static expeditions. All team members, including local employees, should be aware of how the clinic is to be accessed and the scope/limitations of available care.

Established expedition clinic times:
- Provide a structured daily timetable for medics and team members.
- Avoid the need to repeatedly open medical kits.
- Enable accurate stock control.
- Encourage self-care outside clinic hours.

It is advisable to structure clinic times around the expedition working day. If involved in non-medical expedition activities, the medic can run a brief clinic in the morning before or after breakfast, during which there can be a review of ongoing problems and also rapid assessments of new issues. Comprehensive clinics can be run at other convenient times. Unless there are issues requiring simple answers or advice, or an emergency, individuals should be encouraged to attend clinics at the allotted times. A situation may arise where individuals wish to discuss a problem without the rest of the team becoming aware. The medic should ensure this is possible and that team members are aware of this option.

Clinic location

Medical clinics should be comfortable and well lit. Ideally they should be away from communal areas and in a location that maximizes confidentiality and privacy. Clinics should not be on major camp thoroughfares where team members continually pass by.

If a dedicated clinic area is not possible, some expeditions may facilitate the medic having a slightly larger or independent sleeping area, e.g. a larger tent, where medical consultations can take place.

Depending on the expedition and camp layout, it may be preferable for the medic to visit individuals. Be aware that tents provide little sound insulation and sensitive information may be overheard.

Clinic layout

The ideal clinic should allow for patient examination to be conducted in a manner that closely resembles that of a healthcare facility at home.

Consider the following:

- Sufficient space for patient examination.
- Sufficient light—especially when assessing wounds/injuries.
- Ease of access –injured patients may struggle to access enclosed spaces.
- Safe and secure storage of medical equipment.
- A method of collecting waste.

Most patients can be examined in a seated position. If possible, a small chair or bench is a valuable piece of clinic furniture. However, if items like this are not present, improvise.

Within the clinic, clinicians should have access to:

- Medical kit.
- Hand washing/cleansing facilities.
- A method of sterilizing equipment.
- Medical notes.
- Basic reference textbooks such as this and, ideally, the Internet or other method of communication.

Clinical areas should be kept as clean and free from dirt/waste as possible—especially food waste that attracts animal life. Surfaces should be wiped down with antibacterial/antiseptic solutions (e.g. Dettol®) after use. Clinical waste should be burned or disposed of appropriately. Sharps must be carefully stored and disposed of appropriately on return from expedition.

Medical kits are expensive commodities and should be kept in as secure location as possible. Access to medical kits should be limited to the clinician and specifically named individuals.

Sanatorium/sick bay

Most individuals suffering from illness or injury on expedition can continue to use their normal sleeping accommodation. Exemptions to this might include:

- Communicable disease requiring isolation.
- Where continual or rapid access to toilet facilities is required.
- Where continual/regular patient monitoring is needed.

In these instances it will be beneficial to create a clinical area sufficient for the medic to provide care as dictated by the illness. This may necessitate the medic moving nearer the patient. In environmental extremes (such as polar blizzards), repeated visits between medic and patient will be impractical, even dangerous.

Sick or injured patients using their own accommodation should have a means of contacting the medic should their condition deteriorate. The medic's accommodation should be clearly marked and easily accessible.

Increased attention should be given to tidiness and hygiene in areas where patients are being looked after. Expedition patients often resort to the easier 'go behind the nearest tree' option, rather than utilize appropriate latrines. This behaviour should be discouraged.

Latrine hygiene is especially important during times of sickness. Creating a rota of cleaning responsibilities may be useful to ensure consistently high standards of hygiene. It is not uncommon for individuals suffering from traveller's diarrhoea to experience bouts of incontinence. In such situations clothes will require careful laundering.

Medicines storage

Expedition environments are unforgiving on equipment, and extremes of temperature and humidity will degrade less robust containers. A balance must be struck between container strength, durability, and weight. Medical kit containers should be strong enough to withstand all the rigors of transport, with delicate items such as glass vials packed in foam within ridged containers. Sterile packaging of items such as intravenous giving sets is particular prone to damage through abrasion or moisture. Labels should be written in permanent ink or laminated, as text can become illegible in damp or humid conditions.

Medicines containers should be sealed sufficiently to keep out moisture, extremes of temperature, and animal or insect invasion. If possible, keep the kits off the ground.

Most oral medications (tablet or syrup) are stable across a broad range of temperatures. Pre-mixed and injectable medicines can be less stable with some requiring refrigeration. Lyophilized (powdered, non-mixed) injectable medications (such as rabies vaccines) are generally very stable outside stated storage temperatures.

Medicine stability information can be found in the Summary of Product Characteristics (SPC), which can be obtained at ℜ http://www.medicines. org.uk. The SPC will also contain a manufacturer's helpline. Pharmaceutical manufacturers will often have extra information not normally found on the SPC.

Certain medications such as snake antivenom or insulin will degrade if stored outside specified temperatures. If refrigeration of these substances is impossible, use a medicine pack designed specifically to insulate medications against extremes of temperatures such as a vacuum flask. In environments where a considerable temperature gradient exists between night and day, the flask can be cooled at night and sealed during daylight hours. Minimize access to these medications during daylight hours to preserve low temperatures.

Medical kits are one of the most important parts of expedition equipment. However, without care and discipline they will soon deteriorate. There have been instances where vital medical kit has been found unusable in emergencies due to poor care and maintenance—an unacceptable scenario. Therefore aim to keep the medical kit in a condition you would like to receive it in.

Field nursing care

Successful management of any illness or injury depends on the harmony between the clinical skills of medicine and the dedicated care and compassion of nursing. Good nursing skills should be employed in every aspect of patient care, for those in the acute phase of patient assessment and treatment as well as those awaiting either evacuation or being nursed back to health in the field.

Nursing care includes providing psychological reassurance, maintaining patient comfort, and ensuring observations and interventions are carried out and well documented.

Nursing a sick or injured patient is not something that comes naturally to everyone. Perhaps the best way of approaching patient care is to remember and emulate the care and compassion you received as a poorly child. Generally speaking, the one individual any ill person wants to see when feeling unwell is their mother. Be their mother.

Psychological support

Being unwell whilst far from the safety and security of a domestic health service can be disconcerting at best, terrifying at worst, particularly for younger or less experienced team members. The knowledge that in-country healthcare systems may be inaccessible or inadequate will add to this stress. From initial assessment the clinician should seek to provide reassurance and encouragement. Keeping patients informed throughout procedures, treatments, and care planning will keep stress levels to a minimum and help patients feel involved.

The reaction of others will affect an individual's perception of the severity of their illness or injury. Looks of terror or disgust are likely to increase feelings of anxiety. This should be considered especially in those with little or no previous exposure to traumatic situations.

The power of touch is frequently overlooked in a modern, busy health service. The calm reassurance of someone holding a hand or stroking hair is often enough to help a patient relax. However, some patients will prefer not to be fussed over.

Cleanliness and hygiene

Expedition members should strive to maintain adequate levels of cleanliness and hygiene. This reduces the risk of becoming unwell and, in the event of illness, reduces the probability of sickness spreading throughout the camp.

If injury or illness prevents a patient from caring for him- or herself, they should be assisted in doing so. Individuals may not be accustomed to the intimacies of washing or helping to wash an individual.

- Do not neglect body areas prone to infection, e.g. groins and armpits.
- Ensure any soap used is rinsed off.
- The patient must be dried thoroughly.
- Do not neglect dental/mouth care.
- Maintain the highest level of dignity possible.
- It may be advisable to have a chaperone.

Cleanliness, hygiene, and care of pressure points are especially important in unconscious patients and those whose movements are restricted, e.g. spinal immobilization. A person lying in one position for too long may develop serious skin sores and muscle injuries that take months to heal. Regular turning and massage can reduce this risk. These patients may also require toileting assistance.

Documentation

> Good notes = good defence.
> Poor notes = poor defence.
> No notes = no defence.

Good documentation is important for the following reasons:
- Allows observation of illness progression/regression.
- Aids diagnosis.
- Increases handover accuracy and safety.
- Provides a record of what has/has not been done.
- Can be a source of reassurance for less experienced medics.

Documentation should include medical assessments, diagnosis, and treatment, along with ongoing care, which will include medicines administered, observations, and interventions. It is preferable to write medical notes as soon as something has been done but do not delay interventions for the sake of documentation. Good medical records will allow a receiving clinician to have a clear understanding of the patient's illness, treatment, and progression, irrespective of their level of involvement.

Clinical observations
Depending on the nature of the illness or injury, regular observations may be indicated (see ➔ Clinical measurements, p. 174). Observations must be documented in a manner that allows rapid interpretation and pattern recognition. Minimum observations should include:
- Respiratory rate (RR).
- Heart rate (HR).
- Temperature (T).

In addition, the following may also be required:
- Blood pressure (BP).
- Blood sugar.
- Pain scores. Use a scale of 0–10 where: 0 = no pain to 10 = the worst pain *the patient* has ever experienced.
- Neurological observations—using either the AVPU ('awake/verbal/pain/ unresponsive') or Glasgow Coma Scale (GCS) (see Box 7.1).
- Fluid intake and output.

Frequency of observations
Injury or illness severity will dictate the frequency of observations. As a basic rule, the further a patient's observations are from normal, or the more acute the injury or illness, the more frequent observations should be.

For example, a patient suffering from shock following a serious injury will require regular observations (e.g. RR, HR, BP, GCS/neurological, pain score, fluid intake, and urine output) approximately every 10–15 minutes, until the shock has been corrected and the patient remains stable. An uncompromised patient suffering from gastroenteritis will require basic observations (RR, HR, T, urine output) once or twice daily.

Charting observations

A model observations chart, similar to that standardized within the NHS, is provided in Fig. 8.7, which includes a scoring system to highlight whether a patient is deteriorating. It cannot be reproduced in full size within this book and all expeditions are recommended to obtain full size, colour reproductions of an observation chart as part of their first-aid kit.

Care of documentation

Ensure any documentation is kept in the best possible condition. This may prove difficult in some environments, such as the tropics, where humidity or dirt invade every aspect of expedition life.

Notes are confidential and should be kept securely and accessible only by those involved directly in patient care. Patient confidentiality extends beyond the expedition and any medical records should be stored securely on return home. Clinicians should retain a copy of the notes for reference purposes.

Giving drugs

Before you give a drug to anyone, you should know about it. Information can be sourced from:
- The Patient Information Leaflet (PIL) supplied with the drug.
- The Summary of Product Characteristics (SPC) available at ℅ http://www.medicines.org.uk/emc
- Freestanding apps such as the *British National Formulary* (BNF) or *Epocrates*.
- Online formularies or the Internet.

Errors in drug prescribing and administration are frighteningly common even amongst trained hospital staff. Fig. 3.1 provides a flow chart of the things that require checking each time a drug is given to a patient.

Any other treatments such as dressing changes should be documented in the patient notes and relevant observations made, e.g. wound granulation, signs of infection. Documentation should be clear and unambiguous so as to avoid confusion and potential drug errors.

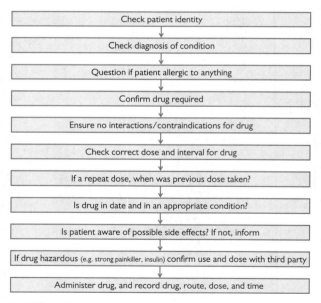

Fig. 3.1 Drug administration.

Treating pain (analgesia)

Ensuring patients are free from pain or discomfort will help them rest. Patients in pain should have their pain score monitored regularly. Before administering analgesic drugs, consider other ways of relieving discomfort:

- Temperature—ensure the patient is not too hot or cold.
- Control of nausea and vomiting.
- Fatigue.
- Psychological stress.
- Other symptoms.

The analgesic ladder

- Current techniques of pain relief depend upon the use of increasingly potent treatments, used in combination until the patient is comfortable (see Table 3.1). A low dose of several different drugs is preferable to a high dose of just one (see Table 3.2).
- *Simple physical measures*: padding, rubbing, supporting, or splinting may reduce discomfort. Heat or cold, depending upon the nature of the injury, can relieve swelling and discomfort.
- A *simple analgesic*, such as paracetamol (acetaminophen) will be safe for most people.
- A *non-steroidal anti-inflammatory drug* (NSAID) such as ibuprofen or diclofenac can be given orally or rectally and may be available as a skin rub. About 15% of the population cannot take NSAIDs—see Table 3.2.
- *Codeine* is a drug that works very well in some people, but leaves others feeling spaced out and dreadful.
- *Tramadol* is a powerful painkiller which is reasonably safe to use as it usually does not cause respiratory depression. It can be taken by mouth or injected. However, it can make some people feel sick, dizzy, or disoriented and initial supervision is required to see if these side effects develop.

Table 3.1 Pain control for adults

Mild pain	Physical measures Paracetamol 1g, 4-hrly (max 4g/day)
Moderate pain	Physical measures Paracetamol 1g, 4-hrly Ibuprofen 400 mg, 4–6-hrly
If moderate pain uncontrolled	As above plus: Codeine 60 mg, 4-hrly or Tramadol 50–100 mg, 4-hrly
Severe pain	Physical measures Paracetamol 1 g, 4-hly Ibuprofen 400 mg, 4-hrly *or* codeine 60 mg 6-hrly Morphine 10 mg, 2–4-hrly

Children and small (<50kg) adults require lower doses.

- *Opiates*, of which morphine is the most common, are very powerful painkillers but frequently produce sedation, dizziness, and nausea.
  A person unused to their effects will need close supervision. Respiratory depression can develop if high doses are given and a casualty given an opiate must be closely observed (➜ Clinical observations, p. 89;
  ➜ Treatment of dental pain, p. 348).

Anxiety and stress make pain worse both psychologically and because muscles tense around the affected part of the body. Small doses of anxiolytics (midazolam, diazepam) can help, but must be used with extreme caution if the patient has received potent painkillers as respiratory depression or deep sedation may result.

Table 3.2 lists only a small range of basic drugs, but used in combination these will be adequate for most situations. A wide range of long-acting oral and transcutaneous painkillers are now manufactured, and if your expedition medical kit contains these, read about their benefits and drawbacks. If painkilling preparations are purchased from a local pharmacist, read the small print carefully to determine what they contain; often it will simply be an expensive combination of the types of drugs listed in the table.

Table 3.2 The analgesic ladder (adult doses only)

		Route	Usual adult dose	Contra-indications	Cautions/side-effects
Physical measures	Pad, support, strap, splint, elevate				Ensure circulation not affected by swelling. Monitor capillary return & colour
	Cold (ice packs)	Skin	Useful for: bruises, sprains, burns		Avoid freezing skin or deep tissues
	Heat	Skin	Useful for aching pains		Avoid burns
Mild pain	Paracetamol Acetaminophen (US)	Oral/ Rectal/IV	1 g 4 times daily	Allergy (rare) Liver disease, Alcoholics	
Moderate pain	Ibuprofen	Oral	400mg 4 times day For short periods: 400mg 6 times daily	Allergy Peptic symptoms Some asthmatics Bleeding tendancy Anticoagulants Renal disease Heart disease	Stomach pain (take with food or milk if possible) Increased bruising
	Diclofenac	Rectal Skin rub IV (diluted)	50mg 3 times day		
	Codeine		30–60mgs 6 times day Max 240mg/day	Allergy	Drowsiness Confusion Nausea Dizziness
Severe pain	Tramadol	Oral, IV, IM	Titrate to pain relief, then: 50–100mg 4 hourly. Max 600mg/day.	Allergy	Drowsiness Confusion Nausea Dizziness
	Morphine	Oral, IV, IM	Titrate to pain relief then: 10mg 2 to 4 hrly	Allergy	Respiratory depression (monitor), drowsiness, giddiness, nausea, vomiting, confusion.

Kitchens and food preparation

One of the greatest contributing factors to the success or failure of an expedition is the standard of the food. Success depends not only on the provision of a nourishing and varied diet, but also on the prevention of diet-related illness and disease, probably the biggest cause of diarrhoea in travellers abroad.

The kitchen

The position and construction of a kitchen will vary according to the type, size, budget, and location of the expedition. The gold standard for a big base camp, one could argue, should be to reproduce a commercial kitchen, with all the regulations required to pass a health and hygiene examination. Ideally the kitchen should be located at least 30 m away from areas of possible contamination such as latrines, wash areas, and equipment stores.

Catering personnel

Some teams will employ local people for this role, whilst others will use expedition members and may opt for a rota system of cooking, cleaning, and washing up. It is important that everyone on the team is clear about their roles and responsibilities.

Beware of illnesses in all members of the expedition team. This might include chronic illnesses carried by locally hired staff such as:

- Diarrhoea or other gastrointestinal upsets.
- Helminth or protozoal infections.
- Carriers of chronic diseases (e.g. *Salmonella typhi* and TB).

Ensure that both catering and expedition teams clearly understand what is required regarding:

- Standards of hygiene and cleanliness within the kitchen.
- Regular hand washing with soap.
- Use of equipment.
- Disposal of refuse.

Basic kitchen rules

- If you are ill, do not go in the kitchen. Do not prepare food until at least 48 h have passed since last vomit or loose stool.
- Wash hands regularly.
- All cooking utensils should be washed, dried, and stored appropriately.

The kitchen should be kept scrupulously clean at all times:

- Clean work surfaces after use.
- Clean storage areas daily and when required.
- Clean and dry equipment immediately after use (including the cleaning equipment itself).
- Restrict the kitchen area to those involved in food preparation.
- Look after the chef, and the chef will look after you.

Food storage

Proper storage of food is of paramount importance, as:

- It prevents gastrointestinal illness through contamination.
- It provides protection against foraging animals.
- Properly stored food lasts longer.
- It is easier to track supply requirements.

Food needs to be accurately labelled and accounted for, preferably managed by a designated quartermaster. Separate cooked foods from raw. If using a fridge, store cooked food above raw.

Food preparation

Gastrointestinal upsets are the commonest illnesses to affect travellers. Minimize problems by ensuring that water is clean (➲ Water purification, p. 102), and that food preparation is as hygienic as possible.

Although without evidence, the saying 'wash it, peel it, boil it, or forget it' is good practice. Common sense dictates that it is not always possible to control the preparation of food whilst on expedition, but the further one strays from this advice, the greater the chance of succumbing to diet-related illness.

Refrain from sharing cutlery, bowls, and other eating or drinking utensils. Sharing is one of the fastest ways of spreading germs around camp. Note that many contagious diseases have an asymptomatic incubation period.

After eating:

- All cooking and eating utensils should be washed, dried, and stored cleanly and away from possible interference by insects and animals.
- Try to use a two-bowl system for washing up: one for washing, the other to rinse.
- Surfaces should be wiped clean, if possible with a disinfectant, as it will reduce the chances of bacteria/viral contamination or build-up.
- Floors should be cleaned of even the smallest crumbs of food.
- Hands should be washed, again.

Cooking in tents

- Avoid cooking in tents or other small enclosed areas if possible.
- Take great care when handling stoves in enclosed spaces—burns and scalds are common.
- Ensure adequate ventilation and consider risk of carbon monoxide poisoning.
- Plan escape route from tent if fire develops.

Diet

Most expeditions involve considerable physical exercise. A balanced and varied expedition diet is essential to enable expedition members to maintain health, fitness, and morale. The choice of foodstuffs will depend upon the:

- Duration of the expedition.
- Environment: energy requirements are greatly increased in cold climates, while travel in hot climates will require increased fluids and electrolytes.
- Availability of local foodstuffs.
- Energy expenditure of the participants.
- Levels of fitness: untrained individuals will take longer to complete a journey and hence have greater total energy expenditure.
- Budget of the expedition.
- Ability to transport food: backpack, porters, pack animals, vehicles, or by air.
- Availability of fuel and water.
- Adolescent teenagers have a high metabolic rate and will have a considerably higher calorific requirement in even the most mundane expedition environment.

Calorific requirements

The basic daily calorific requirement for a 75-kg person doing little physical work is 1500–1700 kcal; additional energy requirements are dependent upon the work undertaken. Fast walking burns 600–700 kcal/h, and running uses around 850 kcal/h. The duration of a task must be considered; working at low intensity for several hours requires more energy than short bursts of high-intensity exercise. The more food carried, the more energy is burnt in carrying food. Climbing carrying loads and man-hauling sledges are amongst the most energetic activities known, with around 10,000 kcal/day expended. On short expeditions, deficits in energy balance can be tolerated healthily; this is not the case on longer expeditions. Highly trained individuals can endure persistent energy deficits but at a cost of up to one-third of their lean body weight, and gradual decline in physical capabilities.

Dietary components

Dietary balance

Individuals tolerate novel food to different degrees, but providing the same menu each day will also discourage healthy eating. Simple sauces or condiments can make basic food more interesting. Fresh fruit and vegetables are always welcome, but are difficult to preserve without refrigeration. Jams and conserves are rich in vitamins and are worth taking. Additional calorie intake is less important in the short term than the quality of nutrition and the distribution of nutrients. (See Table 3.3.)

Table 3.3 Food types: pros and cons

Food type	Advantages	Disadvantages
Prepared food, e.g. sandwiches	Pleasing to the palate	Requires prior preparation Not practical on longer expeditions. Short shelf life
Tinned produce	Very long shelf life High liquid content Can be eaten cold	Bulky and heavy Non-biodegradable waste product
Local produce	May be readily available Part of cultural experience of travel	Risk of infections and gastroenteritis Longer preparation time
Dried produce, e.g. pasta and sauce	Pleasing to the palate	Time-consuming Requires large amount of fuel to prepare Bulky compared to finished product
'Boil in the bag' or MRE (meal ready to eat)	Easy to prepare Can taste good Long shelf life Can be cooked in dirty water or even eaten cold Requires no pan washing	Expensive: £3–4 per meal Limited choice of meals Lower energy density than dried products
Dehydrated meals	Some can be made with hot water added to bag and not prepared on a stove Energy-dense	Others require cooking over stove for 6–8 min Uses significant amounts of water
Powdered synthetic foods, e.g. sports drinks	Easy to prepare. No cooking utensils required Energy-dense (several thousand kcal can be carried in under 1 kg)	Taste Unbalanced diet, lack of fibre

Protein

Proteins enable muscle strength and allow repair and regeneration. Animal protein sources are better balanced than lactovegetarian sources; vegetarians can sustain high daily activity but their diet is bulkier. Protein intake should be greatest during rest periods and evenings, as protein consumed during exercise is largely burned to provide energy. Studies have shown that low protein consumption leads to a decrease in exercise potential over time. The recommended daily intake to minimize losses in lean body mass should be 1.5–2.0 g/kg. Roughly 15% of total calorific intake should be protein.

Carbohydrate

Carbohydrates are the main energy substrate for exercise. Simple sugars (sweets and glucose drinks) are rapidly absorbed, requiring little or no digestion. They should be consumed during exercise to provide the body with a constant source of energy. Complex sugars (pasta, rice, bread) are digested slowly, and must be metabolized to simple sugars before they can act as an energy substrate. Consuming complex sugars during exercise will have the detrimental effect of diverting blood flow to the gut from exercising muscle. They should therefore be ingested before and after exercise to replenish glycogen stores. Body glycogen stores are exhausted after just 2 h of strenuous exercise. In the absence of further intake, the body will begin to break down muscle and fat stores.

Fat

Fatty acids cannot be metabolized sufficiently rapidly to be used as an energy substrate during high-intensity exercise, but fats provide a useful substrate during prolonged low-intensity exercise. Fat is three times more energy-dense than carbohydrate and on expeditions a high-fat diet reduces the bulk and weight of food needed. Fat metabolism pathways must be enhanced prior to departure; this process can be achieved by 1 or 2 h of low-intensity (and hence low lactate production) training early in the day before breakfast, when glycogen stores are already depressed. Caffeine increases fatty acid utilization during exercise. Eating a high-fat meal immediately after exercise delays glycogen store replenishment and muscle regeneration, and hinders recovery for the next day. In hot climates and at altitude, high-fat diets can be unpalatable, but hungry travellers will enjoy a high fat-content, high-calorie diet in cold climates.

Water purification

Water purification

A safe water supply is essential. Adults in temperate conditions need to drink about 3 L a day, but in very hot climates an individual can lose up to 15 L of fluid a day. If walking all day in the desert up to 10 L of water may need to be carried per individual. A further 4 L of clean water per person per day will be needed for cooking and washing up. Sufficient safe water must be provided both at base camp and for use by field parties. Often water from taps and wells, as well as that from rivers, lakes, and ponds, can be contaminated. Spring water, i.e. clear 'pristine water collected away from human habitation' may be safer, but it is still sensible to treat it.

Water must be treated:
- To remove silt.
- To remove harmful organic matter and other pollutants.
- To kill all forms of organism.

Sediment must be removed initially if sterilization procedures are to be effective. Removing silt can pose considerable problems if you are trying to obtain supplies for a large expedition, and sedimentation tanks may be required. If the expedition is close to mines or factories, chemical pollution must be foreseen and appropriate filtration methods used.

Some methods of water purification are more suitable for base camp and others for field workers. Before choosing a system, consider the likely infective organisms and the risk posed by them.

Transmission of disease by water

Organisms such as bacteria, viruses, protozoa, and other parasites (including schistosomes, guinea worm larvae, and leeches) can transmit infections. Two types of organisms contracted through drinking surface waters which are of particular concern are:

Giardiasis

This is caused by the protozoan *Giardia lamblia*, part of whose life cycle involves faecal–oral transmission. The organism is consumed together with contaminated food or water, and then cysts—which are viable for a long time—are deposited from faeces into water or food to infect another host. Humans and animals, both domestic and wild, can host the infection and contaminate water; it only takes a few cysts to lead to a harmful infection.

The symptoms of giardiasis may be debilitating and develop 1–4 weeks after ingestion. Symptoms largely result from malabsorption of foodstuffs, and produce a frothy foul-smelling diarrhoea, in addition to nausea, abdominal discomfort, flatulence, and bloating. Symptoms usually last for 1–2 weeks, but sometimes a persistent chronic disease develops.

Metronidazole or tinidazole are effective treatments; in resistant cases albendazole has proven effective.

The cysts are relatively large and are quite easily removed by filter systems but are resistant to all but the highest doses of chemical agents and then still require prolonged contact times (➋ Methods of water purification, p. 104).

Cryptosporidium

Cryptosporidium spp. cause a very severe diarrhoea and, like *Giardia*, this organism is spread by the faecal–oral route, although ingestion of low numbers of cysts may not always result in infection. The organism is chiefly spread by humans and domestic livestock, either directly or through contaminated water. The spore of the organism can remain dormant in the soil for many years. The main danger for expeditions is surface waters close to human habitation with poor sanitation systems, or where water is washed down from grazing fields. Cases have been reported after swimming in infected waters, as well as from consumption of contaminated food and water. *Cryptosporidium* outbreaks occur from time to time in developed countries when sanitation systems break down.

Symptoms occur 2–14 days after contact and consist of a very profuse watery diarrhoea, abdominal pain, low-grade fever, and cramps, which last around 7 days. Sometimes the disease relapses after about 14 days. The biggest danger is to those with impaired immune systems, e.g. those with HIV/AIDS or those taking immunosuppressive drugs, where complications can be fatal. The very young and the elderly may also be at greater risk. There is no specific treatment other than aggressive rehydration.

A complication for expeditions is that the cysts are resistant to chlorination so filtration or the use of chlorine dioxide remain the most viable options if this disease is perceived as a potential problem.

Removal of sediment and organic matter

If water is cloudy or contains suspended matter it must be cleared before further treatment.

Settling tanks

Cloudy water can be left to stand for some hours for solids to settle, either in a jerry can or in sedimentation tanks depending on the volume to be treated. Very fine particles, such as 'rock flour' in glacial outflow and mica flakes, are gastrointestinal irritants and must be removed by a ceramic filter. Simply clearing water does not sterilize it and further treatment will be needed before it may be drunk.

Fabric pre-filters

A convenient method for removing sediment in relatively small volumes is to pass the water through a tight woven cloth material. The popular Millbank bag, a sock-shaped bag woven so that solids are retained but water flows by gravity through the weave, is the most well-known device of this kind. The bags can be found in army surplus stores, 'bushcraft' shops, or on the Internet, and are well worth hunting down.

Coagulation–flocculation

Small amounts of certain chemicals can be added to cause an aggregation of particles which will sink to the bottom of the container. The flocculate is then strained off through a tight woven cloth or Millbank bag. A potential advantage is that larger organisms such as *Giardia* or *Cryptosporidium* are removed by this technique, although it is not as reliable as an appropriate mechanical filter. The most easily obtained chemical is alum, of which about an eighth of a teaspoonful is added to 4 L of water, more if it remains cloudy. The water is then stirred for 5 min and allowed to settle for 30 min.

Methods of water purification

Boiling
This is undoubtedly the best method, but is often inconvenient and wasteful of fuel supplies or natural resources. Water should be kept boiling continuously for 5 min, which is sufficient at any altitude, although some experts state that 1 min is adequate. The water must be covered when cooling to prevent recontamination.

Chlorine
Chlorine is effective against a wide range of organisms, although it is less effective for amoebic cysts and *Giardia*, and is ineffective against *Cryptosporidium*. The effectiveness of chlorine is reduced by several factors that may not be easy to control, such as alkaline water, very cold water, or the presence of organic matter—hence the need for prior filtering.

Aquatab™ tablets are the most widely available method of chlorination, and one tablet of the maxi-size will treat 25 L. For very large tanks some expeditions prefer to use a substance called chloramine T, where 5 mg is added to each litre of water. Treated water should be left for at least half an hour before drinking and longer if it is very cold.

Sodium thiosulphate will improve the taste but will inactivate the chlorine, so it should be added by individuals only at the time the water is drunk. It should never be added to a storage receptacle such as a canteen or jerry can.

Iodine
Iodine has been a popular choice of chemical for water purification for wilderness travellers for many years, being more tolerant to the presence of organic matter than is chlorine. However, due to lack of commercial interest no company has registered an iodine-based product in Europe following the introduction of the EU Biocide regulation and it is therefore not now available. It remains on the market in non-EU countries such as the USA.

Chlorine dioxide
This has been widely used in water purification plants and is effective against *Cryptosporidium*. It has now largely replaced iodine as one of the most popular chemical methods for sterilizing water amongst wilderness travellers and expeditions. Unlike chlorine it does not impart a taste to water, though it should be used on water free from organ matter and particles requiring similar contact times for sterilization. It is, though, considerably more expensive than chlorine products. There are two forms available in the UK under the brand name Biox Aqua™; tablets and a two-stage solution. There is little specific evidence regarding differences in efficacy between the various chlorine dioxide products. Against *Cryptosporidium* and cyst-forming organisms it may not be as reliable as boiling or effective filtration systems.

Silver compounds
Micropur™ tablets contain a compound called Katadyne silver that is effective against *Amoeba*, *Giardia*, and viruses. It does not impart a bad taste and it is claimed to be able to prevent recontamination by bacteria of water for many weeks. Micropur™ tablets should not be added to water previously treated with chlorine or iodine.

Filters and pumps

There are many mechanical devices available for purifying water. Some devices employ a simple filtration method (microfiltration), in which water is pumped through tiny holes that organisms are unable to pass through. Ceramic filters (pore size 0.2µm) will remove bacteria and protozoans, but not the smaller viruses (0.02–0.2µm). Other devices employ both a filter and chemical treatment with an iodine resin which strains and sterilizes in one go but again due to the new EU biocide laws these are not available in the UK. Choosing the right device is important, so here are some tips:

- Manufacturers often say how many litres of pure water a device will produce. However, this can be drastically reduced if the water is silty and not pre-filtered.
- If heavy use is expected, make sure that the purifier can be taken apart, cleaned, and reassembled in the field to prevent blockages.
- Check the pump rate as some can take a lot of effort to produce a small amount of water.
- Many manufacturers of pumps go to great lengths to state what they will remove, while keeping quiet about what is not removed. For example, pumps will not remove chemical effluent, such as mercury in the tributaries of the Amazon river, without the addition of a carbon filter. For those visiting areas where there is mining or factories up-river this may be important.
- Water storage time is also important; ideally after sterilization the water should be used within 24 h.
- Although a filter plus iodine resin may appear the ideal solution for treating water in all circumstances, this system has been known to fail and, in the US, some have been withdrawn from the market.

Other potential methods of water purification

Coagulation–flocculation with disinfection

A newer system developed by Proctor and Gamble, consists of sachets containing chemical disinfectant and substances that cause flocculation of particles. This has been very effective in field trials and may also be useful against *Cryptosporidium*. The product goes under the name of PUR™ and each sachet treats 10 litres of water.

UV radiation

There are a number of devices available that have claimed efficacy, including against *Cryptosporidium*. Water must be clear before treatment and power requirements may limit their viability. A handheld device called Steripen™ is available that has a good efficacy if used correctly. It relies on batteries and units are quite expensive. Steripen™ now has a version that can be powered by solar panels or dynamos.

Reverse osmosis filters

These are highly effective membrane filters that will remove all micro-organisms and have the additional advantage of being able to desali-nate seawater. The small hand-pump versions are expensive but a useful survival aid at sea.

Drinking bottle filters

These are bottles with filters attached to the top. The most well-known is the Aqua Pure Traveller™. The bottle is filled with the water to be treated and then squeezed into a drinking cup for purification or drunk straight from the bottle. In low-risk areas this may be acceptable but in a high-risk area, the water should be squeezed out of the bottle into a suitable container and chemically treated. Filters are now available for the popular water bladder and tube type bottles, such as the Camelbak; again, in high-risk areas chemical treatment should still be considered.

These filters have also been adapted for group use and to an extent can replace the function of the Millbanks bag. Large 4–10L bladders are filled with collected water, suspended over a receptacle and the water allowed to pass through a tube leading to the filter by gravity. The bladder can be topped up constantly to produce large amounts of filtered water.

Choice of water purification system

The choice of technique will depend on the size and circumstances of the expedition.

If practicable, a large pot should be put on to boil at the end of an evening meal to allow preparation of water for the following morning. In addition, all members should have some method of sterilizing their own drinking water. Boiling large volumes of water consumes considerable fuel.

If not relying on boiling, consider the sources of water likely to be used. Either mechanical filtration or chemical methods can be used to purify clear, pristine surface waters. However, near human habitation or agricultural areas a combination of methods may be required to give maximal protection. Filters are not as effective as the chemicals at removing viruses, but on the other hand chemicals are not generally effective or reliable against *Cryptosporidium*. So, with potentially contaminated water one should either use an effective one-step device which can remove all types of organisms, or use a two-step process involving both chemicals and filtration.

Possible methods include:

- For large groups: chlorination provided that the condition of the treatment tanks can be carefully monitored.
- For smaller groups: chlorine dioxide, particularly if on the move: strain water through a cloth and provide members with their own small bottle of chlorine dioxide or chlorination tablets to treat water after drawing it off into their own water bottles. The strained water could be used for boiling water, e.g. for beverages.
- Using one of the new generation of water bottles with a filtration/purification method attached (e.g. Aqua Pure™). Their ease of use helps the user to keep up a constant intake of water. However, in high-risk areas it is suggested that the water be squeezed through and chemically treated.

Camp water purification arrangements

Providing enough treated water from a natural source for a camp of 20 people is time-consuming, but exceedingly important. The best approach is to incorporate a strict regime from the start by appointing one person as 'water chief' to supervise the sterilization, safe storage, and use of the water. The appointed person should also make sure that every member of the expedition is capable of sterilizing his or her own drinking water.

Rigid plastic containers with a tap and handle are the best for water. These come in 10- or 25-L sizes, but the larger size container is heavy when full of water so keep in mind distances to water source and terrain. If you do not have a method of removing the taste of chemicals, water will taste better when cold. Storing water in special canvas bags will keep it cool through evaporation from the small pores of the canvas. If they can be obtained, army surplus bags are excellent and come in sizes suitable for storage of large volumes in camp or for tying to the back of a vehicle.

If a daily average of 6 L per person is required for drinking and 4 L for cooking/washing up, containers holding 10 L per person per day will be required. Water treatment could be split into sessions if it is necessary to reduce the number of containers in use. To avoid confusion, have a good system of marking containers for the three different types of water treatment:

- Untreated for storage, sedimentation, or settling process.
- Strained ready for treatment.
- Fit for drinking.

Field parties

Each field party member should carry personal equipment for sterilizing water; metal cups are preferable to plastic as the latter often break.

If travelling by vehicle, do not use one large container for storing water; a single puncture may have disastrous consequences. Jerry cans or the canvas bags as described earlier are the best option, but try to adopt the same system of markings as employed in base camp.

See also:
Fluids and electrolytes, p. 760;
Diarrhoea and vomiting, p. 398.

Sanitation and latrines

See also ➜ Water and sanitation in tropical forests, p. 781.

The health and hygiene surrounding the waste that we generate is as important to the prevention of illness as are the standards of cleanliness we apply to the preparation and consumption of food.

The management of waste on an expedition is a balancing act between factors such as location, available facilities, and personal adherence to standards or procedures, with an overall aim to minimize ecological and environmental impact.

Latrines

The disposal of human waste on expedition can be separated into its two forms:

Urine disposal

Unless infection is present, urine is sterile and therefore provides less of a problem in its disposal. However, large quantities of urine can smell offensive in a short space of time, and affect fragile ecosystems.

When siting a urinal:

- Choose an area 50–100 m from the camp.
- Make sure it is downstream of any water collection point.
- Avoid caves or other areas where urine will remain stagnant.
- Avoid rocks or gravel, where urine lingers.
- Clearly mark the path to the urinal and the urinal itself.
- Re-site the urinal on a regular basis to avoid large collections of urine.

Latrine placement

The latrines have to be far enough from camp to pose no infection or contamination risk, yet close enough to be used with convenience. Thus:

- Place it 100 m from the camp.
- Place it 100 m from any lakes, rivers, or streams:
  - Look for high water marks.
  - Consider local water tables.
- Consider water run-off channels in the event of:
  - Heavy rain.
  - Flash floods.
- Mark a path to and from the latrine.
- Consider hazards posed by fauna and flora—especially at night.
- Include a system of notifying people when it is in use.
- Identify latrine boundaries clearly.
- Ensure that everyone is familiar with latrine etiquette.

Other human waste disposal options

Some national park authorities now recommend urinating into fast flowing rivers or the saturated river banks. This avoids unpleasant odours and damage to sensitive ecosystems.

Burying
This is only an option in environments where there is enough bacterial activity within the soil. Bacterial activity normally occurs only within the first 10 inches (25 cm) of topsoil, therefore only a shallow scrape is required.

When re-filling the scrape, use a stick to 'stir' in faeces, ensuring greater contact with soil enzymes, and then cover over with topsoil.

Group latrines should consist of a long trench, approximately 6 inches (15 cm) wide and 8 inches (20 cm) deep.

When the first trench is filled in, site another one.

Treating/sterilizing
Chemically treating faecal waste on expedition is a complicated process. It can be costly, and requires equipment and proper faecal storage facilities.

In strictly limited circumstances where expeditions find themselves in remote locations away from human or animal populations, it is possible to use the sun's ultraviolet rays to break down faecal matter with a method known as 'frosting a rock' or 'icing a cake'.

Carrying out
• The last method requires a suitable container which should be either disposable or re-usable (and therefore cleanable), durable, portable, an appropriate size for expedition length, and size of the expedition population.
• There should be a definitive plan regarding final disposal of effluent. 'Carrying out' is sometimes used for forward camps in ecologically sensitive environments. On return to a base camp in a more hospitable environment, the waste can be disposed of appropriately.

Sanitary towels/tampons and toilet paper
These should never be buried as they do not biodegrade effectively in the wild. Store them with used toilet paper, then burn at the end of the day, or carry out to dispose of after the expedition. For alternatives to sanitary towels/tampons, see ➔ Logistics, p. 411.

Hand hygiene
This is without doubt the most important part of personal hygiene. At the latrine entrance there should be facilities for hand washing, which include:
• Water container/bucket with lid.
• Water (clean but not sterile).
• Scoop or ladle.
• Soap/disinfectant.
• Nail brush (optional).

Water should be scooped out with a ladle to prevent dirty hands contaminating the container. Hands should be washed and rinsed away from the container. In addition to soap and water, consider the use of an alcohol-based hand rub.

Chapter 4

Ethics and responsibilities

Section editors
Shane Winser and James Moore

Contributors
Jim Bond
Rebecca Harris
Amy Hughes
James Moore
Nick Lewis (1st edition)

Ethics of expeditions *112*
Clinical competence *116*
Care of local staff *118*
Interacting with local communities *120*
Working with other expeditions *124*
Environmental impact *124*
Assessing an expedition's environmental footprint *125*
Working with the media *126*
Disaster medicine *130*

Ethics of expeditions

Ethics and medicine are intrinsically linked, and the importance of ethical considerations and behaviour on an expedition cannot be overstated. Despite its achievements—be they adventurous goals or scientific discoveries—an expedition is often remembered according to how appropriately it has been planned, and how well it has behaved towards people in its host country.

Consideration of the ethical principles surrounding an expedition may be superficial, or involve much heart-searching. Each of us should be individually guided by a conscience and a sense of social responsibility. However, at least four other sets of ethical standards should influence policies and decisions on an expedition:

- The personal ethics of other individuals.
- The group ethics that the team adopts, deliberately or subconsciously.
- The religious beliefs, values, and cultural mores of the people in whose territory you are journeying.
- Universal human rights.

Principles

The 'four principles plus scope' model of biomedical ethics[1] is a recognized framework that helps make some of these standards explicit—and defendable. It should be familiar to most recent medical graduates and can, if thought through, be applied to almost any situation.

> *The 'four principles' of ethical debate and behaviour*
> 1. *Respect for autonomy*: the right to individual self-determination.
> 2. *Beneficence*: the doing of good.
> 3. *Non-maleficence*: the avoidance of doing harm.
> 4. *Respect for justice*: equity, fairness.

Autonomy (A)

Autonomy involves respecting an individual's right to choose treatment or refuse it. Respect for the autonomy of others carries with it the moral obligation to maintain (appropriate) confidentiality, to keep one's promises, not to deceive one another, and by extension, to communicate well at all times.

Beneficence (B) and non-maleficence (N)

Beneficence ('doing good') and non-maleficence ('not doing harm') are complementary obligations. Examples include ensuring that all team members, including the expedition medic, have adequate training for what they would reasonably be expected to do, and providing clear information about the risks that people will be encountering.

---

1 Beauchamp TL, Childress JF (1989). *Principles of Biomedical Ethics*, 3rd edn. Oxford: Oxford University Press.

Empowerment

Whether of individuals or local communities (see ➲ Scope, p. 113), empowerment can be seen as an overlap of the first three principles (A, B, and N). Arguably, it is a core function within any expedition.

Justice

Respect for *justice* is the moral obligation to act on the basis of fair adjudication between competing claims. This can be to do with:
- The fair distribution of scarce resources (distributive justice).
- Respect for different peoples' rights (rights-based justice).
- Respect for morally acceptable laws (legal justice).

Scope

When applying the four principles, you need to determine the boundaries within which your ethical issues lie.[2] A basic ethical review would consider how your journey could impact—either positively or negatively—on those who will come into contact with you, but your scope may need to be much broader if, for instance, you plan to travel in sensitive wilderness areas and need to consider the environmental impact of your travels.

There are often no easy or absolutely right answers for what constitutes ethical practice; individuals' viewpoints may vary as a result of professional, personal, cultural, financial, educational, or religious differences. It will be impossible to satisfy everyone all the time, but it is important to attempt to understand others people's views—especially if these views are strongly held. Part of the fun of an expedition is the new and unexpected challenges that make you think about, or re-think, your position. Acknowledge your mistakes, apologize if you have got it wrong, and learn from them.

Cultural clashes

Cultural clashes occur surprisingly often, both within expeditions and between expedition groups and the local communities. The issues with expeditions, who may be embedded within a community for weeks or months, can be greater than the problems caused by tourists behaving in a similar way, but who are perceived by the locals as passing through, or simply 'doing their own thing'.

Any situation where a mixed group of people is working together under arduous conditions has some potential for a clash. Cultural miscommunication, leading to loss of mutual respect and trust may be exacerbated by:
- A history of colonialism in either the host or guest peoples.
- Apartness (or apartheid), in eating, sleeping, or travelling arrangements.
- Inappropriate behaviour including arrogance, inappropriate dress, or failure to respect local customs or religious codes.

The ethical situation can become very complex if, for instance, customs and behaviour towards women or children in the local community are perceived by the visitors to be wrong.

2 Gillon R (1994). Medical ethics: four principles plus attention to scope. *BMJ*, 309, 184.

The hazards of such situations can be minimized by effective communication including:
- Awareness that you are operating in a different cultural norm.
- Good translation skills that, for instance, make implicit meanings explicit.
- Good listening skills, including body language.
- Serious efforts to understand socially and culturally determined references and attitudes.
- Openness, honesty, good humour, and inclusiveness at all times.
- Appropriate behaviour: especially the avoidance of drugs, alcohol, and sexual licentiousness.
- Appropriate personal values: such as humility, respect for differing beliefs and taboos, and a strong work ethic.

At the very least, cultural clashes have the potential to cause upset. In extremes, they can wreck an entire expedition.

Personal and professional clashes

Even with the best of intentions and a shared common purpose, people do not always get on well with each other during expeditions. Hardships, close working conditions, and interdependency may turn minor irritations into resentments, and lead to arguments. If everyone on the team has a clear role to play, it may be easier to respect each other's contribution, while accepting joint responsibility for helping out in any way possible when things are not going well.

Causes of interpersonal disharmony
- Poor communication: both expressive and receptive.
- Unrealistic expectations: which may in themselves be a result of poor communication.
- Conflict based on pre-conceived ideas/notions surrounding professional hierarchies and relationships.
- Personal clashes sometimes masquerade as professional clashes and vice versa.

Leadership styles vary, and people respond in different ways to the same style. Usually inclusive leadership styles in which problems are talked through in groups are more likely to lead to effective understanding and solution of problems. However, some people are more comfortable with hierarchical leadership and perceive inclusive leadership as being weak.

Regular group meetings to discuss progress and effective debriefing after activities can bridge gaps. Such meetings should ensure that everyone continues to support the goals of the expedition and feels that risks are being minimized in the most effective manner.

Regardless of any personal views, the medic should try to remain removed from interpersonal conflicts so that everyone on the expedition remains able to communicate their concerns and worries, confident that they will be listened to sympathetically.

Preventing interpersonal disharmony

- *Before setting off*: choose your team carefully. Consider team-building exercises, e.g. imaginary worst-case scenarios. Ensure there are clear and unambiguous leadership roles, especially within the medical and leadership team.
- *At the start*: establish ground rules, e.g. no criticism of people behind their backs; respect for personal space. Acknowledge the potential for falling(s) out and work out clear ways in advance to air grievances and resolve disputes early.
- *During*: aim to build on shared group values and develop a sense of group responsibility. Communicate with each other; no one should be expected to carry all the weight of their particular role alone.
- *In a crisis*: depending on the particular hazards of the expedition, you may ultimately need to have a formal chain of command.
- *After*: be self-critical and prepared to learn from your mistakes for next time.

Management of disputes

Although the management of disharmony should ideally be a group responsibility, it often falls on the leader or the expedition medic (in his or her confidential capacity) to sort such conflicts out. Allowing everyone to have their say is important; however, 'time-out' may need to be called first before a resolution is attempted. In some instances it may be useful to use an arbitrator external to the expedition, perhaps via satellite phone, which can make the final decision, redirecting conflict away from the clinician or leadership team. See also ➔ Creating expedition teams, p. 26.

Clinical competence

As in other areas of professional practice, there is pressure to improve the defined clinical competencies of those providing medical support to expeditions. Individual clinicians have a responsibility, both professional and ethical, to ensure they are capable of providing appropriate medical expertise in an autonomous, decision-making situation far removed from the support systems present at home.

As a sole or lead clinician you may find yourself dealing with a serious clinical or logistical problem, without recourse to senior support, with few or no diagnostic adjuncts to aid decision-making, which is further complicated by hostile environmental conditions. This is a level of responsibility and stress often not anticipated in the initial excitement of joining an expedition.

Medics should ensure they are appropriately qualified for the anticipated role, and have completed appropriate training. Hosting organizations and distant advisers should be aware of the level of medical expertise able to be provided by the clinician, and expedition members need to know what sort of medical support they can expect whilst abroad, both from staff on the expedition and from the local medical services.

By itself, the label 'expedition medic' does not explain one's level of competency and it would be misleading to use this title—giving the impression of great competence—if one only has minimal medical, knowledge, skills, or experience in the field. See also Role of the expedition medical officer, p. 20.

Decision-making

The combination of unfamiliar medical pathologies, difficult logistics, and lack of diagnostic aids on an expedition can make medical decision-making incredibly difficult. Inexperienced clinicians will not have the scope of knowledge to make informed choices, and may struggle with decisions such as:

- How and when do you decide to medevac a patient?
- When do you stop a group ascent or jungle trek if you think that environmental conditions are inappropriate, or the journey will exceed an individual's capabilities?
- How and when do you remove an individual from an expedition if they have health issues, are physically unable to cope, or do not gel with the rest of the group?
- How do you manage communication both with the group, with local people, and with those back home?

Medics may be pressurized by an individual or the whole team to take decisions based on factors beyond the purely medical situation. For instance, clinical judgements about whether to evacuate a patient following an injury might be being influenced by issues such as:

- The proximity of the expedition to its goals (e.g. a summit within reach).
- Financial implications—loss of sponsorship, or film rights.
- Logistic difficulties in evacuating the individual.
- The continuing viability of the team having lost a key member.

In addition to such external pressures, the medic may be taking decisions based purely on clinical judgement, lacking the usual diagnostic equipment available at home. Given the numerous unknowns, medics should usually err on the side of caution, assume the worst, and arrange evacuation. They ought not be criticized for this, even if the eventual diagnosis is of a benign rather than a serious medical condition.

Throughout, the responsibility lies with the clinician and the aftermath of a wrong decision can be catastrophic both for the patient, and for the medic who may suffer professionally, personally, and medico-legally. Clinical experience, appropriate training, familiarity with the 'pre-hospital' environment, and time spent in remote environments travelling or in global health settings eases the path to decision-making and most likely improves outcome for all those involved. See also ➔ Legal liabilities and professional insurance, p. 76.

Obtaining experience

Expedition medicine can be without doubt one of the most exciting clinical areas in which to practise. As such it often attracts young, enthusiastic healthcare professionals who, unhindered by the responsibilities of marriage, mortgage, and multiple offspring, find it easier to take time out of regular career pathways. Whilst in an ideal world one would prefer expedition medics to have many years of experience in an acute specialty, preferably with pre-hospital experience, this is not always possible. Enshrined within their prospective codes of conduct[3,4,5] clinicians from all disciplines are expected to work within their known scope of competency. Therefore medics should constantly check the levels of autonomy and judgement required of them, against the standards of their education, training, and experience. For first expeditions, junior medics will benefit from:

• Completing a good quality course on expedition medicine, relevant to the environment that they will visit (see ➔ Medical and first-aid training, p. 44).
• Shadowing experienced doctors, nurses, paramedics, or rescue teams.
• Working on less remote expeditions.
• Ensuring they have access to good communications and telemedicine (see ➔ Telemedicine and communications, p. 160).

It is worth remembering that good clinical skills make up about only one-third of the skills required to be a good expedition medic; personal and expedition skills are just as important. As one gains experience and knowledge, the boundaries can be pushed—the moral responsibility of the medic is to know when and how hard to push. See also ➔ Joining an expedition, p. 16.

3 ⌕ http://www.gmc-uk.org/guidance/good_medical_practice/knowledge_skills_performance.asp

4 ⌕ http://www.nmc-uk.org/Publications/Standards/The-code/Provide-a-high-standard-of-practice-and-care-at-all-times

5 ⌕ http://www.hpc-uk.org/assets/documents/1000051CStandards_of_Proficiency_Paramedics.pdf

Care of local staff

Duty of care

An expedition's 'duty of care' extends to all participants. A participant should be defined as 'anyone who would not be in a given situation if it were not for the expedition', e.g. local drivers, porters, guides, and cooks. Factors that should be considered include:

- The basic essentials of life: are your local staff appropriately fed, watered, clothed, shod, and sheltered at night?
- The right to be consulted, and to say no.
- Fair recompense for any work carried out, or extra risks taken. Payments should be commensurate with local wages and costs, so as not to distort the local economy completely.
- Health and safety:
  - Is there enough basic protective gear such as life jackets and helmets to go round, and does everyone know how to use one?
  - Are some participants expected to take greater risks than others; e.g. local people riding in the back of a pick-up?
  - Access to appropriate medical attention: standards of medical care for everyone on the expedition should be similar. This does not necessarily mean expatriation for treatment of serious injury or illness, but could well entail having to arrange casualty evacuation for local personnel to appropriate in-country medical facilities.
  - Respect for home and family life. Setting off at a certain time may mean a man can't milk his goats and he has to arrange someone else to do it for him.
- Respect for feast days, providing time to pray, etc.
- Long-term consequences for local participants.
- Are you empowering them?
- Is anything you're asking them to do (e.g. to translate) likely to compromise their social standing in the community?

Good practice

Duty of care, whether moral or legal, is only a minimal requirement. Good practice, enabling you and your team to get the most out of the expedition, demands a lot more. When an expedition is embedded within an isolated community for an extended period of time, the boundaries between expedition participants, their dependents, and the rest of the local population may become rather blurred at times. The limits to this need to be defined as the expedition may find that large numbers of people become dependent upon it—potentially a huge drain on resources.

Interacting with local communities

Understanding the life of those who live in the areas visited by an expedition can be very rewarding, and some researchers rely almost exclusively for their data on what they can learn from working with local guides and their communities.

General approach

The wisdom of being open, honest, warm-hearted, and respectful in all your dealings cannot be overstressed; people hate it if they think you are trying to deceive them. Local customs and hierarchy should be observed. For example:

- Avoid arriving at a village at daybreak.
- Wait to be properly introduced and accepted by the headman and elders.
- Seek permission before taking any photos.
- Do not assume ignorance of the outside world; TV, the Internet, and cellular communication networks are influencing all but the most remote areas.

Put yourselves in their position:

- How would you wish to be treated by a group of wealthy foreign visitors who decide to come and spend some time in your community? Would you wish to be ignored, kept at a polite distance, or invited into their camp?
- How would you respond to their curiosity about your way of life?
- Would you prefer them to have at least mastered a few basic civilities in your language, such as greetings, 'thank you', 'delicious', etc.?
- How would you feel if they were overpaying staff and upsetting the economy of the village?
- Hospitality is very important to most societies and is never to be abused.

Treating local people, not part of the expedition

In many parts of the world expeditions are perceived by local people to be rich and endowed with clinical skills and drugs. The apparently universal human desire to take medication may be stimulated by the arrival of the expedition, and the slightest hint that you will treat people in the local community may produce a flood of 'ill' people. It is tempting to try to 'help' and to establish goodwill by offering medicines to all but, before you do, consider the potential harm:

- You may not understand local people's health problems and therefore misdiagnose.
- You may endanger your own expedition members by using drugs intended for them.
- You may be blamed unreasonably for adverse outcomes.
- You may offend local healers (and health services).
- Treatment may be incomplete and thus ineffective or harmful.
- You might be exploited for your novelty value.
- You may not be in a position to follow up treatment.
- You may encourage expectations among local people that the local medical services cannot meet.

Nevertheless, sometimes you cannot, and should not, avoid doing what you can to help other people. If you have appropriate time and facilities it could appear churlish not to see and examine anyone who presents, if only to reassure yourself and others whether it is a genuine emergency. Ethically, and in some jurisdictions legally as well, clinicians have an obligation to act as 'Good Samaritans' in situations where there is an acute emergency and when setting off to work in very remote communities, it may well be worth budgeting a little extra for such scenarios when preparing the medical kit. Local people, particularly children, who are severely ill or injured, should be treated, but not necessarily by you; evacuate these patients if possible. Your authority may help to achieve this.

> *Examples of emergency situations encountered on expeditions in Madagascar*
> - A villager with cerebral malaria.
> - An infant of a nomadic forest people, with a severe chest infection.
> - A fisherman, stung by a stonefish, who had a necrotic dorsum of foot, requiring surgical debridement and antibiotics to help it heal.

As the expedition medic, you should not treat chronic disease. You will not have the resources or the time, and it will be better for everyone if patients are treated by the local health service. You also have an ethical duty to empower people, i.e. to manage their own illness, wherever possible, and to strengthen, rather than undermine, existing healthcare systems, including traditional healers (see ➲ Working with local healers, p. 122).

What if things go wrong?

As medical practitioners, we should be used to taking appropriate risks for our patients, with their full and informed consent. Good communication is thus paramount, particularly when warning of possible adverse effects. Know and admit your limitations; don't attempt heroic procedures when you're out of your depth. A useful maxim is 'always treat each patient as you would if they were a member of your own family'.

Public health

Occasionally, it may be clear that the whole population of a village or surrounding area could potentially benefit from an intervention to address a common threat to health, e.g. dirty water, malaria, trachoma.

Public health interventions, working with a local population, can appear seductively simple, but should not be undertaken lightly. They require a good deal of sensitive groundwork to work well. An ongoing project in the same area has many advantages over a 'one-off' expedition, by being able to build up trust and demonstrating commitment. It may be more empowering and effective in the long term to sow the seed of an idea, rather than to raise false expectations.

Working with local healers

Indigenous healers provide roughly 80% of the medical services used world-wide.[6] Beyond their wealth of local knowledge, they usually have a strong sense of clinical duty toward their constituency, and a great deal of influence. This is an often-overlooked potential resource, particularly in public health (see Box 4.1).

As an expedition medic, working in the territory of a local healer, one might anticipate that you could be viewed as competition, or worse, a threat. This should not put you off going the extra mile to seek out and pay one's respects to a fellow healthcare professional. You might be surprised at the reception and level of cooperation you subsequently receive for showing this simple courtesy.

Box 4.1 Case study: Project Renala—community-led TB treatment in SW Madagascar

On an ethnobotanical research project, working with the Mikea, an elusive, forest people, the expedition doctor/botanist was approached by local healers to advise on how to deal with an outbreak of TB, which was affecting their (apparently TB-naïve) population. Because of cultural differences, a nearby mission's TB programme was finding it hard to reach the Mikea people effectively in their forest home.

Over the next few years, the project helped to bridge the gap between the two healthcare systems, by providing backup and training. A special, fully ambulatory TB treatment regimen/arrangement for the Mikea was worked out with traditional healers and other notables taking full responsibility for initial case detection, and treatment supervision in the forest, and the mission's healthcare workers confirming diagnoses and managing any complications.

In this way, a responsible DOTS-TB treatment programme was extended to include the Mikea on their terms, but without compromising their semi-nomadic, hunter-gatherer lifestyle, and without undermining the authority or undervaluing the clinical acumen of either set of healers.

---

6 Green EC (1999). *Indigenous Theories of Disease*. Walnut Creek, CA: Sage.

Working with other expeditions

The same basic rules about ethical conduct apply when interacting with other expeditions; for instance, avoid negative criticism of another expedition's methods or style, etc.

In the field, your expedition will inevitably be scrutinized and compared with others by local people. Overt displays of friendliness towards another group, e.g. of the same mother tongue/nationality as your own, that is different from your interactions with local people, will not go unnoticed.

Expeditions are not competitions. If you hear, in advance, that another expedition is planning something similar, or might coincide with yours, the 'right' thing to do is to take the initiative and start talking things over with them. You might find that the ground you are each planning to cover is actually somewhat different, or even complementary, from a research perspective. Aside from the possibility of sharing data, there may be the opportunity to pool certain resources, such as medical expertise or use of a satellite phone for medevac. For obvious reasons, this kind of arrangement is preferably discussed in advance.

If another expedition has already set up camp at the site you had intended to use, normal etiquette would be for your, second group, to find another suitable location at a comfortable distance, if possible. Establishing good relations should be a priority, once local formalities have been completed.

Your interaction with other expeditions visiting the area may continue long after the expedition is over. Keep in contact, learn from each other's successes and mistakes, never misrepresenting others' efforts, and share your expedition findings.

Environmental impact

Environmental management requires you to analyse and then minimize whenever possible the consequences of an expedition's activities. Larger expeditions inevitably have a greater environmental impact as a result of increases in:

- Transportation requirements.
- Quantities of supplies.
- Need for local staff.
- Requirement for water.
- Amount of waste and sewage produced.

Economic effects can be complex and are largely dependent upon how much money an expedition spends locally.

Assessing an expedition's environmental footprint

Ideally, each group should appoint an environmental manager, whose responsibilities should include:
- Researching the environmental requirements of the host country.
- Ensuring that these are taken into account during permit and grant applications.
- Looking into the specific environmental issues of the expedition, including areas such as path erosion, sensitive areas, problems from existing waste accumulation, etc.

The environmental manager should work closely with the other members of the expedition to consider:
- Transport options to and from the destination: can public transport be used?
- Accommodation options: do the hotels or guesthouses subscribe to a reputable environmental initiative?
- Local employment cooperatives: will the expedition's employees get the best deal?
- Expedition support agencies including guides, trekking companies, and boat charters: what is their environmental policy?
- Waste management procedures during the expedition, including the packaging on food and equipment, the type of waste-handling structures available in the expedition area, and any documentation required for waste disposal in the country.

Everything should be considered from the point of view of reducing the amount of unnecessary resources that the expedition will use. Good use of locally provided, sustainable resources can also benefit the local economy.

Making an environmental mitigation plan

An environmental plan needs to be drawn up to explain how the impacts already highlighted will be mitigated. The environmental plan should include the following:
- The expedition's environmental statement. Say what it is you are trying to achieve from an environmental point of view.
- A summary of the environmental problems that may already be present in the area.
- The impacts that will be generated by you.
- How you will mitigate them, listing the different responsibilities.
- The waste management options available to you.
- What environmental permits or applications are required to visit your area.
- Your arrangements for local employment: you need to educate any local expedition employees (e.g. cooks and porters) sympathetically and diplomatically about the importance of avoiding environmental damage. For example, use wood fires as little as possible, as deforestation is a serious problem in many expedition areas. Supply fuel-efficient stoves and encourage their use.
- Any reporting requirements upon completion of the expedition.

The plan should be succinct and easy-to-understand. Try getting it onto one side of paper.

Working with the media

Providing medical support alongside a film or television production company can offer exciting opportunities for an expedition medic. These include paid employment whilst doing a 'glamorous' job, the chance of working on location in remote and exciting settings, possibly with celebrities, and even the opportunity to appear on-screen.

However, the appealing nature of these opportunities often belies the very real and unique risks associated with working in this field. Before signing up as a medic for a television or media company, it is important to consider these risks and obtain a comprehensive understanding of the situations likely to be encountered and the probable ability of the production company to deal with them.

Medics are only likely to be recruited if filming will involve a remote or dangerous assignment, where if something were to go wrong the harm would be considerable. Although most production companies undertaking this type of work are well informed and produce detailed risk assessments, such attention to detail isn't guaranteed. Remote filming trips often experience 'expedition' conditions, yet some media companies, often more through inexperience than malpractice, do not do the detailed planning one would expect. This despite the strict health and safety regulations governing their business.

Regardless of personal performance, the high-profile nature of these trips means that should something go seriously wrong, the medic is as risk not merely of questions from the regulatory authorities, but could end up experiencing 'trial by media', which can be immensely stressful and equally damaging.

There are various types of media production styles. These include:
- Documentaries.
- News/current affairs.
- Reality TV.
- Feature films.
- Advertising (commercials).

Having an understanding of the aims and goals of the programme will give an indication as to potential health risks involved. For example, news and current affairs programmes might film in areas of conflict or famine where there is the ever-present risk of physical and psychological trauma, whereas reality TV programmes potentially place contributors in increasingly hazardous or challenging situations in an attempt to obtain exciting TV.

Risks can broadly be considered in terms of those affecting the medic, the film crew (behind the camera), presenters/contributors (in front of the camera) and the production team (director/producer and so on).

Medic-specific risks

- Limited involvement in pre-travel team screening, leading to:
  - Unknown pre-existing medical problems.
  - Reduced appropriate team medical preparation.
- Limited involvement in pre-travel risk assessment, including:
  - Little/no knowledge about in-country medical facilities.
  - Little/no knowledge about emergency procedures.
  - Limited knowledge of insurance cover details—such as casevac for remote locations (e.g. is it only available from major cities?).
- Unclear definitions of roles and responsibilities, including:
  - When medical intervention is deemed appropriate.
  - Levels of control and input into decision making, particularly in relation to schedules, filming locations, and leadership.
- Lack of personal knowledge about the illnesses/injuries likely to be encountered (including psychological stress).

Production crew risks

Although all crew are issued with a Production Risk Assessment prior to filming, to protect them on location, sometimes they overlook their own personal safety:

- Media crews are focused on filming and less on personal day-to-day health issues such as hydration, hygiene, sun-exposure and protection against vector-borne diseases such as malaria.
- Whilst filming, camera operators have a narrow field of vision. If mobile, they will not see physical hazards such as uneven ground, dangerous flora, e.g. rattan, or dangerous fauna, e.g. snakes/spiders.
- The nature and pressure to achieve the 'once in a career' shot can place crew in harm's way with limited chance of regress, e.g. in exposed, hazardous positions, even whilst being swarmed by insects or charged by larger animals.
- Camera crew carry heavy kit, for long periods of time, in all weathers and terrains and so are occupationally vulnerable to certain types of injury, e.g. back, shoulder, and knees.

Contributors/presenter healthcare risks

- Tight production schedules increase pressure on both contributors and presenters to 'deliver', despite the presence of illness or injury.
- Contributors take part without the skills/expertise required of the film location.
- Contributors are placed in situations hazardous to their physical/mental well-being in order to obtain exciting TV.
- Production crews are often used to working in difficult conditions, whilst contributors can have little/no experience—leaving them physically and mentally vulnerable in demanding situations.

Production team risks

- Tight filming schedules caused by budgetary constraints, permits/ visas, and availability of crew/presenters lead to reduced environmental acclimatization. This in turn results in an increased risk of health issues such as heat exhaustion and acute mountain sickness.
- Poor preparation for living and working in hostile environments.
- The production team (director/producers) are often the 'silent' workers—continuing to work when the crews, presenters, and contributors have finished filming. Tiredness can make them vulnerable to health risks.
- Regular health risks associated with working in foreign/hostile environments.

Issues with working in television

Certain types of programme, such as reality TV, can raise ethical concerns for a medic as their objective is often to stress participants to breaking point, through physical and mental challenges, or in some cases use the rigours of expedition life to deal with traumatic personal issues not being faced at home. As a medic, you are responsible for both the physical and psychological well-being of the team.

Before embarking on such a project ensure you are clear in your own mind as to where your boundaries lie, and how far you are willing to let individuals be pushed. Your ethical standards may well differ from those of the production team. Whilst filming, there is a risk that film crews focus more on production, schedules, and personal needs, rather than the welfare of porters, staff, and local communities. Medics have the advantage of being separate from the filming process and can help to prevent this from happening.

Teamwork

An alert and attentive expedition medic will predict and prevent problems before they materialize. For the majority of the time the medic will not be involved in providing medical care. However, on a daily basis, a medic can have a valuable role as a 'second pair of eyes' for the health and safety of the team. It is important that the medic is seen as an active member of the team, contributing to the smooth running of the production.

The nature of filming can result in excessive periods of waiting; for particular filming conditions/subjects to appear or during repeated takes of the same shot. Keeping alert during these periods will help ensure the medic is not caught out.

Celebrities

It should go without saying that a strict professional duty of confidentiality should apply to all personal insights gleaned from working alongside a celebrity presenter: it is as ever the medic's role to show a good example. This is particularly worth noting after the expedition, when no longer in the professional bounds of the production and support team.

Disaster medicine

Disasters can occur anywhere in the world, often having the greatest impact on a community and country infrastructure in low-income countries, where needs significantly outweigh resources.

To many, they appear exciting and often appeal to a medic's natural instinct of wanting to help others and utilize skills less frequently used in the UK. Raw and emotive media coverage helps fuel this desire to travel to catastrophes across the globe, from providing relief work after natural disasters with organized agencies, through to leaving a postgraduate training programme and travelling independently to a war zone.

Although opportunities to provide assistance in a disaster are frequent, there are many ethical issues that surround this type of medical provision. Medics travelling independently to disaster zones, even with the best intentions, are at great risk of becoming a hindrance to local and international healthcare efforts, In addition they can be a drain on local resources and an infrastructure already under great pressure. Issues that often draw criticism include:

* *Language:* Western healthcare workers have been found providing medical care without interpreters or the ability to communicate effectively with the local population.
* *Continuity:* teams provide treatment e.g. basic surgical procedures, splinting of fractures, but with no regress to follow-up care.
* *Documentation:* care is often provided without medical records.
* *Coordination:* there is often little or no coordination between various healthcare providers; a situation made worse with multiple, international teams.
* *Credentials/suitability:* independent workers may provide care unsupervised and without any formal checking of credentials, or lack any authority to practise in a country.

Historically there has been a trend for medics embarking on disaster relief projects to be more junior and less experienced. As such, not only are they likely to lack the relevant clinical competencies and accountability required for such work, they are likely to be unaccustomed to the scale and magnitude of suffering visited on populations during periods of disaster. This inexperience can place personal health and well-being at risk, as well as that of the local population.

Being part of a team providing medical care following natural or man-made disasters is exciting, challenging, and incredibly rewarding. However, it is also a complicated, multifaceted process, in which even global governmental and non-governmental organizations sometimes struggle. It is now widely accepted that professionally, clinically, and perhaps even ethically, the most appropriate way to become involved is through well-established and regulated bodies that can provide suitable training and direction.

The UK International Emergency Trauma Register (UKIETR)

UKIETR has been established as a register aiming to draw together clinicians interested in deploying as part of a team in response to sudden-onset disasters and humanitarian emergencies. Its aim is to provide structured and standardized training to individuals and teams, promoting a governed, coordinated, accountable, clinically competent, and guided approach to medical and logistical team response in disasters. For more information see ✆http://www.ukmed.org

Chapter 5

Crisis management

Section editors
Shane Winser and Chris Johnson

Contributors
Kristina Birch
Rose Drew
Peter Harvey
Stephen Jones
Clare Morgan
Marc Shaw

Medical crisis management 134
Emergency response plan 136
Missing persons 140
Scene management 144
Evacuation 146
Moving an injured person 148
Repatriation 158
Telemedicine and communications 160
Sexual assault 165
Death on an expedition 166

Medical crisis management

A medical crisis on an expedition can result from illness, injury, or accident to team members. The expedition planning team has a duty to foresee and try to prevent a crisis by developing a *risk analysis and safety management system* (RAMS). If an emergency develops, a comprehensive *emergency response plan* (ERP) will provide the team with the information and resources necessary to manage the situation effectively.

Medical aspects of the safety management system include:
- Organizing medical training for all participants.
- Providing appropriate medical kits (Chapter 28).
- Organizing medical insurance with full emergency evacuation cover (◆ Medical insurance, p. 74).
- Planning for evacuation and repatriation of a severely ill or injured person (◆ Evacuation, p. 146; ◆ Repatriation, p. 158).
- Preparing a communication network in case of evacuation (◆ Emergency response plan, p. 136; ◆ Telemedicine and communications, p. 160).
- Investigating medical facilities and support available both locally and remotely (e.g. using telemedicine, ◆ Telemedicine and communications, p. 160).
- Maintaining medical records and compiling accident reports.

During an emergency the team are likely to be involved in:
- Locating the ill or injured parties.
- Preventing additional illness or injury.
- Providing care to the ill or injured (Chapter 7).
- Expediting evacuations using effective logistics and communications.
- Managing and supporting the rescue team.
- Communicating accurately and effectively with key individuals.
- Considering how to minimize long-term psychological effects on casualties and other team members (◆ Psychological reactions to traumatic events, p. 526; ◆ Post-traumatic stress disorder, p. 530).

Emergency response plan

Emergency response plan

Associated with each phase of the expedition should be an ERP, a reference document that includes information to enable any member of the team to respond appropriately to an emergency. Elements of an ERP are summarized in Fig. 5.1.

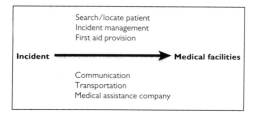

Search/locate patient
Incident management
First aid provision

Incident ➡ **Medical facilities**

Communication
Transportation
Medical assistance company

Fig. 5.1 Elements of an emergency response plan.

All these elements are important in expediting an evacuation. A rapid and timely response to a crisis may save a life; prior research, training, and resourcing are vital. Global communication is now relatively easy and satellite phones enable medical consultations from the field, so long as the medic has ready access to a medical specialist.

The most reliable source of help in an emergency is your expedition team. As far as possible be self-contained. Reliance on third parties in home countries is not robust and the best solutions are often local and simple. Therefore, do your research and know the transport, medical, search and rescue (SAR) options for the region in which you are working. Once collated, everyone involved in the expedition should know the plan, and their responsibilities in implementing it:

- All participants.
- On-call contacts in the home country and host nation.
- Support organizations (e.g. medical assistance company).
- Insurance company.

Components of an emergency response plan

An ERP should include as a minimum:

Section 1: roles and responsibilities in an emergency situation
This should clarify roles and responsibilities, focusing on the initial priorities as outlined in Table 5.1. Simplicity is critical. Consider who is trained and competent for each nominated role.

Section 2: initial response steps
Ensure that the initial response of the team is quick and effective. The generic steps outlined here can be applied to diverse situations:

- S.T.O.P.—Stop, Think, Observe, and Plan.
- Manage the scene.
- Remain calm.

Table 5.1 Roles and responsibilities in an emergency situation

Role	Tasks
Leader	Overall coordination
Incident manager	Scene safety
Logistics	Evacuation/transportation
Communication	Radio/telephone links and information transfer
First aid	Provision of temporary immediate care

- Assess hazards.
- Preserve life and prevent further injury.
- Minimize damage to property/environment.
- Delegate roles.
- Inform expedition leader.
- Ask expedition members not to contact home or use any social media.
- Contact appropriate medical assistance company.
- Contact on-call team with details, location, and contact number.

An example of an initial response plan is given in Fig. 5.2.

Section 3: emergency services—contact numbers

This should contain important telephone, email contacts, and addresses, and include:

- All team members' mobile/satellite phone numbers.
- 24-h on-call contact details.
- In-country contact details.
- Emergency medical support company details.
- Insurance companies.
- Response organizations you may need to call on, such as air charter companies, the host country air force, police, air ambulance, local mountain rescue teams, coastguard, etc. The more information that is available, the better.

Section 4: medical facility information

This section should list in-country medical facilities to enable effective evacuation of ill or injured participants. Each facility should be listed with its name, address, directions (including maps), telephone numbers, capabilities, and hours of operation. Hospitals and clinics vary around the world and it is important to assess what capabilities exist in the area of your expedition. People are not always safer in a local clinic or hospital.

Screened blood

In countries where blood is unavailable or there are concerns over its quality, arrangements can be made to obtain supplies of blood in an emergency. The Blood Care Foundation states that it is able to provide screened blood, in an emergency, to its members in any part of the world. Further information can be found at ℘ http://www.bloodcare.org.uk

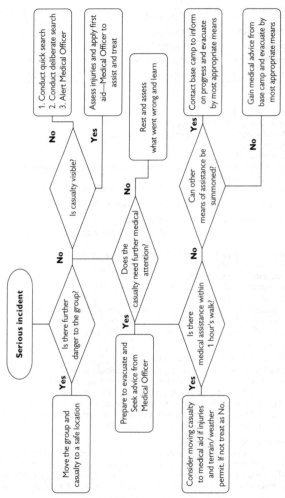

Fig. 5.2 Initial response plan.

Section 5: trip itinerary and evacuation options

This section enables the on-call contact to locate the group if there is an emergency at home or a breakdown in communications. The itinerary should include enough detail and contact numbers to enable the on-call contact to locate the group. As a minimum this must include a list of dates of where the group will be staying, including addresses and phone numbers.

In addition, this section should briefly outline the emergency evacuation route for an injured participant from each phase of the expedition.

Section 6: participant emergency contact list

In emergency situations it may be necessary to contact a participant's next of kin. To enable this, each participant will need to supply a minimum of two contact names and numbers to be stored in the ERP.

Section 7: plans to deal with death or critical injury

These are discussed in Fig. 5.2 and ➜ Death on an expedition (p. 166).

Section 8: media plan

The media plan needs to establish the procedures and resources needed to respond to the press in the event of a serious incident and/or death. It might include a draft Press Release outlining the intentions and purpose of the expedition, the framework for reporting the incident and who to contact for further information.

Search and rescue

Searching involves looking for a person whose location is unknown; rescuing is the evacuation of someone from a known location, generally a more straightforward task.

SAR services typically consist of groups of volunteers supported by logistics from police, ambulance or coastguard, and may be integrated into the national civil defence system. The volunteers usually have extensive local knowledge and may have specialist skills in marine, cliff, mountain, or cave rescue. Effective SAR systems will bring manpower, communications, appropriate transport, and tools such as thermal imaging, sniffer dogs, and rescue stretchers. Equipment and personnel have to be transported to site in a manner appropriate to the terrain; this could involve the use of boats, four-wheel drive, superjeeps, tracked vehicles, skidoos, hovercraft, or animals. Casualty evacuation may eventually involve a helicopter, fixed wing or float plane, but one cannot rely on aerial support as it may be restricted by range, height, or weather conditions. Casualties may have to be transported to a suitable landing zone.

SAR services are expensive, sometimes hazardous for the personnel involved, and take time to assemble. The quality and availability of service varies worldwide; in developing countries expeditions may have to be fully self-sufficient. Risk management plans should include determining the capability of SAR services available, methods of contact, and insurance requirements—as aerial support is frequently charged to the user. In some countries (e.g. Pakistan) payment of a bond in advance is required if there is a possibility that air evacuation will be requested.

Missing persons

Finding that an individual or small group are not where they should be, is worrying. The cause may be innocent—poor timekeeping or an unexpectedly arduous trip—but the concern may be that someone has become injured, lost, or detained. Anxieties will be heightened if those missing are young, elderly, or unfamiliar with terrain and conditions. People are more likely to become separated in dense vegetation, fog, or driving rain, or if leaders set a very fast pace. Navigation is harder in snow which masks the contours, and shifting desert sand.

Don't get lost

- Avoidance is always best.
- Teach survival skills. Maps and compasses are invaluable, but only if you know how to use them.
- GPS is nowadays readily and cheaply available on phones and cameras, equipping everyone is worthwhile, but once again only if people can use the resulting information.
- Ensure everyone in the group knows the plan for the day.
- Designate a leader and back marker, keep everyone else between the two. Do not permit weaker members of the party to drop behind. Ensure the back marker can communicate with the leader.
- If groups separate: designate obvious rendezvous places and specify time.
- Some countries with comprehensive cellular networks provide Apps (e.g. *112 Iceland*) that can link travellers direct to SAR services.

Initial actions

- Ensure main party remains safe: seek shelter, fluids, and warmth wherever possible.
- Attempt to make contact with missing persons by phone, radio, visual or auditory signals.
- Ensure searchers are properly equipped, have means of communication, and a rendezvous place and time.
- Retrace route, most people will be found close to last known position.

Lost persons

If an initial search fails, a more comprehensive search will be needed. Time is important, external SAR agencies using appropriate technologies will be able to cover the ground more quickly and effectively. Analysis of rescues have indicated common patterns of behaviour, which while not individually predictive, give an indication of how individuals may behave.[1] Skilled SAR leaders use knowledge of the situation and locality to plan their search strategy. The International Search & Rescue Database collects data on missing persons, the terrain and methods of search.

Search scenarios can be categorized (Box 5.1).

---

1 Koestler RJ (2008). *Lost Person Behavior*. Charlottesville, VA: Dbs productions.

Box 5.1 Causes of missing persons

- Avalanche
- Immersion and drowning
- Despondency
- Overdue, but unharmed
- Criminal activity including abduction
- Medical problems
- Evasion
- Stranded
- Trauma
- Lost

Becoming lost and disoriented is not unusual; even highly experienced ori-
enteers and backwoods travellers will admit to becoming lost on occasions.
A lost person may adopt one of a number of strategies to re-locate:

- *Random travelling.* Confused and frightened, the lost person moves
  around randomly taking the apparently easiest route. An ineffective
  strategy, most people other than youngsters try to adopt a more
  purposeful method.
- *Route travelling.* The lost person follows a linear feature such as path,
  trail or drainage, even though the route and destination are unknown.
  This is not usually an effective method.
- *Direction travelling.* Travellers aim in a particular direction and persist on
  this route. Direction travelling may be worthwhile if a major target such
  as a road or river is well-used, but following a compass bearing may lead
  to cliff top or impassable terrain.
  - *Backtracking.* The traveller attempts to follow their exact route back
    to its origin. This can be very effective, especially for those with good
    terrain memory, but requires skill, patience,, and an acceptance of
    delay. Surprisingly few people follow this strategy.
- *Route sampling.* The lost person starts at a path junction and samples
  each track in the hope of finding a more familiar or obvious feature,
  returning to the junction and trying again if a path fades away or proves
  unfamiliar. Technique may be used in conjunction with backtracking.
- *Direction sampling.* Similar to route sampling, but in featureless terrain.
  Beginning at a unique feature such as a hill or obvious tree the traveller
  heads out on compass bearings until all main directions have been
  tested. If original base point proves valueless, the person moves to a
  second base and repeats the process.
- *View enhancing.* Heading uphill permits a better view of the surrounding
  terrain and may enable acquisition of a mobile phone signal. It is a
  popular way to attempt to re-locate, especially amongst those able to
  read a map, but is an unpredictable strategy. Weather conditions may be
  worse and it can take you away from water.
- *Heading downhill.* Following a valley or watercourse downhill works
  well in some terrain, especially in areas of high population density
  as habitation clusters around water. However, in remote areas it is a
  hazardous strategy as streams may go over falls or enter gorges before
  possibly terminating in a trackless bog, muskeg, or dry wadi.

- *Staying put.* Survival teaching emphasizes the benefits of staying put especially in thick terrain or if a vehicle has broken down in a remote area; it is often an effective strategy provided that the climate is benign. But few active people have the patience to simply stay put and wait to be rescued, and most move around for at least the first 24 h after becoming lost. Many SAR call-outs in urban areas of Scandinavia and North America involve people suffering from depression or dementia who move less than more active individuals.

Understanding how people may respond to being lost helps limit the area that needs to be searched. Offering a sensible strategy in advance aids decision-making. Generally this will involve 'staying put', but might, for instance state 'head due south until you reach the road, then walk east'.

Making contact
Mobile phones are a great help if within range of masts. Police or SAR services may be able to obtain an approximate fix on a casualty by triangulating their signal or interrogating their position. Some helicopters have the ability to locate and fly down to a mobile phone signal. Elsewhere – especially in thick terrain such as the New Zealand bush—lost individuals have phoned for help and then directed a helicopter to directly above their location—saving rescue groups from much effort struggling through thick vegetation. When possible maximize battery life by turning off unused apps, wi-fi and bluetooth. Extra batteries may be very helpful.

Satellite rescue beacons (➲ Emergency beacons, p. 163) aid location in remote areas and are most likely to be carried on vessels, or by experienced backwoods travellers in remote areas.

Avalanche transceivers (➲ Avalanche transceivers, p. 644) should be worn during winter travel in backcountry mountain areas.

The rescue
Even if uninjured, a person lost for some time is likely to be frightened, cold, hungry, and thirsty; they need appropriate support. Occasionally, individuals on adventure treks appear totally naïve to hazards and must to be watched to ensure they do not get into further difficulties.

Scene management

Management of a serious wilderness incident may be complex. Excellent leadership, teamwork, communications, and forward thinking are necessary. If resources allow, the expedition leader should stand back from the actual rescue and coordinate the overall situation, dynamically assessing and managing potential hazards.

Patients who have been injured are often in hazardous environments. The safety of the rescuers should have paramount importance. Stop and assess the risks of the situation. A minute spent on this task is vital for the safety and efficiency of the rescue operation, and the delay rarely leads to an adverse outcome for the patient.

In *steep ground* place a belay (anchor) above the incident to secure both patient and rescuers. Consider the potential for rock fall or avalanche.

At *road traffic collision* (RTC) sites deploy two members of the team to stop the traffic in both directions. To protect rescuers from further collisions, park vehicles back from the site at an angled 'fend-off' position. Once the crash vehicle can be approached (danger of fire, explosion, rollover, etc.) the vehicle ignition should be turned off and the handbrake applied. Vehicle stabilization procedures should be improvised as soon as possible.

If there is a continuing significant risk to rescuers or patient it may be necessary to extricate the patient rapidly from the hazardous zone before a primary survey has been completed and, in some cases, before spinal immobilization has been optimized (➔ Neck and other spinal injuries, p. 198).

Equipment should be organized in a kit dump a few metres from the accident scene. This ensures the equipment is readily located when needed but does not create a trip hazard to those managing the casualty.

Whenever possible, external help should be sought. While the casualty is being assessed and treated, ideally by medics, the leader should plan the different stages of the evacuation; effective logistics facilitate rapid and effective evacuation.

Meanwhile the rest of the group will also need to be supported and cared for (particularly true with commercial and youth expeditions). Whilst ensuring their safety, try to involve those nearby as much as possible in the rescue. Keep everyone informed about what is happening, even if they were not directly involved.

Structured communications

Effective succinct communications reduce misunderstandings. The nature and position of an incident must be accurately reported (see ➔ Telemedicine in the field, p. 161.

ETHANE report
- Exact location.
- Hazards.
- Access.
- Number of casualties.
- Emergency services on scene and required.

ISOBAR
- I Identify yourself and patient.
- S Situation.
- O Observations.
- B Background.
- A Agreed plan.
- R Read back (so I know you have understood me).

Evacuation

Medical evacuation (medevac) is defined as the movement of a sick or injured expedition member to appropriate local medical facilities. Transfer may be by land, water, or air. Repatriation is the return of an expedition member home following initial treatment. About 10% of expeditions will have to evacuate someone who requires medical assistance, while 3% will need to repatriate a team member.

Advance planning reduces the stress of a difficult situation and should allow an evacuation to proceed as smoothly and safely as possible, with minimum risk to the sick or injured person and their companions. The aim is to get the casualty to the right care at an appropriate speed; too much haste may increase hazard without benefit to the victim.

Many expeditions visit areas with sophisticated SAR facilities. If visiting such areas, determine the capabilities of the local rescue services, their requirements, and costs. Night-time evacuations can be particularly difficult, so alternative ERPs for day and night are recommended.

Considerations in planning a specific evacuation

- Is the patient's condition time-critical?
- Can the patient receive further treatment in their current location?
- Can care be provided in a local clinic or hospital, or should they be transferred to a major hospital?
- Might they be able to rejoin the expedition after treatment?
- What is the capacity, availability, and suitability of procurable local transport?
- Could the patient survive a road/water journey or is air transport a better option?
- Is the patient safe to travel by air at the altitudes involved?
- Is medical supervision available for the journey?
- Can the evacuation be completed in daylight, and if not what are the relative risks of delaying evacuation until next morning, or travelling at night?

The answers to these questions vary depending on the location of the incident, the nature of the injuries and the treatment required. A serious head injury, for example, will require a different response from a fractured wrist.

Moving an injured person

Incidents often occur at locations remote from good transport links; initially the patient must be transferred to a location from which evacuation is possible. Anyone in danger should be moved at once by whatever means possible. Patients not in immediate danger should first be stabilized and positioned to prevent aggravating their injuries during transport. Once a safe location is reached, fully assess their condition to determine the urgency of evacuation.

Urgent movement

If an injured person must be moved immediately from a life-threatening situation (damaged building, fire, avalanche or rock fall), the greatest danger is the possibility of aggravating a spinal injury or compromising the airway. Try to pull the patient in the direction of the long axis of the body to provide as much protection to the spine as possible.

If on the ground, pull the patient's clothing in the neck or shoulder area. If available, log-roll the patient onto a sleeping bag, blanket, or air mattress (Fig. 5.3) and drag material head first with the patient's head and shoulders off the ground to prevent further injury. If nothing is available to support the patient, place your hands under the armpits (from the back) and grasp the forearms to drag the patient (Fig. 5.4).

If not on the ground, move the patient by any means possible, but do not pull a patient's head away from the neck or the rest of the body.

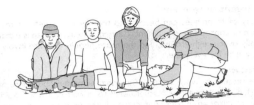

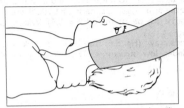

Always support the neck (never release)

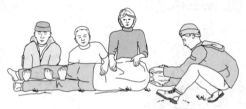

Everyone works together, with the person
at the head directing movement

Fig. 5.3 The log-roll method of turning a casualty with a suspected spinal injury.

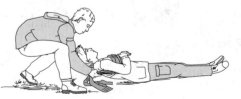

Fig. 5.4 Reverse drag.

Non-urgent movement

A variety of techniques can be used to transfer the patient to the nearest piece of appropriate equipment. Carrying a heavy human is exhausting, especially over rough ground, and the more people who are involved the safer it will be for everyone.

Single rescuer

A single rescuer is always at risk of injuring themselves, but there may be circumstances where a lone rescuer needs to move a casualty. Traditionally the way to carry an unconscious person is the fireman's carry, but there is a high risk of back injury to the rescuer and it should be avoided if the injuries involve the arms, legs, ribs, neck, or back. If the patient is able to assist, a sling carry may be attempted (Fig. 5.5). Walking poles may assist with balance.

The tied hands crawl (Fig. 5.6) may be used to drag someone who is unconscious under low structures. The injured person's head is not supported.

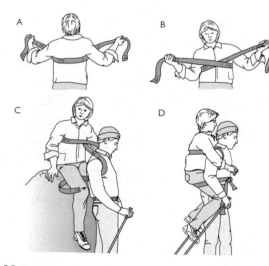

A B C D

Fig. 5.5 Single-person sling carry.

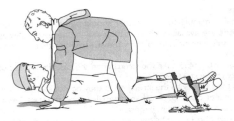

Fig. 5.6 Tied hands crawl.

The chair carry is good for going up or down stairs or down narrow passages. This should not be attempted in a patient with neck, back, or pelvic problems. Variations of this lift can be used without a chair with two rescuers.

Rope sling (Fig. 5.7) using two rescuers relieves some strain over longer distances, but increases the risk of falling in rough ground.

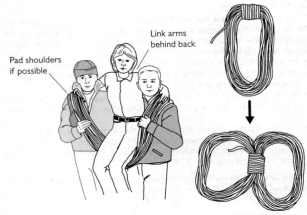

Link arms behind back

Pad shoulders if possible

Split coil of climbing rope

Fig. 5.7 Two-person sling carry.

Stretchers

If available, a manufactured stretcher should be used to transport a casualty. If none are available, improvisation may be necessary. Always ensure there are sufficient people to carry the stretcher so that you do not drop the casualty.

- Whenever possible, take the stretcher to the casualty instead of the casualty to the stretcher.
- Fasten the casualty to the stretcher so they do not slip, slide, or fall off.
- Use blankets, clothing, or other materials to pad the stretcher and protect the casualty from exposure.
- Try to splint broken limbs before movement and provide appropriate pain relief (➜ Treating pain (analgesia), p. 93) to minimize distress and reduce shock.
- Lay the casualty on their back for transport unless this may cause further injury.
- Ensure that the airway will remain open and unblocked.
- Move the casualty feet first so that the rear bearer may watch the patient for signs of difficulty or distress.
- Always brief the personnel carrying the casualty and the casualty themselves, if applicable, about the procedure to be employed. Ensure one person is designated as team leader.

Improvising a stretcher

If a custom-made stretcher is not available, a stretcher may be improvised by using available materials such as boards. Always attempt to secure the casualty to the makeshift stretcher to prevent the risk of further injury. Other methods for manufacturing a stretcher include:

- *Blanket stretcher*: the casualty is placed on their back in the middle of a blanket, tent or similar fabric material. Four people roll the side edges towards the casualty and lift.
- *Blanket and poles stretcher*: a blanket may be wrapped around two poles (approximately 7 ft in length) to make a stretcher that two persons can carry.
- *Jackets and poles stretcher*: button or zip two or three jackets together and turn them inside out with the sleeves on the inside. Pass the poles through the sleeves after making holes in the shoulder areas to allow the poles to pass through (Fig. 5.8).

Most improvised stretchers give inadequate support to permit the evacuation of a casualty with fractures or extensive wounds.

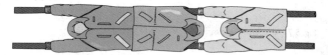

Fig. 5.8 Improvised jacket and poles stretcher.

Priority for evacuation of a casualty

A system commonly used to communicate the priority required for evacuation of the patient is outlined in Table 5.2.

Table 5.2   Priority classification

Priority 1A	Immediate evacuation of the casualty required, if possible from the accident site
Priority 1B	Immediate evacuation required but the casualty can be moved from the accident site
Priority 2	Evacuation required within 12 h
Priority 3	Evacuation required within 12–24 h
Priority 4	Evacuation required but is not time-sensitive

Evacuation transport and considerations

Evacuation may be by:
- Air—fixed wing or helicopter.
- Land—usually motor vehicle, but mules or porters can be better over rough ground.
- Water—boat or raft.

Evacuation of a casualty by air

Advantages of air evacuation
- Casualty can be transported relatively long distances quickly.
- Sophisticated medical care can be accessed quickly.
- Air transport allows difficult terrain to be traversed safely.
- Rotary wing aircraft can reach areas inaccessible to ground or water transport, especially if they have winch facilities.

Disadvantages of air evacuation
- Aircraft are very expensive to run.
- They cannot fly in adverse weather conditions.
- Fixed wing aircraft require a landing strip, while helicopters usually require a suitable landing zone (LZ), unless they are equipped with winching facilities.
- Noise and vibration may make monitoring of and communication with the casualty impossible. Ear defenders for the patient and any person accompanying them are preferable. Diagnosis is difficult.
- Air sickness can be a significant problem.
- Helicopters work inefficiently at high altitude and trade payload for altitude. Do not rely on helicopter rescue from high altitudes; it will only be possible in ideal weather using the best available aircraft.
- Altitude: as altitude increases and pressure decreases, air will expand. If air is trapped in a confined space, severe problems may result. At 18,000 ft (5500 m) the atmospheric pressure is half that of sea level, but the drop is not linear, with the decrease in pressure greater closer to sea level.

Creating a temporary helicopter landing zone
- A LZ may have to be improvised if casualty evacuation by rotary wing (helicopter) aircraft is planned.
- Try to keep the LZ at least 150 m downwind of base areas or the casualty to prevent blowing dust and debris affecting the patient or operations. The LZ should be level and free of obstacles such as cables, wires, rocks, or ruts. Obstacles that cannot be moved should be clearly marked with items that cannot be affected by prop wash or gusting winds. Mark the wind direction to assist the pilot in landing into wind.
- Light signals should be planned. For example, the head lights of two downwind vehicles converging on the LZ, or four people with flashlights marking each corner of the LZ. The lights must be bright enough to be visible during the day, but not so bright they blind the pilot.
- A designated person should guide the aircraft in with land-to-air communication and direct the pilot by standing with their back to the wind and arms outstretched to indicate the LZ.
- Never approach a helicopter unless signalled to do so by the crewman. If a crewman is not on board, only approach in the pilot's field of frontal vision so they may indicate when and how to approach the aircraft.

Potential problems include:
- Development of tension pneumothorax.
- Distension of gas in stomach or bowel.
- Intracranial air expansion if pneumoencephaly.
- Over-pressure of air in endotracheal tube cuffs.
- Ambient temperature falls by about 2°C per 1000 ft increase in altitude.
- Hypobaric hypoxia: the reduction in partial pressure of oxygen in inspired air produced by ascent to altitude is a serious potential risk during flight at high altitude, particularly if the patient's oxygenation is critical. (See ⊕ Humans at altitude, p. 650.)

Helicopter evacuation from offshore craft
See ⊕ Helicopter evacuation, p. 722.

Evacuation of the casualty by land
Advantages of evacuation over land
Vehicles, either propelled mechanically or by animals, are usually more available than aircraft, and in locations with road access permit immediate evacuation to medical facilities. Vehicles can travel in conditions that impede boats and aircraft.

Disadvantages of evacuation over land
Speed and range may be limited. Rough terrain and winding roads may prevent immediate access to the casualty and make evacuation a slow, painful or nauseating journey for the casualty.

Evacuation of the casualty by water

Advantages of evacuation by water

In tropical forests and marine archipelagos, water is the main communication route. Evacuation by boat or seaplane becomes possible. Boat transport can be quite quick and smooth, with good access to the patient during transfer. Care must be taken to ensure that a restless or confused patient does not upset the boat or plunge overboard.

Disadvantages of evacuation by water

Boats must be big enough and stable enough to be capable of transporting a patient. Weather, geographical, and biological hazards must be considered before the evacuation begins.

Documentation for a medevac

It is desirable that a companion travels with a casualty to ensure that they are properly supervised and to enable their condition to be communicated back to the expedition and to relatives at home. However, there are circumstances such as helicopter transfers where this will not be possible and it is essential that appropriate paperwork travels with the casualty. This should include:

- Passport and travel documents.
- Expedition and next of kin contact details.
- Insurance documents.
- Copy of any medical documents (e.g. pre-expedition medical questionnaire, and any assessment notes). (See ➲ Documentation, p. 89.)
- Incident report.
- Medical assessment and records of external advice received.
- Record of procedures.
- Medication chart and history of allergy.
- Investigations (e.g. malaria rapid diagnostic test).
- Observations and fluid balance chart and pain charts.
- Written instructions to accompanying personnel (if relevant).

Other evacuation considerations

- Ensure you know the whole evacuation plan, from the patient leaving your location to arriving at a facility that can offer adequate care. Ensure any escort is aware of the planned destination. If possible, try to confirm the arrival of the casualty at a medical facility.
- If accompanying the patient, try not to do so alone. It can be a long and very tiring process. Try not to leave the casualty alone if medical facilities are basic. Carry enough money or credit cards with you to cover accommodation and travel; you can always be reimbursed later and, if possible, take communications such as a radio or mobile phone.
- Take a translator with you if available and required.
- Take a medical kit.
- Take a snatch bag with food, water, spare clothes, and wash kit. This may make the journey more comfortable.

Nursing and emotional care awaiting evacuation

Patients requiring evacuation need nursing care which might include:
- Clinical observations and patient monitoring.
- Assistance with personal hygiene.
- Assistance with nutrition/fluids.
- Pressure area care for unconscious/spinal injured patients.
- Dressing changes.
- Administration of medicines or IV fluids.
- Psychological and emotional support.

When nursing patients, try to provide care in a structured routine or way, as this is both reassuring for the patient and helpful clinically.

Clinical observations should be taken and documented as dictated by the severity of the illness/injury.
- Adhering to regular daily patterns, such as washing and mealtimes normalizes the daily routine.
- Time the administration of medicines to maximize their clinical effectiveness, e.g. providing analgesia and antiemetics prior to sleep, or avoiding acetazolamide (Diamox®) before bedtime, as it is a diuretic.
- Administration of fluids is generally easier when patients are awake.

Medical evacuation from an expedition has the potential to be a psychologically stressful event, for both patient and clinician. Stress can be caused by:
- Medevac method.
- Delays.
- Duration.
- Sick or unstable patients.
- Discomfort during medevac (e.g. overland transfers for patients with fractures).

Patients being evacuated from an expedition may feel dismayed over the prospect of permanently leaving the project site. Contributing to an expedition may have considerable financial implications and this financial loss may compound feelings of distress or frustration. In some instances patients will dispute the need to be evacuated, or even refuse to leave (e.g. patients with psychosis or more determined personalities). Do not let these issues cloud clinical judgement or distract from the need for evacuation. Inexperienced medics or those providing care in 'high-pressure' situations should be especially aware of the potential for this issue.

Patients should be made as comfortable as possible during the evacuation. Keeping patients well informed will generally reduce stress levels, as will honesty over events, conditions, and treatment. Where appropriate, facilitating communication with home may help lessen fear and anxiety whilst at the same time provide reassurance through contact with loved-ones. However, this should be balanced with minimizing the psychological stress likely to be caused to friends and relatives at home who are unlikely to know the full clinical picture.

During a medical evacuation the overall aim is to maximize a patient's clinical condition and comfort, minimize or eliminate clinical deterioration, and ensure a thorough handover to definitive care.

See also ➔ Field nursing care, p. 88.

Repatriation

Repatriation may use a dedicated air ambulance or a commercial airline. The patient will usually need to be escorted by an experienced aeromedical doctor or nurse. Such transfers are very expensive and it is essential that insurance covers this possibility.

Medical assistance companies

Because they will not start an evacuation or repatriation without guarantee of payment, most expeditions will initially contact a medical assistance company through their insurers. Most of the work of medevac organizations involves tourists and businessmen in destinations with good travel links rather than expeditions in remote regions, so their databases may not contain information on the capabilities of remote clinics/hospitals, or on the logistical solutions to remote evacuations. Medevac organizations should be relied upon as a third level of support after help has been sought from the group's own medical expertise and the medical resources in-country.

Expeditions should do their own research on local medical facilities and the logistics and transport necessary to ensure a patient can get to an internationally recognized airstrip capable of receiving a medical team via Learjet.

> *Medical assistance companies include:*
> - International SOS: ℘ http://www.internationalsos.com
> - Royal Flying Doctor Service of Australia:
>   ℘ http://www.flyingdoctors.org
> - AMREF: ℘ http://www.flydoc.org
> - CEGA: ℘ http://www.cega-air-ambulance.com
> - Healix: ℘ www.healix.com
> - International Assistance Group:
>   ℘ http://www.international-assistance-group.com

Establishing a direct relationship with a medical assistance company is recommended, although this can be difficult as one normally is forced to negotiate through the insurance company. Once in direct contact, it is important to confirm the organization's capabilities and limitations. Check all contact numbers before departing on the trip and consider running a test to ensure the system works.

Telemedicine and communications

Telemedicine and communications

Telemedicine refers to the use of information and communication technology (ICT) to facilitate in the delivery of healthcare between two people at a distance from each other. It can be as simple as a phone call between medical practitioners about a case. Other examples include live videoconferencing between a patient and specialists, or a specialist remotely analysing a MRI scan sent by email from the other side of the world.

Telemedicine is a rapidly evolving area of medicine as access to the Internet increases globally, the cost of ICT reduces, and more types of media can be digitalized. It has well-established uses in remote and developing areas of the world where healthcare is hard to access. Telemedicine can avoid the cost of patient transfers and specialist travel expenses, while in technologically advanced areas of the world patients can now have their blood sugar levels or cardiac rhythms monitored from home by specialists.

Telemedicine relies on having a reliable means of communication, which can be a problem if there are poor radio links or a very slow Internet connection. There may also be problems maintaining equipment and finding adequately trained staff. Patient confidentiality may be hard to guarantee.

Telemedicine has exciting possibilities and it is conceivable that it will result in many more aspects of healthcare delivery moving away from clinical settings and into patients' homes.

Uses of telemedicine in expedition medicine

Telemedicine has obvious advantages for expeditions. Its use may avoid the cost of an evacuation and the disruption that arises from potentially losing key members of the expedition. It can reassuringly support relatively inexperienced doctors acting as expedition medics by giving them access to senior and specialist advice. The reality for most expeditions is that the budget and location will mean that the options for telemedicine will involve a relatively low-tech approach. Examples of its use in the field include:

- A non-medic on the expedition radioing from a satellite camp back to base camp to get advice from the expedition doctor.
- The expedition doctor emailing a specialist back home with a photo attachment for help with diagnosis.

Telemedicine: preparations before departure

A contact point for obtaining senior or specialist advice should be organized before departure. It may be a personal contact, ready made in the form of a senior medic that works for the expedition company, or from a commercial company that provides a telemedicine service. It is important that the person giving advice understands the nature of the expedition and what facilities are available to you on the expedition. It is unhelpful being advised to get a computed tomography scan as the investigation of choice by a specialist when you are a week away from the nearest hospital.

It may be worth setting up an agreement with a company that provides telemedicine support, bearing in mind the cost paid to the company may be considerably less than the cost to the expedition of having to undertake a medevac. World Clinic[2] and Talk to a Doctor[3] are both online telemedicine companies.

2 🔗 http://www.worldclinic.com

3 🔗 http://www.talktoadoctor.co.uk

Before departure, ensure that the communication equipment that you are taking is working, and that you know how to use it. Consider battery life and whether it is robust enough for the environment and expedition. Ensure that you understand and can use any medical equipment supplied to you for the expedition in case you are advised to use it. It is worth training up at least one other member of the expedition to use the kit in case of your absence, or if you become the patient. Leave a definitive list of your equipment and medicines with your home base or telemedicine contacts so they can advise you knowing your actual resources, e.g. list of the antibiotics you have.

Telemedicine: in the field
Once you have arrived in country, test the systems that you have put in place—checking both that the communication equipment works and that your telemedicine contact is contactable.

Ensure that non-medics who might have to contact you for advice have a guide to assist in their questioning and examination of patients (see Chapter 6) and that, to avoid unnecessary delay during the radio session, they know what sort of information you will seek from them.

Arranging a set report format makes communications as efficient as possible. This may be useful for getting information to telemedicine contacts as well as receiving information from non-medics on expedition. Keep good records of telemedicine consultations; consider recording the call if able to do so. Remember the issue of confidentiality and think about what methods of communication are secure and which are not. Note what advice was given and by whom. These are as important as any other clinical record. The use of 'prowords' (professional words to help an operator to understand a message) can be useful.

Examples of prowords
- *Medevac*—urgent assistance required for medical evacuation.
- *Alpha*—location including grid reference or latitude and longitude.
- *Bravo*—nature of injury.
- *Charlie*—name of injured person.
- *Delta*—treatment given.
- *Echo*—details and time of incident.
- *Foxtrot*—assistance required and when will they next communicate.
- *Golf*—date and time of report.
- *Hotel*—are the next of kin to be informed?

Contact with seniors back home may be on an as-required basis only, or it may be that a regular time is set to report back. Ensure both parties know what frequency of communication to expect and what to do in the event of a scheduled communication being missed.

Technologies for telemedicine

Radio

Likely to only be of use within the expedition itself but a useful way for the expedition medic to communicate with other parties in the expedition. Readability is not always reliable so it is important to have a pre-formatted report procedure to avoid loss of information. Radio use requires training and is not a secure method of communication, with other members of the expedition and outside parties potentially able to listen in.

Telephone

Could be landline, mobile, or satellite (SATCOM). Has the advantage of familiarity of use and with increasing global coverage likely to be the first port of call for many telemedicine consultations especially for when emergency advice is needed. As with talking to specialists on the phone at work back home, remember to orientate the caller to who you are, why you are calling, and keep information succinct.

Email and Internet

May be an option out in the field and likely to be available from fixed base camps. Good option for when routine advice is required that can wait a day or two before a reply. Not all email accounts are secure so consider anonymizing information about individuals.

Attaching photos to emails is an excellent way to get information across for another opinion:

• Consider compressing photo files to reduce the time it takes for the recipient on the other end to download the attachment. However, ensure enough detail is left for them to study the photo properly.
• If photographing an injury or rash, for example, consider using a hand, ruler, or familiar object to portray scale to the reviewer.
• Plain X-rays can be photographed easily with a camera to create a digital form that can be emailed on for further opinion.
• In dental cases, the use of mirrors is invaluable in allowing the most hidden of tooth surfaces to be photographed.

If the Internet bandwidth is wide enough, video files can be shared. This can be a useful way for someone to demonstrate how to perform a procedure to an expedition medic. Remember that there are many clinical demonstrations on video sharing websites.

Satellite phones

Satellite phones work in remote locations beyond the coverage of normal telephony and cellular networks. Satellite phones complement the use of international roaming on GSM cellular phones or the use of locally bought SIM cards to access in-country cellular networks.

Satellite phones work with one of three basic systems. A stationary phone can be aligned with a specific satellite (Inmarsat, BGAN); a mobile satellite phone can communicate with a specific satellite overhead (e.g. ACeS, GlobalStar, and Thuraya); or a satellite phone can transmit and receive to an array of orbiting satellites to give global coverage (e.g. Iridium).

Considerations before rental or purchase of satellite phones include:

- Location: compare the coverage maps to see which system will work where you are going.
- Applications: decide what you need, from two-way voice communication to email and video conferencing, and then see which are supported.
- Accounts structure: decide on pre-pay or on account options, and check how easy it is to top up a prepaid SIM card whilst you are away.
- Running cost: compare the airtime costs per minute.
- Power supply: plan a recharging system suitable for your planned area of usage, such as solar panels or lithium batteries in areas where mains electricity is not available.

Plan to protect your equipment from water, dust, and shock hazards with padded or waterproof cases. Pelican Products® cases and micro-cases are excellent.

If your project is dependent on satellite phone communications take more than one, and spare ancillaries.

Improve the functionality of email over slow satellite phone connections by using a specialist satellite email service such as UUPlus or other compression service. Check before departure whether the expedition is equipped to use a satellite phone as a modem to send emails or pictures so you know in advance the telemedicine capabilities.

Satellite phones are subject to restriction or additional controls in some countries, check before leaving home.

Emergency beacons

Beacons for expedition use divide into two categories: emergency beacons that alert government-run Rescue Control Centres in the COSPAS-SARSAT system, and tracking beacons that report position and messages to the owner's choice of recipients such as home base and website. The COSPAS-SARSAT SAR satellite system is for emergency use only, whereas tracking beacons can be used for non-emergency reporting and to provide location updates to maps on websites. Both types have roles as useful items of expedition equipment.

The joint American–Russian SAR satellite system called COSPAS-SARSAT provides an international SAR network with global coverage for transmission-only emergency beacons. They use the 406 MHz frequency and the frequency is a useful way of identifying the type of beacon. The technology has a different name depending on where it is used:

- Aircraft carry emergency locator transmitters (ELTs).
- Ships carry emergency position indicating radio beacons (EPIRBs).
- People on the ground carry personal locator beacons (PLBs).

When a beacon goes off its signal is transmitted to a network of Mission Control Centres and then on to a Rescue Control Centre near the beacon's location. In some cases no action will be taken so it is critical to ascertain what action will be taken and by whom in advance.

Along with location information, 406 MHz beacons transmit *information on* the type of beacon, the country code, and identification of the beacon.

Using this information, SAR bodies can access contact details and information on the aircraft/ship from a beacon database.

An earlier generation of 121.5 MHz beacons is being phased out of satellite reception. Most current beacons transmit on 406 MHz and model options include GPS.

406 MHz emergency beacons need to be registered before use. In the UK this is to the EPIRB Registry of the Maritime and Coastguard Agency. For countries that do not have a registration system, beacons can be registered at the International Beacon Registration Database (IBRD).[4]

PLBs should only be used for life-threatening emergencies, as no qualifying information can be added. They are a useful item of last resort as a back-up to satellite phones.

Tracking beacons, where the recipients of messages and data are selected by the user, can be used for non-emergency use such as position tracking, message sending, as well as emergency alerts.

VHF and HF radios

Two-way voice communications by radio are an important part of the communications system on many expeditions. VHF radios are for short-range local use; the range can be extended by using a more powerful base station at one site with handheld radios being used to call back to base, or to shore. VHF radios require little training, and some are licence-free in many countries. HF radios can be used over very large distances but require more training to operate and licensing.

If the expedition involves mobile sub-groups working in the same area then VHF radios will be very useful. In some situations, such as mountaineering on a peak with more than one team present at the same time, it is good practice to have a shared radio frequency so different teams can alert everyone on the mountain about a problem and a response can be coordinated.

Radio communications are not private, anyone in range on the same frequency can listen, so for medical communications or for passing confidential information it is useful to be able to switch to satellite phones which in normal use are more secure.

Sexual assault

A sexual assault is defined as any type of sexual act committed without the informed consent of one of the parties. Incidents of this type are highly distressing to all involved. Both men and women can be subject of an assault, which may come from within the expedition group or occur during travel.

Expeditions—especially those involving groups of teenagers or young adults—should consider how they would respond if a member of the group claims to have been sexually assaulted. The response of local authorities in different jurisdictions can vary considerably and may not always be sympathetic to the complainant.

Management
Consider the 4 Ps (Table 5.3).

Table 5.3 The 4 Ps—management of sexual assault

Four Ps	Consider
Police	If patient wants police involvement this *must* be done first (any examination may compromise forensic examination). Report to local police—see ℘ http://fflm.ac.uk/library for timescales for forensic testing, maximum 7 days
Pregnancy	Emergency contraception: Levonorgestrel 1500mcg (Levonelle®) as soon as possible (up to 72 h). Ulipristal acetate (EllaOne®) as soon as possible (up to 120 h). Emergency IUCD fitted up to 5 days (or day 19 of 28-day cycle).
Prophylaxis	Post-exposure prophylaxis following sexual exposure (PEPSE) for HIV (see Table 15.5 and ➔ Post-exposure prophylaxis, p. 513). Start within 72 h. Consider prophylactic antibiotics to cover chlamydia, gonorrhoea, and *Trichomonas*. Doxycycline 100 mg twice daily for 1 week *or* azithromycin 1 g PO stat. Ceftriaxone 500mg IM stat (or other 3rd-generation cephalosporin) *or* cefixime 400 mg stat *or* ciprofloxacin 500 mg stat but beware of high resistance worldwide. Metronidazole 400 mg twice daily for 5 days *or* metronidazole 2 g stat. If not vaccinated against hepatitis B, first dose can be given within 3 weeks to cover retrospectively. Rapid course of vaccine preferred (0, 7, 21 days, and 6 months).
Psychological	Strongly consider repatriation owing to likely physical and emotional trauma. Ongoing counselling may be required (➔ Psychological reactions to traumatic events, p. 526; ➔ Post-traumatic stress disorder, p. 530).

Death on an expedition

Although death during an expedition is rare, expeditions need to have a plan for this eventuality included in their ERP (➋ Emergency response plan, p. 136). If an expedition member should die, then it is important that the death is dealt with sensitively, expeditiously, and in accordance with the legislative requirements of both the deceased's home country and the country where the incident occurs. Local police and judiciary should be informed as quickly as possible—in some countries the location of an unexpected death will be considered to be a potential crime scene until the circumstances have been confirmed. Your local embassy or consulate may be able to offer support, advice, legal assistance, and communication links. The psychological sequelae following the death must be considered, with all the surviving team members involved in measures to prevent their long-term distress.

Following the death, a designated person within the group, in all likelihood the expedition MO, should coordinate the necessary actions:

- *Ensure there are no further injuries.* Make sure that the team are at no increased risk as a result of the death. If the death has occurred in a difficult physical location, then retrieval of the body may be necessary, but there should not be any undue risk to the rest of the team in attempting recovery of the body.
- *Find out what happened.* Record the details as they are given and then check with all available sources to establish any other details that are known or gradually learned, and compile these together into an accurate 'diary of events'.
- *Locate the body.* Take responsibility for locating the body and, if retrieval is possible, collect it and deliver it to the appropriate authorities to obtain a death certificate. This may involve packaging and transporting the body some considerable distance, a process that should be done quickly and with dignity. Other expedition members will be noting the response of the medical team to the event.
- *Prevent possible infection.* If the person died of an infectious (or potentially infectious) disease, or if the cause of death is unknown, handle the body in a manner that minimizes the risk of infection spreading to other members of the expedition.

Practical considerations following the death

Once death has been confirmed

A signal or message needs to be sent to the expedition's headquarters informing them of the tragedy. Importantly for the families of other surviving members of the expedition, the information needs to note that other team members are safe and well.

Other expedition members need to be informed of the death (see Box 16.1).

The next of kin must be notified at the earliest opportunity. This should be done in person by two people representing the expedition; two people because the person advising of the death will need support and both together have a greater chance of giving support to the deceased's relatives. In many cases, police in their home country will inform the next of kin.

The family of the deceased should be offered immediate access to practical and social support; whether this be psychological to deal with the event, practical help with the funeral or, where possible, financial assistance.

Legal responsibilities
- Urgently inform the embassy or consulate representative of the deceased person of the circumstances surrounding the death.
- Inform the embassy or consulate representative of other expedition members' situation and safety.
- Inform the police, particularly if there are legal issues about the death.
- Obtain a police report, if necessary.
- Organize an autopsy, if required.
- Contact insurance companies.
- Issue an appropriate report on the tragedy, for insurance purposes. This will need to be done in conjunction with the expedition leader.
- Develop contacts between the insurance company and the local authorities who can organize repatriation.

Repatriation of the body
- Often the local embassy or consulate will assist with this process.
- It will include negotiations with local authorities, insurance, and transport companies.
- Keep an accurate diary of all events, the persons who were communicated with, and the times of these communications.

Dealing with the media
Prepare a statement or press release that can be used to respond to any media enquiries and prevent any incorrect reportage.

Caring for the group
(See also ➲ Reactions to traumatic events or bad news, p. 528.)
- Consider needs of surviving team members and their families.
- Consider needs of concerned outsiders.
- Ensure regular opportunities for communication between team members and their families whilst on the expedition, but try to discourage use of social media. It is better for families to receive information in a controlled and supportive manner than through poorly regulated social media.

After the expedition, ensure members are followed up to ensure that there are no adverse psychological responses. Screen for symptoms of depression, excessive arousal, avoidance behaviours, intrusive phenomena, and dissociation. The emphasis here is on recognizing 'at-risk' individuals. If involved in the care of the deceased, the medic may have particular feelings of responsibility, guilt, or failure that need to be recognized.

Chapter 6

Emergencies: diagnosis

Section editor
Jon Dallimore

Contributors
Edi Albert
Jon Dallimore
Charlie Siderfin (1st edition)

History and examination: an introduction
for non-clinicians 170
Clinical measurements 174
Illness assessment form 176

NB This guide to the medical history-taking, examination, and measurement of vital signs is designed to assist someone without medical training to obtain the necessary information to communicate effectively with a doctor over the radio or telephone.

For information on the initial management of an injured person see Chapter 7.

For the initial management of serious medical conditions see Chapter 8.

History and examination: an introduction for non-clinicians

There are three important aspects to the assessment of the ill patient.

- History—an account of how the illness developed.
- Examination—three modalities are used to examine:
  - Look.
  - Feel.
  - Listen.
- Monitoring—'vital signs' are measured to assess an individual's status and progress.

History

- Patient details.
- Clearly identify the patient and time of examination.
- Write down the main problems.
- Use the patient's own words. Avoid technical medical terms—there is a danger of them being used incorrectly.
- Short history of the illness – a description of how the illness evolved over time. Start from when the patient was last completely well and relate each symptom to time. For instance:
  - Last completely well yesterday.
  - Started to vomit 3 h ago. Vomited five times—initially food.
  - Last vomit 15 min ago—yellow fluid.
  - Abdominal pain for 2 h.

Apparently unrelated symptoms can be important in reaching a diagnosis. A list of important questions can be found in the illness assessment form, ➲ Illness assessment form, p. 176.

Examination

Answer these questions from your own observations, not by asking the patient. Prior to the expedition, obtain training in the techniques of examination. Practise examining normal individuals so you can recognize abnormality. Try not to feel shy or embarrassed—you will do a sick person no favours if you fail to spot an important sign when examining. Examine the whole person carefully in the following order:

- General appearance.
- Hands.
- Face.
- Neck.
- Chest.
- Abdomen.
- Limbs.
- Nervous system.
- Look:
  - General well-being. A subjective assessment as to whether the patient is generally well or unwell. Expose the patient and observe. Compare the left and right side of the body for any asymmetry.

- Feel:
  - Warm your hands, be gentle but firm. Whilst feeling, watch the patient's face for signs of pain.
- Listen:
  - Use a stethoscope or put your ear on the body to listen for breath and bowel sounds.
- Measure:
  - You may be able to make simple measurements to indicate the patient's condition. These include measuring temperature and respiratory rate, taking the pulse and blood pressure, and observing capillary refill time (see ➋ Capillary refill time, p. 175). A small pulse oximeter may be useful on high altitude expeditions.

General appearance

- Look:
  - At patient's expression: in pain, anxious, frightened, or confused.
  - At body posture.
  - Colour of skin.
  - Whether they are sweating.
  - Assess breathing effort.
- Feel:
  - Skin temperature and dampness.

Hands

- Look:
  - Sweating.
  - Temperature.
  - Tremor.
- Measure:
  - Radial (wrist) pulse for rate, rhythm (regular or irregular), and character (bounding or thready).

Face

- Look:
  - For abnormal colour or swelling of face and lips.
  - Inspect mouth and throat for ulcers, blisters, and redness.
  - Look at the tongue: is it dry, coated, or moist?

Neck

- Look:
  - For distended neck veins.
- Feel:
  - For lymph nodes and swellings in neck, cheeks and back of head.
  - For position of the trachea (windpipe).
- Listen:
  - For abnormal sounds associated with breathing.

Chest

Examine front and back of the chest:
- Look:
  - Breathing rate.
  - Compare chest movement on both sides.
  - Check for injuries to the chest wall.

- Feel:
  - Irregularities or crepitus (grating) of chest wall indicating broken ribs.
  - Chest wall tenderness (be gentle!).
  - For lymph nodes in axilla (armpit).
- Listen:
  - Place stethoscope under the collar bone and then outside each nipple. Compare the sounds on each side.
  - Listen over the lungs at the back with the stethoscope and compare the sounds.
  - Breath sounds:
    —Normal.
    —Absent.
    —Added sounds—wheeze or crackles?

Abdomen

Make sure that your hands are warm. Ensure the patient is relaxed, lying on his back, head on one or two pillows, and the abdomen exposed:
- Look:
  - Swelling, discoloration, or bruising (especially over flank), scars.
- Feel:
  - Place hand flat on abdomen and gently apply pressure with all four fingers by bending at the knuckles, keeping the fingers flat and straight.
  - Begin away from region of tenderness and move towards the area. Move methodically around the entire abdomen.
  - Feel for tenderness whilst watching the patient's face. Facial expression will signal tenderness.
  - Tensing of the abdominal muscles (guarding) sometimes occurs with tenderness.
  - Ascertain if guarding is localized or generalized. In severe cases, the abdominal wall will be rigid, implying inflammation within the abdominal cavity (peritonitis) owing to bowel perforation or bleeding.
  - Test for rebound tenderness. Gently feel the abdomen and then rapidly remove your hand, without warning. Pain with this procedure implies peritonitis.
  - Be gentle but firm. If the patient is unable to relax his abdominal muscles, ensure your hands are warm and ask him to bend his knees up to relax the abdominal muscles.
  - Feel in groin creases for enlarged lymph nodes.
- Listen:
  - Place the stethoscope 1 cm below the umbilicus (belly button) and listen for bowel sounds for 1 min.
  - Normal—gentle gurgling a few times per minute.
  - Increased—overactive bowel, e.g. diarrhoea or bowel obstruction.
  - Absent—the later stages of peritonitis.

Limbs
- Look:
  - Areas of redness, swelling, or bruising.
  - Deformity.
  - Joint swelling.
  - Pain on movement.
- Feel:
  - Tenderness.
  - Creaking or grating sensations.

Nervous system
- Look:
  - Assess AVPU (awake, verbal, pain, unresponsive) and GCS (Box 7.1).
  - Check both eyes can move in all directions.
  - Assess pupils for size, asymmetry, and reaction to light.
  - Test power and sensation in all limbs. Place your hands in the patient's hands and ask them to squeeze your hands. Assess the strength of grip on each side. Ask the patient to press up and down with their feet and again assess the strength of movements. Check that they can feel you touching their arms and legs.

Clinical measurements

Measuring body temperature
- Normal temperature: 36.5–37.5°C.
- Hypothermia: <35°C.
- Significant fever: >38.5°C.

See also ➲ Hypothermia, p. 622.

Taking the pulse
Press gently with the pulp of the middle and index fingers. Count beats for a timed minute or half a minute and multiply by two. Evaluate whether regular or irregular and note the pulse strength.
- Normal adult pulse at rest = 60–90 beats per min.

Radial (wrist) pulse
Feel with the fingers on the thumb side of the wrist.

Carotid (neck) pulse
Locate the larynx (Adam's apple) with your fingertips. Move your fingers across the neck until reaching the groove between the trachea (windpipe) and muscle edge. *Press gently.* Never feel the pulse on both sides of the neck at the same time as this will reduce the blood supply to the brain.

Femoral (groin) pulse
Press in the skin crease at the top of the leg halfway between the midline and the iliac crest (front of the pelvis).

Blood pressure
There is large variability in BP between different situations and individuals. It is an important measurement for monitoring a patient's progress over time.

Use of the sphygmomanometer
Automated BP measuring devices are reasonably inexpensive and widely available. However, basic versions of such machines will struggle to measure the BP if a patient has low BP or a slow pulse.

For those who have been taught how to use a manual sphygmomanometer the following will act as a reminder:
- Wrap the sphygmomanometer cuff around the upper arm.
- Straighten the arm, palm up and locate the brachial pulse on the inner aspect of the front of the elbow.
- Inflate cuff 20–30 mmHg above the point that the pulse disappears. Hold the stethoscope gently over the pulse. Listen for pulse and release cuff 3–5 mmHg per second:
  - Systolic pressure = level when pulse first heard.
  - Diastolic pressure = level when pulse muffles and disappears.

Estimating blood pressure using peripheral pulses
- Radial pulse palpable: systolic BP >80 mmHg.
- Femoral pulse palpable: systolic BP >70 mmHg.
- Carotid pulse palpable: systolic BP >60 mmHg.

Capillary refill time
Firmly press your thumb on a fingernail, toenail, or bony prominence for 5 s. When the thumb is removed, the area will appear white. If it takes >2 s for the colour to return, reduced circulation is implied. NB This is not reliable when the patient is cold (compare with your own finger).

Measuring respiratory (breathing) rate
Count the breathing rate over 1 min. Feel the pulse at the same time as the respiratory rate may alter if the patient is aware the respiratory rate is being measured.
• Normal adult respiratory rate at rest = 12–18 per min.

Reduced level of consciousness
In the case of head injury the AVPU scale (◑ Disability, p. 202) is a rough initial assessment. To monitor a patient's progress chart the GCS (Box 7.1). Minimum GCS score is 3, with maximum score of 15.

Three areas of basic brain function are tested and scored: eye opening, speech, and movement:
• Use increasing level of stimulus to obtain response.
• Speak.
• Tap the shoulders gently.
• Apply pain—press firmly over the inner aspect of the eyebrow along the eye socket.
• For scoring see Box 7.1.

A fall in the GCS score indicates deterioration in the patient's condition. Causes include:
• Bleeding.
• Brain swelling.
• Infection.

Remember, if the patient deteriorates during your assessment *immediately* re-check the ABC and rectify any life-threatening problems.

Monitoring
• Keep timed, written notes of the patient's condition.
• Chart vital signs hourly or more frequently. If very unwell monitor every 15 min.
• Pulse.
• Temperature.
• BP.
• Respiratory rate.
• GCS—if previous head injury or concerns about level of consciousness.
• A model chart is given in Fig. 8.7.

Illness assessment form

Date/time:

Name and date of birth:

Main complaints:

History of illness (in the patient's own words):

Past medical history (serious accidents/illnesses, operations, high blood pressure, heart disease, diabetes, asthma, epilepsy):

Drugs (including oral contraceptives, inhalers, antimalarials):

Allergies:

Family history (any significant illnesses in the family, causes of premature death, high blood pressure, heart disease, diabetes):

Social history (tobacco, alcohol, recreational drugs, recent foreign travel and immunizations):

Direct questions

Cardiovascular
- Chest pain.
- Shortness of breath.
- Palpitations.
- Ankle swelling.

Respiratory
- Cough.
- Wheeze.
- Sputum.

Gastrointestinal
- Appetite.
- Weight.
- Nausea/vomiting.
- Indigestion.
- Abdominal pain.
- Bowels (blood, diarrhoea, constipation).

Urogenital
- Pain on passing urine.
- Need to pass urine frequently.
- Loin pain.
- Genital discharge.
- Date of last menstrual period . . . .

Nervous system
- Headache.
- Problems with eyes or ears.
- Weakness/numbness.
- Fits/faints.

Examination

General comments (unwell, rashes, sweating, dehydration):
- Temperature . . . .°C
- Pulse . . . ./min
- Breathing rate . . . ./min
- Blood pressure . . . ./. . . . . mmHg.

Chest
- Laboured breathing.
- Symmetry of chest movements.
- Breath sounds (wheezes/crackles, normal, absent).

Abdomen
- Distended.
- Bowel sounds.
- Tenderness.
- Guarding.

Nervous system
- Level of response:
  - Alert.
  - Verbal—normal speech.
  - Pain.
  - Unresponsive.
- Pupils:
  - Equal size.
  - React to light.
- Limbs:
  - Movements:
    —Right arm.
    —Left arm.
    —Right leg.
    —Left leg.
  - Sensation:
    —Right arm.
    —Left arm.
    —Right leg.
    —Left leg.

Possible diagnosis

1.
2.
3.

Management plan

Signed   Date

Chapter 7

Emergencies: trauma

Section editor
Jon Dallimore

Contributors
Edi Albert
Spike Briggs
Jon Dallimore
Sundeep Dhillon (1st edition)
Stephen Hearns (1st edition)
David Lockey (1st edition)
Julian Thompson (1st edition)

Initial response to an incident *180*
Triage *182*
Assessment of a casualty *185*
Airway *186*
Breathing *190*
Circulation *194*
Neck and other spinal injuries *198*
Disability *202*
Exposure and environmental control *203*
Secondary survey *204*
Continuing care *206*
Blast injuries *207*
Lightning *208*

Initial response to an incident

(See also Chapter 5.)

The ABC approach to patient assessment ensures that the most important life-threatening conditions are dealt with in the correct order.

- Ensure safety of scene, self, and casualty.
- Triage casualties if multiple victims.
- Airway (and cervical spine control where appropriate).
- Breathing and ventilation.
- Circulation.
- Disability.
- Environmental control and evacuation following proper preparation of patient for travel.

Triage

A major incident involving several casualties, e.g. an avalanche or RTC, stretches the resources of fully equipped emergency services. In the wilderness it is easy to feel overwhelmed and helpless. However, developing and practising an effective triage and treatment system will enable as many people as possible to be treated and give later reassurance that everything possible was done.

The triage process aims to prioritize patients according to their medical needs given the resources available. This approach ensures that those requiring immediate treatment receive appropriate care, but also that limited resources are not diverted to treating an irrecoverable condition at the expense of other casualties. Triage principles should be applied whenever the number of casualties exceeds the resources of skilled rescuers available. It is a dynamic process where the state of the patient may change and the environment and available equipment will dictate the level of care available.

Priorities

Several systems are used internationally. The four priority groups are defined as follows:

- P1. Immediate priority—casualties who require immediate life-saving interventions.
- P2. Urgent priority—casualties who require surgical or medical intervention within 2–4 h.
- P3. Delayed priority—less serious cases whose condition can safely be delayed beyond 4 h.
- P1 Hold. Expectant priority—casualties whose condition is so severe that they cannot survive despite the best available care and whose treatment would divert medical resources from salvageable patients who may then be compromised.

When multiple casualties occur remember that it is usually the still and silent person that needs the most urgent attention. Someone who is noisy or hysterical may be distressed and in pain, but at least is conscious and has a clear airway.

Triage classifications

Priority	Description	Label colour
P1	Immediate	Red
P2	Urgent	Yellow
P3	Delayed	Green
P1 Hold	Expectant	Blue
Dead	Dead	White or Black

Casualties should, if possible, be regularly re-triaged. Triage categories can change at any time and are not fixed.

Triage sieve
- This is a rapid, simple, safe, and reproducible method of prioritization based upon the Airway, Breathing, Circulation (ABC) approach of resuscitation. (See Fig. 7.1.)

Mobility
- Walking patients are initially categorized as P3, delayed priority.
- If the patient is not walking then apply the ABC approach.

Airway
- Patients who cannot breathe despite simple airway manoeuvres (chin lift or jaw thrust) are dead.
- If breathing starts on opening the airway, the patient is P1, immediate.

Breathing
- Check respiratory rate (RR). If RR >30 or <10 then patient is P1, immediate.

Circulation
- Check capillary refill time (CRT) (see → Capillary refill time, p. 175).
- If >2 s then patient is P1, immediate.
- If CRT <2 s then patient is P2, urgent.
- Cold conditions may prolong CRT and comparison with the rescuer's CRT will allow adjustment.
- In extreme conditions or in the dark, CRT may be impossible to assess and a pulse rate of 120 beats per minute can be used as the circulatory assessment. Heart rates exceeding this at rest in adults give cause for concern.

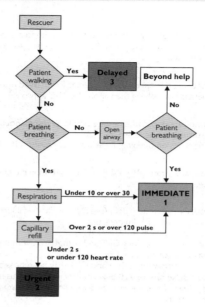

Fig. 7.1 Triage sieve.

Assessment of a casualty

Once the incident scene has been made safe, approach and evaluate the casualty. If you have the skills, follow Advanced Trauma Life Support (ATLS) guidelines. This text offers guidance to those without advanced resuscitation skills, and suggests courses of action appropriate to the wilderness setting.

Assessment of the trauma victim

The assessment and management of the seriously injured patient in remote wilderness environments is extremely challenging. Problems include:

- Lack of equipment.
- Lack of skilled assistance.
- Prolonged transfer times to definitive care.

It should be made clear to everyone in the expedition group that the clinical interventions possible in remote environments are extremely limited compared to those that one would expect in urban environments in a developed country.

The key to managing any pre-hospital trauma is to perform basic assessments and interventions well and then transport the casualty safely and rapidly to a centre capable of providing definitive surgical and critical care. A properly prepared evacuation plan (medevac) will facilitate this process (➔ Evacuation, p. 146).

Airway

Assessment and management of the airway is the first priority in the management of an injured casualty, except in the rare situation of life-threatening haemorrhage from a limb, when bleeding should be controlled first (➲ Control of haemorrhage, p. 196).

The main causes of airway obstruction are:

- Loss of muscle tone owing to reduced conscious level, which can lead to the tongue falling back and blocking the throat.
- Blood and/or vomit in the airway.
- Anatomical distortion or swelling caused by direct facial trauma or burns.
- Trismus (tightly clenched jaw) during seizures.
- Initially ask the patient a question or get them to stick their tongue out. If they can speak or protrude their tongue then the airway is patent and protected; and usually no further intervention is required. If you think there is a problem with breathing:
  - Look.
  - Listen.
  - Examine.

Inspection of the chest and neck may reveal that the patient is working hard to move air through a partially obstructed airway. If the airway is seriously blocked, the casualty, particularly their lips, may appear blue from cyanosis.

When *listening* to the airway one may hear gurgling or stridor (noise on breathing in). If the airway is obstructed and the patient is unconscious the first thing to do is attempt to clear the obstruction with a jaw thrust. With both thumbs on the patient's cheek bones insert the index fingers of both hands behind the angle of the jaw. Firmly lifting the jaw upwards will move the tongue away from the back of the throat, opening the airway. Try to minimize neck movements during this manoeuvre (Fig. 7.2).

Examine the airway. If there is fluid or vomit in the mouth or throat, this should be gently removed using a portable suction device. Alternatively, the patient should be log-rolled onto their side (see Fig. 5.3) whilst maintaining in-line cervical spine immobilization, to allow the fluid to drain with gravity. Inspect the mouth to see if there is foreign material in the throat.

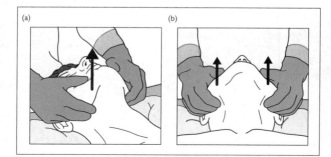

Fig. 7.2 Opening an obstructed airway.

Maintaining an open airway

Oropharyngeal airways (OPAs)

Two types of basic airway adjuncts can be used to keep the airway open. The Guedel OPA is inserted into the mouth with the tip lying between the tongue and the back wall of the throat. An airway of this type is measured by placing it against the side of the patient's face before insertion. The length of the airway should be the same as the distance from the central incisor teeth (mouth in the midline at the front) to the corner of the jaw under the ear. Slide the curve of the airway over the tongue until the flange is against the lips. Do not trap lips or tongue between teeth and airway. If the victim's mouth is dry it may be easier to insert the airway inverted, and then rotate gently as the tip reaches the back of the mouth. A size 2 (9 cm) is usually appropriate for adult females and a size 3 (10 cm) for males. A semi-conscious patient may not tolerate an OPA; do not persist in trying to insert the device as it may cause the patient to vomit. Consider removing the OPA and placing the patient in the recovery position, or use a nasopharyngeal airway instead.

Nasopharyngeal airways (NPAs)

Such airways are ideal during seizures when the teeth are clenched, preventing the use of OPAs. A 6-mm internal diameter airway is appropriate for adults (use the size of the patient's nostril as a guide). The packet includes a safety pin which should be pushed through the NPA flange. Lubricate the tube well before insertion and apply gentle continuous pressure straight towards the back of the head, not upwards parallel to the ridge of the nose. Insertion can cause bleeding, but this should stop once the airway is in place. If one nostril seems very tight, try the other as nasal cavities are rarely symmetrical, or use a smaller size. Gentle rotation may help if the airway gets stuck at the back of the nose. Tape a safety pin to the skin to fix the NPA. The NPA is extremely useful in semi-conscious patients who will not tolerate an oral airway. Insertion of an OPA or NPA does not guarantee that the patient's airway will remain clear. Jaw thrust may be needed in addition.

Endotracheal tubes and supraglottic airways (LMAs, i-Gels™, etc.)

Airway manoeuvres and basic adjuncts help to maintain the airway in the majority of seriously injured patients, but do nothing to prevent aspiration of regurgitated stomach contents. Definitive airway maintenance and protection can only be achieved by the insertion of a cuffed endotracheal tube, or to a lesser extent, by the insertion of a laryngeal mask airway or other supraglottic device. If an injured patient is so obtunded that an endotracheal tube or supraglottic airway can be inserted without the use of anaesthetic drugs, the patient's chance of survival is very low. Endotracheal tubes and supraglottic airways can be misplaced, lead to airway obstruction, spasm of the vocal cords, vomiting, bradycardia, and raised intracranial pressure.

Only personnel who both understand and can correct these problems should use these airway adjuncts.

Surgical airways
Surgical cricothyroidotomies, or tracheostomies, are indicated in patients whose upper airway obstruction cannot be relieved by other means, e.g. victims of burns or serious facial injuries. Cricothyroidotomy should only be performed by appropriately trained personnel but its need can be anticipated in circumstances where the clinical situation typically deteriorates steadily, such as serious airway burns. An expedition medical kit is unlikely to include a cricothyrotomy kit; in dire circumstances consider using a narrow bladed knife or scalpel, together with the barrel of a ball-point pen or the sharp end of an IV fluid-giving set.

Breathing

Chest injuries are common in serious trauma. Some are rapidly life-threatening but amenable to treatment if detected and acted upon in the early stages of resuscitation.

During assessment look for the following:

- Respiratory rate: one of the most important clinical indicators of significant chest injury. Count over 30 s and record regularly. Normal respiratory rate is 10–20 breaths per minute.
- General condition: severe respiratory distress suggests a tension pneumothorax. Look for cyanosis and swollen neck veins.
- Inspection: look for bruising, swelling, abrasions, wounds, flail segments. Examine the back and front of the chest.
- Palpate the chest: in a noisy pre-hospital environment, palpation is often more practical than auscultation. Feel the back as well as the front for crepitus and tenderness over fractured ribs. Feel for surgical emphysema which could indicate pneumothorax.
- Tracheal position: deviation is difficult to feel and is a late sign in tension pneumothorax. The diagnosis is usually evident from other more reliable clinical features.
- Auscultation: listen in the axillae, not the front of the chest to compare air entry effectively. There is decreased air entry with pneumothorax and haemothorax.
- Percussion: dull with haemothorax. Hyper-resonant with tension pneumothorax.
- Saturation: if a pulse oximeter is available—should be >98%, but decreases with increasing altitude.
- High-flow oxygen (via a reservoir) should be administered to all patients with serious chest injuries if it is available. If a small supply of oxygen is available then lower inspired concentrations for a longer time are probably better than a short burst at high flow rates. Start with a high flow rate and then decrease until the reservoir bag is almost completely deflated at the end of inspiration.

Pneumothorax

This refers to air in the pleural space between chest wall and lung. Air leaks into the pleural cavity either from a damaged lung or through a hole in the chest wall. It is typically caused by blunt or penetrating chest injury or as a result of barotrauma from rapid ascent when diving (see ➋ Barotrauma, p. 740), but occasionally—typically in tall, lean men—it may develop spontaneously. There is decreased air entry on the affected side. Chest drainage will be required if breathing is compromised and a chest drain must be inserted before aeromedical evacuation (➋ Moving an injured person, p. 148; ➋ Repatriation, p. 158).

Tension pneumothorax

This is as for pneumothorax, but with ongoing increase in volume and pressure of trapped air. Pressure causes the opposite lung to be compressed and pushes the heart across the chest, compromising its venous inflow from the vena cava. The clinical features are:

- Severe distress—'air hunger'.
- Increased heart rate.

- Reduction in BP, the pulse strength may vary with each breath.
- Hyper-resonance when percussing the affected side.
- Cyanosis may develop when the condition is severe.

Tension pneumothorax requires urgent needle decompression followed by formal chest drainage.

Needle decompression of tension pneumothorax

Use a large-bore cannula attached to a syringe partially filled with fluid. Insert the cannula at right angles to the skin, through the second intercostal space in the midclavicular line, just above the third rib, so as to avoid the vessels and nerve that run immediately below the second rib.

Aspiration of air indicates that the cannula tip has entered the pneumothorax.

If no air is aspirated:
- Either the diagnosis was wrong.
- Or the cannula has been occluded by a 'fat plug' (blow a few millilitres of air through the cannula).
- Or the chest wall is deeper than the needle is long. If the diagnosis is still suspected then try again in the fifth intercostal space in the anterior–axillary line.

After aspiration of air remove the syringe and tape the cannula in position. If available, insert a formal chest drain attached to an underwater seal or a Heimlich valve (Fig. 7.3).

ThoraQuik® is a purpose-built device for decompressing a tension pneumothorax in the pre-hospital environment. This may be available in certain situations and is straightforward to use after very little training.[1,2]

A tension pneumothorax can often redevelop, especially when the patient is moved, and may require further decompression—leave the original cannula *in situ*.

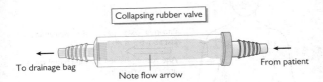

Fig. 7.3 Heimlich valve.

1 http://boundtree.co.uk/thoraquik-chest-decompression-device
2 http://www.youtube.com/watch?v=4aAXDbOUCeg

Chest drain insertion

(See Fig. 7.4.)

This procedure should only be undertaken by those with prior training and experience.

- Equipment required: local anaesthetic (LA) (lidocaine 1%), syringes, needles, scalpel, antiseptic solution, sterile gloves, artery forceps for blunt dissection, adhesive tape, chest drain (size 28–32), Heimlich valve or underwater seal set with water, suture material.
- Place the patient at 30–60° with patient's arm above head.
- Identify the site for incision—the fourth or fifth intercostal space in the anterior axillary line. Avoid breast tissue.
- Clean the skin and infiltrate local anaesthetic down to the pleura.
- Using the scalpel make a 3-cm incision directly above the rib.
- Bluntly dissect down to the pleura with artery forceps and insert a gloved finger through the pleura.
- While keeping the finger in the hole, slide the chest tube beside the finger (trocar removed). This is easier if the end of the chest tube is attached to one jaw of an artery forceps.
- Push the tube into the chest and direct the tip towards the apex of the lung. Ensure all the drain holes are in the pleural cavity.
- Attach the Heimlich valve or underwater seal. Look for condensation in the tube or swinging of water in the underwater seal apparatus.
- Fix the tube firmly to the skin using sutures. Avoid a purse suture which may cause unsightly scarring.
- Apply gauze swabs to the skin at the base of the tube and tape in position.

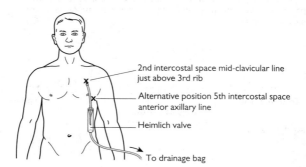

2nd intercostal space mid-clavicular line just above 3rd rib

Alternative position 5th intercostal space anterior axillary line

Heimlich valve

To drainage bag

Fig. 7.4 Chest drain with Heimlich valve.

Haemothorax

Following blunt or penetrating chest injury, blood leaks into the space between chest wall and lung, usually from damaged intercostal vessels. The bleeding often stops following formal chest drainage and re-inflation of the lung. The bleeding may be associated with a pneumothorax—the chest will be dull to percussion over the blood-filled area; bleeding can be massive and lead to hypotension.

Flail chest

If multiple adjacent ribs are fractured in two or more places there is a free-floating segment of chest wall that moves inwards with inspiration instead of outwards (paradoxical movement). This injury is typically caused by blunt chest trauma and is always associated with significant underlying pulmonary contusion.

Clinical features:
- Increased respiratory rate.
- Visible flail segment (may not be obvious clinically).
- Palpable crepitus.
- Painful breathing—use paracetamol and NSAIDs for background pain relief and titrate an opiate if available.

Splinting the flail segment with tape may improve both discomfort and breathing.

Urgent evacuation from the field will be required as bleeding and lung infection are common.

Sucking chest wound

This refers to an open wound through the chest wall as a result of penetrating chest injury. Air preferentially moves through the hole rather than the trachea with inspiration if the diameter of the hole is ≥2/3 of the diameter of the trachea (typically around 1 cm).

Clinical features:
- Sucking wound.
- Decreased air entry on the affected side.
- Severe respiratory distress.

Cover the wound with an occlusive dressing sealed on three sides to prevent tension pneumothorax developing. The Bolin®[3] and Asherman®[4] chest seals are designed for sucking chest wounds in the pre-hospital environment.

Insert a chest drain then seal the wound completely.

All patients with suspected or actual chest injury will require evacuation. *All patients with a real risk of pneumothorax must have a chest drain inserted before air evacuation.*

3 http://boundtree.co.uk/bolin-chest-seal
4 http://www.ashermanchestseal.com

Circulation

Major haemorrhage in the seriously injured casualty can be from any of five places: 'blood on the floor and four more', i.e. external bleeding or bleeding into the chest, abdomen, pelvis, or thighs. Much can be done to arrest bleeding from wounds or closed long bone fractures but little can be done outside of the operating theatre to arrest haemorrhage in the other three sites. Rapid evacuation to a hospital with surgical facilities is therefore essential in these patient groups.

Assessment of circulatory status:
- Heart rate: may be raised with blood loss (≥120 bpm) but may be raised in the absence of blood loss due to pain or anxiety.
- BP: owing to compensatory mechanisms in young healthy adults, there may be significant blood loss before the BP falls. Beware of a false sense of security with a normal BP.
- Peripheral perfusion: very useful in a warm environment to indicate circulatory failure. It is not as useful in cold environments as this may be a response to the environment rather than any blood loss.
- Peripheral pulses: absence of a palpable radial pulse indicates significant blood loss.
- Mental status: hypovolaemia leading to reduced cerebral perfusion leads to confusion and reduced conscious level.
- Bleeding source: look for wounds and haematomas. Examine chest, abdomen, and pelvis. Examine long bones, especially femurs. Don't forget the back and scalp.

All patients should receive oxygen if available. Minimize movement by planning the 'patient packaging' process in advance. Unnecessary movements may cause blood clots which have formed to dislodge, worsening haemorrhage. Most clotting factors are used in the formation of the initial clot. Give adequate pain relief and attempt to reassure the patient; this will reduce catecholamine release. Keep the patient warm. Hypothermia worsens clotting and increases haemorrhage.

Arrest external haemorrhage with direct pressure, dressings, and elevation (see ➋ Control of haemorrhage, p. 196). Bleeding wounds, especially scalp wounds, may require urgent suturing. In cases of life-threatening bleeding from limb injuries, initially apply very firm pressure over the wound but, if this fails to stem the flow, apply a proximal tourniquet such as the Combat Application Tourniquet (CAT®). A number of commercially available compounds are available which can be applied to wounds to promote clotting. They are currently in use with many military medical services and may be of use in certain remote expedition settings, e.g. Celox® and QuickClot®.

Limb injuries should be splinted to promote clot formation and decrease pain. Femoral fractures can result in up to 1.5 L of blood loss. Traction splints act to reduce haemorrhage by reducing soft tissue damage and reducing the volume of the thigh compartment, hence increasing pressure and tamponading bleeding.

Open fractures should be reduced if possible. They should be covered with Inadine® dressings and broad-spectrum antibiotics administered, e.g. co-amoxiclav or ceftriaxone. See Table 28.1.

Pelvic fractures can cause fatal haemorrhage. Examination and movement should be minimized to promote clot formation. A splint should be applied to stabilize the fracture. These can be commercially designed splints (e.g. SAM Pelvic Sling®) or improvised with a sheet wrapped firmly around the pelvis. The aim is to return the pelvis to its normal anatomical position, not to tighten the splint as much as possible. The knees should be slightly flexed and tied together (with padding between). If a pelvic fracture is suspected it should be treated as such, splinted, and not re-examined until the patient reaches hospital.

Over the past decade there has been a shift away from routinely administering large amounts of IV fluids to injured patients. A normal physiological response to bleeding is for the BP to fall, reducing flow through damaged vessels and tissues and so allowing clots to form. The remaining blood circulating has a high concentration of haemoglobin and may be sufficient in volume to allow perfusion of the vital organs if peripheral vasoconstriction has occurred. Administering IV fluids does not increase the oxygen-carrying capacity of the blood but does increase the BP. This may dislodge clots which have formed, causing further loss of haemoglobin. IV fluids, especially colloids, also adversely affect coagulation, again increasing bleeding.

Established pre-hospital trauma management practice is not to administer fluids if the patient has a palpable radial pulse. If the radial pulse is not palpable, normal saline is titrated in 250 mL boluses until the radial pulse returns (NICE guidelines 2004). The evidence supporting this 'permissive hypotension' is mostly based in urban environments with short times from injury to definitive surgical care to arrest bleeding. Its use in remote environments is not proven but is likely to be appropriate when blood transfusion is not available and fluid supplies are limited.[5]

Tranexamic acid has been shown to reduce mortality in major trauma provided that it is administered in the first 3 h after injury. Do not give to children under the age of 12, to a casualty with isolated head injury, or to anyone with known sensitivity to the drug. Give a loading does of 1 g (10 mL) 1 mL at a time over 10 min. Faster injection can cause nausea, vomiting, or convulsions. Subsequent doses may be given by infusion, but seek advice from a base hospital as the casualty will require urgent evacuation.

5 ✎ http://www.nice.org.uk/guidance/ta74

Control of haemorrhage

1. Direct pressure to the bleeding point

This should be tried first for all external bleeding and is effective in most cases. It may be ineffective if the bleeding vessel is not 'within reach' of pressure (e.g. deep in a wound). In this case, consider 'packing' the wound firmly from the base upwards using gauze/sterile bandage material.

2. Elevation of the affected limb/site of bleeding may also slow flow

Elevation helps less if bleeding is arterial rather than venous and is less effective when big vessels are damaged. Avoid raising legs if there are suspected pelvic, lumbar spine, or leg fractures/injuries.

3. Pressure on a direct arterial pressure point upstream of the site of bleeding

For bleeding from leg wounds, use the femoral pulse (middle of the groin); for arm wounds, grip the brachial artery firmly over the middle of the medial surface of the upper arm.

4. Using a tourniquet

A tourniquet is indicated when direct pressure to a bleeding point may be ineffective for any reason. It can be used to 'free hands' from having to apply such sustained direct pressure. It is generally used when major arteries have been severed and have retracted beyond reach or where the area of tissue disruption in a limb is extensive (e.g. avulsions or ballistic injury).

Always apply above the knee (for lower limb injuries).

You can increase efficacy by helping apply directed pressure (i.e. a packed pad over the artery). Pad a little beneath the tourniquet to prevent skin damage.

Use a commercial tourniquet or improvise:

• A strip of cloth 5–10 cm wide.
• Tie around limb loosely, and tie a half-knot.
• Slip to 5–10 cm above the wound (and above the joint if the injury is distal).
• Put a stick over the half-knot, and complete the tie.
• Rotate the stick as a 'windlass' until the bleeding stops.
• Leave on for at least 30 min. Use this time to try to identify the bleeding point and directly pack/compress. Do not 'dig and dab'; clot must be left to stabilize.
• Slowly release the tourniquet and observe. If bleeding continues, reapply the tourniquet.

Neck and other spinal injuries

Neck and other spinal injuries

Suspected spinal injuries cause great anxiety for mountain rescue teams and during expeditions to remote areas. Data from the Bangor Mountain Medicine Project indicate that half of mountain trauma casualties in Snowdonia, Wales, have a mechanism of injury that would mandate spinal immobilization in urban pre-hospital practice. However, only about 2% of mountain casualties *found alive* after a significant mechanism of injury had an unstable spinal fracture.

Spinal cord injury is a relatively rare, but potentially devastating injury. However, irrational fear should not overrule clinical judgement and the use of common sense. There are a number of key messages that any practitioner in a remote or wilderness setting must understand.

- 'Neck injury', 'broken neck', and 'spinal cord injury' are not synonymous.
- Most victims sustaining a neck injury will simply have a soft tissue injury (→ Acute neck sprains, p. 305).
- A small minority may have a stable compression or avulsion type fracture with no threat to the spinal cord.
- An even smaller proportion (19 per week in the UK) will have an unstable fracture that has caused damage to the spinal cord.

Spinal injuries most frequently occur at junctions of mobile and fixed sections of the spine (C6,7/T1, T12/L1). In patients with multiple injuries who have a spinal injury, over half will have a cervical spinal injury. Approximately 10–15% of patients with one spinal fracture will be found to have another.

Spinal cord injury must be considered in the following circumstances:
- High-speed injuries (RTCs, falls, or falling objects striking the victim's head).
- Patients with multiple injuries.
- Patients with head injuries.
- Unresponsive patients who have suffered trauma.

It is now known that damage to the spinal cord takes place either at the time of the injury or during a later phase as a result of bleeding and soft tissue swelling at the site of the fracture. Whilst victims with suspected spinal injury must be handled carefully, unfounded fears of making the damage worse should not prevent the rescuer or medic from making sensible on-site decisions. In an expedition or wilderness setting the decision to immobilize and evacuate a patient should not be made lightly as it can have significant resource and safety implications for the patient's companions and for organized rescuers. The patient may initially be treated for a spinal injury, but this can be reviewed once other injuries have been treated and the patient is warm and comfortable. However, clearing the spine clinically, especially in the higher-risk patients, must not be undertaken lightly.

Assessment

Assessment of the cervical spine in a conscious patient takes place as an extension of the primary survey described on ➲ Initial response to an incident, p. 180 to ➲ Control of haemorrhage, p. 196. Remember that ATLS guidelines clearly state that airway management takes precedence over cervical spine control. Two prospectively validated decision making tools are commonly used to assess the cervical spine: Canadian C-spine and NEXUS guidelines. Whilst the former have been shown to have a slightly higher sensitivity in a conventional setting, the more restrictive criteria, and the differing context and population make the latter the more logical choice for the expedition or wilderness context. (See Fig. 7.5.)

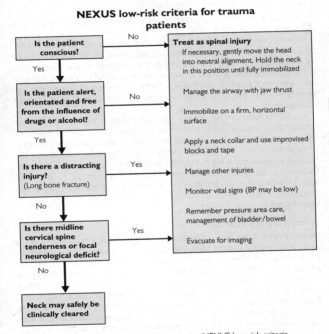

Fig. 7.5 Assessment of patients with trauma using NEXUS low-risk criteria.

Using the NEXUS low-risk criteria

- Exercise extreme caution using this approach in young children or the elderly.
- Distracting injury means an injury where the pain is sufficiently severe that it distracts the patient from the assessment process. If the patient can cooperate with your assessment without difficulty then no distracting injury is present.
- Often it is the 'mid-line tenderness' criterion that clinicians find the most difficult to assess. Many patients with neck pain will have tenderness in the para-spinal muscles. Ensure that it is mid-line bony tenderness that you are testing. If in doubt act conservatively and reassess later.
- Neurological assessment for NEXUS purposes is limited to assessing upper and lower limb motor function.

Patients who are clinically cleared should be managed as for a neck sprain (➲ Acute neck sprains, p. 305).

Patients who fail the NEXUS criteria must be assumed to have a cervical spine injury. Avoid turning these patients unless penetrating trauma or significant haemorrhage is suspected as the outcome of the examination will not change management in which case they should be log-rolled with neck alignment carefully maintained. Further neurological assessment can be delayed until the patient reaches definitive care as it does not change management.

In patients who can be cleared clinically, the question of a thoracic or lumbar spine fracture is still valid. Patients with a fracture will complain of severe pain in the back, and those with lumbar spine fractures may have complained of pain and difficulty performing a straight leg raise during the NEXUS assessment. A log roll should be performed unless pelvic or femoral fractures are suspected. Midline bony tenderness would be expected with a fracture, but may be absent in anterior wedge fractures of the vertebral body. Patients with neurological signs or suspected fracture must be immobilized on a firm surface.

Spinal immobilization

Ideally cervical spine immobilization should consist of a proprietary semi-rigid collar, blocks or sand bags, and tape, with the patient lying supine on a firm surface. A Stifneck select™ is ideal as one collar may be carried and adjusted to fit different sized patients. It should be realized that even a well-fitting collar will only reduce neck movements by 50%. A poorly fitting collar will irritate the patient and may result in increased neck movement. Rigid spine boards are for short-term use to transfer patients only. They should not be used for long-term transport or ongoing patient care as they are uncomfortable and may cause pressure areas. In a wilderness setting a collar may be improvised using closed cell foam mat cut to shape, a SAM splint, or a padded rucsac hip belt. The patient's boots can make improvised blocks for either side of the head. Improvised splinting must be effective and perform the required immobilisation—inadequate splinting is falsely reassuring for rescuers.

Hazards of spinal immobilization

Spinal immobilization has been a component of immediate aid protocols for many years and in some circumstances may be entirely appropriate. However, an evidence-based review by the Wilderness Medical Society (2013) has highlighted the paucity of evidence for its benefits, and the potential risks of the procedure in remote areas when transfer to hospital care will take time. A spinal board or neck collar may force a casualty into inappropriate positions, and increase the risks of inhalation of vomit, pain, pressures sores, and breathing problems. These risks should be weighed against the possible benefits and immobilization not seen as a gold-standard treatment. Those interested in learning more should read the full guidelines.[6]

Disability

Assess the casualty's level of consciousness (disability) using the AVPU scale:
- Awake and alert.
- Verbal—responds to voice ('Squeeze my hand').
- Pain—responds to pain.
- Unresponsive—no response to painful stimulus.

To monitor a patient's progress, chart the GCS (see Box 7.1). Minimum GCS score = 3, with maximum score of 15. Three areas of brain function are tested and scored: eye opening, speech, and movement. Use an increasing level of stimulus to obtain a response:
- Speak: 'Are you okay? What's your name?'
- Tap the shoulders gently. 'Squeeze my hand'
- Apply pain: press firmly over the inner aspect of the eyebrow along the eye socket (supraorbital nerve).

A fall in the GCS score of two or more is significant and may indicate deterioration in the patient's condition. Causes include:
- Bleeding.
- Swelling.
- Infection.

Remember, if the patient deteriorates during your assessment *immediately* re-check the ABC and rectify any life-threatening problems.

Box 7.1 Glasgow Coma Scale

Eye opening	Score
Open spontaneously	4
Open to verbal command	3
Open to pain	2
No response	1
Verbal response	
Talking and orientated	5
Confused, not orientated	4
Inappropriate words	3
Incomprehensible sounds	2
No response	1
Motor response	
Obeys commands	6
Localizes pain	5
Flexion/withdrawal	4
Abnormal flexion	3
Extension	2
No response	1

Reproduced from *The Lancet*, 304:7872, Teasdale G, Jennett B, Assessment of coma and impaired consciousness, pp. 81–84, Copyright (1974), with permission from Elsevier.

Exposure and environmental control

It is important to examine the patient thoroughly and protect them from exposure to the elements.

A seriously injured patient, especially one with a reduced conscious level, may have life-changing injuries which are not obvious during the initial stages of resuscitation. This is because pain from them may be masked by more serious injuries, or the clinician involved is concentrating on immediately life-threatening problems. Such injuries might include peripheral joint dislocations or eye injuries which may lead to lifelong disability if not detected and corrected in the early stages. A systematic head-to-toe examination ('secondary survey') is necessary to seek and identify these injuries.

At this stage it may be appropriate to insert a urinary catheter if the patient is to be transferred by stretcher. Remember to exclude possible injury to the urethra by seeking signs: scrotal bruising, blood from the tip of the penis, and a high riding prostate on rectal examination.

During and after the secondary survey the patient should be adequately insulated and protected from the external environment.

Secondary survey

The aim of primary survey is to simultaneously identify and treat life-threatening problems. Secondary survey is a methodical head-to-toe search for all the injuries that may be present. It may be possible to conduct a full secondary survey where the patient is found, but in a wilderness setting it is likely that the patient will need to be protected from the environment using a group shelter or tent. If the patient must be moved remember the possibility of spinal injury and try to conduct a limited secondary survey first.

In injury cases take a brief history. Remember:

AMPLE

- A—Allergies.
- M—Medicines.
- P—Past medical history.
- L—Last meal time.
- E—Events leading to the injury.

Examination

The casualty should be undressed to enable a complete head to toe examination. Examine the whole body, front, sides, and back, in the following order:

1. Head including nervous system.
2. Neck.
3. Chest.
4. Abdomen.
5. Pelvis.
6. Legs.
7. Arms.
8. Spine.

General appearance

- Skin colour—pale or blue (cyanosed).
- Dehydration.
- Sweating.
- Body temperature.

Examination of the head

- Scalp: bleeding, swelling, bruising.
- Conscious level: assess AVPU or measure the GCS score (see ➜ Disability, p. 202).
- Eyes: pupil size and reaction to light.
- Nose: look for deformity, discharge (?CSF leak), bleeding. See ➜ Facial injuries, p. 302.
- Ears: discharge (?CSF leak), bleeding.
- Face: feel face on both sides looking for deformities and tenderness. Is there a fractured jaw?
- Mouth: does the breath smell (alcohol)? Any broken teeth?

Examination of the neck
- The patient may complain of limited or painful neck movements or limb tingling/weakness.
- Look and feel for any 'step', swelling, or tenderness.

Examination of the chest
- Look for tracheal deviation, asymmetrical chest movements (flail chest), open wounds, bruising, impaled objects, or signs of a tension pneumothorax (see → Pneumothorax, p. 190).
- Is there tenderness on rib springing? Only do this if there is no obvious external injury.
- Listen for reduced air entry—listen under the collarbone and outside the nipple on each side.

Examination of the abdomen/pelvis
- Look for bruising, open wounds.
- Feel in all four quadrants for localized tenderness, particularly *rebound* tenderness.
- Listen for bowel sounds.
- Gently feel the pelvis *once only* to elicit pain/movement.

Examination of the limbs
- Look for bruising, swelling, deformity, wounds, shortening, crepitus.
- If injuries are found check Movement, Circulation (pulses), and Sensation—M, C + S.

Examination of the spine
- If a spinal injury is suspected do not move the patient unnecessarily—log roll and use neck immobilization. See Fig. 5.3; → Spinal immobilzation, p. 200.
- Look for loss of movement or sensation. Feel for swelling, tenderness, 'step'.
- In high neck injuries diaphragmatic breathing may be present and in males an involuntary erection of the penis (priapism) indicates a high-level spinal injury.

Continuing care

(See also Chapter 3 and Chapter 5.)

Subsequent care will depend upon:
- Severity of the injuries.
- Condition of the patient.
- Urgency of evacuation.
- Ease of evacuation.

Isolation or adverse weather conditions will mean that the expedition team may have to care for a casualty for several days. During this time you will have to provide effective nursing care:
- Regular observations to give warning if patient's condition deteriorates and they develop shock (➔ Clinical observations, p. 89).
- Pain relief (see ➔ Treating pain (analgesia), p. 93).
- Nutrition and fluids as possible.
- Warmth.
- Personal needs and hygiene, including toileting (➔ Nursing and emotional care awaiting evacuation, p. 156).
- Good nursing to avoid pressure areas (➔ Field nursing care, p. 88).
- Psychological support (➔ Psychological support, p. 88).

Blast injuries

Blast and gunshot injuries are common in some parts of the world. Explosions can be caused by vehicle accidents, gas cylinders, in some industrial environments (e.g. mining), or, more commonly, in wars and acts of terrorism. There may be multiple casualties after an explosion.

Explosions cause injury in six ways:

1. Blast wave.
2. Blast wind.
3. Fragmentation.
4. Flash burns.
5. Crush.
6. Psychological.

Blast wave

This is a momentary front of overpressure formed by compression of air at the interface of the rapidly expanding sphere of hot gases. Injuries are caused by a combination of body compression followed by disruption of tissues at air/tissue interfaces—particularly in the lungs, gut and ears. The lungs are commonly affected in two ways—intra-alveolar haemorrhage and pneumothoraces (➔ Pneumothorax, p. 190). These can be rapidly fatal or lead to adult respiratory distress syndrome. Bowel haemorrhage and perforation may develop several days after the initial injury. The ear drums are often ruptured but will depend on the angle of the blast wave.

The overpressure can be multiplied several times over when the pressure wave is reflected by walls, ceilings, or water.

Air can enter the pulmonary circulation and result in fatal air emboli.

Blast winds

These are rapidly moving columns of air which follow the blast wave. They can be powerful enough to dismember or even disintegrate a person close to the explosion. Casualties further away can sustain traumatic amputations and can be thrown against solid objects which will cause deceleration injuries and fractures from the impact.

Fragmentation missiles

Most injuries after an explosion are caused by fragmentation. The missiles are primary (from the bomb casing or nails, bolts, nuts packed around the explosive) or secondary (stones, glass or wood from the environment). These missiles can cause lacerations, fractures, contusions, and penetrating wounds.

Flash burns

The hot gases from the explosion can cause smoke inhalation injuries to the airway and exposed skin may be burned. Burns tend to be superficial. For management of burns, see ➔ Burns, p. 280.

Crush injuries

Falling debris and building collapse can cause crushing injuries (see ➔ Crush injuries, p. 277).

Psychological injuries

These may be the main objective in terrorist attacks. Explosions result in panic, fear, and widespread destruction. In the long term, some will experience post-traumatic stress disorder (see ➔ Post-traumatic stress disorder, p. 530).

Lightning

The voltage in a bolt of lightning is between 200 million to 2 billion volts of direct current. A bolt of lightning can reach temperatures approaching 28,000°C and lasts microseconds. Lightning strikes can injure humans in different ways:

- Direct strike—where the electrical charge hits the person.
- Splash hits—the lightning jumps from a nearby object and strikes the victim on its way to ground.
- Ground strike—the lightning bolt lands near to the victim and is conducted through the ground. The energy transmitted depends on the resistance of the ground material—dry sand is a poor conductor and wet spongy earth is a better conductor.
- Electromagnetic pulse—a burst of electromagnetic energy which produces high currents and voltages.

720 people were affected by lightning strikes in the UK between 1988 and 2012. 21% were killed and 7% had CPR and survived. 16% had serious injuries (fractures, burns and unconsciousness) and 56% had minor injuries (minor burns, temporary damage to eyes or ears, transient numbness). Most survivors have no significant long-term disabilities. Similar figures have been found in studies of lightning injuries in the US.

Lightning injuries

- Cardiopulmonary arrest. Cardiac arrest tends to be brief because of the heart's intrinsic automaticity; however, paralysis of the respiratory centre in the medulla may lead to prolonged respiratory arrest.
- Burns. There may be characteristic feathering burns (Lichtenberg figures) or linear or punctate burns.
- Neurological injuries. Victims may be confused, have convulsions, paralysis, or amnesia.
- Ear and eye trauma. Tympanic membrane rupture is very common (>50%) and blindness occurs. Cataracts can develop as a late complication.
- Other injuries. Fractures, muscle aches, chest pains, and contusions may be seen and clothing/footwear can be damaged.
- Long-term injuries. These are usually neurological, including memory problems, sleep disturbance, dizziness and chronic pains.

Treatment

Some victims suffer immediate cardiac arrest and will not survive without immediate emergency care:

- Assess ABC and commence CPR if indicated. Prolonged resuscitation may be required because of temporary damage to the respiratory centre in the medulla.
- Consider the possibility of spinal injuries as the victim may have been thrown a considerable distance by the strike.
- Reduce and splint any fractures.
- Evacuate for cardiac monitoring and observation. Cardiac failure can occur as a late complication.

Prevention of lightning injuries

- Avoid power lines, boat masts, ski lifts, and wire fences.
- If in a tent, stay away from the poles and wet canvas.
- Avoid tall trees in open areas or hilltops and ridges.
- Move away from open water and metal boats.
- Stay away from isolated small structures in open areas.
- In forests, seek low areas under small trees.
- Do not shelter in the entrances of caves.
- If in the open, seek low ground and stay away from single trees. Do not lie flat on the ground. If possible insulate yourself from the ground with sleeping mats and bend forwards on your knees keeping hands off the ground.
- Hair standing on end, blue haloes around objects, and crackling noises all indicate an imminent strike. Leave the area if possible or crouch down on the balls of your feet with head tucked down.

http://www.sciencedirect.com/science/article/pii/S0169809500000831

Emergencies: collapse and serious illness

Section editors
Jon Dallimore and Chris Johnson

Contributors
Edi Albert
Spike Briggs
Jon Dallimore
David A. Warrell
Sundeep Dhillon (1st edition)
Mike Grocott (1st edition)
Stephen Hearns (1st edition)
Hugh Montgomery (1st edition)
Julian Thompson (1st edition)

The collapsed patient 212
Medical emergencies 214
Resuscitation in the wilderness 216
Basic life support (CPR) 220
Choking 224
Recovery position 226
Shock 228
Management of the shocked patient 230
Types of shock 234
Chest pain 242
Shortness of breath (dyspnoea) 246
Coma 248
Headache 250
Delirium/confusion 252
Convulsions 254
Diabetic emergencies 256
Gastrointestinal bleeding 260
Fever 262

The collapsed patient

Management of injured patients follows a well-established sequence (see Chapter 7). However, when an individual suddenly becomes unwell ('collapses'), their basic life functions must be supported, a diagnosis made, the appropriate treatment instituted, and the patient stabilized before evacuation can be considered.

Collapse in young adults is very rare, but is generally very serious; infectious disease or environmentally induced conditions are the most likely causes. Psychological causes must be considered, but only after medical ones have been excluded. In older travellers, the likelihood of cardiovascular disease increases.

Medical emergencies

Medical emergencies

Before attempting to examine any seriously ill person look for life-threatening hazards so as to avoid further injury to the patient and any danger to the rescuers. If absolutely necessary, rapidly and carefully move the casualty to a place of safety.

Rapid primary assessment and resuscitation

This is the simultaneous assessment, identification, and management of immediate life-threatening problems. Rapid primary assessment should follow the ABC model.

- **A** Assessment whilst approaching the casualty.
- **A** Airway (with neck control if there is a history of injury).
- **B** Breathing.
- **C** Circulation (control bleeding and manage shock).
- **D** Disability of the nervous system.
- **E** Exposure and environmental control.

Primary assessment should be repeated following any change in the patient's condition.

Assessment and approach

When it is safe to approach, check the casualty's level of responsiveness. Tap or gently shake the shoulders and say 'Are you OK?' If there is no response call for help and proceed to check the airway.

Airway

- Assess without moving the neck more than necessary—particularly if the patient has fallen and might have injured the head or neck. Remember, airway takes precedence over neck control.
- Open the airway using chin lift or jaw thrust (**➲** Airway, p. 186).
- Look for, and remove any obvious obstruction, consider the use of airway adjuncts such as nasopharyngeal or oropharyngeal airways (**➲** Maintaining an open airway, p. 187). Remember that oropharyngeal airways can provoke vomiting, and nasopharyngeal airways cause nosebleeds.

Breathing

- Once the airway has been checked and opened, assess breathing.
- Look, listen, and feel for breathing (10 s); if the patient is hypothermic then extend this period to 30 s.
- Give oxygen if available, particularly to those who are shocked, bleeding, or who have breathing difficulties.
- If respiration is absent, impaired, or inadequate, commence CPR (**➲** Resuscitation in the wilderness, p. 216).
- Is the breathing rate normal?
- Can the patient count to ten in one breath?
- If you suspect a chest problem, examine the chest for movement and breath sounds; normal, crackles, wheeze, or absent?

Circulation care with haemorrhage control

The aim is to detect and treat shock. Look for and control any external bleeding (consider direct pressure and elevation). Consider the possibility of internal bleeding.

- Look at the patient's skin colour and assess the skin temperature.
- Measure pulse rate and assess pulse character (normal, thready, or bounding).
- Estimate the BP by feeling the pulse:
  - Carotid (neck): systolic BP >60 mmHg.
  - Femoral (groin): systolic BP >70 mmHg.
  - Radial (wrist): systolic BP >80 mmHg.
- Capillary refill should be <2 s in a warm casualty (➲ Capillary refill time, p. 417).
- Treat shock:
  - Lie the patient flat, elevate legs on pillow or rucksack.
  - Keep warm and reassure.
  - Consider IV fluids—replacement amounts and rate will depend upon the cause of the shock.

For management of other causes of shock see ➲ Shock, p. 228.

Disability
- Assess the patient's neurological status using the AVPU scale:
  - A Alert.
  - V Responds to verbal command.
  - P Responds to pain.
  - U Unresponsive.
- Pupils—assess size and reaction to light.
- Look for neck stiffness.
- Check blood glucose levels if possible.
- If the patient is fitting, place them in the recovery position.

Exposure and environmental control
Where possible, examine the patient in a warm, light environment such as a tent or group shelter. Be gentle; unnecessary roughness may aggravate the problem. Examine the patient carefully but always prevent the development of hypothermia which will worsen shock. Measure body temperature and look for a rash.

Rapid history
The patient or bystanders may be able to give brief details to aid diagnosis:
- Events leading up to the illness, any history of injury.
- Past history, particularly known cardiac or respiratory illness, diabetes, epilepsy, alcohol/drug abuse, head injury.
- Medication taken on a regular or occasional basis.
- Allergies.

Secondary assessment
(See also ➲ Secondary survey, p. 204.)
Secondary survey is a methodical search for all signs of disease which may be present. On an expedition this should be delayed until the casualty is in a warm, dry environment such as in a tent or building or under a group shelter, lying on a mattress, airbed, or sleeping bag.
History-taking and examination are covered in Chapter 6.

Resuscitation in the wilderness

Survival from a cardiac arrest depends upon the cause of the arrest, the previous health of the patient, the rapidity of the initial response, and the availability of medical and transport facilities to ensure *the chain of survival* (Fig. 8.1).

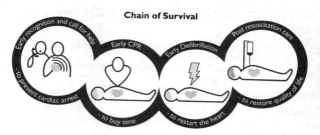

Fig. 8.1 Chain of survival. Reproduced from fig 1.1 in JP Nolan et al.: *Resuscitation* Vol 81 (2010) p1223. ERC Guidelines 2010, with permission.

The basic life support (BLS) algorithm (Fig. 8.2) remains the default response for a collapsed, unresponsive patient. However, current BLS and ALS guidelines have been developed for the patient who has had a cardiac arrest, most likely due to a myocardial infarction, and who collapses in an environment where early defibrillation and timely transfer to a facility for post-resuscitation care are possible.

Resuscitation in the wilderness presents issues that do not normally need to be considered in a conventional healthcare setting, and may require some difficult decision-making. Rescuers must consider their own safety both at the time of arrival on scene and for potential dangers arising during the resuscitation and rescue process, and be prepared to either not commence resuscitation, or abandon it. The expedition leader must consider not only the medical needs of the victim, but also recognize that there is a duty of care to other expedition members. A prolonged resuscitation and rescue may expose others to unacceptable environmental risks, especially if the other members are children. The physical location of the victim and the available rescue equipment may mean that it is not possible to rescue the victim *and* continue CPR effectively.

Special circumstances[1]

Rescuers must consider if the following circumstances apply and modify their approach accordingly:

- *Hypothermia* (➔ Hypothermia, p. 622)—airway protection and CPR should be commenced as soon as possible. However, CPR *must* be continued until the patient is either 'warm and dead', or return of spontaneous circulation (ROSC) occurs. If this cannot be guaranteed then CPR should be withheld and the patient handled very carefully.
- *Avalanche burial* (➔ Avalanches, p. 642)—follow the algorithm in Fig. 21.3. CPR should not be continued in buried victims with a blocked airway on extrication and a burial time >35 min.
- *Snake bite or marine envenomation*—prolonged CPR is sometimes successful.
- *Electrocution* (lightning strike) (➔ Lightning, p. 208)—prolonged CPR is worthwhile, especially after lightning strike. Late defibrillation may be successful.
- *Drowning, including cold water immersion* (➔ Immersion and drowning, p. 688)—commence CPR, but discontinue after 30 min unless timely evacuation to a medical facility is possible.
- *Cardiac arrest secondary to trauma/haemorrhage* (➔ Hypovolaemic shock, p. 234)—mean survival rate in conventional practice is 5%. Survival in a wilderness setting is extremely unlikely.

If none of these circumstances apply then conventional BLS and ALS guidelines should be followed where possible. Recovery from a ventricular fibrillation arrest requires timely defibrillation. If defibrillation occurs in a pre-hospital setting within 4 min of arrest with subsequent transfer to hospital, then long-term survival is 60%, at 20 min it is <1%.

Automated external defibrillators

Automated external defibrillators (AEDs) are compact, light, and relatively inexpensive; they can be used by lay people with little additional training, and in theory could be carried on many types of expedition. However, there are two major potential breaks in the chain of survival that render this approach of little value in most expedition contexts. Firstly, it is unlikely that the victim will have their cardiac arrest close to the medical kit where the defibrillator is kept. Secondly, long-term survival is usually dependent on the ability to identify and correct secondary complications such as arrhythmias, acidosis, and electrolyte disturbance.

---

1 Soar J, Perkins G, Abbas G, Alfonzo A, Barelli A, Bierens JJ, *et al*. (2010). European Resuscitation Council Guidelines for Resuscitation 2010: Cardiac arrest in special circumstances. *Resuscitation*, 81, 1400–33.

Do not initiate CPR
- If there is danger to the rescuers.
- Obvious lethal injury, e.g. decapitation.
- Rigor mortis.

Discontinue CPR
- If spontaneous pulse and breathing return.
- Rescuers become exhausted.
- Rescuers are placed in danger.

Dangers of resuscitation

There is understandable concern about the possibility of transmission of blood-borne diseases during resuscitation—particularly HIV and hepatitis B and C. Although viruses can be isolated from the saliva of infected persons, transmission is rare and there are few cases of CPR-related infection in the literature. To minimize the risk of acquiring infection, rescuers should wear gloves and use barriers whenever possible, and great care must be taken with sharps.

Basic life support (CPR)

'For any seriously ill or collapsed patient it is important to assess for level of response and to start cardiopulmonary resuscitation (CPR) if breathing is abnormal or there is no palpable pulse.' (From the *Resuscitation Guidelines* 2010).[2]

Initial management of adult patients
(See Fig. 8.2.)

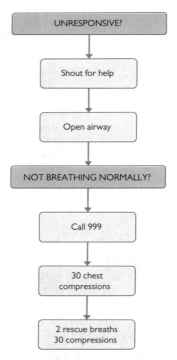

UNRESPONSIVE?

↓

Shout for help

↓

Open airway

↓

NOT BREATHING NORMALLY?

↓

Call 999

↓

30 chest compressions

↓

2 rescue breaths 30 compressions

Fig. 8.2 Adult basic life support algorithm. Reproduced from the Resuscitation Council (UK) Guidelines 2010, with permission.

2 🖰 http://www.resus.org.uk/pages/guide.htm

- Check for a response:
  - Gently shake the shoulders. Ask loudly 'Are you alright?'
- If patient responds:
  - If the individual is able to speak the airway is open and maintained.
  - Leave him in the position you find him, provided there is no further danger.
  - Stabilize the head and neck if there is a possibility of injury (Fig. 5.3).
  - Find out what is wrong and get help (ideally via radio, telephone, or written message), if available.
  Reassess regularly.
- If patient is unresponsive:
  - Shout/call for help.
  - Turn the casualty on his back, whilst maintaining neck control.
  - Institute life support measures.

Assess, open, and manage the airway as described in ➲ Airway, p. 186. Check the airway for 10s.
  If the casualty is not breathing *normally* start CPR (Fig. 8.3):
- Start with 30 chest compressions at a rate of 100–120/min:
  - Kneel beside victim.
  - Place heel of one hand in centre of victim's chest.
  - Place heel of other hand on top of the first hand.
  - Interlock fingers of your hands and ensure pressure is not applied over the victim's ribs, upper abdomen, or bottom end of the bony sternum.
  - Position yourself vertically above the victim's chest and, with straight arms, press down on sternum 5–6 cm.
  - Release pressure without losing contact between your hands and the sternum. Compression and release should take equal time.
- After 30 compressions give two rescue breaths:
  - Open airway with chin lift and head tilt.
  - Pinch soft part of the victim's nose closed with the index finger and thumb of your hand on his forehead.
  - Allow his mouth to open whilst maintaining chin lift.
  - Take a normal breath and place lips around his mouth. Ensure a good seal.
  - Blow steadily into his mouth for about 1 s and watch the chest rise.
  - Maintaining head tilt and chin lift take your mouth away and watch for the chest to fall as air comes out.
  - Take another normal breath and blow into the victim's mouth to give two effective rescue breaths. Immediately return your hands to his sternum and give a further 30 compressions.
- If rescue breaths do not make the chest rise and fall, before next attempt:
  - Check victim's mouth and remove any visible obstruction.
  - Recheck there is adequate head tilt and chin lift.
  - Do not attempt more than two rescue breaths before returning to 30 chest compressions.
- Chest compressions: rescue breath ratio 30:2.

Continue CPR until:
- Normal breathing resumes.
- You become exhausted.
- A more experienced doctor tells you to stop.

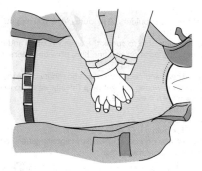

Fig. 8.3 Hand position for CPR.

Core rules of CPR
- Call for assistance.
- Push hard (effective cardiac compressions).
- Push fast (maintain regular cardiac compressions).
- Breathe slowly (excessive ventilation is unnecessary).
- Don't stop (gaps in compression reduce survival).
- Obey automated defibrillator (if available).

Choking

Recognition

Foreign bodies may cause either mild or severe airway obstruction. It is important to ask the conscious victim 'Are you choking?'

General signs of choking
• Attack occurs while eating.
• Victim may clutch his neck.

Signs of mild airway obstruction
Response to question 'Are you choking?':
• Victim is able to speak, cough, and breathe.

Signs of severe airway obstruction
Response to question 'Are you choking?':
• Victim unable to speak.
• Victim unable to breathe.
• Breathing sounds wheezy.
• Attempts at coughing are silent.
• Victim may become unconscious.

Management
(See Fig. 8.4.)

Mild airway obstruction
Encourage him to continue coughing, but do nothing else.

Severe airway obstruction
• Give up to five back blows.
• Stand to the side and slightly behind the victim.
• Support the chest with one hand and lean the victim forwards.
• Give up to five sharp blows between the shoulder blades with the heel of your other hand.

If five back blows fail to relieve the airway obstruction, give up to five abdominal thrusts:
• Stand behind the victim and put both arms round the upper part of his abdomen.
• Lean the victim forwards and clench your fist and place it between the umbilicus (navel) and the bottom end of the breastbone.
• Grasp hand with your other hand and pull sharply inwards and upwards. Repeat up to five times.
• If the obstruction is still not relieved, continue alternating five back blows with five abdominal thrusts.

If the victim becomes unconscious:
• Support the victim carefully to the ground.
• Begin CPR (see ➋ Basic life support (CPR), p. 220).
• If this is unsuccessful, consider a surgical airway (➋ Surgical airways, p. 188).

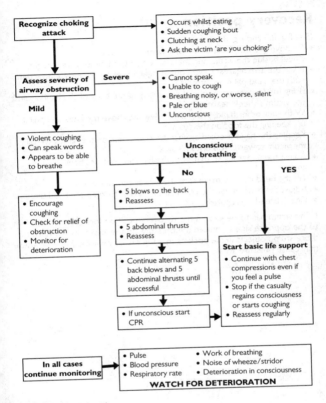

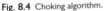

Fig. 8.4 Choking algorithm.

Recovery position

(See Fig. 8.5 and Fig. 8.6.)
- Remove the victim's spectacles, if worn.
- Kneel beside the victim and make sure that both his legs are straight.
- Place the arm nearest to you out at right angles to his body, elbow bent with the hand palm uppermost.
- Bring the far arm across the chest, and hold the back of the hand against the victim's cheek nearest to you.
- With your other hand, grasp the far leg just above the knee and pull it up, keeping the foot on the ground.
- Keeping the hand pressed against the cheek, pull on the far leg to roll the victim towards you onto his side.
- Adjust the upper leg so that both the hip and knee are bent at right angles.
- Tilt the head back to make sure the airway remains open.
- Adjust the hand under the cheek, if necessary, to keep the head tilted.
- Check breathing regularly.

If the victim has to be kept in the recovery position for >30 min turn him to the opposite side to relieve the pressure on the lower arm. Ensure that there are no objects in the pockets that the casualty will be lying on—these may cause pressure areas.

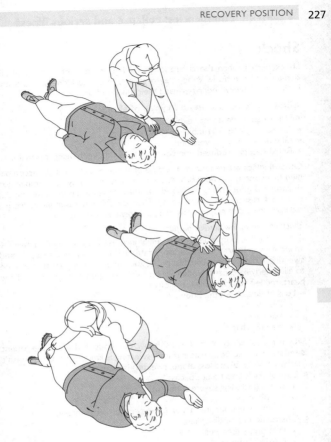

Fig. 8.5 Turning into the recovery position.

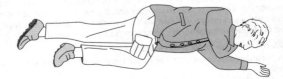

Fig. 8.6 The recovery position.

Shock

Shock occurs when the circulation is inadequate to meet the metabolic demands of the body. When key organs such as the kidneys, heart, and brain are relatively under-perfused their function fails.

Clinical presentation and types of shock

All 'shocked' patients may exhibit:
- Cerebral effects—irritable, drowsy, yawning.
- GI effects—nausea, vomiting.
- Renal effects—reduced urine output (>0.5 mL/kg/h being 'normal').

Other findings will depend on the type of shock. Shock is usually accompanied by hypotension (low BP). Arterial BP is governed by the combination of cardiac output driving the blood into the arteries and peripheral vascular resistance resisting its forward flow. Thus low BP may result either from a *reduction in cardiac output* or from a *fall in peripheral resistance*.

Shock caused by low cardiac output

A fall in cardiac output leads to a reflex increase in sympathetic activity—an increase in heart rate, respiratory rate, peripheral vasoconstriction, and sweating. Cold, clammy skin, fast pulse, and rapid breathing will be common to all underlying causes. Under-filling of the main pumping chamber of the heart, the left ventricle, may result from:
- Loss of fluids from the body:
  - Diarrhoea.
  - Vomiting.
  - Haemorrhage.

Skin turgor (elasticity of the tissues) is low, the mouth is dry, and the patient is thirsty. If whole body water is low, sweating is limited (i.e. the skin isn't 'clammy'). With blood loss alone, sweating is expected.
- Loss of fluids into tissue spaces:
  - Burns (including severe sunburn).
  - Anaphylaxis.
  - Profound hypoproteinaemia (as may occur in dysentery).
- Obstruction to cardiac filling.
  - Pulmonary embolus.
  - Cardiac tamponade.

When fluids have been lost from the body or moved into tissue spaces, neck veins will be empty: when there is obstruction to blood flow from pulmonary embolism or cardiac tamponade, the neck veins will be full and jugular venous pressure will rise with inspiration. Breathlessness may be most profound with pulmonary embolism (as hypoxia contributes).

Shock caused by low peripheral resistance

This occurs in anaphylaxis, or any major systemic inflammatory response, including:
- Severe infection (septic shock).
- Toxins (stings, venom) and/or anaphylaxis.
- Severe sunburn.

Blood vessels vasodilate, peripheral resistance decreases, and therefore BP falls. The inflammatory response directly affects the peripheral blood vessels and so the compensatory sympathetic response cannot cause the blood vessels to constrict; BP remains low. The skin may be warm, hot, or 'patchy'. In sepsis, such 'patchiness' may alter with time (legs freezing one minute, and warm the next). Neck veins will be collapsed, and the skin may sweat due to fever but will not be 'cold and shut down' (i.e. clammy). Pulse rate and cardiac output will be high.

Catches in the wilderness

- The young and fit can maintain BP for a very long time through sympathetic activity. In some cases BP may not fall until around 50% of the circulating volume has been lost.
- Underlying dehydration may be common.
- Urine output may already be low.
- Sweating responses may be reduced—sweating thresholds are altered by acclimatization to ambient temperature and to exercise loads (➔ Acclimatization to heat, p. 754).
- In the heat, most people are vasodilated. In 'heat stroke' (➔ Heat-related illnesses (HRIs), p. 748), severe inflammation coupled with volume loss may lead to a 'shivering clammy' patient, despite a very high central temperature.
- In the cold, most are vasoconstricted.

Management of the shocked patient

- Identify the type of shock.
- As for all major emergencies—make sure that the environment is safe, summon help, and attend to *Airway*, *Breathing* and then *Circulation* (see Chapter 7).
- Control the source of any massive haemorrhage first. Apply direct pressure to the bleeding point and/or use pressure points. Use a tourniquet where necessary and consider Celox® or Quik Clot® (➔ Circulation, p. 194; ➔ Control of haemorrhage, p. 196). Pack deep large wounds and bind firmly.
- Consider IV tranexamic acid, see ➔ Circulation, p. 194.
- Treat anaphylaxis at once (➔ Anaphylaxis and anaphylactic shock, p. 236; Fig. 8.8). Look/listen for signs of airway obstruction such as wheeze, stridor, facial and neck swelling, or/and urticarial (nettles-type) rash.
- If the patient is more than mildly unwell, establish venous access at once. You may find it a lot harder later!
- Stop the losses and treat the causes:
  - Stop all sources of loss (e.g. use antidiarrhoeals, antiemetics, cooling with sponging and fanning, keeping in the shade, light-reflective clothing if sun unavoidable).
  - If septic, seek the source (including the rare, but often missed, retained tampon) and treat at once with broad spectrum antibiotics.
  - Give fluids. Most wilderness victims will be depleted of intravascular volume, as will most with shock of any cause (see ➔ Types of shock, p. 234). The rate and route will be determined by a number of factors: if you have an uncontrolled source of blood loss, internal or external, give fluids cautiously until the source of bleeding is controlled. Raising pressure by rapid resuscitation will make bleeding worse. If fluid supplies are limited, use 'permissive hypotension' (maintain a just palpable radial pulse).
  - If the patient is conscious and able to swallow (without GI tract injury), let the patient drink as a means of conserving IV fluids.
  - No data, beyond anecdote, support the rectal administration of fluids in this context. However, this may be considered in the absence of other means of resuscitation.[3]
  - Consider intraosseous administration if oral or venous routes are unavailable, and you have the kit (and are trained to use it!).
  - During fluid resuscitation, give fluids by 'bolus' of 250 mL, and observe response, especially heart rate. For maintenance, calculate losses (blood loss, diarrhoea, vomiting, from skin in burns), including insensible losses (sweating and breathing, 10–20 mL/kg/day). Once resuscitated with boluses, spread this 'maintenance' over 24 h.
- Treatment endpoints:
  - Control of fluid losses.
  - 'Organ survival and function': urine output >0.5 mL/kg/h; patient is alert and orientated.
  - Improvements in observations—heart rate within normal range and respiratory rate falling, BP rising.

3 Grocott MPW, McCorkell S, Cox ML (2005). Resuscitation from hemorrhagic shock using rectally administered fluids in a wilderness environment. *Wilderness Environ Med*, 16(4), 209–11.

Additional specific treatments depending upon the type of shock are described in Fig. 8.9.

Remember to put this treatment in the context of what is available to you. If you have only 2 L of IV fluids, then you must use them with care to resuscitate fast (e.g. if massive bleed now stopped) or gently (e.g. minor hypotension with continuing losses).

Remember, too, to call for help/evacuate fast. Prompt and sustained resuscitation is vital to survival.

Monitoring shock in the wilderness

BP may be well maintained at first. Look for trends over time and any postural drop (measured while lying then sitting or standing). If in doubt, use sitting BP as standing can provoke loss of consciousness.

● Are heart rate and respiratory rate rising?
● What is happening to:
   ● Skin perfusion (skin colour/temperature)?
   ● Brain (alert/orientated)?
   ● Kidney function (urine output)? Consider a urinary catheter (if you have one) and measure hourly urine output. You can measure with a cup or Nalgene® bottle if no measuring jug.
   ● Breathlessness (reflecting sympathetic activity, and clearance of lactic acidosis through respiratory compensation)?
   ● Record the above on a chart to give a visual display of changes (➔ Documentation, p. 89).
● Fig. 8.7 reproduces the NHS observations chart including the National Early Warning Score (NEWS). Patients whose observations fall outside the normal range require increased monitoring, and deterioration in the score will highlight the need for increased frequency of observations and may guide urgency of a medevac. Expeditions are recommended to obtain equivalent charts to these at full size and in colour as part of their medical stores. Online instruction of the use of NEWS can be found at: ⅏ http://tfinews.ocbmedia.com/#home

Prevention and preparation

● You cannot prevent a fellow traveller becoming seriously ill. However, you can take appropriate equipment.
● Decide on the volume of fluids you will carry, depending on logistic constraints (weight, bulk), duration of trip, evacuation times.
● Take antibiotics for infections and adrenaline (epinephrine), steroids, and antihistamines for anaphylaxis.
● Find out how safe or dangerous local blood sources may be.
● Avoid GI tract infection if possible (➔ Camp health and hygiene, p. 22), and all the other recognized environmental causes.
● Know the arterial pressure points.
● Make sure your cannulation skills are updated.

Observation chart for the National Early Warning Score (NEWS)

| | | NEWS KEY 0 1 2 3 | NAME: | | D.O.B. | | ADMISSION DATE: | |

RESP. RATE			
	≥25		3
	21-24		2
	12-20		
	9-11		1
	≤8		3

SpO₂			
	≥96		
	94-95		1
	92-93		2
	≤91		3
Inspired O₂%	%		2

TEMP			
	≥39°		2
	38°		1
	37°		
	36°		
	≤35°		3

NEW SCORE uses Systolic BP — BLOOD PRESSURE			
	230		3
	220		
	210		
	200		
	190		
	180		
	170		
	160		
	150		
	140		
	130		
	120		
	110		1
	100		2
	90		
	80		
	70		3
	60		
	50		

HEART RATE			
	>140		3
	130		2
	120		
	110		1
	100		
	90		
	80		
	70		
	60		
	50		
	40		1
	30		3

Level of Consciousness	Alert		
	V / P / U		3

| BLOOD SUGAR | | | |

| TOTAL NEW SCORE | | | |

| | Pain Score | | |

Urine Output			
Monitoring Frequency			
Escalation Plan Y/N n/a			
Initials			

National Early Warning Score: July 2012

Please see next page for explanatory text about this chart.

 Royal College of Physicians

NHS
Training for Innovation

© Royal College of Physicians 2012

Fig. 8.7 Observations chart including National Early Warning Score (NEWS).
℗ https://www.rcplondon.ac.uk/sites/default/files/documents/news-observation-chart-with-explanatory-text.pdf; ℗ https://www.rcplondon.ac.uk/sites/default/files/documents/national-early-warning-score-with-explanatory-text.pdf.
Reproduced from Royal College of Physicians. *National Early Warning Score (NEWS): Standardising the assessment of acute illness severity in the NHS.* Report of a working party. London: RCP, 2012 (Review date 2015).

National Early Warning Score (NEWS)*

PHYSIOLOGICAL PARAMETERS	3	2	1	0	1	2	3
Respiration Rate	≤8		9–11	12–20		21–24	≥25
Oxygen Saturations	≤91	92–93	94–95	≥96			
Any Supplemental Oxygen		Yes		No			
Temperature	≤35.0		35.1–36.0	36.1–38.0	38.1–39.0	≥39.1	
Systolic BP	≤90	91–100	101–110	111–219			≥220
Heart Rate	≤40		41–50	51–90	91–110	111–130	≥131
Level of Consciousness				A			V, P, or U

*The NEWS initiative flowed from the Royal College of Physicians' NEWS Development and Implementation Group (NEWSDIG) report, and was jointly developed and funded in collaboration with the Royal College of Physicians, Royal College of Nursing, National Outreach Forum and NHS Training for Innovation

Fig. 8.7 (Contd.)

Types of shock

Hypovolaemic shock

Causes
- Blood loss:
  - External and visible (e.g. external wound).
  - Internal and invisible (e.g. into gut, into muscle around a fractured bone, into chest or abdominal cavity, into tissues behind abdominal contents).
  - Low fluid intake (usually when combined with high losses).
- Loss of fluid from the body:
  - Gut (diarrhoea, vomiting).
  - Skin (extensive grazes, burns).
  - Sweat (fever, environmental heat).
  - Breathing (dry air, high respiratory rates).
- Loss of fluid into tissues:
  - Anaphylaxis.
  - Crush injury.
  - Severe systemic inflammation and sepsis.

Signs
Those of 'low cardiac output shock' (➔ Cardiogenic shock, p. 235).

Specific treatment
Stop losses, fluid challenges of 250 mL IV, calculate daily maintenance and administer over 24 h.

NB Crush injury leads to loss of volume into the tissues, and low output shock. Tissue damage may worsen the inflammatory state and the muscle damage worsens kidney function. Maintain a high urine output if possible. Do not use diuretics (as this will worsen volume depletion). Check for compartment syndrome (as this may be causing low perfusion every bit as much as a fall in systemic perfusion pressure). Fasciotomies (➔ Compartment syndrome, p. 443; ➔ Crush injuries, p. 277) may be needed but beware: fluid losses will be massive. Have you enough IV fluids to keep up?

Septic shock

Causes
Infection in the bloodstream. Sometimes this may be from a wound that is hard to see. In women, ask about possible retained and infected tampon. Urine infection may be a source.

Signs
Those of 'low peripheral resistance shock': tachycardia, high volume pulse, warm skin (or patchy skin temperature distribution which changes), low BP, sweating/sweats. Rigors (severe 'bone-shaking' shivers) may occur.

Specific treatment
- IV fluid challenges of 250 mL IV to resuscitate; calculate daily maintenance and administer over 24 h
- Administer IV broad-spectrum antibiotics (e.g. ceftriaxone 1–2 g IV twice daily)
- Evacuate as soon as possible.

Cardiogenic shock

Causes
- Acute impairment of heart contractile function. In expedition teams, most commonly an acute myocardial infarction.

Signs
- Generally preceded by history of classic cardiac pain (tight across chest, to shoulders, jaw, or down arm(s).
- Signs are those of 'low cardiac output shock': tachycardia, low volume pulse, cold clammy skin, and low BP. Breathlessness. Inspiratory crackles at bases, spreading throughout lungs. (NB At altitude, consider high-altitude pulmonary oedema.) Neck veins may be elevated if right side of heart involved. (NB Consider pulmonary embolus.)

Specific treatment
- This is life-threatening. Arrange evacuation at once. Give oxygen if available.
- Sitting upright may help relieve breathlessness.
- Fluids only if jugular venous pressure not elevated and chest clear (suggesting isolated right heart infarct). Unguided IV fluids may make matters worse.
- If stabilizes over time, may need cautious fluids (100 mL challenges maximum).
- Powerful analgesics to relieve chest pain.
- Aspirin 300 mg to reduce progression of infarct.
- A diuretic may relieve breathlessness if the jugular venous pressure is raised.

Pulmonary embolus

Blood clot impacts in pulmonary arterial circulation. Most commonly originates in leg veins, often after prolonged flight/coach journey/immobility. The risk rises when blood viscosity is high (dehydration, altitude).

Signs
Those of 'low cardiac output shock': tachycardia, low volume pulse, cold clammy skin, low BP. Neck veins may be distended. Look for unilateral (occasionally bilateral) lower limb swelling—may be confined to calf.

Specific treatment
- IV fluid challenges of 250 mL IV to resuscitate.
- Low molecular weight heparin (e.g. enoxaparin) 1.5 mg/kg subcutaneously once daily.

Neurogenic shock

Neurogenic shock is a very rare situation, in which severe damage to the spinal cord disrupts the transmission of 'tightening up' nerve impulses to the small arteries. The blood vessels therefore dilate, and 'low resistance shock' results.

Causes
Spinal cord injury (usually trauma, although inflammatory/infective causes are possible).

Signs

Those of 'low peripheral resistance shock': tachycardia, high volume pulse, warm skin, low BP. Casualty may develop priapism—an involuntary erection of the penis in males (seen with high spinal cord injuries above T6). Other signs of spinal cord injury (sensory loss, weakness or paralysis).

Specific treatment

IV fluids (as the intestines usually stop moving with high spinal cord injury) using 250 mL fluid challenges. Calculate daily maintenance and administer over 24 h. Evacuate as soon as possible. May need a nasogastric tube. Remember pressure area care and immobilization of the entire spine.

Anaphylaxis and anaphylactic shock

Anaphylaxis is a rapidly evolving and often dramatic clinical syndrome, usually precipitated by recent exposure to a substance (allergen) to which the patient is allergic, e.g.:

- Drugs: any, especially penicillins.
- Foods: any, especially nuts, fruits, sea food.
- Environmental factors: animal venoms (e.g. wasp, hornet, bee, ant, or snake), plant substances (latex).

Examination

Anaphylaxis is characterized by one or more of the following features in any combination:

- Rash and/or mucous membrane involvement: urticaria ('hives', 'weals', 'welts'), flushing, itching, generalized erythema and swelling owing to massive extravasation of fluid and swelling of the lips, tongue, gums, and uvula.
- Life-threatening circulatory collapse ('anaphylactic shock') caused by vasodilatation and/or hypovolaemia: premonitory features include dizziness, loss of vision, tachycardia, falling BP, and loss of consciousness.
- Life-threatening airway obstruction: lower airways— bronchoconstriction/ asthma or, less often, upper airway— angio-oedema of the larynx. The signs include wheeze, tachypnoea, stridor ('croup'), and cyanosis.
- GI symptoms (vomiting, diarrhoea, retrosternal pain, abdominal colic).

Patients look and feel severely unwell, are usually anxious, and may have a feeling of impending doom. In extreme cases, they may collapse and lose consciousness within minutes of allergen exposure. Some present with shock and hypotension alone.

Worrying features

- Upper airway obstruction.
- Wheeze.
- Systolic BP <90 mmHg.

Differential diagnosis
- Asthma.
- Heart attack or pulmonary embolism (chest pain, shock, respiratory distress).
- Faint, panic attack.
- Vasovagal attack precipitated by injections, stings or sharp trauma (but this will be associated with bradycardia).

Prevention and risk management
- Those with known allergy should carry an adrenaline (epinephrine) auto-injector such as EpiPen®, Jext®, or Emerade®.
- Companions should know the location of the auto-injector and how to use it (Fig. 8.8).
- Ensure cooks are aware of food allergies.

Further treatment
(See Fig. 8.9.)
- Maintain BP >90 mmHg systolic. Give IV fluids as required.
- *If bronchospasm is severe/persistent* despite adrenaline, give bronchodilator by inhalation (salbutamol, ipratropium).
- *If cardiac arrest occurs*: follow guidelines for cardiopulmonary resuscitation. Early advanced life support is essential. IM adrenaline is unlikely to be beneficial in this setting so try an IV route or intraoral/intra-airway.
- Monitor urine output.
- Continue chlorphenamine 4 mg/8 h PO.
- Consider a short course of steroids—prednisolone 40 mg/24 h for 5 days to prevent recurrent anaphylaxis.

The patient may require evacuation for further investigation.

Resources
Association of Anaesthetists of Great Britain and Ireland: ℘ http://www.aagbi.org
British Society for Allergy and Clinical Immunology: ℘ http://www.basci.org
European Academy of Allergology and Clinical Immunology: ℘ http://www.eaaci.net
European Resuscitation Council: ℘ http://www.erc.edu
Resuscitation Council UK: ℘ http://www.resus.org.uk

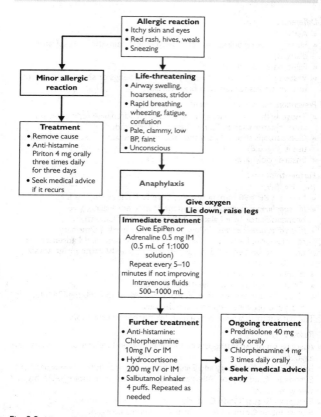

Fig. 8.8 Allergy and anaphylaxis algorithm.

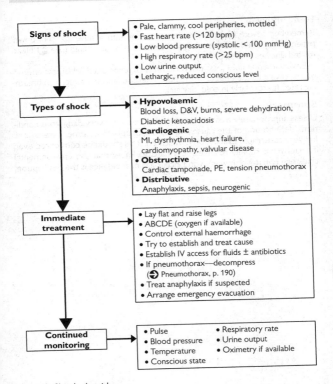

Fig. 8.9 Shock algorithm.

Heat injury

Remember, severe hyperthermia may present with a shivering 'shut-down' patient. They need active cooling and sometimes a lot of fluid (see ➔ Heat-related illnesses (HRIs), p. 748).

Environmental fluid loss: dehydration is *common in all wilderness environments*, owing to the effects of the heat, exercise, and sweating, high breathing rates (particularly in cold, dry air).

Summary

Unless appropriately treated, shock of any cause is a very dangerous condition. Identification of the cause and rapid appropriate treatment are crucial. In every case, rapid evacuation is indicated. This should be considered even if anaphylaxis rapidly resolves: it is hard to know that the environmental challenge (whatever it was) won't occur again; avoidance is the best option.

Chest pain

History
- *Site* of main pain and any radiation to arms, neck, jaw, or back.
- *Character* of pain—heavy, sharp, tight, pleuritic (worse on inspiration).
- *Severity*—out of ten.
- *Onset*—at rest or during exertion.
- *Nature*—whether constant and aggravated by exertion, position, eating, breathing, or relieved by analgesics, antacids, or GTN.
- *Associated symptoms*—sweating, breathlessness, nausea, palpitations.
- *Trauma*—nature of any injury.
- *Past history*—cardiac or respiratory problems, acid indigestion.
- *Drugs*—cardiac or respiratory drugs, antacids.
- *Social and environmental factors*—alcohol/drugs, smoking status, recent stressors.

Cardiac disease risk factors
- Previous ischaemic heart disease (IHD).
- Smoking.
- Hypertension.
- Obesity.
- Diabetes.
- Family history of IHD.
- Hypercholesterolaemia.

Venous thrombosis or pulmonary embolism risk factors
- Previous thromboembolic disease (DVT or pulmonary embolism).
- Smoking.
- Immobility.
- Dehydration.
- Pro-thrombotic conditions.
- Oestrogen containing medication—HRT/OCP.
- Recent surgery/long travel/leg injuries.

Gastrointestinal risk factors
- Gastro-oesophageal reflux disease (GORD).
- Previous peptic ulceration.
- Alcohol excess.

Examination
- Temperature, pulse, respiration rate, BP in both arms, GCS score.
- General condition—cyanosis, pallor, sweating.
- Pulse rate, rhythm, character, BP, look for elevation and dilatation of the neck veins, listen to the heart sounds (any murmurs?), look for signs of cardiac failure (basal crackles in the lungs and swelling of the ankles), look for calf swelling or redness/tenderness.
- Feel for position of windpipe, and assess for chest wall tenderness.
- Feel the abdomen for localized tenderness or a pulsatile mass (abdominal aortic aneurysm).
- Check blood glucose.

See Fig. 8.10 for management.

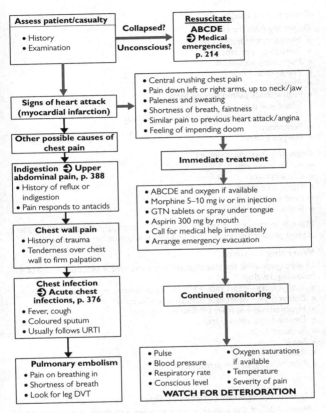

Fig. 8.10 Management of chest pain.

Differential diagnosis

Originating from the chest
- Myocardial infarction/angina.
- Tension pneumothorax.
- Pulmonary embolism.
- Pneumonia.
- Pleurisy.
- High altitude pulmonary oedema.
- Chest wall pain.
- Gastro-oesophageal reflux disease (GORD).
- Pericarditis.
- Herpes zoster.

Originating from the abdomen
- Aortic aneurysm.
- Cholecystitis.
- Peptic ulceration.
- Pancreatitis.
- Sickle cell crisis.

Make a 'best guess' diagnosis and treat accordingly. Observe the patient closely, record the details on a TPR chart, and monitor urine output.

Worrying features

Urgent evacuation for investigation and treatment is indicated if any of the following develop:
- Tachycardia—heart rate >100 bpm persistently or irregular rhythm.
- Bradycardia—heart rate persistently <50 bpm.
- Hypotension—systolic BP <90 mmHg.
- Elevated respiration rate.
- Reduced GCS.
- Sweating.
- Vomiting.
- Pain radiating to jaw, arms, or back.

Urgent treatment (of chest pain)

Assess ABC. If the patient is unresponsive and there is no respiratory effort and/or no palpable pulse, commence CPR.

If the patient is conscious:
- Sit patient up.
- Give high-flow oxygen if available.
- Consider aspirin, GTN, and IV analgesia if cardiac cause seems likely (Fig. 8.10).
- Monitor pulse, BP, and respiratory rate.

Shortness of breath (dyspnoea)

(See Fig. 8.11.)

History

- *Dyspnoea*—speed of onset, cough, wheeze.
- *Sputum* (colour, quantity, any blood).
- *Chest pain*—characterize any pain (see ➔ Chest pain, p. 242).
- *Associated symptoms*—sweating, nausea, palpitations.
- *Trauma*—nature of injury if present.
- *Past history*—cardiac or respiratory problems.
- *Drugs*—inhalers, respiratory or cardiac drugs.
- *Allergies*—medication and environmental, food, other allergens.
- *Social/environmental*—smoking status, travel history (➔ Fever, p. 262).
- *Risk factors for pulmonary embolism/DVT*—previous thromboembolic disease, smoking, obesity, immobility, dehydration, high altitude, pro-thrombotic conditions, HRT/OCP, recent surgery/long travel, leg injuries.

Examination

- Temperature, pulse, respiratory rate, BP, GCS score.
- General condition—confusion, cyanosis, pallor, cool peripheries, sweating, tremor, use of accessory muscles. Can the patient count to ten in one breath?
- Pulse rate, rhythm, BP, look for elevation and dilatation of the neck veins. Measure peak expiratory flow rate if possible, look for tracheal tug/deviation, percuss the chest, listen for air entry and breath sounds—normal, crackles, wheezes or absent. Look for calf swelling/redness/tenderness or ankle swelling (DVT)
- Feel the abdomen for localized tenderness or a pulsatile mass (abdominal aortic aneurysm).

Differential diagnosis

Wheeze present:
- Asthma or chronic obstructive pulmonary disease (COPD ➔ Asthma, p. 380).
- Anaphylaxis (➔ Allergy and anaphylaxis, p. 54; ➔ Anaphylaxis and anaphylactic shock, p. 236).

No clinical signs:
- Pulmonary embolism.
- Hyperventilation (➔ Anxiety disorders, p. 522).
- Diabetic ketoacidosis (➔ Diabetic ketoacidosis, p. 258).

Crackles audible:
- Pneumonia (➔ Acute chest infections, p. 376).
- High-altitude pulmonary oedema (➔ High-altitude pulmonary oedema, p. 661).
- Heart failure.

Stridor present:
- Foreign body (➔ Shortness of breath (dyspnoea), p. 246).

Absent breath sounds:
- Pneumothorax (➔ Pneumothorax, p. 190).

Make a 'best guess' diagnosis and treat accordingly. Observe the patient closely; record the details on a TPR chart.

Worrying features

Urgent evacuation for investigation and treatment are indicated if any of the following develop:

- Respiratory rate >30 breaths/min.
- Tachycardia or bradycardia.
- Core temperature >39°C.
- Hypotension.
- Reduced GCS (see Box 7.1).
- Exhaustion.

> ### Urgent treatment of shortness of breath
>
> Assess ABC. If the patient is unresponsive and there is no respiratory effort and/or no palpable pulse, commence CPR (🠊 Basic Life support (CPR), p. 220).
> If the patient is conscious:
> - Sit patient up.
> - Give high flow oxygen if available.
> - Monitor pulse, BP, and respiratory rate.

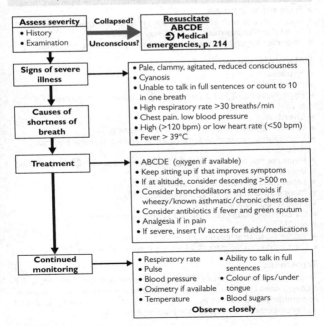

Fig. 8.11 Shortness of breath algorithm.

Coma

Unrousable unresponsiveness. (See Fig. 8.12.)

History (from bystanders)

- How/where found.
- Sudden or gradual onset.
- Seizure.
- Any trauma.
- Recent illness—headache, chest pain, breathlessness, palpitations, fever, confusion, depression, sinusitis, seizures, vomiting.
- Past history—cardiac, respiratory, diabetes, hypertension, psychiatric illness.
- Drugs—overdose? Sedative or hypnotic medication.
- Social/environmental—alcohol, illicit drugs, travel to malarial area.

Examination

- GCS score.
- Check pupil responses frequently.
- Smell the breath—alcohol, ketones.
- Rashes, signs of dehydration, cyanosis, pallor, needle injection marks.
- Signs of external head injury—bruising, haematoma, CSF from ears/nose.
- Fever and neck stiffness.
- Localizing signs such as increased tone in limbs, asymmetrical reflexes.
- Heart/lung for murmurs, rubs, wheeze, crackles.
- Abdomen for organomegaly, aortic aneurysm, bruising, melaena.

Differential diagnosis

- Hypoxia.
- Hypotension.
- Hypoglycaemia (➔ Diabetes, p. 50; ➔ Diabetic emergencies, p. 256; Fig 8.16).
- Overdose.
- Epilepsy (➔ Blackouts, syncope, and epilepsy, p. 316).
- High-altitude cerebral oedema (➔ High-altitude cerebral oedema, p. 664).
- Hypothermia/hyperthermia (➔ Hypothermia, p. 622; ➔ Heat-related illnesses (HRIs), p. 748).
- Sepsis (pneumonia, uro-sepsis, toxic shock).
- Meningitis/encephalitis (➔ Meningitis, p. 473).
- Malaria (➔ Malaria, p. 480).
- Carbon monoxide poisoning (➔ Carbon monoxide poisoning, p. 735).
- Subdural/ subarachnoid haemorrhage, stroke.
- Decompression sickness (➔ Decompression sickness, p. 736).

Treatment

Treat any identifiable cause. Monitor vital signs and urine output. If full recovery does not occur, evacuate for further investigation and treatment. Remember pressure area care, maintenance fluids, and temperature control during evacuation. Catheterize the bladder if possible.

Urgent treatment

- ABC.
- Consider oropharyngeal or nasopharyngeal airway.
- Give high-flow oxygen, if available.
- Stabilize the cervical spine if there is a history of trauma.
- Measure blood glucose and body temperature.
- Obtain venous access and consider IV fluids.
- Control seizures, treat hypoglycaemia (BM <4).
- Treat life-threatening infection if suspected.
- Monitor vital signs: pulse, BP, respiration rate, GCS.

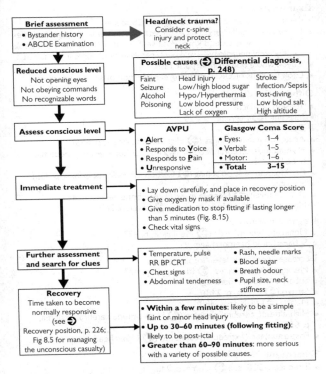

Fig. 8.12 Loss of consciousness algorithm.

Headache

(See Fig. 8.13.)

History

- Headache—severity, location, character, speed of onset, nausea/vomiting, head injury?
- Direct questions—dizziness, blackouts/fits, visual changes.
- Past history—previous headaches, migraine.
- Drugs—recent change in medication.
- Social/environmental—alcohol/drugs, recent stressors, post-diving or change in elevation.

Examination

- Temperature, pulse, BP, blood sugar, GCS score.
- Evidence of head injury? Neck stiffness, photophobia, Kernig's (fully flex hip and passively extend knee. Positive if painful in head or neck). Look for any focal neurology—weakness/paralysis or changes in sensation.
- Check whole body for purpuric rash.
- Look for signs of URTI, including ear infection or sinus tenderness.

Differential diagnosis

- Tension headache.
- Migraine (➜ Migraine, p. 320).
- Dehydration.
- Acute mountain sickness (➜ High-altitude illness, p. 656).
- High-altitude cerebral oedema (➜ High-altitude cerebral oedema, p. 664).
- Carbon monoxide poisoning (➜ Carbon monoxide poisoning, p. 735).
- Sinusitis.
- Dengue fever (➜ Dengue fever ('break bone' fever), p. 465).
- Malaria and other febrile illnesses (➜ Fever, p. 262).

If signs of meningism:
- Meningitis/encephalitis (➜ Meningitis, p. 473).
- Subarachnoid haemorrhage.

Decreased conscious level/localizing signs:
- Meningitis/encephalitis (➜ Meningitis, p. 473).
- Subarachnoid haemorrhage.
- Stroke (➜ Coma, p. 248).
- Malaria (➜ Malaria, p. 480).
- High-altitude cerebral oedema (➜ High-altitude cerebral oedema, p. 664).
- Post-traumatic (extradural, subdural) (➜ Open head injury, p. 314).

Treatment

- If reduced GCS, see ➜ Coma, p. 248.
- Focal neurology or possibility of meningitis/encephalitis: give oxygen, broad-spectrum antibiotics such as IV ceftriaxone or oral ciprofloxacin, evacuate urgently.
- Give fluids and regular analgesia. Advise rest. Observe closely.

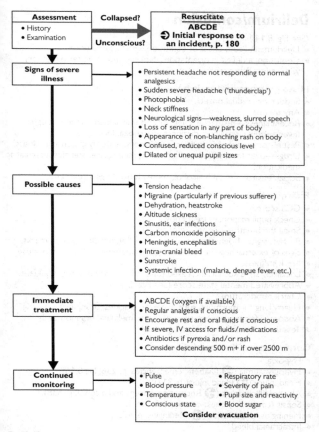

| Assessment
• History
• Examination | Collapsed?

Unconscious? | Resuscitate
ABCDE
⤷ Initial response to
an incident, p. 180 |

| Signs of severe illness | → | • Persistent headache not responding to normal analgesics
• Sudden severe headache ('thunderclap')
• Photophobia
• Neck stiffness
• Neurological signs—weakness, slurred speech
• Loss of sensation in any part of body
• Appearance of non-blanching rash on body
• Confused, reduced conscious level
• Dilated or unequal pupil sizes |

| Possible causes | → | • Tension headache
• Migraine (particularly if previous sufferer)
• Dehydration, heatstroke
• Altitude sickness
• Sinusitis, ear infections
• Carbon monoxide poisoning
• Meningitis, encephalitis
• Intra-cranial bleed
• Sunstroke
• Systemic infection (malaria, dengue fever, etc.) |

| Immediate treatment | → | • ABCDE (oxygen if available)
• Regular analgesia if conscious
• Encourage rest and oral fluids if conscious
• If severe, IV access for fluids/medications
• Antibiotics if pyrexia and/or rash
• Consider descending 500 m+ if over 2500 m |

| Continued monitoring | → | • Pulse • Respiratory rate
• Blood pressure • Severity of pain
• Temperature • Pupil size and reactivity
• Conscious state • Blood sugar
Consider evacuation |

Fig. 8.13 Headache algorithm.

Delirium/confusion

(See Fig. 8.14.)
- Delirium: an acute onset of confusion with hallucinations.
- Confusion: a deficit in orientation, thinking, and short-term memory with reduced awareness.

History (from bystanders)
- Sudden or gradual onset.
- Any trauma.
- Recent illness—headache, chest or abdominal pain, dysuria, cough, fever, seizures, vomiting, dizziness, diarrhoea, incontinence.
- Past history—diabetes, cardiac, respiratory, epilepsy, psychiatric illness.
- Drugs—overdose, sedatives/hypnotics, mefloquine, steroids, psychiatric medication.
- Social/environmental—alcohol, recreational drugs, usual state.

Examination
- GCS score.
- Check pupil responses frequently.
- Smell the breath—alcohol, ketones.
- Rashes, signs of dehydration, cyanosis, pallor, needle injection marks.
- Signs of external head injury—bruising, haematoma, CSF from ears/nose.
- Neck stiffness.
- Localizing signs such as increased tone in limbs, asymmetrical reflexes.
- Abbreviated mental state score (see Box 8.1).
- Check temperature.
- Heart/lung for murmurs, rubs, wheeze, crackles, or injuries.
- Abdomen for tenderness, signs of injury, melaena, organomegaly.
- Test the urine and check blood glucose.

Confusion—differential diagnosis
- Hypoxia.
- Hypoglycaemia (➔ Diabetic emergencies, p. 256; Fig 8.16).
- Head injury (➔ Head injury, p. 312).
- Alcohol/illicit drugs (➔ Recreational drugs and alcohol, p. 538).
- Sepsis (commonly chest or urine infection).
- Meningitis/encephalitis (➔ Meningitis, p. 473).
- Intracranial bleed.
- Stroke (CVA) (➔ Coma, p. 248).
- Drug toxicity.
- Malaria (➔ Malaria, p. 480).
- High-altitude cerebral oedema (➔ High-altitude cerebral oedema, p. 664).
- Post-ictal (➔ Epilepsy, p. 318).

Treatment
Treat any identifiable cause. Do not leave patient alone. Sedate only with great caution: lorazepam 1–2 mg PO/IM/IV. This may allow more detailed examination if the patient is very agitated/confused. Observe closely and evacuate for further investigation/treatment if complete recovery is delayed.

Box 8.1 Abbreviated mental test score (AMTS)

Age	1
Date of birth	1
Repeat 42 West Street	0
Year	1
Time (nearest hour)	1
Current location	1
Recognize two people	1
Year World War II ended	1
Name of the monarch	1
Count backward from 20 to 1	1
Recall 42 West Street	1
Total	10

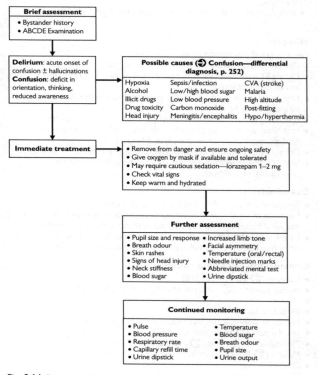

Brief assessment
- Bystander history
- ABCDE Examination

Delirium: acute onset of confusion ± hallucinations
Confusion: deficit in orientation, thinking, reduced awareness

Possible causes (⊖ Confusion—differential diagnosis, p. 252)

Hypoxia	Sepsis/infection	CVA (stroke)
Alcohol	Low/high blood sugar	Malaria
Illicit drugs	Low blood pressure	High altitude
Drug toxicity	Carbon monoxide	Post-fitting
Head injury	Meningitis/encephalitis	Hypo/hyperthermia

Immediate treatment
- Remove from danger and ensure ongoing safety
- Give oxygen by mask if available and tolerated
- May require cautious sedation—lorazepam 1–2 mg
- Check vital signs
- Keep warm and hydrated

Further assessment
- Pupil size and response
- Breath odour
- Skin rashes
- Signs of head injury
- Neck stiffness
- Blood sugar
- Increased limb tone
- Facial asymmetry
- Temperature (oral/rectal)
- Needle injection marks
- Abbreviated mental test
- Urine dipstick

Continued monitoring
- Pulse
- Blood pressure
- Respiratory rate
- Capillary refill time
- Urine dipstick
- Temperature
- Blood sugar
- Breath odour
- Pupil size
- Urine output

Fig. 8.14 Delirium/confusion algorithm.

Convulsions

(See Fig. 8.15.)

Urgent treatment

- Airway: roll patient into the recovery position, protect from further harm but do not restrain. Consider oxygen and a nasopharyngeal airway.
- Breathing: if no respiratory effort commence CPR.
- Circulation and drugs: attempt venous access. Measure blood glucose; if <3.5 mmol/L give 100 mL glucose 10% by infusion. Recheck levels subsequently. Give lorazepam 4 mg IV over 2 min or diazepam 10 mg PR if no IV access.
- If fits continue for >20 min, consider diazepam by infusion 100 mg in 500 mL of 5% glucose; infuse 40 mL/h. Phenytoin is unlikely to be available.
- If seizures continue, make arrangements for urgent evacuation.

History

Get a detailed description of the seizure or fit:
- Onset—activity, position, warning, tonic, starting in one limb?
- During fit—sounds, cyanosis, breathing, eye, facial and limb movements, incontinence, duration.
- Post-fit—tongue injury, post-ictal state, limb weakness, muscle pain/ injuries, headache.
- Preceding illness—headache, chest pain, palpitations, dyspnoea.
- Past history—previous seizures, diabetes, alcoholism, pregnancy, cardiac, respiratory or renal disease. Head injury.
- Drugs—antiepileptics, oral hypoglycaemics, medication compliance.
- Social/environmental—alcohol/drugs, recent feverish illness, post-diving, high altitude.

Examination

- Temperature, pulse, BP, blood sugar, GCS score.
- Evidence of head injury? Sweating, neck stiffness, photophobia. Look for any focal neurology—weakness/paralysis or changes in sensation.
- Check whole body for injury—posterior dislocation of the shoulder is often missed (check for full, pain-free movements of both shoulders).

Convulsions—possible causes

- Epilepsy (➔ Epilepsy, p. 318).
- Hypoglycaemia (➔ Diabetic emergencies, p. 256; Fig. 8.16).
- Hypoxia.
- Alcohol withdrawal.
- Metabolic (low calcium, hyponatraemia/hypernatraemia).
- Head injury (➔ Head injury, p. 312).
- Meningitis/encephalitis (➔ Meningitis, p. 473).
- Malaria (➔ Malaria, p. 480).
- Drug overdose.
- Hypertension/eclampsia.

Treatment after convulsion
- If reduced GCS see ➋ Coma, p. 248.
- Focal neurology or possibility of meningitis/encephalitis evacuate urgently.
- Otherwise give fluids and regular analgesia. Advise rest. Observe closely. If a first fit, evacuate for hospital investigations.

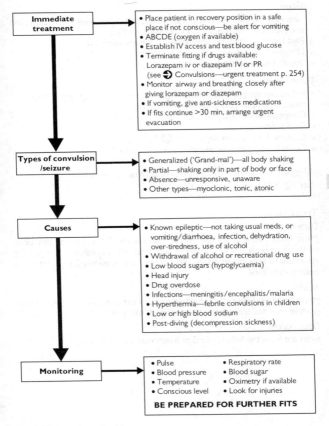

Immediate treatment	→	• Place patient in recovery position in a safe place if not conscious—be alert for vomiting • ABCDE (oxygen if available) • Establish IV access and test blood glucose • Terminate fitting if drugs available: Lorazepam iv or diazepam IV or PR (see ➋ Convulsions—urgent treatment p. 254) • Monitor airway and breathing closely after giving lorazepam or diazepam • If vomiting, give anti-sickness medications • If fits continue >30 min, arrange urgent evacuation
Types of convulsion /seizure	→	• Generalized ('Grand-mal')—all body shaking • Partial—shaking only in part of body or face • Absence—unresponsive, unaware • Other types—myoclonic, tonic, atonic
Causes	→	• Known epileptic—not taking usual meds, or vomiting/diarrhoea, infection, dehydration, over-tiredness, use of alcohol • Withdrawal of alcohol or recreational drug use • Low blood sugars (hypoglycaemia) • Head injury • Drug overdose • Infections—meningitis/encephalitis/malaria • Hyperthermia—febrile convulsions in children • Low or high blood sodium • Post-diving (decompression sickness)
Monitoring	→	• Pulse • Respiratory rate • Blood pressure • Blood sugar • Temperature • Oximetry if available • Conscious level • Look for injuries **BE PREPARED FOR FURTHER FITS**

Fig. 8.15 Convulsion algorithm.

Diabetic emergencies

Hypoglycaemia
- Coma or low GCS with blood glucose <4 mmol/L.
- Can occur in non-diabetics—sepsis, alcohol excess, liver failure, malaria, quinine therapy.

History
- Sweating, hunger, anxiety, inappropriate behaviour, exercise, seizure, last meal, previous hypos, usual blood sugar levels.
- Past history—diabetes, liver disease. Recent infection.
- Drugs—insulin dose, oral hypoglycaemics.
- Social/environmental—alcohol excess.

Examination
- Pallor, sweating, tremor, slurred speech, confusion/aggression, focal neurology, poor coordination, convulsions.
- Check observations: pulse, BP, respiratory rate.
- GCS score.
- Examine for cause of sepsis: see ⊃ Fever, p. 262.
- Consider card test for malaria such as Rapimal®.

Urgent treatment of hypoglycaemia
See Fig. 8.16.

Treatment
Diabetes

Most likely cause is excess insulin, particularly if the patient has been undertaking unusually high levels of activity on the expedition. If hypos are recurrent reduce insulin doses. Monitor blood glucose regularly, preferably before each meal.

Alcohol

Hypoglycaemia may recur if further excess alcohol is taken. Monitor blood glucose until patient is sober and eating/drinking normally.

Other causes

Evacuate from the field for further investigations/treatment.

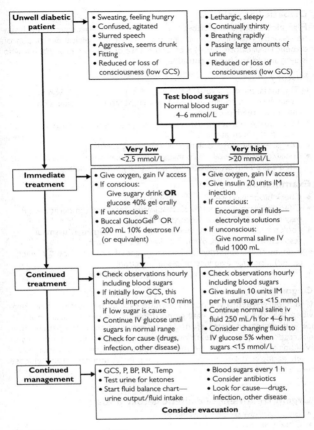

Unwell diabetic patient	• Sweating, feeling hungry • Confused, agitated • Slurred speech • Aggressive, seems drunk • Fitting • Reduced or loss of consciousness (low GCS)	• Lethargic, sleepy • Continually thirsty • Breathing rapidly • Passing large amounts of urine • Reduced or loss of consciousness (low GCS)

Test blood sugars
Normal blood sugar
4–6 mmol/L

	Very low <2.5 mmol/L	**Very high** >20 mmol/L
Immediate treatment	• Give oxygen, gain IV access • If conscious: Give sugary drink **OR** glucose 40% gel orally • If unconscious: Buccal GlucoGel® OR 200 mL 10% dextrose IV (or equivalent)	• Give oxygen, gain IV access • Give insulin 20 units IM injection • If conscious: Encourage oral fluids—electrolyte solutions • If unconscious: Give normal saline IV fluid 1000 mL
Continued treatment	• Check observations hourly including blood sugars • If initially low GCS, this should improve in <10 mins if low sugar is cause • Continue IV glucose until sugars in normal range • Check for cause (drugs, infection, other disease)	• Check observations hourly including blood sugars • Give insulin 10 units IM per h until sugars <15 mmol • Continue normal saline iv fluid 250 mL/h for 4–6 hrs • Consider changing fluids to IV glucose 5% when sugars <15 mmol/L
Continued management	• GCS, P, BP, RR, Temp • Test urine for ketones • Start fluid balance chart—urine output/fluid intake	• Blood sugars every 1 h • Consider antibiotics • Look for cause—drugs, infection, other disease

Consider evacuation

Fig. 8.16 Diabetic emergencies.

Diabetic ketoacidosis

High blood sugars in a diabetic patient with poor glycaemic control may be secondary to infection or steroids. The classical clinical description of diabetic ketoacidosis (DKA) is of a comatose or pre-comatose patient who is dehydrated and hyperventilating.

History

- Tiredness, thirst, polyuria, frequency, dysuria, weight loss, vomiting, breathlessness, cough, sputum, fever, chest/abdominal pain, skin infections, teeth problems.
- Past history—diabetes, date of diagnosis, complications such as neuropathy, ulceration.
- Drugs—insulin dose, oral hypoglycaemics, steroids.
- Social/environmental—alcohol consumption, change in usual diet— often a problem on expeditions, particularly while travelling.

Examination

- Check blood glucose.
- Check observations: pulse, BP, respiratory rate, and temperature. BP may be low. GCS score. Record on chart.
- Look for facial flushing, dry mouth, and rapid breathing (Kussmaul respirations), 'pear-drop' smell of ketones on breath.
- Examine chest, abdomen, and skin for signs of infection (see ➋ Fever, p. 262). Look for evidence of dental infection.
- Test the urine for ketonuria or evidence for infection.

Ongoing treatment

Mild hyperglycaemia will not necessitate evacuation from the field, provided that the patient is eating and drinking and blood sugars normalize with increased doses of insulin and rehydration. If the patient does not respond rapidly to treatment, evacuate urgently; limited amounts of IV fluids will be available on most expeditions. Change to usual insulin when eating and ketonuria <1+. Continue to monitor blood glucose regularly, preferably before each meal.

Urgent treatment of diabetic ketoacidosis

- Give high-flow oxygen, if available.
- Obtain venous access.
- Insulin: give 20 units soluble insulin IM followed by 10 units IM/h. When patient has improved and is eating change to insulin SC
- Fluids: give 1L normal saline IV, then 250 mL/h for 4–6 h.
- When blood glucose <15 mmol/L change to glucose 5% 250 mL/h for 4–6 h (continue insulin 10 units IM/h).
- Start a fluid balance chart and measure urine output.
- Start antibiotics if any cause for infection identified.
- Monitor blood glucose hourly.
- See Fig 8.16: diabetic emergencies algorithm.

Gastrointestinal bleeding

History

- *Vomit*—colour, quantity, blood mixed in, frequency, onset, pain on vomiting.
- *Stools*—onset, quantity, colour (red, black, clots), pain on opening bowels, constipation, diarrhoea, change in bowel habit.
- *Other*—appetite, dysphagia, weight loss, dyspnoea, palpitations, tiredness, dizziness, fainting, sweating, abdominal/chest pain.
- *Past history*—previous bleeding, clotting problems, inflammatory bowel disease, liver disease (varices?), peptic ulceration, heartburn/indigestion.
- *Drugs*—aspirin, NSAIDs, steroids, warfarin, clopidogrel, dabigatran, iron, PPIs/antacids.
- *Social/environmental*—alcohol/drugs, smoking status, recent stressors.

Examination

- Temperature, pulse, BP, blood sugar, GCS score.
- Look for ongoing bleeding, evidence of shock, abdominal distension/tenderness/rebound/masses. Bowel sounds. PR examination for fresh blood/melaena/palpable mass/haemorrhoids.

Gastrointestinal bleeding—differential diagnosis

Upper GI

- Gastro-duodenal ulceration (⊃ Peptic ulcer disease, p. 388).
- Mallory–Weiss tears (⊃ Upper gastrointestinal bleeding, p. 396).
- Oesophageal varices.
- GI malignancy.

Lower GI

- Haemorrhoids/anal fissure (⊃ Haemorrhoids, p. 397).
- Inflammatory bowel disease.
- Diverticular disease.

Treatment

- Keep nil by mouth for 24 h. Maintain BP >90 mmHg systolic by cautious use of fluids. Give analgesia as required (not NSAIDs or aspirin!). Monitor urine output. Consider PPI/antacids. Avoid spicy food. Observe regularly and evacuate for further investigation.
- See Fig. 8.17: GI bleeding algorithm.

Urgent treatment

- Place the patient supine with legs elevated. If vomiting, place in the recovery position.
- Give high-flow oxygen.
- Check observations: pulse, BP, respiratory rate, and temperature.
- Obtain venous access.
- Consider IV saline depending on pulse and BP.

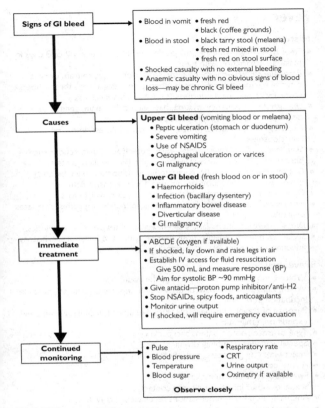

Fig. 8.17 Gastrointestinal bleed algorithm.

Fever

History

- *Fever type*—high swinging, low grade, periodic (i.e. every 2 or 3 days in malaria), association with rigors.
- *Respiratory/ENT*—cough, wheeze, stridor or croup, sputum or nasal catarrh, haemoptysis, dyspnoea, chest pain, otalgia, sore throat, hoarse voice, facial pain, or tenderness (sinusitis), coryzal illness.
- *Urinogenital*—frequency, dysuria, haematuria, loin pain, genital discharge/ulceration, suprapubic pain.
- *Neurological*—headache, photophobia, neck stiffness, impaired consciousness.
- *Skin/mucous membranes/joints*—rash, petechiae, skin infections such as bites/ulcers/sores, mucosal lesions, arthralgia, swollen joints.
- *Gastrointestinal*—vomiting, haematemesis, abdominal pain, bloating, diarrhoea, blood in stools or melaena, foul/excessive flatus.
- *Other*—changes in appetite, aching, night sweats, weight loss.
- *Past history*—previous similar symptoms, immunocompromise, diabetes mellitus.
- *Drugs*—steroids, antimalarials taken regularly, antipyretics, antibiotics.
- *Social/environmental*—infectious disease contact, detailed travel history, adequacy of pre-travel vaccinations.

Travel history

- Which countries and which parts of the countries?
- When? Length of trip, date of arrival, and departure (estimate possible incubation period).
- Purpose of travel—business, pleasure, family visit, military, airline crew, expedition, emigration?
- Type of travel, hotels, safari, backpacking.
- Special activities (climbing, diving, caving)?
- Insect bites/stings (tsetse, ticks, fleas).
- Animal contact.
- Swimming in fresh water lakes.
- Sexual or other infectious disease contact.
- Antimalarials taken/immunizations received pre-travel.
- Illness among other members of the family or party.

Examination

- Temperature (chart if possible), pulse/respiratory rate, BP, GCS score, urine output.
- Warm or cool peripheries, capillary refill time (➜ Capillary refill time, p. 417), sweating, rash, mucosal lesions, wounds, abscesses, insect bites, ulcers, eschar, buboes, cellulitis, or other focal skin infection (examine the entire body surface, including the scalp, axillae, and perineum). Look up the nose and at throat, tonsils, tongue, and buccal mucous membrane. Look in the ears with an auriscope. Examine chest for breath sounds and heart murmurs; abdominal tenderness, bowel sounds, lymphadenopathy; joint pain or swelling, external genitalia (retained tampon) and rectal examination if relevant.

Investigations

Usually impossible. The macroscopic appearance and odour of vomitus, stool, and urine may be helpful (e.g. obvious blood; cloudiness and foul fishy smell of urine suggest infection). Consider dip testing urine, microscopic examination of blood, sputum, urine, stool (experience required). Rapid antigen tests for malaria (see ➜ Malaria, p. 480).

Possible diagnoses

- *URTI*—viral coryza, sinusitis, otitis media, tonsillitis, 'strep' throat.
- *Chest*—bronchitis, pneumonia, tuberculosis.
- *Gut*—gastroenteritis, dysentery.
- *Urinary*—UTI, pyelonephritis.
- *Neurological*—meningitis/encephalitis.
- *Tropical infections*—malaria, dengue, typhoid, legionella, leptospirosis, hepatitis, rabies, typhus/other rickettsiae, viral haemorrhagic fevers.

Treatment

- If reduced GCS, see ➜ Coma, p. 248; Fig. 8.12.
- Focal neurology or possibility of life-threatening sepsis: give oxygen, broad-spectrum antibiotics, evacuate urgently.
- If malaria is a possibility treat urgently (➜ Malaria, p. 480).
- Reduce fever with regular paracetamol and/or ibuprofen.
- Encourage oral fluids and monitor urine output; start a fluid balance chart.
- Advise rest in a cool place. Observe closely, evacuate if not improving.
- Empirical antibiotic therapy:
    - *Urinary tract infection*—trimethoprim 200 mg/12 h PO (or ciprofloxacin 250 mg/12 h PO) 5-day course.
    - *Cellulitis*—flucloxacillin 1 g/6 h IV + benzylpenicillin 1.2 g/6 h IV 7-day courses.
    - *Wound infection*—flucloxacillin 500 mg/6 h PO 7-day course.
    - *Meningitis*—ceftriaxone 2 g/12 h IV 5-day course.
    - *Septic arthritis*—flucloxacillin 2 g/6 h IV 7-day course.
    - *Pneumonia*—amoxicillin 500 mg/8 h PO or clarithromycin 500 mg/12 h PO 7-day course.
    - *Intra-abdominal sepsis*—ceftriaxone 2g/12 h IV + metronidazole 500 mg/8 h IV. 7-day courses.

Penicillin allergy

For many infections a penicillin is a sensible first-line antibiotic of choice. If an expedition member is known to be allergic to penicillins then the medical kit should contain additional quantities of a suitable alternative. Depending upon the nature of the infection, clarithromycin, metronidazole, or doxycycline may be appropriate; consult a pharmacopoeia.

Chapter 9

Treatment: skin

Authors
Jon Dallimore and David A. Warrell

Reviewer
Edi Albert

Solar skin damage 266
Wounds 268
Wound types and management 272
Wound infections 278
Burns 280
Insect bites 284
Ectoparasitic infestations 286
Tropical ulcers 292
Other infective skin lesions 293
Marine wound infections 294
Minor skin conditions 296

Solar skin damage

Introduction

Many travellers harbour the unstated aim of acquiring a 'good' tan. However, excessive exposure to solar radiation is damaging and may cause skin cancers:

- Basal cell carcinoma.
- Squamous cell carcinoma.
- Malignant melanoma.

In the UK, incidence of all skin cancers has increased—doubling between 1980 and 1990, with a 5% annual increase in tumours. Chronic sun exposure is also associated with skin thickening, pigmentation, and increased wrinkles. A number of skin conditions are triggered by exposure to sunlight and some people are sensitive to the effects of sunlight, e.g. sufferers from polymorphic light eruption (PMLE).

Solar radiation

Sunlight is the commonest source of ultraviolet radiation (UVR). UVR is subdivided into UVA (320–400 nm), UVB (280–320 nm), and UVC (100–280 nm). UVC is potentially very damaging to human skin but is normally absorbed by ozone in the earth's atmosphere. UVB plays an important role in sunburn, carcinogenesis, skin ageing, and vitamin D synthesis. UVA is responsible for tanning, ageing changes, and may be involved in carcinogenesis. Between 10 and 20 times more UVA reaches the earth's surface than UVB.

Intensity of sunlight increases nearer the equator, at increasing altitudes, and in polar regions where the protective atmospheric ozone layer may have thinned. It is also greatest when the sun is highest in the sky, between 10 am and 3 pm. UVR is reflected by water, white surfaces (such as snow and sand), and glass.

Sunburn

This follows acute, excessive exposure to UVR. It is an important risk factor for the development of malignant melanoma. Mild sunburn is characterized by skin redness, local heat, and pain. Severe sunburn may result in swelling, blistering, and generalized symptoms such as malaise, nausea, and rigors.

Treatment of sunburn

Sunburn is much easier to prevent than treat. Anti-inflammatories and paracetamol can be used for pain relief. 'Aftersun' creams containing *Aloe vera* are controversial but may help. Hydrocortisone 1% cream also helps to reduce inflammation but should not be applied to large areas or to broken skin. Blisters should not be drained unless very large.

Susceptibility to solar damage

People with different skin types are more or less likely to burn in the sun. Generally, females with pale skin, red hair, blue or green eyes, and freckles are most susceptible to solar skin damage. Those with a personal or family history of skin cancer or PMLE should be particularly careful to avoid excessive sun exposure.

Prevention of sunburn
- Avoid mid-day sun.
- Beware of bright hazy weather—UV can penetrate cloud.
- Use natural shade.
- Cover up with hats and clothing (some have a sunlight protection factor rating).
- Use a sunscreen that protects against UVA and UVB, is water-resistant, and has a sun protection factor (SPF) >15.

Sunscreens

There are two main types of sunscreen:
- Physical
- Chemical.

Physical sunscreens contain zinc oxide or titanium dioxide. They are highly visible on the skin and are very effective at blocking UVA and UVB but may be cosmetically unacceptable to some. However, over the past few years these have become available in dayglo colours and as a result have become fashionable among younger people.

Chemical sunscreens contain para-aminobenzoic acid or cinnamates, and protect against UVB. Some newer compounds also protect against UVA. Chemical sunscreens sometimes cause allergic or irritant reactions. Waterproof sunscreens are available for aquatic/marine use.

Sun protection factor
This is a guide to the ability of a sunscreen to protect the skin from UVB. A star system, 1–4, where 4 is the strongest, indicates the capacity to block out UVA. In theory, the SPF increases the amount of time that can be spent in the sun by the factor quoted. However, variables such as the time of day, the amount of cloud cover, time of year, and the amount of reflection all affect the protective ability of the sunscreen.

Wounds

Minor wounds are common on expeditions but some wounds are life-threatening. An ABC approach should be used (see ➲ Initial response to an accident, p. 180; ➲ Triage, p. 182). All wounds need careful assessment, thorough cleaning, then closure and dressing. Wounds that involve tendon, nerve, or blood vessel injuries cannot be managed in the field—the patient will need to be evacuated.

Immediate assessment and treatment

See ➲ Assessment of a casualty, p. 185.

Take a focused history

- How did the injury occur? (Mechanism is all important; was it an insect, mammal, or snake-bite?)
- Where did it occur (clean, contaminated, or marine environment)? (See Fig. 9.1.)
- When did it occur? (Old wounds >12 h should not be sutured and are more likely to become infected.)
- Was the wound caused by broken glass or other foreign body? (Will need careful examination or preferably X-ray).
- Was the limb trapped or crushed? (Swelling and compartment syndrome are possible; see also ➲ Crush injuries, Crush injuries, p. 277).
- When was the last tetanus booster? (Particularly for deep, penetrating wounds.)
- Is the patient allergic to anything?
- Does the patient take any medication?

Examine the wound

- Measure wounds and consider drawing, using a diagram (Fig. 9.1), or taking a digital photograph using a camera or smartphone/tablet.
- Look for contamination and foreign bodies.
- Check for signs of infection (red, hot, swollen, blistering, painful, tenderness, crepitus, lymphangitis, enlarged regional lymph nodes, fever). The earliest signs may develop after 8–12 h (mammal bites), but there is usually a delay of 2–7 days post injury.
- Check for pulses and capillary refill time (➲ Capillary refill time, p. 417).
- Re-examine carefully for signs of nerve damage—change in sensation, weakness, or paralysis.
- Look for evidence of damage to deep structures—examine the wound, preferably under local or regional anaesthetic.

General wound care

All wounds should be managed using the following principles:

- Stop bleeding.
- Clean carefully to reduce the risk of infection.
- Dress the injury to keep it clean.
- Promote healing and restore function.

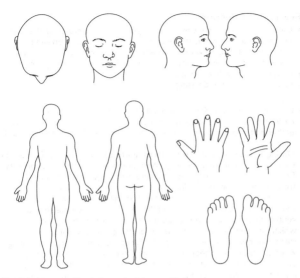

Fig. 9.1 Diagram of body for noting injury or skin feature.

Stopping bleeding

All wounds bleed to a greater or lesser extent; sometimes bleeding may be life-threatening:

- Apply direct pressure over the wound with a clean dressing.
- Lay the casualty down.
- Raise the wounded limb above the level of the heart (but not excessively).
- Apply a further dressing to control the bleeding on top of any original pad. If bleeding persists, remove the dressing, open the wound, and apply pressure deep in the wound (see ➲ Control of haemorrhage, p. 196).
- Bandage firmly to hold the dressing in place.

All wounds swell to some extent; watch for tourniquet effect.

When there are very deep wounds it may not be possible to control bleeding by applying pressure on the surface of the skin. The only way to stop severe, persistent bleeding from deep inside a wound may be to remove the dressings, open the wound, remove clots and debris, and to pack the wound open with sterile gauze or by placing haemostatic sutures using an absorbable suture material. The use of artery forceps should be avoided as they may damage important structures that follow the line of blood vessels such as tendons and nerves.

In torrential haemorrhage, e.g. following a landmine injury or traumatic amputation, it may be necessary to use other techniques such as a tourniquet (which should be released and reapplied every 30 min) or the use of pressure points. For those working in areas where ballistic trauma is a possibility, haemostatic agents such as Quik-Clot® or Celox® may be life-saving (➲ Circulation, p. 194).

Wound types and management

Lacerations are caused by a blunt injury and the skin is torn with irregular wound edges. There is often evidence of bruising in the surrounding tissues.

Cuts or incised wounds are a result of sharp edges such as knives or glass. They have clean-cut edges. Stab wounds are deep and slash wounds are long and superficial.

Closing cuts and lacerations

Gaping wounds will heal more quickly and result in a better scar if the skin edges are brought together.

Steri-Strips™

(See Fig. 9.2.) Steri-Strips™ are paper stitches that come in a variety of lengths and widths. They are placed across a laceration and, if left in place for a week or so, result in a clean, neat scar. Steri-Strips™ do not stick near moving joints, on the palms of the hands and soles of the feet, or on the scalp. However, they are excellent for finger lacerations and facial wounds. In humid or wet environments, such as the jungle or at sea, consider applying tincture of benzoin (Friar's Balsam) to the skin—this helps the Steri-Strips™ to adhere to the skin.

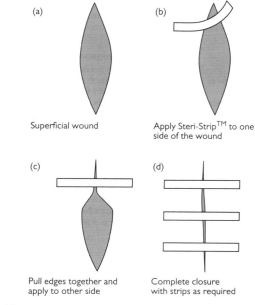

(a) Superficial wound

(b) Apply Steri-Strip™ to one side of the wound

(c) Pull edges together and apply to other side

(d) Complete closure with strips as required

Fig. 9.2 Applying Steri-Strips™.

Suturing

(See Fig. 9.3.) Steri-Strips™ should be used where possible. If Steri-Strips™ will not close the wound, suturing should be considered. Only clean wounds that are <12 h old are suitable for suturing. Deep wounds should be closed in layers by an experienced surgeon in an operating theatre because of the risk of wound infection. If this is not possible, clean the wound, pack with sterile gauze soaked in saline, and re-dress daily until definitive care is reached. Sutures should never be used to close deep or dirty wounds, particularly animal or human bites. Suturing should only be attempted by those who are adequately trained.

Important points when suturing a wound
- Most inexperienced people use too many stitches, too tight, too close.
- Lay the wound edges together to allow healing to occur—do not use tension.
- Use toothed forceps to hold the skin edges and pass the needle close to the part of the skin which is being held with forceps.
- Match up wound edges with strategically placed sutures along irregular wounds then close the gaps.
- Do not be afraid to remove sutures and try again.

Choice of suture material: the skin should be closed with non-absorbable suture material such as Prolene® or nylon on a curved reverse cutting needle. Experienced operators may consider carrying absorbable suture material (such as Vicryl®) to close deep tissue layers and this will help to reduce the risk of haematoma formation and subsequent infection. Vicryl® can also be used to close wounds inside the mouth. Use 4/0 sutures for most parts of the body, 5/0 on fingers, and preferably 6/0 for the face.

Removal of sutures: sutures should be removed after 7–10 days except on the face where earlier removal results in better healing with less scarring when the foreign material is removed. Sutures can be replaced by Steri-Strips™ after 3–4 days.

Staples

These are easy to use with minimal training and may be used in particular to close scalp wounds rapidly. If carried, a staple remover must also be available.

Tissue glue

May be useful for superficial face and scalp wounds, particularly in children. When bleeding is controlled, clean and dry the wound edges and place glue on the skin edges, not in the wound. Hold the wound edges together for 1 min to let the glue set.

Histoacryl tissue glue is used commonly for closing small lacerations and is particularly useful on the head and other areas where there is little skin movement during normal activities. On an expedition the 'super glue' in a repair kit can be used quite safely. Ensure the wound edges are dry, gently bring the edges of the wound together, squeeze a bead of glue along the surface of the wound and wait for 20 s before releasing. Make sure the part of the body with the wound on it is horizontal as glue has a tendency to run, and you don't want it to end up in the patient's eyes or gluing the medic's fingers to the patient!

1

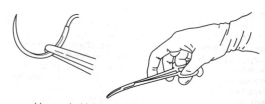

How to hold the needle and surgical instrument

2

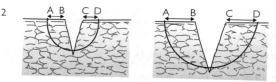

Distance from needle entry/exit points to wound edge. The greater the distance from the wound edge to the needle entry point, the deeper the bite of the needle. AB must equal CD, otherwise a step will occur

3

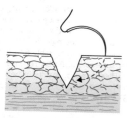

Depth of suture. Aim to close the wound fully by placing the suture to the deepest part of the wound

4

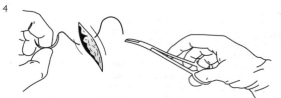

Instrument tie knot. Starting position, needle in left hand, needle-holder in right hand

Fig. 9.3 Skin suturing technique.

5

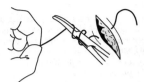

Wrapping the suture around the needle-holder.
Do this TWICE

6

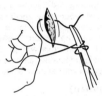

The first throw: take the loose end of the suture in the
jaws of the needle-holder

7

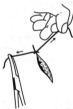

To tighten the first throw, cross the hands, needle-holder
going to the left, and the left hand going to the right

8

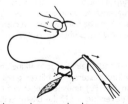

The second throw: the suture has been wrapped over the
needle-holder in the opposite direction and this time the
hand does not cross when tying the suture. Repeat this stage
to complete the surgical knot.

Fig. 9.3 (Contd.)

Abrasions

Abrasions are grazing injuries where the top surface of the skin is removed. They should be cleaned carefully and a non-adherent dressing applied. Ingrained dirt, if not removed, will result in tattooing and makes wound infection more likely. Dressings may require changing once or twice daily in some environments such as the jungle. If dressings stick they can be soaked off with warm, clean water or saline.

Puncture wounds

Infection may occur at the base of deep, penetrating wounds. Tetanus is a significant risk in the anaerobic conditions found deep in puncture wounds, and all expedition team members should be immunized before travel (see Table 2.1). Clean puncture wounds by encouraging bleeding, irrigate the wound using a syringe, and prevent the skin surface sealing over by placing a small sterile gauze wick into the wound. The wick encourages healing to occur from the bottom of the puncture wound upwards, otherwise abscess formation may occur. If deep infection in a puncture wound develops, evacuate the casualty for surgical exploration and cleaning.

Bites (animal and human)

Human bites carry a high risk of bacterial infections such as *Staphylococcus aureus* and *Eikenella corrodens*. Mammal bites should always raise the question of rabies, including the rabies-related bat lyssa viruses (**⊃** Rabies, p. 461; **⊃** Rabies immunization, p. 36) and there is a range of other special pathogens such as *Pasteurella multocida* (dog and cat bites), *Capnocytophaga canimorsus* (dogs), *Bartonella henselae* (cats), and *Streptobacillus moniliformis* and *Spirillum minus* (rodents). Bites should be cleaned as a matter of urgency with liberal amounts of soap and water followed by an antiseptic such as povidone-iodine or alcohol. Tetanus risk should also be considered. (See also Chapter 17.)

Bruises

Contusions or bruises are caused by a blunt force applied to the tissues. Bleeding under the skin gives the bruise its characteristic coloured appearance. Large muscle haematomas may cause hypovolaemic shock. Rest, ice, compression, and elevation (RICE) all help to reduce swelling and pain. Compression may be achieved by applying a crepe bandage firmly around the affected area. Anti-inflammatory drugs such as ibuprofen or aspirin may also help but are not good for haemostasis. After a day or two the affected part should be mobilized to reduce stiffness. (See **⊃** Physiotherapy, p. 452.)

Blisters

Blisters are best prevented. Ideally, stop walking and cover any 'hot spots' before they develop into blisters. If a blister does form, the fluid may be drained using a clean (sterile) fine needle and the area covered with an adhesive plaster but never 'de-roof' the blister unless pus is accumulating. Moleskin®, Compeed®, and Spenco Second Skin® are dressings designed to relieve the discomfort. Simple zinc oxide tape may be effective. Blisters may become de-roofed; in this case treat with a non-adherent dressing. A thin application of Friar's Balsam at the edge of a blister or swathes of zinc oxide tape over the dressings may help to keep protective coverings in place. Healing is rapid if friction at the blister site can be eliminated. Try to correct the cause (faulty footwear). Where possible, leaving the blister uncovered will assist healing by allowing the area to dry out.

Crush injuries

Large amounts of tissue may be damaged in crushing injuries and the potential for infection is high. The crushed part should be carefully cleaned and then elevated. Swelling of muscles in the affected part may cut off the blood supply to the limb beyond the injury, a condition known as compartment syndrome. If the injury is severe there may be a risk of losing the limb and acute kidney injury. Evacuate the casualty urgently for expert assessment; try to ensure casualty maintains a good urine output during the evacuation. Under surgical operating conditions, the pressure may be released and circulation restored by splitting the sheath around the damaged muscles, a fasciotomy, but this is not a procedure to attempt in the field. (See ➔ Compartment syndrome, p. 443.)

Amputation

A digit or limb may be replaced by microsurgery if the patient and the amputated part can be delivered to a surgeon in <6 h. The amputated part should be kept cool, preferably in a container with ice, but not in direct contact with the ice. In an expedition setting it is highly unlikely that such surgical facilities will be available; in this case, treat the bleeding with direct pressure and elevation. The stump should be cleaned gently and then covered with a non-adherent dressing such as paraffin gauze. People with these injuries need to be evacuated to allow surgical treatment to shorten any bone ends and cover the stump with a flap of skin so that healing can take place. Knife injuries that remove a chunk of palmar tissue such as the finger pulp are best treated by re-applying the excised tissue to the wound under a firm dressing or taking the tissue with the casualty.

Splinters

Splinters can usually be removed using a fine pair of tweezers (the ones on Swiss Army knives are good) or a sterile needle. For more stubborn splinters, soaking may help. Spines from sea urchins are easier to remove after a couple of days when the wound becomes inflamed, or after softening the skin by soaking or applying salicylic acid ointment (see ➔ Sea urchin and starfish injuries (echinoderms), p. 570).

Wound infections

Any wound can become infected; bites, dirty wounds, and deep wounds are more likely to become infected. Infections typically appear 2–7 days after the injury but, in the case of mammal bite wounds (*Pasteurella multocida*), all the signs of inflammation may develop in as little as 8–12 h. Signs and symptoms of a wound infection are pain, redness, heat, swelling, and loss of function. In the later stages, red lines may be seen running from a limb wound up towards the trunk (lymphangitis). Lymph nodes in the armpit, groin, or neck may become enlarged and fever may develop.

Abscesses

An abscess is a collection of pus or a 'boil', and is usually caused by a bacterial infection (see ➔ Other skin infections, p. 293). As pus accumulates, the skin over the abscess thins ('pointing'). Once the pus discharges through the skin the throbbing pain rapidly resolves. If an abscess develops during an expedition, applying local heat and oral antibiotics (e.g. flucloxacillin) may help. However, once pus is present it is quicker and kinder to drain it. Exceptions include those affecting the face, genital and anal areas, and breast—abscesses in these areas should be referred for specialist treatment. Local anaesthetic is less effective in the presence of infection because of localized high tissue acidity. Regional nerve blocks such as a digital nerve block (see Fig. 14.6 and ➔ Local infiltration anaesthesia, p. 590). An elliptical cut over the abscess must be large enough to let the pus drain. A small piece of gauze soaked in saline inserted into the incision will act as a wick and stop the roof of the abscess healing over before all the pus has drained. In this way the abscess cavity will heal from the bottom upwards. The wick should be changed daily until the abscess has healed. If there is evidence of spreading infection, antibiotics should be considered.

Cellulitis

Cellulitis refers to a bacterial infection of the skin (usually staphylococcal or streptococcal). Small lesions on the feet or athlete's foot between the toes may provide the portal of entry, but there may not be an obvious source of infection. The signs are the same as for a wound infection; that is, circumscribed redness with a raised edge, heat, pain, swelling, tenderness and fever with rigors which may precede the appearance of the skin lesion. Look for lymphangitis and lymphadenopathy. Treat with oral antibiotics initially (flucloxacillin or clarithromycin). Consider IV antibiotics if the infection is spreading or there are blisters or features of generalized infection such as fever and rigors. Ceftriaxone is a useful broad-spectrum antibiotic for a range of serious problems and can be given IM (made up with lidocaine to reduce pain) if IV access is too difficult.

Burns

Burns may be caused by dry heat, chemicals, electricity, friction, or hot liquids. On expeditions, open fires and fuel stoves commonly cause injuries, particularly when people refuel lighted stoves or burn rubbish with petrol.

Assessing the severely burned patient

Use an ABC approach:

- Ensure a safe approach for rescuers. Disconnect the electricity supply in electrical burns. Smother flames with a blanket or roll the victim on the ground. Remove any source of heat and remove any clothing that is not adherent to the skin.
- *Airway*—look for signs of potential problems—hoarse voice, burning or soot around mouth and nose, difficulty swallowing, singed nasal hair. A surgical airway may be necessary (➔ Surgical airways, p. 188) but the outlook on an expedition is likely to be very poor if evacuation times are long.
- *Cervical spine*—there may be other injuries, particularly if the patient jumped from a building to escape the fire. Immobilize the neck and spine if injury is suspected.
- *Breathing*—severe circumferential burns on the chest may require rapid surgical treatment (escharotomy) and are likely to be fatal in a very remote area.
- *Circulation*—shock is a feature of severe burns and large quantities of fluids may be needed. For fluid resuscitation see ➔ Assessing burns, p. 280 (see also ➔ Management of the shocked patient, p. 230).

History

Establish:

- Did the fire occur in an enclosed space?
- What was the burning material, if known?
- Was the patient unconscious at any time?
- Was there an explosion?

Examination

Assessing burns

The severity and extent of burns is often underestimated, even by doctors and nurses, and extensive burns need specialist assessment and treatment. The 'rule of nines', which divides the surface area of the body into areas of ~9%, is one method used to calculate the proportion of the body which is burned and so helps determine treatment (see Fig. 9.4). It may be easier to remember that the patient's palm (excluding the fingers and thumb) represents ~1% of the body surface area.

Burns may be divided into superficial and full-thickness burns:

- Superficial burns: characterized by redness, swelling, and pain (first degree). Deep partial thickness burns (second degree) are blistered and do not blanch on pressure.
- Full-thickness (third-degree) burns: characterized by pale, leathery, and sometimes charred skin with a loss of sensation. There are no blisters.
- Photographs taken at the time of the initial assessment provide an effective record and may be very helpful to those providing definitive care.

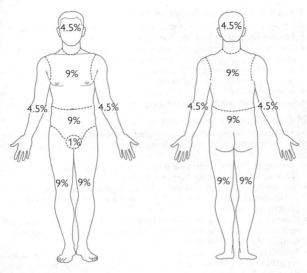

Fig. 9.4 Burns 'rule of nines'.

Consider:
- On an expedition it is important to differentiate between deep partial-thickness and full-thickness burns, although this may be difficult initially. Full-thickness burns need skin grafting, so evacuation to specialist medical help will be necessary.
- Fluid resuscitation for patients with >15% burns.
- Insert a cannula away from the burned areas and give 2–4 mL 0.9% saline/kg per % body surface area burned (excluding areas of erythema). This is the total volume to be given in the first 24 h; half of this volume should be given in the first 8 h.
  Example:
  - 70-kg man with 30% burns.
  - $4 \times 70 \times 30 = 8400$ mL/24 h. Give 4200 mL in the first 8 h.
  - Cover burned areas with cling film.
  - Monitor pulse, BP, respiratory rate, and body temperature.
  - Measure urine output.
  - Arrange urgent evacuation to hospital.

Treatment of severe burns and scalds

- Ensure scene safety to prevent other people becoming burn victims
- Remove the patient from the burning environment.
- Halt the burning process and relieve pain by applying cold water and cover burned areas with cling film or clean sheets.
- Irrigate chemical burns with copious tepid water.
- Leave any adherent burnt clothing.
- Give oxygen and IV analgesia if available.
- Give adequate analgesia, ideally using opioids.

Management of minor burns

As with severe burns, minor burns should be treated promptly to prevent the burning process, to cool the burn, control pain, and apply a suitable dressing.

- *Stopping the burning process*—the heat source should be removed. See ➔ Assessing the severely burned patient, p. 280.
- *Cool the burn*—immerse in tepid water or irrigate. Cooling large areas of skin can cause hypothermia. Chemicals, particularly alkalis, need prolonged irrigation – at least 30 min.
- *Control pain*—covering and cooling burns reduces pain. Strong painkillers such as tramadol or opiates may be required initially; later co-codamol or ibuprofen may be sufficient.
- *Suitable burn dressings*—cling film is ideal and has many other uses on an expedition. Cling film is essentially sterile if the first few centimetres are discarded. It is transparent, stretchy, and impermeable. Hand burns may be treated in a plastic bag. Cooling gels such as Burnshield® are useful to cool the burn and provide good pain relief.

Key facts for burns
- Burns to significant areas such as hands, feet, face, and genitalia should be assessed by a specialist.
- >10% body surface area burns need evacuation as many burns become infected.
- Full-thickness burns will almost certainly require skin grafting and should be evacuated early.
- Blistered burns: do not de-roof; however, large blisters may be aspirated with a sterile needle and syringe.
- In general, avoid prophylactic antibiotics.
- Mupirocin (Bactroban®) cream helps to prevent infection during evacuation and can be placed under cling film or inside a plastic bag in the case of hand burns. Paraffin gauze is very useful to dress burns as it is less likely to adhere to the burn.
- Granuflex® (a hydrocolloid dressing) is adhesive and waterproof, and may be used for awkward areas which are difficult to dress. Change every 3–5 days.
- Elevate limb burns to reduce swelling.
- Early physiotherapy helps to maintain mobility (➔ Physiotherapy, p. 452).
- Regular ibuprofen is usually sufficient analgesia for a dressed burn.
- On an expedition, burns should be re-dressed every 24–48 h. Look for signs of infection (➔ Immediate assessment and treatment, p. 268). Healed burns should be protected from the sun for 6–12 months.

Insect bites

Bites by blood-feeding insects such as mosquitoes, midges, black flies, sand flies, tabanid flies (horse, deer, and stable flies), tsetse flies, and triatomine 'kissing' bugs pose a common irritation and nuisance during expeditions. These 'micro-predators' make brief blood-sucking attacks on humans and animals which can result in persisting medical problems. (See also ➔ Venomous land animals, p. 550; ➔ Arthropods, p. 560.)

Clinical features

Consequences of bites:

- Allergic reactions.
- Secondary infection of the bite site.
- Acquisition of systemic infections transmitted by the insect (see ➔ Arthropods, p. 560).

Bites may be immediately painful and traumatic (horse flies) but the commonest problem is delayed local swelling and itching from hypersensitivity to insects' salivary allergens incurred by previous exposure. A small, intensely itchy, reddish lump with a central (haemorrhagic) punctum develops immediately or after a delay of 24–48 h. A papule, urticarial weal, blister, or bulla may develop even after bites by tiny blackflies (*Simulium*), or bites may provoke a more generalized erythema multiforme or, especially in children, papular urticaria. Systemic anaphylaxis may be provoked (➔ Anaphylaxis and anaphylactic shock, p. 236). Scratching may lead to secondary infection, an inflamed, painful pustule or carbuncle (e.g. Lord Carnarvon's fatal septicaemia from an infected mosquito bite on his cheek near the tomb of Tutankhamun), or a demarcated, hot, bright red, raised area of erysipelas or cellulitis. Causative bacteria include *Staph. aureus* and *Strep. pyogenes*. The risk of secondary infection seems to be higher under humid tropical conditions. Triatomine bug bites are usually multiple, often near the eye or angle of the mouth, and are painful, swollen, ooze blood, and may be surrounded by black staining from the bug's faeces (see ➔ American trypanosomiasis (Chagas' disease), p. 493).

Treatment

- Apply a cooling antiseptic solution, cream, or ointment (e.g. triclosan, Savlon®) to sooth irritation and prevent secondary infection. Reduce itch with counter irritants such as crotamiton (Eurax®) cream/lotion, with or without hydrocortisone.
- Topical corticosteroids (e.g. hydrocortisone 0.5–1% can be purchased over the counter in the UK as creams or ointments) can be tried but topical antihistamines are not recommended as they may be light-sensitizing and are ineffective.
- For severe pruritus use oral antihistamines. Try full dose, non-sedating anti-H1 drugs such as cetirizine (adult dose up to 10 mg twice a day) during the day and chlorphenamine (Piriton®) 4 mg at night.
- Early systemic symptoms of anaphylaxis should be treated with adrenaline (epinephrine) 0.1% (1:1000) 0.5 mL by IM injection (adult dose). This dose may be repeated after 5–10 min if there is no response (Fig. 8.8).
- If inflamed pustules develop, apply a topical antibacterial such as mupirocin (Bactroban®). Multiple infected bites may warrant a course of oral antibiotic such as flucloxacillin or erythromycin.

Prevention

Be prepared for insect bites, not only in tropical rain forests and beaches but also in the arctic and in cool mountainous terrain such as the Californian Sierra Nevada, Italian Dolomites, and Scottish Highlands. The risk of getting bitten varies geographically, seasonally, and diurnally. Seek specific advice.

- Clothing should be as ample and protective as comfort allows.
- Long sleeves and long trousers should be worn after dusk.
- Light colours are less attractive to mosquitoes than dark ones. Blue colour attracts African tsetse flies (see ➔ African trypanosomiasis (sleeping sickness), p. 492).
- Hats and face veils may protect against assaults on face and scalp by swarms of Scottish midges (*Culicoides*), tropical black flies (*Simulium*), or sand flies (*Phlebotomus, Lutzomyia*).
- Effective repellents include diethyl-toluamide (DEET)) and *p*-methane-diol (Mosiguard®)-containing preparations applied to exposed skin or impregnated into cotton clothing or forehead, wrist, and ankle bands. Beware that some preparations of DEET can dissolve plastics and synthetic fibres, causing damage to spectacles and clothing.
- Clothes can be impregnated with pyrethroid insecticides at the expense of waterproofing.
- Protect sleeping quarters. Mosquito proofing of sleeping quarters and insecticide spraying at dusk reduces the risk. Night bites by mosquitoes that transmit malaria (Box 15.3), cone-nosed (triatomine) 'kissing' bugs (Central and South America) that transmit Chagas' disease (➔ American trypanosomiasis (Chagas' disease), p. 493), bed bugs, ticks that transmit tick-borne encephalitis and tick-borne relapsing fever (➔ Ticks, p. 288), and even vampire and other bats that transmit rabies (➔ Rabies, p. 461) and venomous snakes can be prevented by sleeping under a pyrethroid-impregnated mosquito net. Burn pyrethroid-releasing mosquito coils or, if there is electricity, plug-in insecticide vaporizers. Ceiling fans deter mosquitoes from biting.

Ectoparasitic infestations

Fleas, lice, mites, ticks, invasive flies (myiasis), and leeches

Some blood-feeding invertebrates take up temporary or long-term residence on the surface of humans' bodies or clothing. Tropical climate, poor socioeconomic conditions, and poor hygiene increase the risk of acquiring ectoparasites from other humans or from the environment. The very thought of these 'bugs' may induce psychosis and their presence, visible or palpable, is irritating, distressing, and embarrassing, but it is only in the past century that Westerners have grown less accustomed to being flea-ridden and lousy. For example, Marie Curie was awoken by a myriad of bed bugs falling off her back as she rolled over in her poor Paris attic bedroom.

The biting and burrowing of these ectoparasites causes pain and irritation, and may lead to hypersensitivity, secondary local infection, or transmission of systemic diseases such as:

• Rickettsioses (typhus) and plague by fleas.
• Viral encephalitides and haemorrhagic fevers, spirochaetoses, rickettsioses, and bartonelloses by ticks.
• Spirochaetoses and rickettsioses by lice.
• Scrub typhus by trombiculid mites.
• Local streptococcal infection leading to acute glomerulonephritis by scabies mites.

Fleas

Humans can be infested and bitten by human fleas (*Pulex irritans*) and by dog, cat, rat, pigeon, and other animal fleas. Direct contact with an infested person or animal is not necessary. Tropical rodent fleas (*Xenopsylla* spp.) transmit plague and murine typhus. The first evidence of fleas is the appearance of small groups of intensely itchy bites (red macule with a central punctum), often in a line a few centimetres apart, especially on the trunk or buttocks. Fleas may not remain on the body after feeding but retreat to bedding or crevices and cracks in the bed or room. Examination of underclothing or quickly turning back the bedclothes may reveal the jumping fleas.

• *Treatment:* itching bites are treated with counter-irritants, topical corticosteroid, or systemic antihistamines (see ➔ Insect bites, p. 284). Domestic animals and the infested environment should be kept as clean as is practicable and treated with pyrethroid or other pesticides.

Lice

Human head lice (*Pediculus capitis*), body (clothing) lice (*P. humanus*), and pubic lice (*Pthirus pubis*) are obligate human parasitic insects that spread through close physical contact.

Head lice: flourish in the human scalp even in hygienic, affluent conditions, especially among teenage schoolgirls. Eggs ('nits') stuck to head hairs are recovered using a fine comb. Itching and scratching may cause secondary infection with occipital lymphadenopathy.

• *Treatment:* repeated application of insecticide lotion (pyrethroid, organophosphate, or carbamate) and combing.
• *Prevention:* avoid head-to-head contact.

Body lice: infestation is promoted by poor hygiene (unwashed clothes and bodies) and crowding, common accompaniments of disasters, imprisonment, wars, forced immigration, and cold, wet seasons as in the highlands of Ethiopia. Lice and their eggs may be discovered on skin, body hair, or in clothing, especially in the seams. More than 21,500 lice have been found on one person. Individual bites look like flea bites but there is no linearity and only mild local irritation.

• *Treatment:* burn clothing or heat-sterilize and impregnate with pyrethroids. Bathe infested people with soap and 1% lysol.

Pubic (crab) lice: sexually transmitted infestation of the pubic hair and also body hair, eyebrows, and eyelashes. They provoke itching, scratching, secondary infection, and curious bluish staining (maculae caeruliae). Eggs are stuck to the hairs.

• *Treatment:* apply insecticides (see ➋ Insect protection and repellents, p. 771) to affected areas and leave on for 1–2 days then repeat after a week. Treat sexual contacts.

Mites

Scabies mites (*Sarcoptes scabei*): burrow under the skin, creating linear papulo-vesicular tracks, typically in the interdigital clefts and skin creases. There is intense itching, especially at night, provoking scratching, excoriation, and secondary infection. Transmitted by close physical contact. Exuberant crusting (Norwegian scabies) develops in immuno-compromised patients.

• *Treatment:* two treatments a week apart of aqueous lotion—0.5% malathion or 5% permethrin. Apply lotion to the whole body surface of all affected people and leave on for 24 h before being washing off. Itching may persist for several weeks and requires topical counter-irritant and corticosteroid (e.g. crotamiton and hydrocortisone) and sedating antihistamine (chlorphenamine at night). Ivermectin (200 micrograms/kg single dose) is used for Norwegian scabies and in patients whose severe excoriations make topical treatment intolerably irritating and painful.

Trombiculid (harvest) mites: sometimes known very misleadingly as 'chiggers' (see 'Tungosis' entry in ➋ Invasive fly larvae (myiasis) and fleas (tungiasis), p. 289), can infest in large numbers, especially under tight underpants, causing multiple, persisting, painful, itchy, blistering bites.

• *Prevention:* use DEET-containing repellents, tuck trousers into boots, and avoid notorious 'mite islands' densely infested with trombiculids in cleared areas of jungle.

Bed bugs (*Cimex*)

At night, bed bugs emerge from cracks and crevices in the bedroom to bite sleeping humans. Insomnia and painful, red papules result.

• *Prevention:* discourage bites by keeping the light on all night, by sleeping under a permethrin-impregnated mosquito net, and putting newspaper under the under-sheet. Eradication is by thorough cleaning of the environment and application of the usual residual insecticides. Sleeping bags should be exposed to the sun (including both outside and inside) and treated with insecticide. However, insecticide-resistance has developed and bed bugs are becoming more abundant.

Ticks

- *Soft (argasid) ticks:* live in animal burrows and human dwellings. They attach briefly at night, engorge rapidly with blood, and then drop off and hide in cracks and crevices. Ticks of the genus *Ornithodoros* transmit relapsing fever.
- *Hard (ixodid) ticks* or their tiny nymphs may be picked up from vegetation or brought into gardens by deer or indoors by dogs. They find a secluded area (groin, perineum, waist, umbilicus, axilla, scalp, even external auditory meatus) and feed for days until they are spherical and engorged. Some species transmit Lyme disease (➔ Lyme disease, p. 472), Rocky Mountain spotted fever (➔ Typhus, p. 478), African tick fevers (➔ Typhus, p. 478; Plate 8), European tick-borne encephalitis (➔ Tick-borne encephalitis (TBE), p. 460), Crimean–Congo haemorrhagic fever (➔ Bunyaviruses: Crimean–Congo, Hantavirus, and Rift Valley fevers, p. 467), Colorado tick fever, louping ill, babesiosis, ehrlichiosis, and other human infections. Some ticks in North America and Australia inject a paralysing neurotoxin (➔ Other venomous invertebrates, p. 565).

Prevention of tick-transmitted infections

Examine yourself at likely tick attachment sites (see ➔ Ticks, p. 288 and use a mirror or a friend) when undressing at night while on the expedition.
- Avoid contact with tick-infested domestic animals.
- Wear light-coloured trousers against which ticks are more visible.
- Tuck trouser bottoms into boots.
- Apply DEET-containing repellents.
- Specific antibiotic chemoprophylaxis against tick-transmitted infections is not justified.

Removing ticks

Grasp the tick as close to your skin as possible with fine curved (iris) forceps (avoid squeezing the engorged body) and pull it out gently *without twisting* (Fig. 9.5). If the mouth parts break off, remove them separately with forceps or a needle. The aim is not to leave the barbed hypostome in the wound as it may provoke inflammation and granuloma formation. Keep the tick for later expert examination in case you become ill.

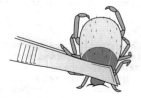

Fig. 9.5 Tick removal using forceps.

Invasive fly larvae (myiasis) and fleas (tungiasis)

Larvae (maggots) of some tropical flies hatch from eggs contaminating human skin and burrow into tissues, creating an uncomfortable, inflamed boil which wriggles, exudes blood-stained pus, and has a definite head through which the larval spiracles may protrude ('myiasis'). Secondary infection may cause fever and lymphadenopathy.

The *human bot fly* (*Dermatobia hominis*) of Central and South America is also known as ver macaque, berne, el torsalo, or beefworm. Eggs are laid on mosquitoes which deposit them on human skin. The larvae grow for 10 weeks.

The *tumbu fly* (*Cordylobia anthropophaga*) of sub-Saharan Africa and southern Spain is also known as putsi fly or ver du cayor. Eggs are laid on sand, stick to clothes (e.g. washing laid out on the ground to dry), and hatch on the skin. Larvae penetrate and grow for 10 days.
- *Treatment:* folk remedies such as raw steak or bacon fat, and occlusion of the maggot's breathing hole in the skin with paraffin, petroleum gel, and candle wax occlusion sometimes work. However, attempts to squeeze them out like giant blackheads make matters worse. Injecting local anaesthetic into the base of the lesion may force the maggot out. The final solution is removal through a small scalpel incision.
- *Prevention:* hang washing to dry on a clothes line in strong sunlight; do not lay clothing on the ground. Iron washing to kill the tumbu fly ova.

Congo floor maggots, larvae of the fly *Auchmeromyia luteola*, live in earthen floors of huts throughout tropical Africa between latitudes 18°N and 26°S. They suck blood from those sleeping on the ground, causing local swelling and itching. Fumigate the hut and treat the bites symptomatically, making sure that no secondary infection is introduced (wipe the skin with tincture of iodine, and give systemic antimicrobials if there are signs of infection).
- *Prevention:* if possible, don't sleep on the ground (there are several other good reasons for this advice—see snake-bites!).

Invasive myiasis, involving wounds, body orifices, and cavities: aggressive larvae of screw worm flies, such as *Cochliomyia (Callitroga) hominivorax* in Latin America and *Chrysomyia bessania* in eastern Europe, Africa, and Asia, hatch from eggs laid on wounds or on healthy mucosae (especially of the eye, orbit, nasal cavity, or external auditory meatus), and invade body cavities, orifices, and living tissue, causing life-threatening destruction and secondary infection.
- *Clinical:* there is pain, irritation, a feeling of wriggling movement, discharge of serosanguineous matter and maggots, obstruction (e.g. of the external auditory meatus causing deafness), and symptoms of secondary bacterial infection.
- *Treatment:* irrigation with sterile saline solution and dilute antiseptic is a first aid measure but eventually, thorough surgical debridement is essential.
- *Prevention:* protect wounds from flies.

Tungosis ('jigger' or 'chigoe' flea) (*Tunga penetrans*) occurs in Latin America and Africa. After fertilization the female flea jumps (feebly) and burrows alongside the nail fold or into the skin of the groin, loses its legs, and produces eggs each night. A painful swelling develops on the foot, typically under a toe nail, and there is a risk of secondary bacterial infection and ulceration.

- *Treatment:* the encapsulated flea must be curetted out (excised, ideally with a small surgical spoon with sharpened edge) and iodine applied. Complete enucleation is required.
- *Prevention:* wear proper shoes; do not walk around bare-footed.

'Creeping eruption' (cutaneous larva migrans): arthropod infestations must be distinguished from creeping eruption (Plate 1) which occurs in tropical countries worldwide. It is caused by larvae of cat and dog hookworms, such as *Ancylostoma braziliense, Uncinaria stenocephala,* and *Ancylostoma caninum.* Contact with contaminated ground (especially from sleeping rough on beaches in Central/Southern America) allows filariform larvae to penetrate the skin. They crawl under the skin a few millimetres each day, causing excruciating itching. Feet, buttocks, knees, hands, and back are commonly affected, sometimes by dozens of worms. The best treatment is 10–15% thiabendazole applied topically in paraffin ointment under occlusion for 1 week or, if that fails, oral albendazole 400 mg daily for 3 days or a single 200 micrograms/kg dose of ivermectin (adult doses).

Leeches

Leeches are blood-sucking ectoparasites that live in the water or on moist land surfaces. Usually those encountered are small, 7–40 mm, but the largest ones are 45 cm long.

Aquatic leeches cause bleeding after entering the nose, mouth, nostrils, ears, eyes, vulva, urethra, or anus of swimmers or being swallowed in water from natural sources. They tend to remain attached for longer than terrestrial leeches.

Land leeches frequent game paths in moist vegetation and may drop onto upper limbs from trees or bushes, or rapidly climb up from the ground, fastening onto the legs. Usually, they are far more upsetting than harmful.

Attachment is via a three- or two-jaw bite giving a Y- or V-shaped incision. There may be a tickling sensation or sharpness as they bite but, as they inject local anaesthetic as well as anticoagulants, bites often go undetected until bleeding is noticed. Bites may ooze for hours, but blood loss from a single bite is insignificant.

- *Prevention:* leeches can squeeze through small gaps such as shoelace eyes, and so boots, socks, or trousers offer little protection. Application of DEET to boots, socks, and skin or coarse tobacco rolled into the top of socks and kept moist is repellent. Take care when swimming and drink only filtered sterilized water. British troops in Malaya wore condoms at night to prevent urethral invasion by leeches while they were asleep in the jungle.
- *Treatment:* if detected before attachment flick or pull off.

Once attached: ripping off can leave the mouth parts behind and predispose to infection. Apply salt (kept dry in a screw-top plastic container), iodine tincture, alcohol, lighted cigarette, tobacco, or other irritant to persuade them to release. This may precipitate regurgitation of ingested blood into the wound and, to avoid secondary infection, treat as an open wound; clean, apply antiseptic, and compression dressing.

If a leech has attached inside the mouth, gargle with strong salt solution but don't swallow as it may induce vomiting.

Leeches will spontaneously release after feeding. Their gut contains symbiotic *Aeromonas hydrophila* which are potentially pathogenic.

Tropical ulcers

Tropical (phagedenic) ulcer

In tropical climates, even trivial wounds seem to heal slowly or persist. Classical tropical ulcers usually affect the shins and occur in 30% of some indigenous communities. They start as minor abrasions (thorn prick, scratch, insect bite, existing skin lesion, pressure blister) that become infected with saprophytic bacteria (e.g. *Fusobacterium ulcerans*, *Borrelia vincentii*) in mud or stagnant water.

Clinical

A pustule appears and after 5–6 days discharges foul-smelling pus. Over the next few weeks a painful, circular ulcer develops with a defined, raised, undermined edge and floor of granulation tissue covered with purulent discharge. Over subsequent months and years the ulcer becomes painless but the infection penetrates to deeper tissue, tendon sheaths, periosteum and bone, becomes gangrenous and may show malignant transformation.

Treatment

In the early stages, high-dose penicillin or erythromycin, preferably parenteral, may promote healing. Later, surgical debridement and reconstruction or even amputation may be needed.

Prevention

In tropical environments, especially in wet conditions, protect legs and ankles from scratches and pricks, and treat any new injury, however trivial, by washing with sterile (drinking) water, applying antiseptic or topical antibacterial (e.g. mupirocin), and protecting with a dry dressing.

Other types of tropical ulcer

(For genital ulcers, see Table 15.3.) Ulcerating skin lesions can be caused by many different tropical pathogens:

- Pyogenic bacteria (*Staphylococcus*, *Streptococcus*, *Berkholderiapseudomallei*—melioidosis).
- Cutaneous diphtheria ('desert' or 'veldt' sore).
- Spirochaetes (yaws).
- Mycobacteria (TB, *Mycobacterium ulcerans*, 'Buruli ulcer').
- Protozoa (leishmaniasis).
- Fungi (histoplasmosis, cryptococcosis, and deep fungal infections).
- Non-infectious diseases such as sickle cell disease, varicose veins, and other vascular problems.

Other infective skin lesions

Pustules, furuncles, boils, styes, abscesses, paronychias, whitlows (felons), cellulitis, erysipelas, ecthyma, and other painful, inflamed, and obviously infected skin and soft tissue lesions should be treated promptly. Depending on their stage of development and severity, they may require only topical antiseptic or antibiotic treatment, but systemic antibiotics and drainage are often needed.

Marine wound infections

Swimmers, scuba divers, fishermen, sailors, wind-surfers, and anyone in contact with marine or brackish water or sea animals are susceptible to wound infections and otitis externa caused by unusual pathogens acquired from salt water. Infective otitis externa should be distinguished from swimmer's ear (see ➲ Ear problems, p. 698; ➲ Otitis externa, p. 742). Heatwaves associated with higher sea temperatures, even in the Baltic and North Seas, increase the risk. Infections complicate injuries such as coral cuts (➲ Prevention, p. 568), skin penetration by fish or sea urchin spines and stings (➲ Sea urchin and starfish injuries (echinoderms), p. 570), and fish hooks, merely handling fish (erysipeloid) and other traumas associated with fishing and boating.

Marine pathogens

- Vibrios: *Vibrio vulnificus* infection starts with local erythema round the wound, followed by swelling, haemorrhagic blisters, necrotic ulceration, and severe systemic symptoms (fever, rigors, septic shock). Case fatality is high, especially in people with chronic debility (immunocompromise, chronic alcoholism, diabetes mellitus). *Vibrio parahaemolyticus* (see also ➲ Diarrhoea and vomiting, p. 398), *V. cholera*, and *V. alginolyticus* can also cause inflammation, sometimes within 8 h of injury, with the risk of deep, severe wound infections and bacteraemia in immunocompromised people.
- *Aeromonas hydrophila*: (brackish and fresh water) can cause muscle damage—myonecrosis and pyomyositis.
- *Erysipelothrix rhusiopathiae* (erysipeloid, 'seal finger', 'whale finger'): demarcated red/violaceous plaques appear on the hands after handling fish. The rash spreads proximally and may be associated with arthritis.
- *Plesiomonas shigelloides*, *Acinetobacter* spp., *Chromobacterium violaceum*, *Flavobacterium* spp., and *Pseudomonas aeruginosa* are commonly cultured from marine wounds.
- *Mycobacterium marinum* causes chronic granulomatous lesions in aquarium keepers and others who are exposed to sea water.
- *Staphylococcus aureus*, pyogenic *Streptococcus*, and enteric pathogens derived from the patient rather than the marine environment. However, the sea water near some popular beaches (e.g. Waikiki Beach, Honolulu) is heavily contaminated with *Staph. aureus*, including MRSA.
- Achlorous algae (*Prototheca* spp.): cause a chronic papule, plaque or ulcer, or olecranon bursitis, and may become disseminated in immunocompromised people.
- Free-living amoebae (*Acanthamoeba*, *Naegleria*, *Balamuthia mandrillaris*): a hazard of tropical ponds, swimming pools, saunas or spas can cause keratitis in contact lens wearers and encephalitis.

Diagnosis

Clinical suspicion based on history of marine exposure and underlying illness is crucial for early antibiotic treatment. Expert microbiology involves special cultures in 3% saline media. Biopsy and histopathology may yield the diagnosis.

Treatment

Urgent surgical debridement is needed if there is any suggestion of necrotizing fasciitis or myositis.

Blind antibiotic treatment:
- For mild lesions: oral doxycycline or co-trimoxazole.
- For severe lesions with systemic illness: combination treatment—tetracycline + aminoglycoside (e.g. gentamicin) + cefotaxime or tetracycline + aminoglycoside + a fluoroquinolone.

Specific treatment
- Marine vibrios: doxycycline, co-trimoxazole, fluoroquinolone, gentamicin, cefotaxime, or co-amoxiclav.
- *Aeromonas hydrophila:* doxycycline, fluoroquinolone, gentamicin, or cefotaxime.
- Erysipeloid: penicillin or erythromycin or tetracycline.
- *M. marinum:* doxycycline or co-trimoxazole for trivial lesions; rifampicin and ethambutol for destructive lesions.
- Others: as directed by laboratory sensitivities.

Prevention

Sensible behaviour, acquisition of technical skills, and appropriate protective clothing may reduce the risk of marine injuries. Beachcombers should not expose open wounds to sea water and should avoid eating undercooked or raw shellfish. Wounds contaminated by sea water should be cleaned immediately with drinking water (not rinsed in the brine). Foreign bodies should be removed and the wound watched carefully for early signs of infection. Start blind antibiotic treatment at the first hint of infection. For those at high risk of invasive marine vibrio infection (see ➲ Marine pathogens, p. 294), prophylaxis with doxycycline or co-trimoxazole is recommended.

Minor skin conditions

Superficial fungal infections (dermatophytosis, ringworm, tinea)

Infection of the skin by *Trichophyton, Microsporum*, and *Epidermophyton* spp. is spread by direct contact with infected humans or animals or from soil saprophytes. It is common in tropical climates.

- *Clinical:* the classic lesion is a circumscribed round or oval scaly patch with vesicles around its border and central clearing (see Plate 2). Scalp, face, body, beard area, hands, nails (➔ Fungal infection of nails (tinea ungulum, onchomycosis), p. 298), intertriginous areas (groins, axillae, 'dhobie's itch'), and feet (➔ Athlete's foot (tinea pedis), p. 298) may be affected. Hyperkeratotosis caused by scratching, and follicular and granulomatous lesions may be present.
- *Diagnosis:* direct microscopic examination of scrapings incubated for 20 min in 5–20% potassium hydroxide may reveal hyphae and spores. *Microsporium* spp. fluoresce green with Wood's lamp.
- *Treatment:* topical creams or ointments containing imidazoles or terbinafine are usually effective (see ➔ Athlete's foot (tinea pedis), p. 298), but nail and scalp infections require systemic treatment with imidazoles (e.g. ketoconazole 200 mg each day), triazoles (e.g. itraconazole 200 mg each day), or terbinafine (250 mg each day) for many months (adult doses).[1]

Tinea (pityriasis) versicolor

Skin infection with the yeast *Pityrosporum orbiculare* (*Malassezia furfur*) spreads by direct contact, affecting half the population in some tropical communities. Scaly macular rashes coalesce over large areas usually of the trunk. They appear hyperpigmented or hypopigmented, or yellowish or brownish. Fine scales can be scraped off these lesions.

- *Treatment:* topical imidazoles, 20% sodium thiosulfate solution, compound benzoic acid (Whitfield's) ointment, or selenium sulfide, or ketoconazole shampoos are applied overnight repeatedly. Relapses are common.

Skin conditions of the hands and feet

Ingrowing toenails

An edge of a big toe nail is forced into the nail fold either by pressure of tight footwear or abnormal growth. This causes trauma, pain, bleeding, or serosanguineous discharge and infection of the nail fold (inflammation, swelling, pus formation, paronychia; see ➔ Paronychia, p. 297; Fig. 9.6) that can make walking very painful.

- *Treatment:* soak in saline, clean with antiseptic, apply antiseptic cream, and relieve compressing footwear. Trimming the nail may make matters worse. Curative treatment of intractable in growing toenails: under digital block (see Fig. 14.6; ➔ Local infiltration anaesthesia, p. 590) incise the side of the nail back to and including the nail bed (Fig. 9.6).
- *Prevention:* cut toe nails straight across and avoid wearing tight footwear, especially brand new boots that have not been worn and thoroughly broken in before the expedition.

1 ⌨ http://www.bad.org.uk/ResourceListing.aspx?sitesectionid=159&itemid=391&q=Fungal%20 infections%20of%20the%20nails%20-%20printable%20version#.VIRB8zGsWSo

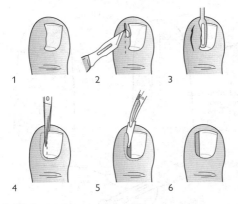

Fig. 9.6 Relief of paronychia or ingrowing nail.

Paronychia

Frequent immersion of the hands in infected water may result in chronic *Candida* and acute staphylococcal nail fold infections. There is painful redness and swelling of the nail fold. Pus may be trapped under the nail. *Pseudomonas aeruginosa* infection causes greenish discoloration of the nail and foul-smelling greenish pus.

* *Treatment:* initially, warm saline soaks, topical antiseptic or antibacterial cream, and drainage of abscesses may be curative. Otherwise, consider systemic antibiotics or removal of the nail edge(s) under digital block (Fig. 14.6) as for ingrowing toe nails.

Whitlow (felon)

Acute swelling, redness, inflammation, and throbbing pain of the pulp space of finger or toe is usually caused by *Staphylococcus* or *Streptococcus* from a splinter or spread from paronychia. Contact with herpes simplex causes a whitlow with painful vesicles. Orf, a sheep virus, causes pustular whitlow. Inflammatory swelling in the pulp space may compress the digital artery, causing necrosis. The terminal phalanx may be infected. Nail biters, especially diabetics, may self-inoculate oral *Eikenella corrodens*.

* *Treatment:* initially try warm saline soaks and antibiotics for suspected pyogenic infection (flucloxacillin or erythromycin) and aciclovir for herpetic whitlow. If tense, painful swelling persists, a relieving incision (Fig. 9.7) may be needed under digital block (Fig. 14.6; ➲ Local infiltration anaesthesia, p. 590). Herpetic whitlows should not be incised as this may spread the infection.

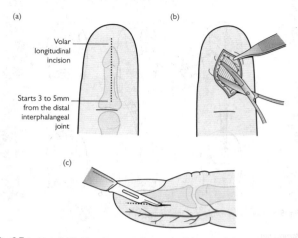

Fig. 9.7 Incisions for draining abscesses in finger pulps (felons or whitlows). (a, b) Incision for abscesses pointing in the central area. (c) Incision for those pointing laterally.

Fungal infection of nails (tinea unguium, onychomycosis)

Initially there is white, yellow, or brown discoloration of the free edge of the nail and later hyperkeratotic thickening of the nail bed, and ridging and crumbling of the nail surface and separation from the nail bed (onycholysis). There is no inflammation of the nail fold (paronychia). Not all the nails are involved but there is usually superficial fungal infection elsewhere.

- *Treatment:* early infection responds to topical amorolfine nail lacquer or tioconazole (Trosyl®) cutaneous solution. Established infection requires systemic terbinafine 250 mg or itraconazole 200 mg each day for 3 months.

Athlete's foot (tinea pedis)

In shoe and sock wearers, skin of the interdigital spaces between the toes, especially the third and fourth, may become greyish white, moist, macerated, fissured, dehiscent, itchy, and sore. An associated vesicular eruption is common. Lesions may become secondarily infected, causing cellulitis of the lower leg.

- *Treatment:* wear sandals at least in camp and keep the interdigital spaces dry and clean. Terbinafine cream applied twice daily for 1 week is the most effective antifungal, but a wide range of cheaper preparations is also effective such as compound benzoic acid (Whitfield's) ointment and -azole creams (e.g. clotrimazole).

Chapter 10

Treatment: head and neck

Section editors
Chris Johnson and Jon Dallimore

Contributors
Alistair R. M. Cobb
Paul Cooper
Daniel S. Morris
Annabel H. Nickol
David Geddes (1st edition)
Stephen Hearns (1st edition)

Anatomy 300
Facial injuries 302
Minor injuries to head and neck 304
Fractured facial bones 306
Head injury 312
Blackouts, syncope, and epilepsy 316
Migraine 320
Sleep disturbances 322
The eye 324
Ear problems 334
Nasal problems 335
Upper respiratory tract 336

Anatomy

The head can be thought of in terms of the neurocranium—the brain box—and the face (viscerocranium). The face acts as a protection to the brain in large impacts—rather like an air bag in a car. The two structures are intimately related to each other and to the neck, which is forcibly extended following a frontal blow to the face. In major facial trauma it is essential to look for signs of cervical spine injury (10% of mid face fractures will have a concomitant c-spine fracture) and start head injury observations.

Areas of the head are described according to their underlying bony parts (Fig. 10.1). The eyes lie protected within the orbit, while the prominent nose is susceptible to injury.

The breathing and digestive passages cross in the oropharynx, requiring complex mechanisms to ensure correct routing (Fig. 10.2). The nose and upper airway form a humidification and filtering mechanism. The opening to the lower airway is the larynx, a complex cartilaginous structure hung from the hyoid bone, which in turn is slung from the base of the skull. When foods or fluids are swallowed, the epiglottis, a roof-like flap, closes over the glottis and protects the trachea. Inside the lower end of the larynx are the vocal cords, used both to provide a watertight seal to the airways and to phonate. The two prominent thyroid cartilages form the anterior border, the 'Adam's apple' of the larynx. Just below these cartilages is an obvious groove, the cricothyroid membrane—the safest location for emergency surgical access to the airway.

The swallowing mechanism primarily involves the tongue and oropharynx. Movement of a food or fluid bolus to the back of the mouth causes reflex closure of the larynx and a peristaltic wave to pass down the oesophagus. Tongue swelling or a sore throat will disrupt swallowing.

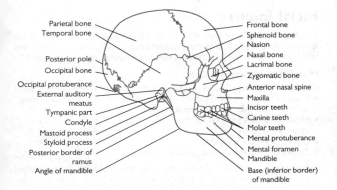

Fig. 10.1 Bony structures of the head.

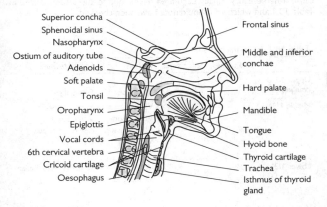

Fig. 10.2 Anatomy of the airway.

Facial injuries

Whatever the outdoor pursuit, the face is an easy target for injuries as it is left uncovered by most protective helmets so that we can see, breathe, and talk. Facial injuries may affect bones, soft tissues and teeth (see Chapter 11).

Maxillofacial examination

Consider the face as divided into equal thirds, plus the inside of the mouth:
- Upper 1/3 is from the eyebrows up to the hairline and when examining we look right over the cranium too.
- Middle 1/3 runs from under the supra-orbital rims to the tip of the upper front teeth.
- Lower 1/3 is the mandible.
- The inside of the mouth is the fourth area to examine.

In each area check the bony tissues for tenderness, mobility, or unexpected steps, the soft tissues for lacerations and bruising, and nerve function. Sensation is conveniently conveyed by a branch of the trigeminal nerve for each of the thirds of the face. Motor function is via the five branches of the facial nerve. Any lacerations which cross the path of these nerves may cause a nerve injury. Finally each area has unique features summarized in Table 10.1 and which you should note have been checked.

Table 10.1 Facial injuries summary

	Hard tissues	Soft tissues	Nerves	Special features
Upper 1/3 & cranium			Va	Battle's sign
			VII temporal	External ear
Middle 1/3			Vb	Eye movements
			VII temporal	Visual acuity
			VII zygomatic	CSF rhinorrhoea
			VII buccal	CSF otorrhoea
				Parotid duct
Lower 1/3			Vc	Temporo-mandibular joint
			VII marginal	
			VII mandibular	
Intra-oral			XII lingual	Dental occlusion
				Salivary flow from parotid duct

Begin by looking at symmetry of the face and any injuries:
- The three thirds should be equal height and if not there might be a fracture dislocation. If the middle third of the face looks elongated or depressed, it could indicate a Le Fort fracture of the maxilla.
- Swellings or bruises may indicate an underlying injury.
- Assess the level of the eyes—are they equal?
- Do the zygomas (cheek bones) look symmetrical?
- Is there any subconjunctival or peri-orbital bruising of the eye?

The upper 1/3 and cranium is best examined from above and behind the seated or lying patient:
- Check over the skull vault for depressions and bruising.
- Palpate the frontal bones and supra-orbital rims.
- Look at the eyes from above—is one more prominent or depressed than the other?
- Curl your index fingers to lie over the zygomatic bones as you look from above down: if asymmetrical the depressed one may be fractured and you may palpate a dent at the fracture site.
- Ask the casualty to open and close their mouth while your fingers feel the temporomandibular joints (TMJs) in front of the tragus of the ear—pain may indicate a mandibular condyle fracture.
- Look for leakage of clear CSF fluid from the ear or bruising behind the ear (Battle's sign—see Plate 22): both signs of possible skull base fracture.
- If any laceration passes over the path of the parotid duct (the middle third of the line from the tragus of the ear to the middle of the upper lip philtrum) check that saliva is milk-able from Stensen's duct which opens opposite the upper second molar tooth and is not evident through the laceration.

Now stand in front of the patient:
- Grasp the front of the maxilla between finger and thumb placed above the incisors in the mouth. Gently see if the maxilla moves.
- Assess the facial and trigeminal nerve function. Does part of the face droop, can the patient smile evenly and close eyes tightly?
- Examine visual acuity (eye sight), pupil reactions, and check for double vision especially in upward gaze—characteristic of an orbital blowout fracture.
- Check the symmetry of the nose and look for blood or clear CSF fluid from the nostrils.

Now look in the mouth:
- Ask the patient to bite their teeth together and if it feels different from normal. Do the teeth close properly and look even, or are there any step defects or gaps?
- Check for lacerations, bleeding, bruising, or broken teeth.

Minor injuries to head and neck

Head injuries such as bruises, black eyes, or lacerations are relatively common; more serious head injuries are fortunately rare, but are an ever-present risk during outdoor activities.

Lacerations

(See ⊃ Wound types and management, p. 272.)

Scalp lacerations tend to bleed a lot initially and can look a lot worse than they really are. Apply firm pressure until the bleeding stops. Small wounds can be closed using cyanoacrylate tissue glue. Conventional superglue has been used for this purpose, but can provoke tissue reactions and is not recommended.[1] Shaving the hair around large lacerations may make wound closure easier.

Simple facial lacerations usually heal well, but it is important to minimize scarring. Clean the wounds carefully and, where possible, use glue or skin fixers (Steri-Strips™, etc.) to bring the edges together. If wounds are deep, try to remove tension from the surface by placing resorbable subcutaneous sutures (e.g.4/0 Vicryl® Rapide) to approximate the edges and then suture the skin itself using a fine suture material (e.g. 5/0 Novafil® on face; 6/0 for lips and eyelids) to finish the job. Ensure that tension is even throughout the wound and that the edges are aligned. When a lip has been cut, make every effort to realign the vermilion edges as even small deviations are very obvious and may require subsequent corrective surgery. Remove sutures after 5 days. Most facial lacerations do not require antibiotics.

Complex or heavily contaminated lacerations will require specialist surgical management. Cover exposed bone with saline-soaked dressing, begin an IV antibiotic such as co-amoxiclav 1.2 g IV three times daily (if no penicillin allergy), and evacuate the casualty urgently for specialist surgical treatment.

Intra-oral lacerations are closed with resorbable 3/0 or 4/0 sutures. Explore them well using suction. If the labial mucosa is involved ask for help from a colleague to pull the lip tightly away from the teeth to give you a flat surface to suture.

Nasal injuries

(See ⊃ Nasal fracture, p. 308 and ⊃ Epistaxis (nose bleed), p. 335.)

Injured noses tend to bleed a lot. Apply cool compresses. Almost all nose bleeds can be controlled by pinching the soft tissues together across the tip of the nostrils, although rarely it may be necessary to pack a nostril using either a nasal tampon or ribbon gauze lubricated with paraffin ointment or a suitable antibiotic ointment.

Tongue

Bitten tongues and burnt tongues are usually made worse by attempting surgical treatment. Provide pain relief, rest, and keep the patient head-up if there is significant airway swelling. Sucking ice, if available, can relieve pain and swelling.

---

1 Cascarini L, Kumar A (2007). Case of the month: honey I glued the kids: tissue adhesives are not the same as "superglue". *Emerg Med J*, 24, 228–31.

Acute neck sprains

Neck sprains most commonly result from low-velocity, rear-end road traffic collisions, but may also occur in other circumstances such as being rolled by a wave whilst surfing. Initial assessment should attempt to eliminate the possibility of a fracture or dislocation of the neck, which can be indicated by the mechanism of injury, usually severe pain, and localized midline tenderness of the cervical spine. Assessment and exclusion without the aid of X-rays is difficult, especially for the inexperienced. If in doubt, immobilize and evacuate for specialist assessment (see ❯ Neck and other spinal injuries, p. 198).

However, if muscular pain predominates without bony tenderness or neurological symptoms, then it is probably that the neck has been sprained with damage to trapezius and sternomastoid muscles. Neck sprains are managed with analgesia and encouragement to mobilize. Immobilization with neck collars causes stiffness and should be avoided.

Fractured facial bones

Detailed diagnosis of facial bone fractures is impossible and irrelevant in a remote environment. Fractures to both the mandible and maxilla will cause pain and swelling, limit diet, and may threaten the airway. The best advice is to arrange early evacuation to specialist care. However, this may take time and in the interim the following can help, assuming there are no other life-threatening injuries:

• Reduce and stabilize the fracture.
• Apply comfortable and supportive bandaging.
• Arrange for a soft food or liquid diet.
• Provide details of the circumstances of the accident, treatment to date, and medication.
• Arrange for a carer to accompany the casualty to specialist care.

Mandibular fractures

The bottom jaw is typically fractured following a fall or punch. Patients complain of sensory loss of the lower lip, pain, and teeth not meeting properly ('deranged dental occlusion'). There may be blood and/ or gaps around individual teeth and step defects along the plane of the tops of the teeth. It may be possible to elicit movement of the mandible between teeth—passive and active on examination.

Broadly speaking we can consider the fractures as being in the tooth-bearing area (a–d in Fig. 10.3) or in the ramus and condyle of the mandible (e–h).

Treatment

• In the tooth-bearing area the fracture is at risk of infection and amoxicillin and metronidazole together or co-amoxiclav should be started (assuming no penicillin allergy; see ➋ Penicillin allergy, p. 263 if allergic).
• If there is a lot of movement at the fracture site the jaw may be very painful. Consider placing a wire or a thick nylon suture around the two teeth either side of the fracture to close and stabilize the fracture. These fractures require surgical fixation with miniplates, ideally within 24 h.
• If undisplaced, ramus or condylar fractures are treated conservatively. There may be swelling and difficulty opening and closing the mouth. They are reassessed at a week after the injury. If displaced they may require surgical reduction.
• Give simple analgesics and a soft diet. Arrange evacuation for surgical management.

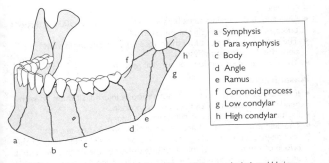

a Symphysis
b Para symphysis
c Body
d Angle
e Ramus
f Coronoid process
g Low condylar
h High condylar

Fig. 10.3 Mandibular fracture sites. Adapted from O'Connor, Isobel, and Urdanq, Michael, *Handbook of Surgical Cross-Cover* (2008), with permission from Oxford University Press.

Maxillary fracture

There are many categories—don't worry about them. Once you have identified the presence of a fracture of the maxilla, check the airway, eyes, and cervical spine (especially in falls from height) and arrange for evacuation. The type of fracture can be determined by the receiving medical team by CT scan. Typically the window for operating is 2 weeks.

Treatment

The airway is very rarely a problem. An awake patient will naturally sit forward to keep their airway patent. But in an unconscious patient with a high fracture, the facial bones may be pushed down and back along the skull base, causing the soft palate to snag on the tongue and so closing the airway. A Guedel airway, laryngeal mask, or endotracheal tube may be required, or, if there is extreme airway swelling or bleeding, a cricothyroidotomy (⊃ Maintaining an open airway, p. 187) could be life-saving. Fortunately such situations are very unusual. Deal with epistaxis if present using pressure or nasal packs.

Zygomatic fractures

Cheek bone fractures can involve either the arch of the zygoma causing a dimple in the skin over the arch and possibly entrapment of the coronoid process of the mandible limiting jaw movement, or the zygomatic body. There may be bruising and swelling in the region with flattening deformity if displaced. Look for bloody injection of the white of eye lateral to pupil: subscleral haemorrhage and paraesthesia of the face below the eye (infra-orbital nerve).

Examine for signs of eye involvement (diplopia, visual acuity loss, or an injury to the globe), a blow out fracture of the orbit, or even retrobulbar haemorrhage (see ⊃ Examination of the eye, p. 325; ⊃ Orbital compartment syndrome, p. 331).

Treatment
- Give antibiotics against sinus bacteria—oral amoxicillin 500 mg three times a day for 1 week (if not penicillin allergic).
- The patient should not blow their nose for 2 weeks to prevent periorbital surgical emphysema.
- There is a 2-week window for surgical reduction.

Nasal fracture

- If the casualty is conscious and not seriously injured, sit them up with head well forward to allow secretions to drain.
- Exclude associated head or cervical spine injury.
- The diagnosis of a nasal fracture is a clinical one. X-rays are not routinely required. Swelling, tenderness, and possibly deformity of the bridge of the nose are visible. Consider whether the nasal injury could be part of a more complicated fracture—involving the orbit, ethmoids, or frontal bones. If it is an isolated injury it may be possible to straighten a deformed nasal bone fracture soon after the injury, although the casualty may be reluctant to permit this.
- It is essential to look for and exclude a septal haematoma—a smooth swelling of the midline of the nose that can develop into septal necrosis. In the wilderness a septal haematoma should be incised under local anaesthetic, and then the nostrils packed to prevent recurrence.
- Swelling often prevents an early assessment of the degree of nasal deformity. Between 5 and 7 days after injury, the nose should be re-examined; if there is evidence of deformity or septal deviation, the patient requires evacuation for specialist surgical assessment and management. Deformities should be corrected operatively within 10 days of injury.
- Open fractures of the nose require prophylactic antibiotics such as co-amoxiclav or clarithromycin.

Blow-out fracture of orbit

Blunt trauma to the globe of the eye (e.g. from a fall or a punch) can cause the weak bony orbital floor to fracture. This may cause prolapse of orbital fat into the maxillary sinus below. Double vision can occur from the swelling, which may be intolerable and require patching of the damaged eye (see Fig. 10.6). Surgical repair, if required, is possible for up to 2 weeks following injury.

In children, the inferior rectus muscle can become trapped and be the cause of diplopia. A simple test to check is to get them to look up and if the globe cannot move, there is entrapment. This can cause malaise, vomiting, and headache, and be confused with a head injury. These children need urgent surgical release—ideally within 24 h—to prevent permanent visual impairment.

Diagnosis is made of the basis of:
- History.
- Pain on eye movement.
- Double vision (diplopia).
- Sunken eye (enophthalmos).

If you suspect this injury:

- Check visual acuity in both eyes ('Can you read this?').
- Feel around the bony margins of the eye socket.
- Make sure that the whole of the globe of the eye is intact.
- If the double vision is intolerable, cover the damaged eye with a patch (see Fig. 10.6).

Injuries of this type may also lead to:

- Corneal abrasion.
- Hyphaema (blood in the anterior chamber of the eye).
- Subluxed lens.
- Vitreous haemorrhage.
- Retinal detachment.
- Posterior globe rupture.
- Surgical emphysema periorbitally—the patient should not blow their nose for 2 weeks.
- Orbital compartment syndrome (➔ Orbital compartment syndrome, p. 331).

If visual acuity is reduced after a blunt trauma, evacuation is essential.

Dislocated jaw joints

The TMJ may dislocate, typically when yawning too wide. The individual may well have a history of this. If dislocation occurs in association with trauma, be wary—fracture dislocations require specialist surgical management.

The TMJ consists of the mandibular condyle (the finer projection up from the mandible) and the glenoid fossa—the dished surface on the temporal bone skull base, in which the condyle articulates. During small movements the condyle just pivots in a fixed position, but when the jaw opens wide it slides forward, down, and out of the glenoid fossa. It soon meets a physical block—the articular eminence, which stops it moving further—but in extremely wide opening it can flip over this eminence and get stuck leaving the mouth fixed open, the lower jaw jutting forward and the chin very prominent.

A *closed* fixed mouth is not a dislocated jaw, by definiton.

Just pushing the mandible backwards will not reduce the dislocation—it simply pushes the condyle straight back into the articular eminence, so the mandibular condyle has to be pushed *down* and over the articular eminence. Attempt relocation as soon as you can before the jaw muscles go into spasm and prevent further movement. Lie the patient flat in a quiet environment. The process is not painful but it can be uncomfortable.

Stand in front of the patient. With gloved hands insert your index finger into the mouth behind the most posterior lower tooth onto the mucosa overlying the bone behind the molar teeth (Fig. 10.4). Do this on both sides if both condyles are dislocated. Make sure that your fingers lie *around* the cheek side of the back teeth and not over them or you will get bitten when the jaw goes back into place! Then curl the thumbs under the chin on each side. Your aim is not to push the mandible straight back as this just pushes the condyle back onto the articular eminence. Instead you have to push the condyle down and back, *over* the articular eminence before it returns to the glenoid fossa. Press down and back with the index fingers and push the chin up with the thumbs. This rotates the mandible making the condyle move down and back more easily. It is not a sudden relocation but instead is a slow sustained pressure for up to several minutes. Usually one condyle returns before the other. Obviously in unilateral dislocation that is enough, but most are bilateral and will require a little more effort. However, once one side is in the other usually swiftly follows. Then advise the patient to rest the jaw joint for a few weeks by stifling yawns by preventing wide mouth opening with a hand underneath the chin and having a soft diet.

Cases which cannot be relocated easily may need sedation, local anaesthetic injections to the muscles around the joint, or evacuation to be relocated under a short general anaesthetic.

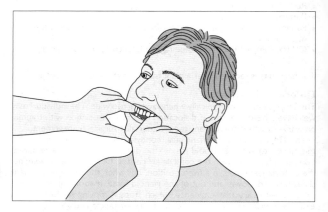

Fig. 10.4 Relocating a dislocated jaw.

Cervical spine

For discussion of the assessment and management of suspected cervical spine trauma see ➜ Neck and other spinal injuries, p. 198.

Head injury

A person should be considered to have a head injury if they have suffered any trauma to the head, apart from superficial lacerations to the face. Head injuries can be:

- Direct or indirect.
- Closed or open.

and may result in:

- Primary or secondary brain damage.

Epidemiology

It is best to avoid a head injury! About 60% of adults with moderate head injuries and 85% with severe head injuries remain disabled 1 year after their accident. Even a minor head injury can ruin a trip: 3 months later, 80% have persistent headaches and 60% have memory problems. Wear a suitable helmet if at risk of head injury.

Causes

- Direct head injuries are caused by a blow to the head of some form; this can result in a closed injury, without penetration of the skull, or an open injury, where the skull is penetrated.
- Indirect injury is caused by a 'whiplash' effect of the brain moving within the skull, though without a direct blow to the head; this can result in brief concussion, but in a young adult is unlikely to cause significant damage.

History and examination

- Ask about amnesia for events before and after the injury. Brief amnesia of <1 min is common with even mild concussion, but any significant amnesia should be a cause for concern. Post-traumatic amnesia (PTA) may be a more reliable marker of severity, and should be taken to end at the point when the victim regains continuous memory, rather than just islands of recollection. Significant head injuries are usually associated with PTA of >30 min.
- Care is particularly needed for high-energy injuries, e.g. a pedestrian struck by a vehicle, any high-speed road traffic collision, or any accident involving motorized off-road vehicles such as snowmobiles, jet skis, or quad bikes. High-energy injuries also include any significant fall from a height, or any rock fall.
- *Assess level of consciousness*, using the GCS (Box 7.1). This is easily and reliably administered with minimal experience and is particularly useful to monitor progress. Failure of the GCS to improve and, in particular, a fall in GCS is of significant concern. The scale has a range of 3–15. A score of 8 or less indicates a very severe head injury, one that, if it were available, would prompt immediate critical care. A score of 12 or less at any point after a closed head injury indicates possible significant injury, but secondary intracranial bleeding can develop even in someone who was fully conscious initially.

- Carry out *careful inspection* of the head, looking particularly for signs of any skull fracture. Classically basal skull fracture may be associated with:
  - CSF fluid leaking from ear (otorrhoea) or nose (rhinorrhoea).
  - Blood behind tympanic membrane ('haemotympanum').
  - 'Battle's sign' (bruising and tenderness over mastoid—see Plate 22).
  - 'Panda eyes' (black eye(s) without orbital injury).
  - However, these signs are often absent.
- Carry out and document a *simple neurological examination*. As a minimum this should include:
  - Examination of pupil size and reaction.
  - Check of visual acuity.
  - Eye movements.
  - Examine tympanic membranes if possible.
  - Always assess hearing and look in the ears.
  - Gag reflex if not fully conscious.
  - Examine for any focal motor deficit, including plantar responses.
  - Check for any sensory loss.
  - Ask about paraesthesia.
  - Look for ataxia.
- Other features may include irritability and/or altered behaviour, persistent headaches, or vomiting. An apparent convulsion at the moment of impact is a well-recognized feature of concussion, often seen in contact sports, and need not be of great significance. Any subsequent seizure is of great concern.
- Do not attribute a depressed conscious level and/or altered behaviour to intoxication with alcohol or drugs unless you are sure that there has been no significant brain injury. Any intoxicated person with a suspected head injury needs close observation.
- Always carefully examine the spine, especially the cervical spine in any significant head injury, particularly those with a dangerous mechanism of injury. Around 10% of those knocked out with a head injury have an associated neck injury (➲ Neck and other spinal injuries, p. 198).
- Document any findings and repeat examination; judgement is needed to determine the frequency and extent of repeat examination, but if you are concerned about a possible significant head injury it would be reasonable to repeat GCS every 30 min for 2 h; by then the GCS should be 13 or better. Continue to repeat hourly for 4 h, then 2-hrly thereafter until the GCS is normal, and do not leave the person alone for 24 h.

Clinical features

Closed head injury

- Results from falls, road traffic collisions, etc.
- Typically high-energy injury.
- No penetration of the skull.
- *Primary* damage tends to be diffuse:
  - Diffuse axonal injury.
  - Some focal damage, particularly to vulnerable areas such as frontal lobes, anterior temporal, and posterior occipital poles.

Open head injury
- Penetrating injury to the skull.
- *Primary* damage is largely focal but the effects can be just as serious.
Secondary deterioration is usually due to:
- *Oedema* (swelling) of damaged tissue, resulting in increased intracranial pressure and possible brain herniation.
- Intracranial haemorrhage (bleeding) from torn vessels, which can be:
  - *Subdural*: between the dura and the brain.
  - *Extradural:* outside the dura, beneath the skull vault.

Swelling inside the closed cranium interferes with blood flow into the brain. Cerebral perfusion pressure (CPP) is the balance of mean arterial pressure (MAP) less intracranial pressure (ICP):

$$CPP = MAP - ICP$$

It is therefore important to maintain BP, with fluid replacement, and minimize ICP. Factors that increase ICP that can be correctable in the wilderness include pain and hypoxia due to altitude.

Management

Management options for a significant head injury in a remote environment are limited:
- Maintain airway and breathing, and replace fluids when possible.
- Assess and manage cervical spine.
- Give adequate analgesia to control pain, and try to be calm and provide reassurance. Opiates, if available, may be needed to control severe pain, but can mask signs of deteriorating cerebral function.
- Elevation of the head to 20° improves venous outflow from the brain and may reduce intracranial pressure. This should only be attempted after any hypovolaemia has been corrected.
- If the casualty is at altitude sufficient to cause hypoxia then, if possible, bring down, and give oxygen when available.
- Steroids should not be given; they have been shown to increase mortality rates.
- Secondary deterioration owing to cerebral oedema may respond to diuretics. Mannitol is preferred because it causes less electrolyte disturbance than loop diuretics, but it is unlikely to be available. Furosemide and other diuretics should be used with care; give sufficient to induce diuresis, but ensure that BP is maintained.
- Deterioration caused by intracranial bleeding is usually untreatable in the wilderness, though a doctor familiar with the technique might in desperation attempt a burr hole to relieve a developing extradural haematoma.
- The major issue is whether to arrange evacuation. This decision depends on the situation and the severity of the injury. Most head injuries do not require neurosurgery, but there are many factors following any significant injury that are better managed in hospital, and secondary deterioration because of intracranial bleeding is potentially correctable. If evacuation is realistically possible, following anything other than a minor head injury it should be arranged.

Complications

- Infection: meningitis is a recognized complication of any skull fracture where the integrity of the blood–brain barrier may be breached. If transfer to hospital may be delayed it is appropriate to give a broad-spectrum antibiotic. There is particular risk if there is a CSF leak, a common presentation of which is the loss of clear, slightly salty, watery fluid coming from the nose or ear.
- Seizures: epileptic seizures can occur early or late. Early seizures, within 24 h, may not require long-term treatment, but in the wilderness any seizure is best treated until definitive care is available. A seizure should be considered a sign of possible intracranial deterioration. Medication available is likely to be limited to a benzodiazepine such as lorazepam or diazepam. The risk of sedation is outweighed by the need to control seizures.
- Neurological symptoms: these can be divided into minor symptoms that can follow any concussion, and more significant deficits. Headaches, unsteadiness, and poor concentration are common after minor head injury; they are likely to last for up to 3 months and possibly longer. Benign positional vertigo can follow any blow to the head; it results in intense vertigo with a sensation of spinning precipitated by movement of the head. Give prochlorperazine or cyclizine and arrange an ENT assessment.

Severe head injuries have many consequences, and may require long-term rehabilitation.

Resource

NICE (2014). *Head Injury: Triage, Assessment, Investigation and Early Management of Head Injury in Children, Young People and Adults*. Available at: ℘ http://www.nice.org.uk/Guidance/CG176

Blackouts, syncope, and epilepsy

An episode of transient loss of consciousness is often referred to as a 'blackout'. Blackouts commonly result from:

- A disorder of the circulation—e.g. syncope (fainting).
- A disorder of the brain—e.g. epilepsy.
- A disorder of the psyche—e.g. psychogenic blackouts.

It may prove difficult, if not impossible, to determine the cause of some blackouts in the wilderness. Any previous diagnosis in an expedition member should be treated with caution, particularly if there are unusual features about the new attack.

Treatment

- Turn patient onto their side in the recovery position (➔ Recovery position, p. 226; Fig. 8.5 and Fig. 8.6).
- Take the pulse; it is quicker and easier to compare the patient's pulse to your own, rather than to try and count it. If the pulse is weak, thready, and particularly if it is slow, it may well be that the person has fainted, but had associated muscle movements.
- Give oxygen if available, particularly if the seizure is prolonged.
- Do not attempt to force anything into their mouth.
- Your choice of available antiepileptic drugs is likely to be limited. Most seizures are self-limiting, and a single seizure does not require treatment unless the seizure is prolonged (over 5 min).
- If the seizure is prolonged, then give any available benzodiazepine IV, IM or PR. It is safest to titrate lorazepam or diazepam IV.
- An alcoholic binge-induced seizure may be complicated by low blood sugar levels. If possible measure the blood glucose level and correct with sugar or glucose gel.

Management

- Question the patient carefully for any prior history. If they are confused, or you doubt their medical history, consider contacting their family or GP if communications are available.
- Carry out as comprehensive a neurological examination as you are able to, looking carefully for papilloedema if possible, and checking for any persisting focal neurological deficit.
- If you believe that a team member has developed epilepsy for the first time in a wilderness environment, particularly if the patient is unwell, if there are any focal features to the seizure, or focal neurological deficit, then evacuate as soon as possible.
- Consider cerebral malaria (➔ Malaria, p. 480) and give therapeutic doses of antimalarials if in doubt.

Seizures may occasionally complicate high-altitude cerebral oedema (HACE ➔ High-altitude cerebral oedema, p. 664.)

Syncope (fainting)

Incidence

Cardiac syncope accounts for most blackouts, and of these the majority of cases are due to reflex syncope, with up to 30% of people suffering reflex syncope during their lives. In contrast, epilepsy only affects ~0.5% of the population at any one time, with a lifetime incidence of 2%, although many of these will develop at one or other extreme of age. Blackouts are also often seen in the absence of organic physical disease; such attacks may be accompanied by apparent convulsive movements, but their origin could be psychological rather than physical, particularly in very stressful circumstances.

The cause of syncope may be either *cardiac* or *vascular*:

- *Cardiac causes* could be due to structural heart disease or an arrhythmia. Sudden death in young people is occasionally associated with a structural cardiomyopathy. An arrhythmia in the wilderness could be a marker of myocardial infarction, although otherwise very fit middle-aged individuals can develop atrial fibrillation and feel awful. Syncope *during* (as opposed to *after*) exercise is potentially serious and may presage sudden cardiac death owing to a familial arrhythmia such as long QT syndrome.
- *Vascular causes* are more likely, and include:
  - Reflex causes, such as vasovagal syncope.
  - Situational causes, such as cough and micturition syncope.
  - Postural causes, such as orthostatic hypotension which may reflect dehydration.
  - Pulmonary embolism.

In hot environments, consider heatstroke (➋ Heat-related illnesses (HRIs), p. 748).

Clinical diagnosis

Diagnosis is made from the history, particularly the circumstances around the blackout. Syncope results in transient self-limited loss of consciousness owing to transient reduction in blood flow to the brain, typically leading to collapse; most attacks, particularly those with vascular causes, therefore occur when patient is standing, although fainting can occur while sitting.

- The patient may recall a brief lightheadedness, when voices sounded distant, and vision faded.
- Onset is rapid; recovery is spontaneous, complete, and usually prompt.
- During the episode the pulse may be slow and BP low, but often the episode is too brief and the bystanders too panicked for either to be reliably measured.
- The patient characteristically appears limp and pale.
- Limb jerks (myoclonus) commonly occur. These are usually brief, but complex movements resembling epilepsy can be seen. This 'convulsive syncope' often results in panic in bystanders and may be reported as an 'epileptic fit' by even medically trained observers unfamiliar with the phenomenon.
- During recovery there may be brief bewilderment, but prolonged confusion is rare.
- If the person gets up too quickly they may collapse again.

Epilepsy

Epilepsy can be classified as idiopathic, a condition in isolation, or symptomatic, resulting from some underlying disease. The resulting seizures are either generalized, involving the whole brain from onset, or focal, starting in one area but then affecting all areas.

- *Idiopathic epilepsy* usually starts in childhood, so is unlikely to be a diagnostic issue in the wilderness; however, some syndromes first appear during adolescence, and could therefore present in a teenager. Idiopathic epilepsies usually cause generalized seizures, tonic–clonic convulsions, myoclonus, and absences; most probably have a genetic basis.
- *Symptomatic epilepsy,* particularly in the context of wilderness medicine, is more likely to result in focal or secondarily generalized seizures. The seizure may indicate an underlying localized brain disorder, and in these circumstances concern should be raised about infection, including cerebral malaria and meningitis.

A separate classification describes the resultant seizures: these are *partial* or *generalized*.

Partial (or 'focal') seizures

- More likely to be caused by a symptomatic epilepsy; that is, where pathology has developed in part of the brain, causing the seizures—this is potentially of more concern in the wilderness.
- Begin in one part of the body, and may then spread.
- Signs are variable: the patient may or may not lose awareness, and may or may not collapse.
- If the attack is witnessed, record its details, which may include automatic behaviour, asymmetrical limb jerking, or a forced turn of the head.
- Afterwards the patient may recall a strong unpleasant smell, or a brief but intense sense of déjà vu.

Generalized seizures

- Involve the whole of the brain.
- Best recognized form is a tonic–clonic convulsion.
- Onset is sudden with an initial tonic phase: all muscles stiffen, the limbs become rigid, and there may be a strangled cry. The person falls to the ground and may become cyanosed.
- The subsequent clonic phase involves rhythmic jerking of the limbs; initially this may be vigorous, but the movements slow and become irregular.
- Victim is then usually unconscious for a period.
- When they come round they may be confused, muscles may ache, and they will usually complain of headache.
- They may have bitten the tongue (usually the side).
- The tonic–clonic seizure itself rarely lasts more than 1–2 min, but post-ictal drowsiness and confusion can be prolonged, with general malaise lasting several hours.
- A generalized tonic–clonic convulsion can also develop from an initial partial seizure, the seizure activity starting focally and then spreading to the whole brain; these are secondarily generalized convulsions.

Other types of generalized seizures include collapse with rigidity (tonic sei-zure) or without change in muscle tone (atonic seizures). These usually only occur in the context of a complex epilepsy associated with learning dis-ability. Generalized seizures also include absences, with preserved posture, and daytime myoclonus, both of which may be seen in previously diagnosed idiopathic childhood and juvenile epilepsies.

Psychogenic blackouts and disturbances

These range from simple panic attacks with hyperventilation, which rarely cause blackout and are usually readily recognized, to a wide spectrum of non-epileptic seizures. Typically occurring in adolescents or young adult women, they can be frequent and without apparent cause. Assessment is very difficult, and it is essential to exclude organic disease. Such behaviour is disruptive, especially in a hazardous environment, so evacuation or repa-triation may be required.

Differential diagnosis of blackouts and seizures

If you consider that the blackout was due to syncope, then check for any predisposing systemic illness:

- Anaemia is likely, particularly in young women who faint; check for blood loss—acute or chronic.
- Dehydration or heat exhaustion.
- Salt deficiency.
- Excess alcohol can predispose to fainting, possibly due to dehydration, but can also be associated with epileptic seizures.
- Hypoxia and HACE (see ➨ High-altitude cerebral oedema, p. 664) may cause fitting.
- An initial epileptic seizure may be the first indication of an underlying neurological disease, especially if the seizure was focal. Possible causes include:
  - *Neurocysticercosis:* the most common cause of new adult-onset epilepsy in rural, developing countries with poor hygiene, where pigs are allowed to roam freely. It results from human ingestion of the eggs from the pork tape worm. Visitors are vulnerable, the condition usually presenting some months after exposure.
  - *Schistosomiasis*, may present with epilepsy.
  - *Bacterial meningitis* can cause seizures. The individual is likely to be very unwell with associated fever, photophobia, and a stiff neck.
  - *Cerebral malaria* should always be considered in malarial zones.

Investigations

Few investigations are possible in the wilderness. Check pulse and tem-perature to check for systemic illness, and check blood glucose if possible. Measure oxygen saturation if a pulse oximeter is available.[2]

---

2 NICE guideline on blackouts:
ℛ http://www.nice.org.uk/guidance/cg109
ℛ https://www.epilepsydiagnosis.org

Migraine

Migraine is a disorder characterized by recurrent, usually unilateral, moderate to severe headaches that may be accompanied by dizziness, nausea, vomiting, or extreme sensitivity to light and sound. Migraine is common in young adults. Most migraine sufferers know they have the condition, so a first attack would be unusual but could be precipitated by, for instance, altitude. The cause of migraine is unknown.

Risk factors

Women may be more prone to migraine if on the combined oral contraceptive pill. Focal migraine is a contraindication to the use of the oestrogen-containing contraceptive pill—it may increase the risk of stroke. Triggering factors include:

- Stress, tiredness, exertion, and menstruation.
- Alcohol, especially red wine.
- Citrus fruits.
- Cheese.
- Chocolate.
- Caffeine.

History and examination

Migraine usually develops in a predictable way:

- *Prodromal:* change in mood, depression or restlessness, tiredness or listlessness.
- *Aura:* including flashes, shimmering, and other hallucinations.
- *Headache*: typically one-sided but may affect both sides of the head. It is usually gradual in onset, moderate to severe in pain intensity, throbbing, and worse with physical exertion, and it can last anywhere from 2 h to 2 days in children and 4 h to 3 days in adults. The headache stage is often accompanied by loss of appetite, nausea, vomiting, sensitivity to light and sound, blurred vision, tenderness of the scalp or neck, lightheadedness, sweating, and pallor. In severe cases there may be visual field defects and unilateral limb weakness; these are very frightening symptoms which should be treated seriously unless the patient knows that they are regularly associated with their migraines.

Treatment

Rest, hydration, and adequate analgesia.

If the individual is known to have migraine they may have brought their medication with them. Otherwise, give 900 mg soluble aspirin, which should be given with a glass of milk, if available, to protect the stomach, and ideally also with an anti-emetic. Metoclopramide or domperidone are particularly useful as they promote gastric emptying, but avoid metoclopramide in adolescents and young adults, as it can precipitate an extrapyramidal reaction. Prochlorperazine is a suitable alternative.

Complications

Complications are unlikely. If migraine develops for first time in women on oral contraception then this should be stopped, particularly if migraine has focal features.

Sleep disturbances

On an expedition many factors may disturb sleep, including time zone shifts, unfamiliar harsh living conditions, physical discomfort, environmental extremes including high altitude, sport-specific disturbances (night watches sailing, pre-dawn starts climbing), and psychological factors such as anxiety about the venture ahead or homesickness. Few things erode team morale and daytime performance as much as disturbed sleep; however, forward planning and simple measures can improve things considerably.

General measures to improve sleep

- Comfortable bed—careful choice of tent site, padded sleeping mat.
- Temperature control—fan, hot water bottle (e.g. tomorrow's boiled drinking water wrapped in a fleece), appropriate sleeping bag and mat.
- Mosquito deterrents—nets and repellents.
- Earplugs.
- Safe environment—away from rock fall, avalanche run out zones, flood pathways, or marauding animals.

Jet lag

Many body functions are under circadian control, including hormone secretion, body temperature, cellular and enzymatic function, and sleep. The natural circadian rhythm approximates 24 h. Rapid travel across time zones is associated with desynchronization between the body's circadian clock and the actual local time, resulting in jet lag. This is experienced as difficulty getting to sleep following an eastward flight, wakening early following a westward flight, disturbed sleep, daytime sleepiness, difficulty concentrating, irritability, depressed mood, anorexia, and nocturia. These symptoms usually only pose a minor inconvenience for travellers; however, performance, including decision-making, may be impaired in the first few days following arrival in a new time zone, and this should be allowed for in the travel schedule.

Decreasing jet lag

- Obtain adequate sleep. Use daytime flights in preference or sleep as much as possible during overnight flights. Use short naps terminated by an alarm clock to improve daytime alertness and concentration. Avoid napping late in the day as this will decrease the ability to sleep at night.
- Adopt the new time frame in the country you are leaving and in transit, including bed and get up times and meal times.
- Optimize light exposure. The light–dark cycle is the principal time cue for resetting human circadian rhythms. Bright light exposure during the daytime for the new time zone and avoidance of bright light at other times of day may have a beneficial effect on the circadian clock and jet lag. This usually means maximizing the exposure to light early in the day after flying eastwards and late in the day after flying westwards.
- Take exercise. Exercise both improves sleep quality and has a minor effect on entraining circadian rhythms, with night-time exercise delaying the circadian clock.

- Avoid excess caffeine and alcohol as these can have a deleterious effect on sleep quality.
- Short-acting hypnotic drugs used on overnight flights and for a few nights after arrival may help. Drug-induced sleepiness carrying over into the next day must be taken into account, particularly after short flights followed by driving.
- Melatonin is a hormone that is secreted by the pineal gland and linked to the circadian rhythm. A Cochrane analysis suggests that taken in doses of 0.5–5 mg at the right time of day, it can be effective at preventing and reducing jet lag. However incorrect timing of doses can cause drowsiness and failure to adapt to the new time zone, and exact dosages are as yet uncertain. Low mood, and even frank depression, is a fairly common side effect of melatonin, and it may therefore exacerbate homesickness. Patients taking warfarin and those with epilepsy should avoid melatonin.[3]

Obstructive sleep apnoea syndrome

Obstructive sleep apnoea (OSA) is a condition in which repeated blockage of the upper airway fragments sleep. It presents with snoring, pauses in breathing, and daytime sleepiness. People with this pre-existing condition should consult their physician prior to travel.

OSA may be treated using nasal continuous positive airway pressure (CPAP) during sleep. If CPAP has to be discontinued briefly, there is some carry forward benefit for 1 to 2 nights before symptoms return. An alternative to CPAP for patients with milder OSA is a jaw advancement device, which has the merits of being small, readily portable, and requiring no electrical power. Interestingly mild OSA improves somewhat on ascent to high altitude, presumably as tone in the upper airway is increased by the additional respiratory effort driven by hypoxia.

3 ᕼ http://summaries.cochrane.org/CD001520/melatonin-for-the-prevention-and-treatment-of-jet-lag#sthash.W7PuPDEg.dpuf

The eye

Ophthalmology is viewed by the general physician with anything from mild boredom to abject fear. Unfortunately, eye problems may occur while travelling and this section is designed to help you assess and treat them. An expedition medic should have some experience of using a magnifying loupe and ophthalmoscope as well as administering eye drops and applying a double eye pad.

Ocular anatomy

It is important to have a basic understanding of ocular anatomy to assess the severity of an injury. Fig. 10.5 shows an external and internal view of the eye; note that the cornea is continuous with the sclera and that the conjunctiva lines both the inside of the eyelids and covers the sclera up to the cornea.

Pre-expedition ocular history

Relevant ocular information can be obtained from the pre-departure health questionnaire (see Box 10.1 and also Box 2.3).

> ### Box 10.1 Ocular history taking
> - Do you wear contact lenses?
>   - If yes, what type are they (e.g. hard/soft, monthlies/dailies)?
> - Have you ever been treated by a doctor for an eye problem?
> - Have you ever had any type of operation on your eyes including laser refraction correction? If so, what and when?
> - Does anyone in your family suffer from glaucoma or other eye disease?
> - Are you diabetic?

Travellers with chronic eye conditions may need to take other precautions and should ensure that they have ample supplies of regular medications.

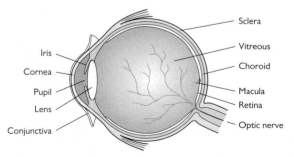

Fig. 10.5 Anatomy of the eye.

Contact lenses

In the wilderness, contact lens users are vulnerable to dry eyes and serious corneal infections, so should be advised on sensible contact lens use (no more than 8 h a day) and strict hygiene when handling lenses. Remind them to bring spectacles as well as plenty of spare contact lenses.

Any potential infection, even an apparently simple conjunctivitis, should be taken very seriously. Contact lens wear should be stopped and intensive broad-spectrum antibiotic drops should be started (e.g. ofloxacin hourly). If no improvement within 5 days, evacuate the patient.

Refractive surgery and high altitude

Refractive surgery is becoming increasingly popular amongst outdoor enthusiasts to decrease dependence on spectacles or contact lenses. During this type of surgery, the refractive power of the cornea is changed either through surgical incisions or laser ablation. However, high altitude can affect the surgical results, causing blurred vision that usually resolves upon descent. Radial keratotomy (RK) has now been superseded by laser *in situ* keratomilieusis (LASIK), laser epithelial keratomilieusis (LASEK), and photorefractive keratectomy (PRK).

RK tends to cause long-sightedness (hypermetropia) at altitude whereas LASIK, LASEK, and PRK may cause short-sightedness (myopia) at altitude. This phenomenon is not predictable and can severely affect vision. Avoid elective refractive surgery within 3 months of an expedition as refraction can be unstable and infection a risk.

Another form of refractive surgery is to have the natural lens removed and replaced with an intraocular lens in a procedure similar to cataract surgery. There is a risk of dry eye and a small chance of intraocular infection after clear lens extraction, but vision is unlikely to change at high altitude.

Any decreased vision, redness, or pain in the eyes of someone who has had refractive surgery should be taken seriously, as they are more vulnerable to infection. If necessary, consider descent and evacuation.

Examination of the eye

- *Visual acuity* is the single most important sign when examining the eye and you do not need a Snellen chart to test it; either compare it with the other eye or simply ask the patient if their vision has changed.
- Do not be afraid to *dilate* the pupil to obtain a reasonable view of the retina. If tropicamide alone is used, it can be easily reversed with pilocarpine in the extremely unlikely event of an acute rise in intraocular pressure owing to angle closure.
- Measurement of *intraocular pressure* does not require specialist equipment. Ask the patient to close their eyes and, with your thumbs, simply press gently on the globe, comparing one eye with the other. This will easily reveal the 'marble' of high pressure from the 'avocado' of normal pressure.
- *Fluorescein* is useful to assess the integrity of the corneal epithelium and the globe. It should only be administered after topical anaesthetic (e.g. tetracaine (amethocaine)). It is best viewed with a blue light in the dark.

Drops or ointment?

Drops are easy to administer but are short lived. Ointments sooth and lubricate, but blur the vision. It is therefore worth having antibiotics in both preparations depending on the patient's needs.

Loss of vision

Loss of vision, even if it is transient, whether or not associated with pain, should be of great concern to the expedition medic especially if no obvious cause such as snow blindness can be found. Always consider evacuating the patient for specialist evaluation.

- Take a full history.
- Evaluate optic nerve function (see Box 10.2).
- Digital intraocular pressure (as described in **⊃** Examination of the eye, p. 325).
- Eye movements.
- Ophthalmoscopy.

Box 10.2 Tests of optic nerve function in the wild

- Visual acuity: compare with the other eye.
- Colour vision: 'How red is my hat compared with the other eye?'
- Visual fields: simple confrontational fields.
- Pupils: check for a relative afferent pupillary defect.
- Ophthalmoscopy: look for optic disc pallor compared to the other eye.

Causes of painful loss of vision

- Snow blindness.
- Orbital cellulitis.
- Bacterial keratitis.
- Acute angle-closure glaucoma.
- Optic neuritis.
- Giant cell arteritis.
- Endophthalmitis.

Causes of painless loss of vision

- Migraine.
- Amaurosis fugax (transient ischaemic loss of vision).
- Cerebral hypoxia.
- High-altitude retinopathy (HAR).
- Hypertensive retinopathy.
- Ischaemic optic neuropathy.
- Retinal artery occlusion.
- Retinal vein occlusion.
- Vitreous haemorrhage.
- Retinal detachment.

Conjunctivitis

Conjunctivitis is the most common eye problem likely to be encountered in the wilderness setting.

Symptoms and signs

One or both eyes are red and painful with pus (bacterial), profuse watering (viral), or itch (allergic) depending on aetiology. Visual acuity is usually unaffected, the conjunctiva red and inflamed, and the cornea clear.

Treatment
Bacterial conjunctivitis should respond rapidly to topical antibiotics, whereas viral conjunctivitis can persist for many days but is eventually self-limiting. If the patient is a contact lens wearer then follow the specific advice earlier in the chapter (see ➲ Contact lenses, p. 325). Allergic conjunctivitis may respond to sodium cromoglicate. Bacterial and especially viral conjunctivitis are extremely contagious so enforce strict hygiene measures.

Dry eyes

Dry eyes can be exacerbated by the dry, windy, bright conditions found at high altitude or in polar regions. Contact lens wearers are particularly vulnerable. The eyes are red, painful, and gritty.

Treatment
- Symptoms are relieved by topical anaesthetic; subsequent fluorescein reveals punctuate staining.
- Use an ocular lubricant frequently.
- Minimize contact lens wear.
- Goggles can decrease tear evaporation.
- Although usually just a nuisance, severely dry eyes can be very painful, vision blurred, and the eyes susceptible to infection.

Corneal abrasion

A tear in the corneal epithelium, usually through mild trauma such as removing a contact lens or perhaps even while asleep.

Symptoms and signs
An acute and exquisitely painful eye. Topical anaesthetic will provide immediate relief, but should not be used as a treatment. Fluorescein will confirm the diagnosis.

Treatment
Prescribe an antibiotic ointment. An eye pad is not usually necessary and can encourage infection.

Snow blindness

Snow blindness is caused by unprotected exposure of the cornea and conjunctiva to ultraviolet light (UVB). Like sunburn, by the time you realize there is a problem, it is too late, and it can be extremely painful. Prevention and treatment are discussed in ➲ Snow blindness (photokeratitis), p. 634.

Corneal foreign body

Occasionally the protective blink reflex fails and allows a foreign body to embed itself into the cornea. This can be metallic or organic; a metallic foreign body will often leave a rust ring.

Symptoms and signs
Red, painful, gritty eye, and foreign body sensation. The foreign body is usually very small, but fluorescein and a magnifying loupe can assist identification and removal. Always evert the eyelid to exclude a subtarsal foreign body.

Treatment
- The foreign body should be removed either with a cotton bud or a needle. Irrigation with sterile saline may assist removal.
- Antibiotic ointment.
- An eye pad is not usually necessary and can encourage infection.
- Remember to ask about the mechanism of injury, as a high-velocity foreign body, such as a shard of metal from an ice-axe, is more likely to penetrate the globe.

Chemical eye injury

Immediately irrigate a chemical injury before any further assessment. A chemical splash can be sight-threatening. It is important to identify the chemical because alkali penetrates the ocular tissues much faster than acid and therefore has a worse prognosis.

Symptoms and signs
- A red irritable eye following chemical splash.
- Visual acuity may be impaired.
- If severe, there may be blepharospasm.

Treatment
- Immediate profuse irrigation, preferably with sterile normal saline and a giving set. If unavailable, use the cleanest water at hand.
- Irrigate for a minimum of 30 min.
- Antibiotic ointment (e.g. chloramphenicol three times a day).
- Ocular lubrication (e.g. artificial tears hourly).
- Cycloplegic drops for pain relief (e.g. cyclopentolate three times a day).
- A white eye following chemical injury can indicate severe ischaemia.
- If there is any concern regarding a chemical injury, especially if visual acuity is affected or there was any delay initiating irrigation, evacuate for specialist treatment.

Eyelid laceration

The eyelids play an important role in protecting the eye and preventing corneal desiccation. If they are damaged, the eye can be rendered vulnerable.

Assessment
- Check visual acuity.
- Assess globe integrity.
- Examine the eyelid carefully for any embedded foreign body.
- Decide whether the eyelid margin is interrupted.

Management
- Remove any foreign body from the eyelid.
- Clean the wound thoroughly.
- If skilled, consider primary repair using a 6/0 non-absorbable suture if the eyelid margin is interrupted and the ends are not opposed. This is especially important for the upper eyelid.
- Antibiotic ointment.
- Broad-spectrum oral antibiotics to prevent orbital cellulitis.
- Patch the eye if there is concern about corneal exposure and to control bleeding.

Complications
- Corneal exposure is a problem, especially after upper eyelid laceration. This can affect visual acuity and encourage infection.
- Lacerations near the medial canthus may involve the tear duct and, if left unrepaired, may cause a permanent watery eye (epiphora).
- A patient with an eyelid laceration with the eyelid margin severed should be evacuated—a primary repair needs to be done properly by an ophthalmic surgeon under magnification. A poor repair performed in the field is likely to result in a permanent defect in the lid margin, which will require revision at a later date.
- Always check that there is no underlying penetrating injury to the globe, especially if the mechanism of eyelid injury was high velocity.

Penetrating eye injury

A penetrating eye injury involves disruption of the globe integrity and is a serious, sight-threatening problem. The mechanism of injury is important in determining whether there could be an intraocular foreign body or a perforating injury (entry and exit).

Symptoms and signs
- Pain.
- Decreased vision.
- Soft watery eye.
- Peaked pupil.
- Expulsion of ocular contents.

Siedel's test involves a drop of fluorescein (after topical anaesthetic) on a suspected corneal penetrating injury. The leak of aqueous fluid out of the wound will dilute the dye, showing up easily with a blue light and loupe. Beware of false negatives, however, as some wounds will seal themselves quickly, potentially leaving an undiscovered intraocular foreign body.

Management
- A casualty with a suspected penetrating eye injury should be evacuated as soon as practical.
- Do not touch any expulsed ocular contents.
- If available, use a topical antibiotic eye ointment.
- Start broad-spectrum systemic antibiotics.
- Both eyes should move as little as possible.
- Protect the injured eye using a double pad and eye shield (Fig. 10.6).
- An increased suspicion of penetrating injury should be maintained in any high velocity eye injury, such as those involving firearms or hammering.

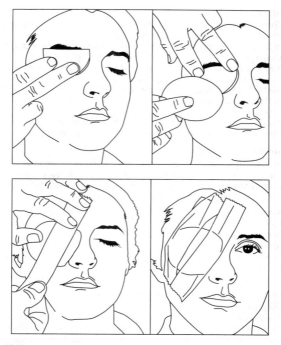

Fig. 10.6 The correct technique to pad an eye

Orbital cellulitis

Orbital cellulitis is a sight-threatening condition that can also be life-threatening if it spreads to form a brain abscess. The infection may originate from an adjacent ethmoid sinus or from mild trauma to the orbital region.

Symptoms and signs
- Pain.
- Reduced and painful eye movements.
- Conjunctival redness.
- Possible visual loss.
- General malaise.
- Pyrexia.

Treatment
- Broad-spectrum antibiotics, preferably IV.
- Optic nerve function should be closely monitored (see Box 10.2).
- Immediate evacuation for hospitalization.

Complications
- Decreased vision owing to optic nerve compression. This can be permanent without rapid orbital decompression.
- Orbital abscess requiring surgical drainage.
- Brain abscess which can be fatal.

Preseptal cellulitis

Preseptal cellulitis involves only the eyelid tissue. There is periorbital inflammation and swelling but none of the other features mentioned in ➲ Orbital cellulitis, p. 330. However, preseptal cellulitis can progress to orbital cellulitis so should be treated with broad-spectrum oral antibiotics and closely watched.

Orbital compartment syndrome

The orbit is a relatively closed compartment with limited ability to expand, so orbital pressure can rise rapidly when an acute rise in orbital volume occurs. This is an emergency where prompt simple treatment can prevent blindness.

The most common cause of orbital compartment syndrome, especially in the wilderness, is retro-bulbar haemorrhage from trauma, but spontaneous retro-bulbar haemorrhage can also occur due to venous anomalies, intra-orbital aneurysms or malignant hypertension. Severe orbital cellulitis with an abscess can also cause an orbital compartment syndrome. Patients with increased orbital pressure present with pain causing vomiting, proptosis, red and swollen conjunctiva, limited eye movements, and decreased optic nerve function (decreased vision and an afferent pupillary defect).

Treatment is with a surgical lateral canthotomy and cantholysis to release the pressure. This is a relatively straightforward procedure that can be performed as an emergency procedure under local anesthesia if evacuation is not possible (see Fig. 10.7).

Following infiltration with local anaesthesia (e.g. lignocaine with adrenaline) the lower eyelid is completely detached from the lateral orbital rim using sharp sterile scissors, first horizontally to cut through the lateral canthal angle (canthotomy) and then vertically to cut the lateral canthal tendon (cantholysis). This may be followed by a gush of blood from behind the eye as pressure is relieved. If the lid is held with forceps it is possible to feel when the tendon has been severed. The patient should then be evacuated for specialist evaluation and treatment.

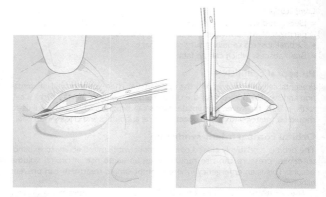

Fig. 10.7 Technique for lateral canthotomy and cantholysis to relieve orbital compartment pressure caused by retro-orbital haematoma. Illustration: Janice Sharp, Snr Med artist, University Hospital of Wales.

High-altitude retinopathy

(See also ➲ High-altitude retinal haemorrrhages, p. 667; Plate 24.)

HAR is defined as 'one or more haemorrhages in either eye of a person ascending above 2500 m'. It is normally asymptomatic but affects around 30% of lowlanders ascending to 5000 m.

Signs
- Retinal haemorrhages (flame, pre-retinal, dot, and blot).
- Cotton wool spots.
- Optic disc hyperaemia.
- Decreased visual acuity (only if the macula is affected).

Aetiology
Retinal vascular tortuosity and engorgement are part of the normal physiological retinal response to the hypoxia of high altitude. However, a combination of factors, including exertion and speed of ascent, cause HAR. It is confusing to include papilloedema in the definition of HAR as this implies raised intracranial pressure; the relationship between HAR and the potentially fatal HACE is not yet known.

Any visual disturbance at altitude is an indication for descent.

Ocular first-aid kit

Appropriate drugs and equipment for an easily transportable lightweight ocular first-aid kit are listed in ➲ Ocular first-aid kit, p. 810.

Ear problems

Ear problems are relatively common, particularly on diving expeditions (→ Barotrauma, p. 740; → Otitis externa, p. 742), owing to pressure changes and prolonged exposure to salt water.

Otitis externa

An infection of the outer ear often associated with constant moisture due to diving, or living in tropical environments. The ear canal itches, hurts, and may discharge; moving the pinna causes pain. The external canal looks swollen and red debris is usually obvious. In severe cases, hearing loss develops if the external canal becomes blocked by debris and swelling. Systemic upset with lymphadenopathy can occur.

Treat by gently cleaning the external canal with saline or clean water. Use a combination preparation of antibiotic and steroid such as Gentisone HC™ four times a day and in severe cases prescribe an oral antibiotic such as co-amoxiclav. Avoid further exposure to water until the condition resolves.

Otitis media

A viral or bacterial infection of the middle ear, often associated with an upper respiratory tract infection. It presents as pain and decreased hearing. The pain is made worse by changes in pressure.

Through an otoscope, the eardrum will usually appear red, but if pus collects behind the drum it can look yellow. Sometimes the drum perforates and pus discharges, with loss of hearing but relief of pain.

Prescribe painkillers and a basic antibiotic such as amoxicillin or erythromycin. A decongestant such as oral pseudoephedrine or nasal drops may help to relieve Eustachian tube obstruction.

Very occasionally, severe cases of otitis media can be complicated by *mastoiditis*, which causes pain, tenderness, and inflammation over the mastoid process, the bony prominence immediately behind and below the pinna. High-dose oral or, ideally, IV antibiotics should be commenced and the patient evacuated for specialist care because there is a small risk that meningitis or cerebral abscess could develop.

Tympanic membrane rupture and barotrauma

Tympanic membrane rupture may be caused by direct trauma or associated with a base of skull fracture. Leakage of blood or clear fluid from the ear may indicate a serious injury (→ Facial injuries, p. 302). The eardrum may also rupture as a result of barotrauma—especially during diving (see → Barotrauma, p. 740). Most eardrum perforations heal spontaneously and do not require specific management. Avoid swimming until the hole has healed.

Inner ear barotrauma is unpleasant. It results from inner ear haemorrhage or a rupture of the oval window. Patients experience vertigo, hearing loss, and tinnitus. Evacuate for examination by an ENT surgeon.

Foreign bodies in the ear canal

On expeditions, these are most commonly insects that have crawled into the external canal. Insects should be drowned in oil and will usually float out. Other foreign bodies may require removal with suitable hooks. If difficulty is experienced in foreign body removal, do not persist at the expense of damage to the tympanic membrane or external canal.

Nasal problems

Epistaxis (nose bleed)

Nose bleeds are quite common in expedition situations, and may be precipitated by the low humidity found at altitude, in cold climates, or aircraft cabin atmospheres. Other associations include direct trauma to the nose and upper respiratory tract infections. Ninety per cent are anterior and 10% are posterior.

First-aid measures are usually effective in controlling haemorrhage. Press on the soft part of the nose with a finger for 15 min. If simple pressure is unsuccessful, try cauterizing off any identified anterior bleeding points with a silver nitrate stick. Before cauterizing the vessel you should apply a topical local anaesthetic such as lidocaine and adrenaline. Look up the nose using a head torch and apply the cauterization stick to the bleeding point for no longer than 5s.

If cautery is not possible or is unsuccessful, then insert a commercially available nasal tampon. Such tampons should be lubricated before insertion. Once correctly positioned, expand the device by dropping saline from a syringe. Often both nostrils have to be packed. They are uncomfortable so prescribe painkillers. If nasal tampons are unavailable, then the nose can be packed with lubricated gauze or a small vaginal tampon.

Nasal packs can precipitate sinusitis and in the expedition setting amoxicillin should be prescribed. Leave the packs in place for 48 h and then remove them.

If bleeding continues despite insertion of a nasal tampon, it is probable that the bleeding point is in the posterior part of the nose. Remove the tampon and insert a deflated urinary catheter along the floor of the nose. Gently inflate the balloon with air and pull the catheter forward until resistance is felt. The pack or tampon should then be re-inserted.

A patient with a persistent nose bleed that does not respond to the measures described will have to be evacuated for further treatment and investigation which must include a blood count and clotting studies. Rarely, transfusion is required.

Nasal fracture

See ➔ Nasal fracture, p. 308.

Nasal foreign bodies

Foreign bodies in the nose need to be removed as they may lead to infection or aspiration. Anterior foreign bodies can be removed with hooked implements or forceps using a head torch to look up the nose.

Upper respiratory tract

Coryza (common cold)

URTIs are very common and often originate before departure. The condition is usually self-limiting and requires only symptomatic treatment. Catarrh may block sinus openings and Eustachian tubes. Pressure differences during flight or ascent may cause ear or sinus pain, which may be severe. Nasal decongestants such as phenylephrine can help. Antibiotics may help if persistent sinus pain and tenderness suggests secondary bacterial infection.

Pharyngitis/tonsillitis

Sore throats with painful swallowing are common in travellers, especially following air travel. The throat infection may be associated with fever and systemic upset. Most are viral in origin. Pus around the tonsils suggests bacterial infection but it is not usually possible to differentiate the two clinically.

Most cases of tonsillitis settle with time and analgesia. In the remote setting, if symptoms fail to improve after a few days then antibiotics should be prescribed. A suitable antibiotic for the most common bacterial pathogen, beta haemolytic *Streptococcus*, is co-amoxiclav 250/125mg three times a day for 7 days. This dose can be doubled if infection severe. Clarithromycin is an alternative in penicillin-allergic patients.

Peritonsillar abscess (quinsy)

Quinsy causes severe unilateral throat pain and dysphagia, with associated pyrexia and systemic upset. Trismus (an inability to open the mouth due to pain) and drooling occur. The tonsil is swollen, inflamed, and deviated medially; the uvula is usually displaced away from the affected side. IV antibiotics are required. In the remote setting the abscess should be drained by needle aspiration rather than incision and drainage.

Throat foreign bodies

These are most commonly fish or chicken bones. The patient complains of pain, especially on swallowing. Foreign bodies stuck in the tonsil or base of the tongue can usually be seen and removed with forceps. If no foreign body is visible it is possible that it may simply have scratched the pharyngeal mucosa on passing. A foreign body stuck out-of-sight in the pharynx may become infected and abscesses can develop, so if symptoms persist the patient must be evacuated.

Equipment

A list of additional drugs and equipment that may assist with ENT problems is given in ➲ Useful equipment and drugs for ENT problems, p. 810.

Chapter 11

Treatment: dental

Section editor
Chris Johnson

Contributors
Alistair R. M. Cobb
Penelope B. Granger
Burjor K. Langdana
David Geddes (1st edition)

Reviewer
Rose Drew

Dental terminology *338*
Pre-departure preparations *340*
Dental work in the field *342*
Toothache and dental swellings *344*
Fillings *351*
Dislodged crowns and bridges *352*
Dental injuries *354*
Dental local anaesthesia *358*
Extractions *364*
Medevac for dental problems *366*

NB Tooth, gum, and mouth problems are common especially on longer expeditions. This chapter offers advice on the prevention, diagnosis, and practical management of dental problems in the field.

On shorter journeys travellers may experience:
- Chips or damage to dental enamel and dentine.
- Broken or lost crowns or fillings.
- Acute oral infections or dental abscesses.

On lengthy expeditions, the risk of dental problems increases due to:
- Changes in diet, especially increased sugar intake.
- Decreased fluid intake, resulting in dry mouth.
- Exposure to extreme temperatures resulting in dental sensitivity.
- Problems with maintaining good oral hygiene.

Dental terminology

Naming teeth

Complete adult dentition consists of 32 teeth, eight per quadrant with the quadrants termed upper and lower, left and right, looking at the patient, with individual teeth named and numbered as in Fig. 11.1. Key dental structures are shown in Fig. 11.2, more detailed terminology is available online.

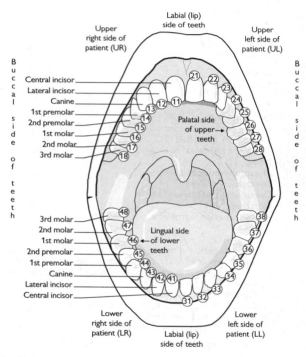

Fig. 11.1 Naming teeth.

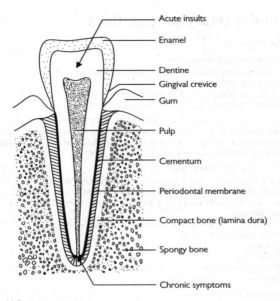

Fig. 11.2 Dental anatomy.

Pre-departure preparations

The traveller

Three months before departure

Travellers should have a thorough dental examination including:

- Bite-wing radiographs.
- Periapical radiographs of all root treated and crowned teeth.
- An orthopantomogram (OPG) if wisdom teeth are present.

The radiographic results determine whether third molar extractions or root canal treatments should be recommended and any existing poor quality dental work should be replaced electively. Preventative care before departure is preferable to treating problems in the field.

Two months before departure

Ensure that appropriate treatments will be completed at least 1 month before departure. Each expedition member should supply a detailed dental chart, together with a copy of their dental radiographs. This should accurately tell you:

- The position of amalgam and white composite fillings.
- Root canal treated teeth.
- Crowns.
- Deep fillings.
- Status of third molars.
- Teeth with cause for concern.

One month before departure

A meeting with expedition members to:

- Explain causes of tooth and gum problems, including dental decay.
- Plan and encourage a sensible diet avoiding too many fermentable carbohydrates, the 'hidden' sugars in processed food, and natural sugars in fruit.
- Reinforce good oral hygiene, interdental brushing, and flossing.
- Recommend brushing twice daily using a fluoride toothpaste, spit but don't rinse after brushing.

During the expedition

- Cold conditions: supply an antisensitivity toothpaste.
- Hot conditions: supply a high-fluoride toothpaste such as Colgate Duraphat™ (available only on prescription in UK).

Preparations by the medic

Field dentistry typically involves the mixing of dental materials to provide a temporary fix. As medic, you will probably be limited to using traditional materials that set by means of a chemical reaction. You should practise the mixing technique. There are two distinct timings:

- *Mixing time* during which the material is workable and will not set, and must be placed in the mouth.
- *Setting time* during which the material needs to be undisturbed, kept dry, and adjusted so that it does not interfere with other teeth or the chewing function.

It is sensible to learn and practise these techniques under supervision. Medics accompanying prolonged expeditions may additionally need to familiarize themselves with the techniques of dental extraction (see → Extractions, p. 364).

Dental work in the field

Effective dentistry requires good lighting and a dry field of work. In the field the necessary equipment may need to be improvised:
- Face sunlight or good artificial light, a head torch is helpful.
- Provide a good backrest for the patient, and ensure that you, your assistant, and the patient are comfortable and that you can work without strain.
- Protect area from wind and insects.
- Familiarize yourself with the dental charting, and keep the patient's dental records to hand.
- Use an assistant to support the patient's head, retract their lips and tongue, and help light the clinical area.

The patient should be appropriately positioned:
- If the lower teeth require examination—seat patient with the lower teeth parallel to the floor and upper teeth at 45° to the floor.
- For the upper teeth the patient lies on their back with their head rotated back for additional direct vision.

It is essential to control saliva so that you work in a dry field:
- Parotid duct—place cotton rolls on cheek side of upper second molars.
- Submandibular duct—place cotton rolls on tongue side of the front bottom teeth.
- Tilt the head to the opposite side so that saliva pools away from working area.

Toothache and dental fillings

Toothache and dental swellings

Dental pain is caused either through direct trauma to the pulp (pulpitis) or by the swelling and pressure affecting the proprioceptors and connective tissues surrounding the tooth, induced by infection (see Fig. 11.3). Whether it originates from the tooth, gingiva, or third molar infections the aim of treatment, in field dentistry, is to reduce this pressure swiftly. Pragmatically, the field medic will be treating the effects of dental disease and not its cause.

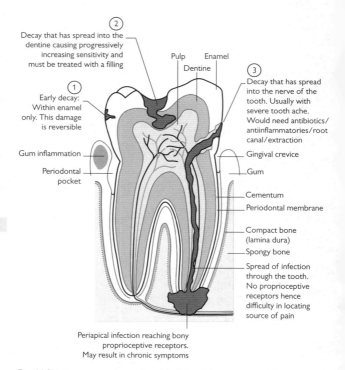

② Decay that has spread into the dentine causing progressively increasing sensitivity and must be treated with a filling

Pulp   Enamel

Dentine

③ Decay that has spread into the nerve of the tooth. Usually with severe tooth ache. Would need antibiotics/antiinflammatories/root canal/extraction

① Early decay: Within enamel only. This damage is reversible

Gum inflammation

Periodontal pocket

Gingival crevice

Gum

Cementum

Periodontal membrane

Compact bone (lamina dura)

Spongy bone

Spread of infection through the tooth. No proprioceptive receptors hence difficulty in locating source of pain

Periapical infection reaching bony proprioceptive receptors. May result in chronic symptoms

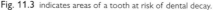

Fig. 11.3 indicates areas of a tooth at risk of dental decay.

Diagnosing dental pain

Use Table 11.1 to make a diagnosis and decide upon the appropriate treatment.

Table 11.1 Dental diagnosis and treatment

Patient complains of	What is likely to be happening	Likely recent history	Plausible previous history	What to do?
Brief twinges from hot, cold, or sweet stimuli, becoming increasingly uncomfortable	Dental nerve within the visible tooth is being insulted by hot, cold, and sweet stimuli. Pulp is not insulated	Broken or lost filling Cracked enamel Undiagnosed decay	Known damaged tooth Recent minor trauma No recent dental care	Avoid the stimuli. Attempt temporary filling to achieve insulation
Twinges from hot, cold, and sweet developing into aching pain of few minutes duration	Dental nerve within the tooth is being insulted and becoming oedematous, but is capable of recovery	Long-term history of reaction to hot, cold, and sweet becoming worse	Known untreated dental damage	Essential to seal the damaged area with an effective temporary filling + NSAIDs
Twinges gradually lessen and replaced by continual aching toothache	Dental nerve is damaged to the point it cannot recover	Long-term history of reaction to hot, cold, and sweet	Known untreated dental damage and history of increasing symptoms	Essential to seal with effective temporary filling, give NSAIDs and consider antibiotics and advise unavoidable need for root canal therapy or extraction
Recent continual toothache from hot, cold, and sweet stimuli, now subsiding to no symptoms	Dental nerve is becoming necrotic but not yet with any abscess symptoms	Long-term history of reaction to hot, cold, and sweet	Known untreated dental damage or history of heavily treated tooth without root treatment	Leave open as blocking with temporary filling will seal in oedematous pressure. Give NSAIDs and antibiotics

(Continued)

Table 11.1 (Cont'd)

Patient complains of	What is likely to be happening	Likely recent history	Plausible previous history	What to do?
Pulsing continual toothache, with little respite, worse on lying down	Dental nerve is necrotic and infected with infection spreading beyond tooth structure and into the periodontal membrane, bone, and main dental neurovascular bundles. Tooth starting to become tender to percussion	Dental symptoms at some time previously, recent upset to immune system	Previous serious restorative dental work close to the dental nerve without root treatment	Leave open as blocking with temporary filling will seal in oedematous and infective pressure. Give NSAIDs and antibiotics and advise extraction is most probably outcome
Pulsing continual toothache, lessening as swelling appears	Dental nerve is necrotic and infected, visible periapical abscess is forming. Tooth is very tender to percussion	Recent continual aching toothache	Previous serious restorative dental work close to the dental nerve without root treatment	Leave open as blocking with temporary filling will seal in oedematous and infective pressure Give NSAIDs and antibiotics and advise extraction is most probably outcome. Attempt to lance swelling if it has started to point
Pulsing continual toothache, lessening as swelling points and discharges pus	Dental nerve is necrotic and infected, periapical abscess is well formed. Tooth is very tender to percussion	Recent continual aching toothache and swelling	Previous serious restorative dental work close to the dental nerve without root treatment Various occasional nagging symptoms	Seriously infected tooth and bone structure spreading anaerobes systemically Heavy dosage NSAIDs and antibiotics and advise extraction inevitable on return. Try to maintain discharge from pointing sinus

| Rapid onset aching toothache with little previous warning plus radiating facial pain, typically involving ear ache for lower molars, temporal ache for upper molars, and lower ache for upper canines or upper premolars. Worse when sleeping prone | Long-term well-formed granulomatous chronic abscess in long-term necrotic tooth, with or without previous root treatment | History of serious dental trauma or treatment in long-term past | Can relate to accident in childhood, or teens, with little intervening symptoms. Patient unlikely to have had regular comprehensive dental care with radiographs | Seriously infected tooth and bone structure spreading anaerobes systemically. Heavy dosage NSAIDs and antibiotics and advise extraction inevitable on return. Try to maintain discharge from pointing sinus. Advise sleeping in a seated position |
| Painful, bleeding, swollen gums around wisdom tooth, bad taste, trismus, submandibular swelling | Food trapped under operculum causing localized infection | Partially erupted wisdom tooth, poor oral hygiene | Previous episodes of pericoronitis | Thoroughly clean under the gum and around tooth, irrigate with chlorhexidine or salty water, improve oral hygiene. NSAID, antibiotics and mouth wash |

Treatment of dental pain

Local measures

- *Antisensitivity toothpastes* help if hot, cold, or sweet stimuli are causing uncomfortable twinges of pain in an area of tooth where placing a temporary filling is impossible. To reduce sensitivity, retain the paste in the affected area for as long as practical.
- *Oil of cloves (eugenol)* is a traditional topical agent that may temporarily relieve pain and reduce sensitivity.
- *Duraphat™ high-fluoride varnish* applied to dry tooth surfaces reduces sensitivity.
- *Local anaesthesia* (LA), either as a nerve block or infiltration around the tooth can provide temporary respite (see **➋** Dental local anaesthesia, p. 358).
- *Temporary fillings* aiming to cover exposed, sharp or sensitive dentine.
- *Ledermix paste*, a mix of antibiotics with an anti-inflammatory agent, can treat an unremitting, pulsating toothache for instance resulting from a large, deep cavity or loose filling. Remove the loose filling and soft debris from the tooth. Apply the paste with a small pellet of cotton wool to the depth of the cavity, which can then be sealed with a temporary dressing such as Cavit™. (See Fig. 11.4.)

Painkillers

- Paracetamol up to 1000 mg four times daily.
- Ibuprofen (NSAID) 400 mg four times daily.
- Diclofenac sodium (NSAID) tablets 50 mg three times daily; also available as rectal suppositories, useful when a patient has difficulty swallowing.
- Codeine phosphate 30–60 mg three times daily.

Avoid NSAIDs if the patient has contraindications to their use such as asthma, a history of peptic problems, a bleeding tendency, renal problems, or is taking an anticoagulant drug. Avoid diclofenac in elderly travellers with heart problems.

Combining paracetamol with ibuprofen and alternating doses every 2 h controls ongoing pain and pyrexia without exceeding the maximum recommended doses. Codeine and paracetamol singly or in combination, are an alternative to NSAIDs, and all three may be used in combination in very severe pain.

When pain is very severe a NSAID such as ibuprofen 400 mg may be given up to six times per day, but this high dose should be reduced after 36–48 h as symptoms decrease.

Pain, loss of sleep, and the stronger painkillers including codeine can slow reflexes and cause drowsiness. Anyone so affected should avoid high-risk activities including climbing and driving. Opiate painkillers and tramadol are not very effective in dentistry other than for the relief of pain from an unreduced facial or mandibular fracture. Pain should settle within a few days, if it does not the condition should be reviewed by an expert as soon as practical.

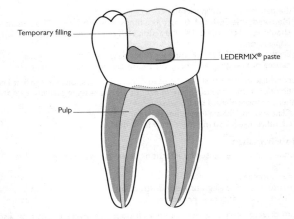

Fig. 11.4 Ledermix cement placement

Antibiotics

Dental infections are typically caused by anaerobic bacteria and require treatment with a broad-spectrum antibiotic. For treatment in remote locations it is often appropriate to use more aggressive antibiotic therapy than that used in general dental practice. Antibiotics will generally reduce swelling and associated pain in 2–3 days.

The principals of controlling dental infection are:
1. Removal of pus (incise and drain either through tooth or by means of gum line incision).
2. Removal of source of infection (extract infected tooth if adequately trained).
3. Antibiotic therapy.

If objectives (1) or (2) cannot be achieved (many medics in the field will be reluctant to attempt drainage or extraction), or there is evidence of cellulitis, spreading infection, or systemic involvement, then begin antibiotic therapy immediately.
- Co-amoxiclav 500/125 mg (adult dose) tablet three times daily for 5 days. If unavailable a combination of amoxicillin 250/500 mg and metronidazole 200/400 mg three times daily for 5 days, can be used.

If the patient is penicillin allergic:
- Metronidazole 200 to 400 mg three times daily for 5 days. The patient should avoid alcohol as its interaction with metronidazole is very unpleasant.
- Erythromycin 250 to 500 mg four times daily for 5 days. May cause nausea or vomiting, and many organisms are nowadays resistant.

Second-line antibiotics should be used if there is no response to the first-line antibiotics, in the case of severe infections with spreading cellulitis, or if the patient cannot tolerate metronidazole:
- Clindamycin 150 mg four times daily for 5 days or
- Clarithromycin 250 mg twice daily for 7 days.

Mouthwashes

Dental pain can be caused by infections of the gums including:
- Gingivitis.
- Periodontitis.
- Acute ulcerative gingivitis (very destructive).
- Third molar infections (pericoronitis).

Gum disease is typically associated with poor oral hygiene, but may also originate around buried or partly erupted third molars. The gums look swollen, reddish-purple in colour, may bleed spontaneously or on touch with an instrument, and may smell foul. Having diagnosed periodontal infection, it is essential to minimize bacteria between the teeth and along the gum margins.

Treatment involves improving dental hygiene with better brushing and flossing and mouthwashes used as an adjunct:
- The patient should be encouraged to brush and floss the painful area. A case of being cruel to be kind!
- Warm salty water: mix a half-teaspoon of salt in a half a cup of tea-temperature water.
- Or Corsodyl® mouthwash: 1 min twice daily.

Acute ulcerative gingivitis/pericoronitis

Local gum disease can be treated by debridement and irrigation together with:
- Metronidazole 200 mg three times daily for 3 days or/and
- Amoxicillin 250 mg three times daily for 3 days.

Fillings

Temporary filling materials are used to insulate the pulp from temperature, hypertonic solutions, chemicals, or irritating foods. If a tooth is damaged—due to a lost or broken filling, decayed dentine, or cracked or broken enamel—but is not giving symptoms, then a temporary filling may be a helpful preventive measure.

Premixed filling materials

Supplied in a sealed tube; squeeze out and apply.

- Premixed materials such as Cavit™ are easy to use but have less structural strength.
- Chemistry is usually a variation on zinc oxide powder and oil of cloves.
- Require a mechanically retentive cavity to stay put.
- Erode and may require replacing as often as every few days.
- Cavity can be damp but not wet.
- Will soothe exposed dentine and reversible dental pulpitis.

Materials that require mixing

Examples include intermediate restorative material (IRM) or any glass ionomer filling material. These materials are more difficult to use, but are very sticky and retentive. Before starting, consider the following:

- Isolating and drying the cavity—the cavity must be protected on either side with absorbent pads or cotton wool.
- A small dry-air aerosol such as that used to clean cameras can be used to dry the cavity or a pledget of cotton wool.
- The exact ratio of powder to liquid is critical.
- The mixing time is about 1 min and the setting time is similar.
- Mix on a glass slab with a flat spatula into a dough-like consistency.
- Apply and compress into a dry cavity, immediately removing all excess material from the biting surface. A Vaseline®-coated finger can help to smooth and shape the filling.
- IRM may be colour-coded: white for a clean cavity, blue for decay present, red for pulpal symptoms.
- The same glass ionomer filling materials, if mixed into a 'double cream-like' consistency, are excellent for reseating and cementing crowns. For greater effectiveness, after removing excess cement, seal the margins of the cement around the crown, whilst setting, with petroleum gel to protect from saliva erosion.

If filling materials are unavailable

Improvisation can be attempted. Dip cotton pellet into oil of cloves or eugenol. Swab the depth of the cavity. Then seal the cavity with candle wax, ski wax, or sugarless chewing gum. Expect limited success of a very short duration.

Dislodged crowns and bridges

Crowns (also often called 'caps') are made of porcelain, sometimes with an inner metal core, used to restore the outer structure of a badly damaged tooth.

Bridges are a series of joined crowns used to support and replace a missing tooth.

Normal crowns rarely dislodge, but you may encounter the following types of dental loss:

- A crown retained by a metal post that inserts into an existing prepared root may displace. The underlying tooth will have already been root-treated (the root tip sealed to prevent bacterial colonization).
- A crown where the cementation has failed or been removed by trauma. In the case of trauma the crown may hold the original, but now fractured, tooth structure.
- An implant-retained crown. The porcelain cap is normally attached to a titanium root surgically implanted into the underlying bone. Implants are a specialist field and you should avoid offering any treatment that tampers with the prosthetics.
- An adhesive bridge fixed onto the hidden surfaces of teeth by metal wings and strong adhesives. The techniques required to restore such bridges are impossible in the field.

Re-cementing a crown with post

Check by carefully flexing the root with a long probe to ensure that the root has not split vertically. If split, then do not re-cement the crown as a gingival abscess may ensue. If the root is intact then:

- Use an aerosol camera cleaner to clean and dry the inside of the root. Maintain moisture control.
- Test, by rehearsing the positioning, the ease of replacing the post.
- Have someone else mix the glass ionomer cement into a thick creamy consistency.
- Apply a little inside the root and most to the clean post.
- Reposition and hold in the correct place until set (2–3 min).
- Remove excess when still soft with the probe, and seal the cement margins with petroleum gel.

Re-cementing a crown with broken core

A problem arises if the core of the tooth breaks off inside the crown.

Tooth previously root-treated

If the tooth has already been root-treated, the crown can safely be left out as the nerves have already been removed. The root treatment is typically seen as pink rubbery material running up the long axis of the centre of the root. Root-treated teeth are brittle and damage of this type is quite common. Temporary filling material placed over the sharp stump, will avoid soft tissue trauma.

No previous root-treatment

If the dental stump has not been root-treated and the exposed nervous tissue is very sensitive, you are duty-bound to try to cover the sensitive area. If there is no damaged tooth core inside the dislodged crown, re-cement the crown using a glass ionomer mixed into cement consistency. The steps are the same as for the post crown. If the core of the tooth bleeds, prescribe antibiotics and NSAIDs to reduce nerve and blood vessel inflammation that could lead to dental pain.

If the tooth has not been root-treated, and the original tooth structure has fractured and remains inside the crown, then attempt the following:

- Remove the fractured tooth substance from inside the crown as best you can.
- Clean and dry the fitting surface of the crown.
- Clean and dry the remains of the tooth.
- Have someone else mix a glass ionomer cement into a wet dough-like consistency.
- Place a slight excess of cement into the crown.
- Press home onto the remaining tooth, seating it down fully.
- Check the patient can bite correctly without impediment from the crown.
- Hold in this position for 2–3 min until the cement begins to set.
- Reduce any excess cement, when still soft, gently with the probe, and seal the margins with petroleum gel. Slight excess cement helps in retention.

Alternatively, preserve the root for future treatment options by sealing the post hole with a temporary filling material. Make sure the patient retains the crown for possible re-use.

It is possible to mistakenly place some crowns back to front. Check the orientation before cementation. A porcelain crown made on a metal base will usually have a shiny metal margin on the palatal/lingual aspect of the tooth.

Dental injuries

Dental injuries may be isolated, or be associated with other facial injuries.
→ Facial injuries, p. 302.

Reduction of tooth luxation

Repositioning a tooth that has been moved by trauma involves the reduction of the fractured alveolar bone immediately surrounding the affected dental roots. This is not difficult and usually not too uncomfortable for the patient, but must be done quickly after an accident to stand much chance of success—certainly within an hour and preferably within 20 min of the injury. One of three situations can occur:

1. The tooth or teeth and bone have been moved a short distance but are reasonably solid. There is a good chance the teeth have retained a functioning blood supply and will survive. The patient, with encouragement, may be able to bite these teeth the short distance back into the correct relationship.
2. The tooth or teeth are very loose, independent of what has happened to the bone structure. If the blood supply has been severed—and there is no way of being sure other than speculating on the looseness—then root treatment will be required soon, and splinting will be required now. Reduce all malpositioned teeth, supporting the teeth by wire and/or glass ionomer cement splinting if you can, and consider evacuation to specialist care.
3. The tooth or teeth are mobile because their roots have fractured. Remove the fractured teeth and leave the roots to be removed by an expert; consider evacuation to specialist care.

In all cases prescribe antibiotics and NSAIDs.

Teeth lying loose in fractured bone can usually be moved quite easily. Typically, frontal trauma will cause upper incisors to be displaced towards the palate. The patient will be unable to close their mouth properly as the front teeth will collide. To reduce the cross-bite:

- Numb the affected area with LA if practical.
- Place yourself above and behind the patient.
- Exert slow but very firm forward pressure from your thumb placed on the palatal aspect of the pre-maxilla and palatal aspect of the loose teeth.
- Maintain the firm pressure until the bone and teeth move back into a normal occlusion.
- The patient will tell you when they can bite together naturally.
- You now need to consider whether the reduction will hold naturally or will need a splint of some type (see → Dental avulsion , p. 354; Fig. 11.5).
- With the best intentions and correct technique, most intrusive luxation will still have a poor prognosis and extrusive/lateral luxation may only have 50% dental survival rate.

Dental avulsion

The repositioning and fixation by splinting of any totally avulsed tooth is getting into the realms of dental heroics, especially in the field. Consider:

- Are there bigger clinical issues that take precedence for triage?
- If the patient requires or may require airway intubation then do not reposition.
- If a dental root is fractured, do not attempt to reimplant the tooth.

Reimplantation stands a worthwhile chance of success if the accident occurred within the past hour. Teeth displaced for more than an hour are much less likely to recover.

Transport of tooth
- Tooth and root must both be clean.
- The best way to carry the tooth after avulsion is in the mouth—saliva is reasonably isotonic, is at body temperature, and the presence of friendly commensal bacteria and protein matrices will help control the risk of infection.
- Never handle the avulsed tooth by touching the root, always handle using the enamel.

Repositioning technique
(See Fig. 11.5.)

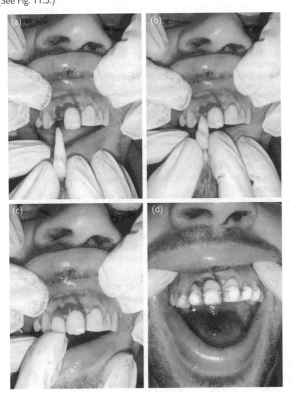

Fig. 11.5 Replacing an avulsed tooth. Adapted from O'Connor, Isobel, and Urdanq, Michael, *Handbook of Surgical Cross-Cover* (2008), with permission from Oxford University Press.

Consider whether you have the necessary equipment and whether the teeth adjacent to the avulsed tooth are solid enough to act as supports. There are two ways to support a tooth:

- Ideally the affected tooth is splinted to the teeth on either side of it by means of a wire stuck on with white filling material. One or more teeth on each side are used to splint the damaged tooth.
- The alternative is a temporary measure—use cyanoacrylic tissue adhesive, with supplementary Steri-Strips™ if needed.

Process

- Numb the affected area with LA if practical.
- Create a splint by cutting a suitable metallic material (a paperclip will suffice if nothing better) to an appropriate length. Its length could equate to one or more teeth on either side of the recently avulsed tooth. If several teeth are loose, use a longer wire. Bend the wire to a suitable curve.
- Remove the displaced tooth from the saliva.
- Rinse the tooth in sterile water.
- Normal haemostasis in a tooth socket occurs within 8 min. This blood clot will have to be removed with a sterile instrument to make way for the root to be firmly embedded full depth into the socket. As the clot is removed gently stimulate the periodontium to bleed again as this will improve the chances of healing.
- Re-insert tooth to its full depth within its socket so that it stands level height with the adjacent teeth.
- Hold in position until haemostasis is re-achieved—typically 4–8 min. This can be achieved by patient biting on a wooden spatula (or ice cream stick).
- Attach the splint wire to the displaced tooth and its neighbours ideally using glass ionomer cement or composite resin white filling materials. Kavit will not work.
- If you have no dental filling materials, an alternative but weaker bond can be made by sticking the tooth to its neighbours with cyanoacrylate tissue adhesive.
- Prescribe NSAIDs and a broad-spectrum antibiotic for at least 5 days (see ➲ Antibiotics, p. 349).
- Ensure diligent oral hygiene after every meal even though it will be difficult and uncomfortable.

Dental local anaesthesia

Being able to apply dental local anaesthetic (LA) accurately is a great boon in many circumstances. LA is useful:

- To enable treatment for painful teeth.
- To permit practical procedures such as dental fillings and fixing dislodged crowns.
- To enable reduction of fractures and splinting.
- To permit dental extractions.
- To give immediate relief from intractable chronic toothache and allow sleep.

Almost all dental LA drugs are premixed in 1.8–2.2 mL cartridges and include a vasoconstrictor that prolongs their duration of action. A well-placed mandibular block will give pain relief for up to 3 h. Check that the syringes you take match the cartridges! The needle gauge will be either 27 or 30, with a length of at least 3 cm.

LAs commonly used in dentistry include:

- *Lignospan®*: 2% lidocaine with 1:80,000 adrenaline (epinephrine) injection solution, used for regional blocks and infiltration. Onset 2–3 min, duration 60 min.
- *Citanest®*: 3% prilocaine hydrochloride with 0.03 IU/mL octapressin (adrenaline free), used for regional blocks and infiltration. Onset 2–3 min, duration 60 min. Used on patients where lidocaine or adrenaline is contraindicated.

Metal dental syringes are heavy; disposable syringes are an alternative, although less easy to handle. If dental LA cartridges are unavailable, other LAs may be used but take care to avoid toxicity from excessive volumes, or accidental intravascular injection.

Three main methods are used to numb the mouth cavity:

- Regional nerve blockade.
- Infiltration.
- Intraligamentary injections.

Different techniques are used to block the upper and lower jaws.

Blocking teeth in the lower jaw

A well-placed inferior dental nerve block will provide pain relief along the whole mandible for up to 3 h and, owing to the density of mandibular bone, is the only effective way to numb the area from the second pre-molar to the third molar teeth at the back of the lower jaw (35 to 38 and 45 to 48). Infiltration techniques in which LA is injected into the gum margins below the roots of mandibular teeth can be used for the front teeth as far back as the first premolar (31 to 34 and 41 to 44).

Regional nerve blockade (inferior dental block)

The mandibular branch of the trigeminal nerve runs down the inside of the mandible and supplies sensation to all the teeth in that half of the mandible. Halfway down the vertical part of the bone the nerve divides into two, with the inferior dental nerve entering a canal within the mandible, and the long buccal nerve continuing outside the bone (Fig. 11.6). You must place the LA drug just above the canal entrance (the lingula):

1. Ask the patient to open their mouth as wide as possible. Stand in such a way that you can see clearly where you need to inject. If right-handed, position yourself behind the patient to anaesthetize the lower left quadrant, and in front of the patient for the lower right. If left-handed, reverse these instructions (Fig. 11.7).

2. Aim the needle point at the mucous membrane on the medial border of the mandibular ramus. The target is the intersection of a horizontal line (the height of injection) with a vertical line (the anteroposterior plane).
   - Height of injection: put your thumb beside the last molar tooth. Feel the jaw bone as it turns upwards to the head. Rest your thumb in the depression there, the coronoid notch. It is about 6–10 mm above the occlusal table of the mandibular teeth. That defines your horizontal plane.
   - Anteroposterior plane: lies just lateral to the pterygo-mandibular raphe—defined as the muscular pillar that connects the lower third molar region to the upper third molar region.

3. Approach the area of injection from the opposite premolar region using your non-dominant hand to retract the patient's buccal soft tissue (your thumb is in the coronoid notch of mandible and index finger on the posterior border of extra-oral mandible). (See Fig. 11.8.)

4. Angle the needle backwards towards and just above the lingula.
   - The needle should touch bone at 3 cm deep; a more shallow touch indicates you are in front of the lingula and in the wrong place. If you don't touch bone once 3 cm of needle have been inserted, your needle point is probably deep to the lingula. (See Fig. 11.9.)

5. Aspirate the syringe to check you are not in a blood vessel. Reposition if necessary. Deliver a full cartridge of LA slowly over 1 min.

6. Continue to inject slowly on withdrawing from injection site to anesthetize the lingual branch.

7. Inject another cartridge into the coronoid notch region of the mandible in the mucous membrane distal and buccal to most distal molar to perform a long buccal nerve block.

8. Wait for a clear indication of anaesthetic effect to the midline of the mandible and full length on the side of the tongue. This may take seconds or minutes. Work should commence only when there is a clear sensory distinction across the mandibular midline.

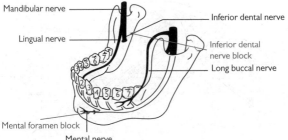

Fig. 11.6 Lower jaw anatomy and nerve supply.

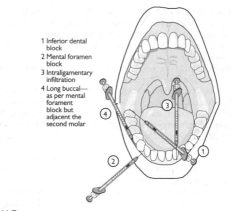

1 Inferior dental block
2 Mental foramen block
3 Intraligamentary infiltration
4 Long buccal—as per mental forament block but adjacent the second molar

Fig. 11.7 Mandibular dental blocks.

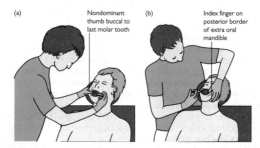

(a) Nondominant thumb buccal to last molar tooth

(b) Index finger on posterior border of extra oral mandible

Fig. 11.8 Inferior dental block—position.

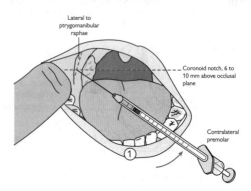

Lateral to ptrygomanibular raphae

Coronoid notch, 6 to 10 mm above occlusal plane

Contralateral premolar

1

Fig. 11.9 Inferior dental block—landmarks.

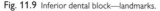

Blocking teeth in the upper jaw

Maxillary alveolar bone is significantly less dense than mandibular bone. This facilitates rapid penetration of anaesthetic around teeth, allowing anaesthesia by simple infiltration injection into the buccal/ labial sulcus adjacent to the affected tooth or teeth. The anaesthetic is placed slightly above the apices of the dental roots. (See Fig. 11.10, Fig. 11.11, and Fig. 11.12.) Most roots can be considered to be about 20 mm from the occlusal surface of the tooth. Upper canines can occasionally be up to 30 mm long.

- Insert the needle into the buccal or labial sulcus and slightly angled towards the facial bone structure.
- Place the needle tip above the level of the root apices.
- Deliver a full cartridge.
- When delivering LA for incisors and canines, place the needle slowly and inject very slowly. The tissue is tight and the nerve plexus considerable. This is a very painful injection if rushed.
- If attempting an extraction, a very small infiltration must also be placed on the palatal side of the tooth until visible blanching is seen. This is also an unpopular injection site.

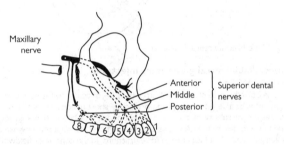

Fig. 11.10 Maxillary division of trigeminal nerve.

Maxillary nerve

Anterior
Middle } Superior dental
Posterior } nerves

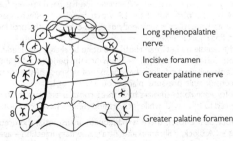

Fig. 11.11 Palatal nerves.

Long sphenopalatine nerve

Incisive foramen

Greater palatine nerve

Greater palatine foramen

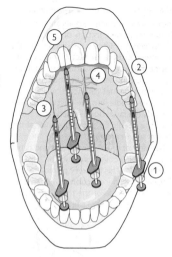

1 Buccal/labial infiltration
2 As per no 1 but go to the level of the lower orbit—suborbital block
3 Sphenopalatine block
4 Incisal papilla block
5 Intraligamentary infiltration

Fig. 11.12 Maxillary dental nerve blocks.

Buccal/labial intraligamentary injection

(See Fig. 11.13.)

The objective is to place a small amount of LA directly into the periodontal ligament with a very fine gauge and preferably short needle. The intention is to use the vascularity of the narrow periodontal attachment between root and bone to deliver the LA to the apical nerve fibres. This approach, when in practised hands, is sufficient even for extractions. In the context of fieldwork it should be considered as an adjunct to block or infiltration to gain profound LA. It is particularly useful when attempting to anaesthetize an area that has been heavily infected or luxated. When infection has been present for some time there is often buffering of the LA which reduces its effectiveness. The intraligamentary approach is sufficiently direct to overcome this problem.

- Select a fine short needle.
- Place the needle tip between tooth and bone by sliding the needle along the tooth surface and inserting 2–3 mm into the periodontal ligament.
- The needle will always follow the long axis of the root of the tooth.
- Using considerable pressure, place about 0.2 mL of LA.
- Repeat for each root—molars have three roots, premolars can be considered to have two, while incisors and canines have one root.

If, after your best efforts, there is inadequate anaesthesia, then repeat all the stages—LA block, infiltration and intraligamentary injection—again and again. Six or seven full cartridges might be considered a maximum dose for a fit young person. Then wait, and wait. For example, it once took 3 h for a field medic to anaesthetize a very badly infected lower wisdom tooth. The tooth was then extracted painlessly and the climber subsequently summited Lhotse Shar.

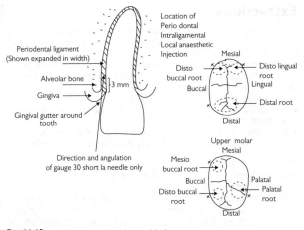

Periodontal ligament (Shown expanded in width)

Alveolar bone

Gingiva

Gingival gutter around tooth

3 mm

Direction and angulation of gauge 30 short la needle only

Location of Perio dontal Intraligamental Local anaesthetic Injection

Mesial

Disto buccal root

Buccal

Disto lingual root

Lingual

Distal root

Distal

Upper molar

Mesial

Mesio buccal root

Buccal

Disto buccal root

Palatal

Palatal root

Distal

Fig. 11.13 Intraligamentary dental nerve block.

Extractions

It is essential that you seek appropriate training before departure if intending to offer extractions as a treatment. Do not attempt dental extractions for the first time in the wilderness.

There are situations where a successful extraction might mean otherwise inevitable evacuation is avoided. Reasons for attempting an extraction in a remote location might be as follows:

- Loose teeth either side of a bone fracture.
- A tooth fractured with the live neurovascular pulp exposed—you will see bleeding from the pulp.
- Intractable toothache which does not respond to antibiotics and NSAIDs, and when the patient is a long distance from expert help.

Principles of tooth extraction

Establish effective LA (see ⟴ Dental local anaesthesia, p. 358) before attempting dental extraction.

During the extraction process you need to both expand and enlarge the socket, thus separating the tooth from its ligament, to the point where it is free to come out. If you have ever tried to remove a tent stake that has been driven deeply into the ground, you know that you can't just pull the stake straight up. Instead, you first have to rock the stake back and forth so to widen the hole in which it is lodged. Once the hole has been enlarged enough, the stake will come out easily.

The bone inside the jaw is relatively spongy. That means, when a dentist applies firm pressure to a tooth (forcing it against the side of the socket), the bone will compress. After repeated application of pressure from many different angles, the entire socket gradually enlarges, and eventually enough space will be created for the ligament to separate from the tooth and the tooth itself can emerge. You are aiming to extract both the tooth and the roots together, without fracturing.

Procedure for dental extraction

- Upper teeth are extracted standing in front of the patient; lower teeth are extracted from a stance behind the patient.
- The jaw and head both need to be immobilized to avoid the extraction force being dissipated. This may necessitate the help of a colleague.
- *Elevators* are levers that look like small screwdrivers. If available it is a good idea to start with them. They are designed to be wedged in the ligament space between the tooth and the surrounding bone. As the elevators are forced and twisted, the tooth is pressed and rocked against the bone. This helps to expand the socket. It also helps to separate the tooth from its ligament. As this work continues, the tooth becomes increasingly mobile.
- You can then switch to *forceps*, which should grip the tooth as far below the gum level as possible—force is never applied in any other way than very precisely along the long axis of the roots. If instead, force is applied tangentially to the root long axis it is likely that the tooth will break leaving its roots in the jaw.

- Never pull a tooth. A great deal of very focused force is slowly and relentlessly applied up or down the long axis of the root. The tooth is then pushed and slowly rotated out using a figure of eight movement and following the line of least resistance, which can be increasingly sensed.
- Once the tooth has been removed check carefully to ensure that all roots have been removed intact.

Extraction aftercare

Once the tooth is out, the bone and periosteum remain exposed and painful infections can develop that last up to 14 days. You should aim for complete coverage of the bone by a solid blood clot. Place a small firm pack of cotton wool roll or absorbent paper over the socket and tell the patient to bite hard onto this. Continual pressure will almost always achieve haemostasis within 5 min. The pack should then be rotated out to avoid lifting the clot. Antibiotics are not usually necessary unless the socket was already badly infected, painkillers (➔ Treatment of dental pain, p. 348) may be needed for the first 12 h. Sometimes the wound requires suturing using 3/0 black silk or Vicryl® sutures on a small curved needle. Black silk sutures can be removed after a minimum of 5 days. Though uncomfortable, thorough oral hygiene is essential.

Advice to patient after extractions

The objective is to avoid further bleeding, returning for further treatment, and infection. The patient should be advised as follows:

- No hot drinks, alcohol, or heavy lifting for 12 h.
- Use a pressure pack to control any subsequent bleeding. Bite hard on this for at least 15 min and then gently rotate out.
- Avoid vigorous rinsing and spitting for 24 h.
- Advise the patient not to smoke for at least 24 h.
- Red-coloured saliva is not a bleed and can be expected; a bleed looks like a substantial mass of 'jelly-like' blood clot.
- Mouth washing and gentle brushing after every meal is essential to limit the food source of damaging bacteria that cause infection.

Final consideration

The extraction of a tooth is irreversible and may have significant long-term health, aesthetic, and financial consequences. Subsequent treatment may be complex, unpredictable, and expensive. So avoid dental extractions if at all possible.

Medevac for dental problems

Indications

Evacuating casualties can be difficult, expensive and may be dangerous. It is not a decision to be taken lightly, but certain circumstances demand it as a precaution. Medevac is indicated for:

- Possibility of airway obstruction from trauma or infection.
- Uncontrolled pain causing severe distress.
- Uncontrollable oral or nasal bleeding.
- Facial fractures (see ➲ Fractured facial bones, p. 306).
- Sepsis not responding to antibiotics.
- Post-septal extension of maxillary abscess (i.e. into eye socket).
- Suspected mediastinal extension of parapharyngeal infection.
- Suspected Ludwig's angina.

Dental pain may result from trauma or infection; individual ability to cope with dental pain varies considerably. Irreversible pulpitis is agony and the only definitive treatment is removal of the pulp (root canal therapy), or extraction of the tooth itself. Pulpal pain is little affected by painkillers, wakes the patient at night and recedes only after 1–2 weeks when the pulp finally becomes necrotic. The pain may then cease for several days because of pulpal necrosis, but if infection develops and extends through the apical foramen the tooth becomes exquisitely sensitive to pressure and percussion. This secondary pain is now of inflammatory origin and can be controlled with antibiotics and NSAID's.

Ludwig's angina

An acute severe diffuse infective cellulitis typically caused by dental or tonsillar infection that spreads rapidly, bilaterally affecting submandibular, sublingual, and submental spaces. Airway compromise is likely. It may be associated with:

- Painful neck swelling.
- Dental pain.
- Dysphagia.
- Dyspnoea.
- Fever and malaise.
- Protruding or elevated tongue.
- Hot potato voice.
- When advanced: oedema and induration of the anterior neck often with cellulitis.

Management

Evacuate the patient as an emergency to a base hospital. Definitive dental and supportive medical therapies are required urgently as the condition rapidly becomes life-threatening.

- Airway management is of paramount importance. If swelling compromises the airway give supplementary oxygen whenever possible. In medical facilities high-flow oxygen or Heliox mixtures are desirable, but such treatments are impractical in the field.

- Initially IV amoxicillin and metronidazole, or co-amoxiclav (➲ Antibiotics, p. 349), definitive treatment requires specialist microbiological input.
- Consider IV corticosteroids if swelling compromises airway. At the time of writing there is no clear evidence for or against their use in the pre-hospital setting. Individual case reports from hospitals suggest that steroids may reduce the risk of airway obstruction and need for intubation, provided that they are used in association with high dose antibiotics, but the literature is very limited.
- Extract the tooth or drain the tonsillar abscess as soon as possible. The patient will require operative drainage under general anaesthetic by a specialist team if pus is present or intubation on an intensive care unit with medical management if no focal sepsis.

Medical supplies

Suggestions for suitable equipment for field dentistry are given in Chapter 28 ➲ Remote dentistry kit list, p. 810. The quantity and extent of this equipment will depend upon the size and duration of the expedition and accessibility of dental help in the local area.

Resources

Atraumatic Restorative Techniques—'ART'—Internet search recommended for a variety of helpful PDF files.
Scottish Dental Clinical Effectiveness Programme: ✍ www.sdcep.org.uk
The Dental Directory: ✍ www.dental-directory.co.uk
The Dental Trauma Guide: ✍ www.dentaltraumaguide.org

Further reading

Andreasen JO, Andreasen FM (1990). *Essentials of Traumatic Injuries to the Teeth*. Copenhagen: Munksgaard.
Wray D, Stonehouse D, Lee D, Clark AJE (2003). *Textbook of General and Oral Surgery*. Edinburgh: Churchill Livingstone.

Chapter 12

Treatment: chest

Section editor
Annabel H. Nickol

Contributors
Jonathan Ferguson
Jonathan Leach
Julian Thompson
Andrew Thurgood
David A. Warrell

Introduction *370*
Chest pain *370*
Myocardial infarction *371*
Rib fractures *372*
Spontaneous pneumothorax *374*
Acute chest infections *376*
Asthma *380*

Introduction

The chest is the region of the body between the neck and the abdomen, along with its internal organs and other contents. It is mostly protected and supported by the ribcage, spine, and shoulder girdle. The chest contains:
- Heart and major blood vessels.
- Trachea, lungs, and pleura.
- Diaphragm.
- Oesophagus.

Also protected by the lower ribs are:
- Liver and gallbladder.
- Spleen.
- Upper part of stomach.
- Upper poles of kidneys.

Injuries to the ribcage may damage the underlying organs. Chest pain may originate from thoracic or intra-abdominal organs.

Chest pain

Chest pain is a relatively common complaint on expeditions. Most chest pain is musculoskeletal in origin and may be treated by analgesics and, where possible, rest. However, severe central chest pains and pleuritic pain made worse by deep inspiration may signal more serious conditions that might require urgent treatment or evacuation. Diagnosis of these conditions is covered in ⟩ Chest pain, p. 242 and the algorithm in Fig. 8.10.

Myocardial infarction

A myocardial infarction or 'heart attack' results from blockage of a coronary artery that distributes blood to the heart muscle. Although this may, especially in those with diabetes, go almost unnoticed, the symptoms and signs are usually obvious. The vascular obstruction can result in failure of the heart to pump properly (cardiac failure) or the development of irregular heart rhythms that can be fatal. Myocardial infarction is more likely to develop in middle- and older-aged people with known risk factors such as previous angina, heart attack, high BP, or history of smoking but occasionally affects young adults.

Symptoms
- Central, crushing retrosternal pain.
- Pain may radiate to shoulder and neck.
- May mimic severe heartburn, but discomfort not relieved by antacids, and may be helped by GTN or oxygen.
- Palpitations.
- Breathlessness.

Differential diagnosis
Causes of chest pain are discussed in ➲ Differential diagnosis, p. 244.

Signs
Patient is anxious, distressed, and often pale, cold, and clammy.

Monitoring
If facilities are available, monitor BP and pulse (by palpation or oximeter). Portable fully automated external defibrillators (AEDs) are becoming cheaper and more widely available; they are located in many transport terminals and large stores. Apply electrode pads and listen to instructions. AEDs are unlikely to contribute to outcome when parties are travelling alone in remote areas, but medics associated with major endurance sporting challenges and those supporting groups of elderly travellers should consider whether having an AED available would be appropriate if support helicopters or land transport could facilitate rapid transfer to tertiary care.

In the wilderness, options are limited:
- Give supplementary oxygen if available.
- Obtain IV access.
- Give analgesia—opiates are valuable both for treating pain and relieving breathlessness. Use tramadol if opiates not carried.
- Give aspirin 300 mg if no contraindication.
- Consider use of GTN as spray or skin patch.
- Inform rescue services of possible diagnosis; in remote areas many paramedics are permitted to administer thrombolytic ('clot-busting') drugs.
- Evacuate as soon as possible to tertiary care hospital.

Rib fractures

Most rib fractures are not dangerous in themselves, but are extremely painful. The pain will probably prevent further participation in the expedition as sleep will be disturbed and carrying a rucksack impossible. Morbidity correlates with the degree of injury to underlying structures. Average blood loss per fractured rib is 100–150 mL.

The pain from a fractured rib can severely restrict breathing and can predispose to reduced movement and infection of the underlying lung. Basic treatment involves managing the pain and monitoring for more serious injuries. When there is evidence of significant injury (as opposed to just chest wall bruising), the patient should be evacuated to definitive medical care as soon as possible.

Signs and symptoms

Suspect a simple fractured rib if any of the following are present:
- Chest wall bruising.
- Tenderness over a specific bony point on the chest.
- Sharp pain when coughing or breathing.
- Deformity of the chest.

Treatment

- If possible, stop all activity, reassure, and try to keep the patient calm to reduce effort of breathing. Assess ABCD (see ➲ Medical emergencies, p. 214). Deal with the identified rib fractures once you are sure there are no other life-threatening problems such as an obstructed airway or bleeding.
- If the patient is compromised with possible underlying organ damage, administer oxygen if it is available.
- Administer ibuprofen 400–800 mg stat (with food) then 400 mg four times a day for pain. If additional pain relief is required add paracetamol 1 g four times a day.
- Encourage the injured person to cough frequently, breathe deeply every hour at least, despite the pain, in order to prevent secretions from pooling in the lung, which could cause chest infection.

Serious fractures

Look for signs that may suggest injury to the lungs:
- Rapid and shallow breathing.
- Elevated heart rate.
- Increased difficulty in breathing.
- Coughing up blood.

The mechanism of injury may indicate serious underlying chest injury, e.g. fall from height, crushing forces, or rapid deceleration injuries in a road traffic collision.
- Place one hand on each side of the injured person's chest and observe the way in which the chest moves with inhalations. If one side of the chest rises during inhalation while the other falls, at least three ribs have been broken on the falling side of the chest—a 'flail chest'. This is best visualized by looking from the patient's feet along the patient's body towards their head, meanwhile watching the chest rise and fall—the 'sunset view' of the chest wall.

- If the casualty is having severe difficulty breathing, or if the chest is rising and falling asymmetrically during breathing, roll them onto the injured side. This makes breathing less painful and helps keep the 'good' lung free of blood. If the patient does not improve try another position.
- Keep the casualty on their side and continually monitor for breathing difficulties. Consider the possibility of a tension pneumothorax (see → Pneumothorax, p. 190).
- Evacuate immediately to a hospital for even the simplest of rib fractures. The injured person must be flown or carried out if there are any signs of respiratory distress (consider chest drain if risk of pneumothorax), but may be able to walk out with simple fractures.
- Morphine or other analgesics: the pain of the fractures may hinder breathing sufficiently for it to be necessary to administer small amounts of an opiate painkiller to enable more effective breathing. Morphine should be administered, ideally intravenously. Give 1 mg doses every 1–2 min and monitor closely the effects of the analgesia. A fit adult may require 20–30 mg and sometimes more of morphine in total to relieve severe pain, but be careful not to give so much that respiration is depressed. Any dose of opiate can cause nausea, reduced awareness and confusion, and can make evacuation more difficult. Tramadol 10–20 mg doses may be similarly titrated to relieve pain. Up to 300 mg may be required. Tramadol is less likely than an opiate to cause respiratory depression, but may cause light-headedness, nausea, and vomiting.
- Traditional firm (not tight) strapping may help pain but, by restricting expansion, encourages infection. Counter-pressure over the affected area before coughing may help reduce pain.

Tips and warnings

- Examine the patient's left and right, front, back, and sides for hidden rib injuries.
- Serious rib fractures will very likely have underlying lung bruising accompanying the condition and this injured lung reduces lung function. The patient must be monitored closely for deterioration and evacuated as soon as possible.
- Older persons are more prone to rib fractures than younger adults owing to weaker bones.
- Position of the fractured rib in the thorax helps identify potential injury to specific underlying organs. Fracture of the lower ribs is usually associated with injury to abdominal organs rather than to lung tissue.
- Fracture of the left lower ribs is associated with splenic injuries.
- Fracture of the right lower ribs is associated with liver injuries.
- Fracture of the floating ribs (ribs 11, 12) is often associated with kidney injuries.

Spontaneous pneumothorax

A pneumothorax is a collection of air or gas within the pleural cavity. (See also ➲ Pneumothorax, p. 190.) Spontaneous pneumothoraces occur more commonly in tall, thin, young males, in conditions where airway pressure is increased (such as during scuba diving or during acute asthma attacks) and in people with underlying lung conditions such as COPD.

Symptoms and signs
- Shortness of breath.
- Increased respiratory rate.
- Lateral sharp chest pain on breathing in.
- If massive: reduced chest movement and air entry on the affected side.
- Hyper-resonant to percussion on the affected side.

Treatment
- Oxygen, if available.
- Pain relief.
- All patients with a pneumothorax require hospital assessment.
- Regularly reassess the patient for the development of a tension pneumothorax.
- Unless the patient is compromised or must be evacuated by aircraft, avoid insertion of needles or drains into the chest. Note that the pneumothorax will expand with gain in altitude. See also ➲ Needle decompression of tension pneumothorax, p. 191; ➲ Chest drain insertion, p. 192.

Acute chest infections

Respiratory infections are a common medical problem on expeditions. Chest infections often follow an initial upper respiratory tract infection (URTI). URTIs, including coryza, sore throat, tonsillitis, quinsy, and sinusitis, are covered in Chapter 10 (➲ Upper respiratory tract, p. 336).

Acute lower respiratory tract infections (ARIs) can be caused by a wide range of pathogens. Those likely to affect members of expeditions include:
- Viruses:
  - Influenza viruses.
  - Measles—rare if immunized.
  - Respiratory syncytial virus (RSV).
  - SARS coronavirus—epidemics only!
- Bacteria:
  - *Streptococcus pneumoniae*.
  - *Haemophilus influenzae*.
  - *Mycoplasma pneumoniae*.
  - *Chlamydia* spp.
  - Q fever—*Coxiella burnetii*.
  - *Legionella*.
  - TB—especially in local populations
- Fungi:
  - *Pneumocystis (carinii) jirovecii*.
  - *Histoplasma capsulatum*.
  - *Cryptococcus neoformans*.

Immunocompromise and underlying chronic illness determines special vulnerabilities, e.g. to *P. jirovecii* pneumonia in HIV-positive patients, to *Strep. pneumoniae* in alcoholics, and to a range of pathogens in smokers and chronic bronchitics.

Transmission is usually by inhaled aerosol from infected people, including asymptomatic carriers and, in the case of some pathogens, from animals (e.g. *Chlamydia psittaci*) and from the environment (e.g. Q fever, fungal pneumonias). Crowded and enclosed areas such as buses, hostels, travel terminals, aircraft, and underground trains increase the risk of transmission.

Symptoms
- Cough with or without sputum production developing after URTI or influenza.
- Fever (sometimes with rigors).
- Breathlessness.
- Exacerbation of underlying asthma.
- Pleuritic chest pain.
- Myalgia.
- Other 'flu-like' symptoms.

Examination

- Temperature.
- Cold sores.
- Upper respiratory tract—catarrh and post-nasal drip from sinusitis.
- Rashes (e.g. measles, *Mycoplasma pneumoniae*).
- Displaced mediastinum.
- Auscultation:
  - Added sounds.
  - Evidence of lobar or patchy consolidation.
  - Pleural friction rub.
- Lobar collapse.
- Pleural effusion.

Lower lobe pneumonia can cause misleading upper abdominal tenderness. Look at the sputum! Yellowish, greenish purulent sputum, sometimes 'rusty' or streaked with frank blood is a typical sign of infection.

Complications include respiratory failure, septicaemic shock, metastatic infection such as meningitis and infective endocarditis, pericarditis and pericardial effusion, pneumothorax, pneumomediastinum, empyema, and lung abscess.

Diagnosis

In the field, diagnosis is made on clinical grounds and can be confirmed later by chest radiography, sputum microscopy, blood cultures, leucocyte count, serology, and antigen detection in urine (*Legionella*).

Antibiotic treatment

Clinically convincing ARI during an expedition in a remote location deserves immediate antibiotic treatment.

If classic pneumococcal lobar pneumonia is suspected, treatment with oral amoxicillin 500 mg three times a day for 5–7 days (or erythromycin 500 mg four times a day/clarithromycin 500mg twice a day for penicillin-hypersensitive patients). In severe cases, or if oral treatment is impossible, start ceftriaxone IV or IM, 2 g once a day.

For broader-spectrum blind treatment (also covering *H. influenzae*, *Legionella* spp., *Mycoplasma, Chlamydia*, Q fever), use oral doxycycline 100 mg twice each day, or clarithromycin 500 mg twice a day.

Supportive treatment

Cough suppressants (cough mixture, linctus) have limited effect but can be soothing, especially if sleep is disturbed. Codeine or pholcodine linctus or sedating antihistamines such as chlorphenamine (Piriton®) may be helpful provided they do not cause respiratory depression.

Asthma exacerbations should be treated with bronchodilators and, in some cases, a short course of oral corticosteroid (see Asthma, p. 380).

Severe pleuritic pain warrants strong analgesia. Start with regular full-dose paracetamol. NSAIDs, tramadol, or opioids may be needed (beware of respiratory depression).

Oxygen (if available, e.g. on climbing expeditions) may relieve severe dyspnoea and hypoxaemia. Affected mountaineers should be moved to lower altitudes as a lower respiratory tract infection may predispose to/or be hard to distinguish from high-altitude pulmonary oedema. Oxygen may be needed for air evacuation of patients with ARI.

Prevention

Vaccination against *Strep. pneumoniae* and influenza viruses (➲ Influenza, p. 34) is appropriate if a high risk of exposure is anticipated; this depends on the expedition's programme, the influenza epidemic status, and the medical history of the expedition member.

Provision of antiviral treatment or prophylaxis (ribavirin for RSV; amantadine for influenza A; zanamivir or oseltamivir for influenza B) would be appropriate only in exceptional circumstances such as unavoidable travel to an area where an epidemic was predicted.

Resources

British Thoracic Society. ✍ https://www.brit-thoracic.org.uk/guidelines-and-quality-standards/community-acquired-pneumonia-in-adults-guideline
Centers for Disease Control and Prevention. *Pneumonia.* ✍ http://www.cdc.gov/pneumonia

Asthma

Asthma affects 10–15% of the population and is becoming increasingly common, especially in the young. It is characterized by recurrent episodes of shortness of breath, cough, and wheeze caused by reversible airway obstruction, often worse in the night and mornings, and sometimes associated with an atopic history with eczema, hayfever or rhinitis. Up to 2000 deaths/year in the UK are caused by asthma, with most occurring outside hospital. Risk factors for death include chronic severe disease, inadequate medical treatment, and those with adverse behavioural and psychosocial factors.

Asthma on expeditions

A person with well-controlled asthma should be able to participate in most expeditions, although any obstructive airways condition except very mild asthma is a contraindication to diving (➔ Fitness to dive, p. 730; Table 24.1). Remote environments restrict the treatment available for severe asthma attacks. Severe or unstable asthma may preclude an individual from joining a trip to a remote area (see ➔ Asthma, p. 50). Any new environment can alter symptoms, either worsening or improving the condition. Emphasis must be placed on the prevention of asthma attacks, and plans made for early evacuation if symptoms develop.

Asthmatics should be identified at the pre-expedition planning stage and efforts made to optimize the condition, assess medication requirements, formulate a plan for an exacerbation, and, if necessary, modify MEDEVAC plans. If space permits they should bring a peak flow meter.

During an expedition, an asthmatic person should note symptoms and, if worsening, record their peak flows regularly. This will identify exacerbations early and prompt the use of prearranged medication increases. Spares of essential medications should be packed separately from regular supplies and a β_2 bronchodilator included in the expedition medical kit.

Altitude

Symptoms may improve in some people at altitude owing to reduced airway resistance and fewer allergens. In others, cold air and exercise may exacerbate it. Peak flow meters may marginally under-read at altitude because of reduced air density.

Prevention of acute asthma attacks

Provoking factors

Cold air, exercise, emotion, allergens (house dust mite, pollen, animal fur), infection, drugs (aspirin, NSAIDs, beta-blockers).

Ensure:
- Medication compliance and good inhaler technique.
- Written asthma action plan for deteriorating symptoms and reduced peak expiratory flow.
- Appropriate preventative treatment, e.g. with an inhaled steroid ± long-acting beta agonist.

Avoid:
- Triggering allergens.
- Smoking.

Symptoms
- Shortness of breath, wheeze, cough and sputum, especially at night or first thing in the morning.

Signs
- Rapid respiratory rate.
- Widespread, polyphonic wheeze.
- Hyperinflated and hyper-resonant chest.
- Diminished air entry.
- Severe life-threatening asthma may have no wheeze and a silent chest.

Assess and record
- Peak expiratory flow rate.
- Symptoms and response to self-treatment.
- Heart and respiratory rates.
- Oxygen saturation (by pulse oximetry if available).

Severity of acute asthma
Moderate asthma
- Peak expiratory flow >50% best or predicted.
- Speech normal.
- Respiration <25 breaths/min.
- Pulse <110 beats/min.

Acute severe asthma
- Peak expiratory flow 33–50% best or predicted.
- Unable to complete sentences.
- Respiration >25 breaths/min.
- Pulse >110 beats/min.

Life-threatening asthma
- Peak expiratory flow <33% best or predicted.
- SpO_2 <92% (caution: saturation may be maintained in severe disease, particularly when supplementary oxygen administered).
- Silent chest, cyanosis, or feeble respiratory effort.
- Bradycardia, dysrhythmia, or hypotension.
- Exhaustion, confusion, or coma.

Differential diagnosis
- Upper airway obstruction.
- Pneumonia/lower respiratory tract infection.
- Hyperventilation.
- Anaphylaxis (➜ Anaphylaxis and anaphylactic shock, p. 236).
- Pulmonary oedema.
- Congestive cardiac failure.
- High-altitude pulmonary oedema (➜ High-altitude pulmonary oedema, p. 661).
- COPD.
- Pneumothorax.

Immediate management

- High-flow oxygen for severe attacks (if available).
- β_2 bronchodilator—e.g. salbutamol.
- 4–6 puffs repeated at intervals of 10–20 min (via spacer or nebulizer if available).
- Hydrocortisone 100–200 mg IV.
- Prednisolone 40–50 mg orally.

If there is acute severe asthma, life-threatening asthma, or a poor response to initial treatment, MEDEVAC to hospital.

If moderate asthma and good response to initial treatment (reduced symptoms, respiratory rate, and heart rate, peak expiratory flow >75%), consider increasing usual treatment and continue oral prednisolone 30 mg for 5 days. Evacuate if any further deterioration.

Life-threatening asthma in remote environment

- Death results from cardiac arrest secondary to hypoxia and acidosis. Give high-flow oxygen if available.
- Consider tension pneumothorax (→ Tension pneumothorax, p. 190).
- Adrenaline (epinephrine) 1:1000 solution 0.5 mL IM may be used to relieve brochospasm if peri-arrest.
- In a resource-poor environment a paper bag or empty water bottle can be used as an improvised spacer for inhalers. Caffeine, a methylxanthine in coffee, tea, and chocolate, is a bronchodilator. Caffeine is readily absorbed from the buccal mucosa and instant coffee granules may be administered in this way.

Resources

The British Thoracic Society publishes comprehensive guidelines for the assessment and management of asthma: ℬ https://www.brit-thoracic.org.uk/clinical-information/asthma

Treatment: abdomen

Section editor
Chris Imray

Contributors
Sarah R. Anderson
Tim Campbell-Smith
Jane Wilson-Howarth

Acute abdominal pain 384
Upper abdominal pain 388
Lower abdominal pain 390
Gastrointestinal bleeding 396
Diarrhoea and vomiting 398
Other gastrointestinal problems 404
Urological problems 406
Acute scrotal pain 408
Gynaecological problems 410

Acute abdominal pain

Mild or moderate abdominal pain or colic is relatively common when exposed to new cultures, diets, and living conditions overseas. Acute abdominal pain can cause great anxiety in a wilderness setting. Often the first thought is of appendicitis; indeed historically, acute appendicitis gave rise to such concern that, until relatively recently, doctors venturing to the Antarctic were offered a prophylactic appendicectomy. In reality, acute surgical emergencies account for only 0.7% of medical problems during an expedition.[1] Although abdominal pain is more common in women, in men abdominal pain is more likely to result from a surgical problem.

When a patient in a remote location presents with acute abdominal pain, the specific diagnosis is less important than the need to decide whether their condition justifies evacuation. Assess on the basis of history, general condition, and examine the abdomen looking for signs of peritonism (see ➲ Abdomen, p. 172; ➲ Lower abdominal pain, p. 390). Peritoneal inflammation suggests a significant surgical problem; resuscitate, provide pain relief and, if appropriate, give antibiotics whilst evacuation is organized.

Managing acute abdominal pain

History
- Age and sex, including menstrual history in women.
- Pain: its onset, location, character, severity, and radiation together with any exacerbating or relieving factors.
- Associated symptoms: vomiting, diarrhoea, fever, melaena, frequency and volume of passing urine, etc.
- Past medical history.

Examination
- General condition including conscious level. Is the patient in pain or distressed, lying still or rolling in pain?
- Flushed or cold, and clammy?
- Cardiovascular system—look for signs of shock—tachycardia, and hypotension.
- Dehydration—assess capillary return, strength of pulse, skin turgor.
- Respiratory system—cyanosis, respiratory rate, and breath sounds (pneumonia can mimic acute abdominal pain).
- Abdomen—note any scars, distension, or tenderness. Is there guarding: a reflex contraction of the abdominal wall muscles on palpation? If present:
  - Is the guarding localized or generalized?
  - Is the guarding distractible (i.e. could it be voluntary)?

1 Anderson SR, Johnson CJH (2000). Expedition health and safety: a risk assessment. *J R Soc Med*, 93, 557–62.

- Is there 'rebound tenderness'?
- 'Percussion tenderness' is more sensitive than rebound. Percuss gently over the abdomen and watch the patient's face for signs of discomfort.
- Listen for bowel sounds (useful if obstructed).
- Signs of chronic liver disease.
- Rectal and vaginal examinations are valuable if appropriate and the situation allows, but always have a chaperone.

Always document consultation findings, differential diagnoses, and your management plan. Begin a chart of regular observations which should include pulse rate, BP, respiratory rate, temperature, fluid balance, and arterial saturations if a pulse oximeter is available. The chart can provide valuable information about whether the patient is improving or deteriorating and may also be medico-legally important.

Management of patient with an acute abdomen
Care will depend upon available equipment, facilities, and skills:
- Good analgesia. Patient may require opiates, IV if possible, particularly if vomiting. Opiates will not mask the signs of peritonitis.
- Antiemetic such as cyclizine.
- Oxygen, if available.
- IV fluid resuscitation with Hartmann's or 0.9% saline. Rectal fluids have been used successfully in the wilderness.
- Nasogastric tube if evidence of obstruction or persistent vomiting. Aspirate gastric contents, or insufflate air and auscultate over the stomach, to check position.
- Consider urinary catheterization (if equipment and skills available). Continued urine output gives a good indication of adequate fluid resuscitation. Not appropriate if patient is to make an ambulatory evacuation.
- Consider diabetic ketoacidosis, check blood glucose.
- Start broad-spectrum antibiotics.
- If available prescribe proton pump inhibitor (PPI) or H_2 blocker—now available as orodispersible preparations.
- If the patient has signs of peritonitis, evacuate urgently.

Differential diagnosis
See Table 13.1.

Table 13.1 Table of differential diagnoses of acute abdominal pain

	Site of pain	Onset and character of pain	Associated symptoms	Examination findings
Perforated pepticulcer	Epigastric. Previous history of ulcer disease	Sudden severe upper abdominal pain. Remains constant	Nausea, vomiting, anorexia (More common in smokers and NSAID takers)	Tachycardic, shocked, dehydrated. Initially upper abdominal tenderness and guarding then becomes generalized. Sometimes RIF pain, as fluid tracks down the right paracolic gutter so may be confused with appendicitis
Biliary colic	Epigastric or RUQ. Radiates to shoulder tip	Gradual. Colicky or constant pain until subsides	Nausea and vomiting. Pain may be precipitated by fatty foods	Mild RUQ tenderness. No guarding
Acute cholecystitis	Epigastric or RUQ. Radiates to shoulder tip	Gradual onset becomes constant	Nausea and vomiting	RUQ tenderness, localized guarding. Murphy's sign positive. Fever
Acute pancreatitis	Epigastric pain radiates through to back	Sudden onset. Severe, sharp pain	Anorexia, nausea, and vomiting Jaundice	Epigastric or generalized tenderness with guarding. Can be shocked and hypoxic
Acute appendicitis	Periumbilical pain which migrates to & localizes in RIF	Gradual onset. Initially vague then sharp pain in RIF	Nausea, vomiting anorexia (common). Occasional diarrhoea	Flushed, fever 38°C, tachycardia. Localized tenderness and guarding RIF. Rovsing sign +ve

	Pain	Onset/character	Associated symptoms	Signs
Intestinal obstruction	Vague central pain	Gradual onset, colicky abdominal pain	Vomiting, absolute constipation	Dehydration. Tachycardia, abdominal distension, vague tenderness. High pitched bowel sound. Evidence of previous abdominal surgery. Hernia.
Acute diverticulitis	LIF pain	Gradual onset, constant or colicky	Diarrhoea	Tenderness in LIF and localized guarding. Occasional mass. Fever
Renal colic	Flank pain radiates around the groin to the penis/labia	Sudden onset, colicky	Nausea and vomiting common Haematuria (on dipstick)	Rolling around in pain. Mild flank tenderness
Acute salpingitis	Bilateral adnexae, suprapubic or iliac fossae	Gradual onset, becoming worse	Nausea and vomiting occasionally	Fever. Vaginal discharge. Cervical tenderness, adnexal mass
Ectopic pregnancy	Unilateral low groin pain early on Shoulder tip pain	Sudden or intermittent, sharp	Often none	Adnexal mass tenderness, hypotension and tachycardia are late signs
Acute retention	Central low abdominal pain	Gradual	Inability to pass urine	Dome shaped swelling arising from pelvis which is dull to percussion
Strangulated hernia	Over the hernia and often generalised colicky abdominal pain	Gradually worsening		Often a red inflamed and tender swelling over the hernia orifice, associated with high pitched bowel sounds

Upper abdominal pain

Common causes of severe upper abdominal pain include:
- Peptic ulcer disease.
- Indigestion and gastro-oesophageal reflux disease (GORD).
- Gallstone disease.

Peptic ulcer disease

Risk factors for peptic ulcer disease include smoking, stress, NSAIDs, steroids, and alcohol. Presentation can be insidious: initially with aching upper abdominal discomfort and irritability, but possibly leading on to severe abdominal pain, bleeding, or perforation.

Symptoms
- Gnawing upper abdominal pain.
- Occurs 1–4 h after eating.
- Relieved by bland foods such as milk and yoghurts which buffer stomach acids.

Examination findings
- Often none, sometimes mild epigastric tenderness.

Management
- Avoid risk factors such as smoking and alcohol—especially binge drinking.
- Antacids.
- H$_2$ antagonists: ranitidine or cimetidine.
- PPI, e.g. omeprazole, lansoprazole, etc.

Indigestion and gastro-oesophageal reflux disease

Symptoms
- Vague upper abdominal fullness.
- Belching.
- Regurgitation of food or stomach acid.
- 'Heart burn'—usually worse after eating.
- Improves about an hour or so later.
- If intermittent, think of gallstones.

Examination findings
- Usually none, patient commonly overweight.

Management
- Avoid smoking.
- Eat smaller meals.
- Antacids and PPI.
- Try low-fat meals (to minimize gallstone colic).

Gallstone disease

Gallstones are common and classically associated with the five Fs: Fat, Forty, Female, Flatulent dyspepsia, Fatty food intolerance. They are found in up to 40% women over the age of 40 years, with symptomatic stones increasingly seen in younger people. Gallstones are initially asymptomatic, but once symptoms develop, they are often recurrent. Conditions caused by gallstones range from 'flatulent' dyspepsia and fatty food intolerance to life-threatening acute pancreatitis and cholangitis. If a prospective member of an expedition to a remote area has recurrent symptomatic gallstones, serious consideration should be given to having a prophylactic laparoscopic cholecystectomy well in advance of departure.

Table 13.2 Differential diagnosis of gallstone disease

	Symptoms	Signs	Management
Biliary colic	Colicky or constant RUQ or epigastric pain Radiates to shoulders, some nausea or vomiting	Mild RUQ tenderness No guarding	Analgesia, rest Avoid fatty foods
Acute cholecystitis	RUQ pain, radiates to right shoulder tip Pain worse on deep breath Nausea and vomiting	RUQ tenderness, localized guarding, fever. Murphy's sign	Analgesia, antibiotics, i.e. co-amoxiclav 375–625 mg three times a day or ciprofloxacin 500–750 mg twice a day Evacuate
Acute pancreatitis	Epigastric or central abdominal pain, radiates through to the back Nausea and vomiting	Central or generalized tenderness and guarding Hypotension and tachycardia, sometimes fever, occasional jaundice	Analgesia, fluid resuscitation, catheter, omeprazole 40 mg and antibiotics* (to treat other possible causes) Evacuate
Ascending cholangitis	RUQ or epigastric pain, rigors	RUQ tenderness, fever, jaundice	Analgesia, resuscitation, broad-spectrum antibiotics (co-amoxiclav 375–625 mg three times a day or ciprofloxacin 500–750 mg twice a day) Evacuate
Obstructive jaundice	May be associated with any biliary condition, itching	Jaundice Pale stools Dark urine	Analgesia if required, broad-spectrum antibiotics (if febrile) i.e. co-amoxiclav 375–625 mg three times a day or ciprofloxacin 500–750 mg twice a day Evacuate

*Acute pancreatitis: antibiotics are not usually part of the acute treatment of mild pancreatitis, but without the ability to confirm the diagnosis, treat as for a perforated viscus.

Lower abdominal pain

Differential diagnosis of lower abdominal pain includes:
- Acute appendicitis.
- Acute diverticulitis.
- GI obstruction.
- Hernias.
- Obstetric and gynaecological problems.

Acute appendicitis

Acute appendicitis is a feared condition to diagnose in the wilderness, and often a cause of anxiety for those going even before the expedition leaves home shores. Appendicitis can occur at any age, but is more common in the young. The diagnosis, even in hospital, is essentially a clinical one, backed up with a white cell count and CRP. *A patient diagnosed with signs of peritonitis requires urgent evacuation.*

Classically, pain begins as a vague central visceral aching pain. Over 12–48 h the pain migrates to settle in the right iliac fossa (RIF), becoming a more focal sharp pain, made worse by moving, coughing, or straining. Anorexia is common, and the most reliable associated symptom. Nausea is common, vomiting less so. Occasionally, patients have diarrhoea (pelvic appendicitis) but this is not profuse as in gastroenteritis. With children, watch them walk; if they limp or bend forward slightly, holding the RIF this is a good indicator of significant pain. Get patients to jump up and down; if they can do this without pain, it is unlikely that they have peritoneal inflammation. Examine them supine. Before even laying a hand, ask them to blow their abdomen up like a balloon and then suck it in. Percuss with your fingers gently throughout the abdomen whilst distracting them with chat, i.e. about the expedition. Both of these manoeuvres will hurt if there is peritonitis.

Symptoms
- Central abdominal pain that migrates to the RIF or solely RIF pain.
- Worse on movement, coughing.
- Occasional loin pain (retrocaecal appendicitis).
- Anorexia (very common).
- Nausea and occasional vomiting.
- Occasional loose stool.

Clinical findings
- Flushed, feverish, tachycardic.
- Furred tongue, fetor oris.
- Tenderness in the RIF with guarding.
- Percussion tenderness (➲ Abdomen, p. 172).
- Pain in RIF when palpating the left iliac fossa (LIF) (Rovsing's sign).
- Pain in RIF when extending or rotating the right hip (psoas irritation).
- Rectal or vaginal tenderness (pelvic appendicitis).
- Feel for cervical excitation (pelvic inflammatory disease—PID).

Management
- Analgesia.
- IV fluids (if available; if not, sip clear fluids slowly).
- Start broad-spectrum antibiotics if >6 h from definitive medical care: cephalosporin and metronidazole, or co-amoxiclav 1.2 g three times a day (preferably IV, or PR metronidazole 1 g twice a day. Check for penicillin allergy).
- Evacuate urgently to base hospital if possible.

If evacuation is impossible, or is likely to be significantly delayed (e.g. over-wintering in polar regions, offshore sailing, prolonged bad weather), then conservative management may need to be considered. When access to safe hospital care is not possible, this approach offers a long-recognized alternative approach and consists of the first three steps listed at the start of this section: pain-relief, fluids, and antibiotics. In a recent meta-analysis, non-operative management of uncomplicated appendicitis with antibiotics was associated with fewer complications, better pain control, and shorter sick leave, but overall had inferior efficacy because of the high rate of recurrence in comparison with appendectomy.[2]

Differential diagnoses
- Mesenteric adenitis (children).
- Meckel's diverticulitis.
- Mittelschmerz (mid-cycle ovulation pain).
- Ovarian cyst (➔ Acute ovarian conditions, p. 394).
- Ectopic pregnancy (➔ Ectopic pregnancy, p. 394).
- Pelvic inflammatory disease (PID) (➔ Pelvic inflammatory disease, p. 395).
- Endometriosis.
- Sigmoid diverticulitis (➔ Acute diverticulitis, p. 391).
- Crohn's ileitis or ulcerative colitis (usually has preceding GI history; loose stools/pain , ➔ Inflammatory bowel disease, p. 54).
- Gastroenteritis (➔ Diarrhoea in children, p. 65; ➔ Diarrhoea and vomiting, p. 398).
- Typhoid (➔ Typhoid and paratyphoid (enteric fevers), p. 477).
- Torsion right testis (➔ Testicular torsion, p. 408).

If in doubt, treat as acute appendicitis and evacuate.

Acute diverticulitis

Diverticulosis is common in developed countries, and increases with age (rare under the age of 40 years), affecting 5% of 50-year-olds and up to 70% of 85-year-olds. Acute diverticulitis is caused by a microscopic perforation of a diverticulum with a resultant surrounding inflammation. This may cause mild systemic upset, which resolves with antibiotics, or can progress to a pericolic abscess, which, if it perforates, leads to generalized peritonitis.

2 Mason RJ, Moazzez A, Sohn H, Katkhouda N (2012). Meta-analysis of randomized trials comparing antibiotic therapy with appendectomy for acute uncomplicated (no abscess or phlegmon) appendicitis. *Surg Infect (Larchmt)*, 13(2), 74–84.

Symptoms
- Lethargy and anorexia.
- Lower abdominal pain, usually localized to LIF.
- Diarrhoea.
- Nausea, vomiting (occasional).

Examination findings
- Pyrexia.
- Tachycardia.
- Tenderness in the LIF ± localized guarding.

Management
- Analgesia.
- Rest.
- Fluid diet for 24–48 h.
- Broad-spectrum antibiotics.
- If signs of peritonitis are present, *evacuate*.

Gastrointestinal obstruction

GI obstruction is a serious condition requiring fluid resuscitation, evacuation, and treatment of the underlying cause. The commonest causes in the UK are adhesional obstruction from previous surgery and strangulated hernias. In the wilderness, making a specific diagnosis is less important than recognizing the problem and initiating fluid resuscitation and evacuation. Fluid losses into the obstructed bowel can be considerable (several litres) and patients can rapidly become dehydrated and shocked.

Symptoms
- Abdominal pain (initially colicky then constant).
- Vomiting, maybe bile-stained (early with proximal obstructions).
- Absolute constipation (no passage of flatus or faeces).
- Abdominal distension.
- Painful swelling (i.e. groin, umbilicus).

Examination findings
- Dehydration (mucus membranes, skin turgor).
- Tachycardia.
- Hypotension.
- Oliguria.
- Distended abdomen.
- High-pitched (tinkling) bowel sounds.
- Hernia (inguinal, femoral or umbilical are most common).
- Evidence of previous abdominal scars.
- Abdominal tenderness (a very worrying sign of possible perforation).

Management
- Analgesia.
- Rest.
- IV fluids.
- Nasogastric tube if vomiting.
- Consider urinary catheter.
- Correct fluid and electrolyte imbalances.
- Evacuate.

Hernias

Hernias should be diagnosed and repaired well before departure. The commonest sites are groin and umbilical. Most hernias will cause discomfort and limit activity, particularly heavy work. If strangulation occurs, urgent evacuation is required. If a hernia becomes apparent on an expedition but is not strangulated it does not require evacuation. Limit the patient to light activities which are comfortable to perform and avoid lifting (particularly rucksacks). Improvised trusses are of little or no value.

Symptoms
- Swelling.
- Discomfort.
- Incarceration: irreducible but not tender ('imprisoned').
- With strangulation:
  - Lump that 'won't go down'.
  - Constant severe pain.
  - Vomiting.
  - Distension.
  - Absolute constipation.

Examination findings
- Uncomplicated hernia:
  - Soft, non-tender swelling:
    —Groin (may extend in to the scrotum).
    —Umbilical.
    —Femoral (higher risk of strangulation).
    —Associated with a surgical incision.
  - Reducible.
- Strangulated hernia:
  - Tender swelling.
  - Hot, erythematous overlying skin.
  - Signs of obstruction.

Management
If uncomplicated:
- Avoid heavy lifting/work/carrying bags.
- Simple pain relief.

Strangulated:
- If presentation is early, it is worth attempting to reduce the hernia using a combination of analgesia, bed rest, and gentle, firm pressure along the axis of the sac (this is obliquely for an indirect inguinal hernia). Even if it reduces, the patient should be evacuated for full assessment and urgent repair.
- As for GI obstruction: *evacuate*.
- IV antibiotics.

Acute ovarian conditions

Acute problems with the ovaries include haemorrhage, rupture of a cyst, and torsion. All these conditions are associated with pain. The time of pain can help distinguish the various diagnoses. Mittelschmerz pain is mid-cycle from ovulatory bleeding and is usually unilateral. Pain from a ruptured ovarian cyst can occur at any time in the cycle. There may be signs of peritonism or the patient may complain of shoulder tip pain if blood tracks up to the diaphragm. Torsion presents as sudden onset of unilateral severe lower abdominal pain and may be accompanied by nausea, vomiting, and diarrhoea. In hospital, these conditions are often thought initially to be appendicitis and are diagnosed at laparoscopy or appendicectomy. These patients, therefore, will commonly be evacuated.

Symptoms
- Lower abdominal/pelvic pain.
- Nausea, vomiting, diarrhoea.
- Shoulder tip pain.
- Examination findings:
  - Low iliac fossa tenderness and guarding.
  - Cervical tenderness and tender adnexae on vaginal examination.
  - Tachycardia but apyrexial.

Management
- Check pregnancy test if possible.
- Analgesia.
- Rest.
- Reassurance with Mittelschmerz.
- If there are signs of peritonism: *evacuate*.

Ectopic pregnancy

All women of childbearing age with abdominal pain should have a pregnancy test performed. The site and onset of pain depends on site of implantation. Pain is usually preceded by a period of amenorrhoea for 6–8 weeks, but patients can still have what appear to be regular periods. Pain is usually unilateral. If there is enough blood, pain is more generalized or may give shoulder tip pain. Vaginal bleeding is scant and usually dark brown, and appears a few hours after the onset of the pain. Risk factors include previous ectopic, progesterone-only pill, IVF and previous pelvic sepsis, i.e. appendicitis or PID, intrauterine contraceptive devices (IUCD). Once suspected, evacuate urgently, as these patients can deteriorate rapidly.

Symptoms
- Amenorrhoea and breast tenderness. 'When was your last period which was normal for you?'
- Previous period atypical.
- Lower abdominal pain.
- Shoulder tip pain.
- Vaginal bleeding (scant and often dark) in <50%.

Examination findings
- Lower abdominal tenderness ± guarding.
- Signs of shock.
- Vaginal bleeding.
- Positive pregnancy test.

Management
- Analgesia.
- Resuscitate.
- IV fluids.
- Evacuate.

Pelvic inflammatory disease

PID is almost always caused by ascending infection from the genital tract. It is acquired as a sexually transmitted infection. The condition used to be commonly gonoccocal; now, up to half of cases are due to *Chlamydia*. Infection usually involves the endometrium and both fallopian tubes. Risk factors include age at first sexual intercourse, number of partners, and presence of an IUCD. The severity is variable, and it may be mistaken for appendicitis.

Symptoms
- Pelvic pain.
- Fever.
- Deep dyspareunia.
- Dysmenorrhoea.
- GI upset.

Examination findings
- Pyrexia.
- Signs of systemic sepsis.
- Bilateral iliac fossa tenderness and guarding.
- Cervical tenderness on vaginal examination.
- Speculum examination may reveal pus from the external os.
- Occasional pelvic mass.

Management
- Analgesia.
- Combination antibiotics.
- Co-amoxiclav or erythromycin + doxycycline.
- Penicillin + metronidazole + doxycycline.
- Evacuate if there are signs of systemic sepsis.

Gastrointestinal bleeding

Upper gastrointestinal bleeding

GI bleeding is a serious problem that even in hospital is associated with significant mortality. Haematemesis (vomit of fresh blood), coffee ground vomiting, or the passage of melaena (black, sticky, offensive smelling, tar-like stools are true emergencies requiring prompt treatment and evacuation. Even if bleeding stops and the patient appears better, they should still be evacuated urgently, as re-bleeding is common and carries a high mortality.

If the expedition is in a very remote location, attempts to carry-out a casualty who is actively bleeding are not recommended. Evacuate by mechanical transport (vehicle, boat, or helicopter) if possible.

Following prolonged, effortful vomiting, minor streaks of blood may be seen in the vomitus. These are caused by small tears in the oesophageal mucosa (Mallory–Weiss tear) and, unlike true haematemesis, are not serious.

History
- There is often a history of peptic ulcer disease.
- NSAID use, smoking, alcohol.

Symptoms
- Haematemesis.
- 'Coffee grounds' vomiting.
- Confusion.
- Passage of malaena or dark blood per rectum.

Examination findings
- Pale.
- Tachycardia.
- Hypotension (a very ominous sign in the young).
- Confusion and agitation.
- Decreased urine output.
- Concentrated urine.
- Melaena on rectal examination.
- Fresh blood per rectum; if from a bleeding peptic ulcer, indicates rapid, life-threatening haemorrhage.

Management
- Rest.
- Place the patient supine with legs elevated.
- IV access and fluids if available.
- PPI or H_2 blockers (orodispersible preparations are available, i.e. Fastabs®).
- Avoid NSAIDs, smoking, alcohol, caffeine.
- Catheterize if possible or measure urine output.
- Evacuate.

Lower gastrointestinal (rectal) bleeding

The passage of small amounts of fresh blood per rectum following defecation is common, and is usually due to haemorrhoids (piles). On expeditions, constipation can be a problem, particularly with dehydration, change in diet, and being confined to a tent in a storm.

Causes of lower gastrointestinal bleeding
- Haemorrhoids.
- Anal fissure.
- Diverticular disease (age generally >60 years; can be copious).
- Acute colitis (stool also contains pus and mucus, usually there is previous history).
- Dysentery (+ diarrhoea and fever) (➲ Diarrhoea and vomiting, p. 398).

Haemorrhoids (piles)

Haemorrhoids are caused by abnormal swelling of anorectal tissue, which may become traumatized during defecation and bleed. They occasionally prolapse, strangulate, and thrombose. This requires pain relief and ice packs and topical analgesia to reduce the swelling, and laxatives to soften the stools.

Symptoms
- Fresh red rectal bleeding following bowel motion (often painless and only seen on toilet paper).
- Perianal itching.
- Prolapsing piles (very painful, if thrombosed).

Examination findings
- Unless prolapsed, haemorrhoids are impalpable.

Management
- Soften stools—high-fibre diet and good hydration, ± laxatives.
- Avoid straining at stool.
- Proctosedyl® or Xyloproct® ointment or suppositories can help.
- Use baby wipes instead of toilet paper.
- If thrombosed, use analgesia and ice packs (not directly on the skin).

Anal fissure

An acute, painful condition where there is a tear/split in the skin lining the anus. It is usually precipitated by an episode of constipation.

Symptoms
- Severe anal pain on defecation (like lemon juice on a cut).
- Small amount of fresh, red, rectal bleeding.

Examination findings
- Soft, non-tender abdomen.
- Rectal examination is usually impossible due to pain and sphincter spasm (and this is diagnostic).

Management
- Soften the stools—high-fibre diet, good hydration, laxative (i.e. lactulose).
- Pain relief—local anaesthetic gel (Proctosedyl® or Xyloproct® ointment).
- Relax the sphincter spasm with 0.4% GTN ointment—shelf-life 3 months (Rectogesic®). Use a pea size amount rubbed on to the perianal skin twice daily for 6 weeks. Can cause headache and postural hypotension.

Diarrhoea and vomiting

Diarrhoea is defined as four or more loose or liquid stools per day. *Dysentry* is acute diarrhoea with blood in the motions.

Diarrhoeal illness causes more than a billion episodes of illness a year worldwide, and in the developing world is a major cause of death in the young and elderly. Up to 1/3 of medical problems encountered on an expedition are related to GI 'upset' or diarrhoea. The conditions may arise as a result of:

- Changes in diet.
- Changes in water supplies.
- Altered schedules.
- Stress of foreign travel.
- Infections.

If diarrhoea has continued for <3 weeks, then infection is the most likely cause.

The commonest route of infection is faecal–oral, caused by poor hygiene or contaminated water (see Table 13.3). Scrupulous hygiene precautions (see Chapter 3) should be maintained throughout the expedition, without this, diarrhoea can be the cause of the expedition failing in its aims or just being a miserable experience. Dysentry = acute diarrhoea with blood.

History

In taking the history ask about:
- Duration.
- Stools: colour, consistency, frequency, blood, or pus.
- Vomiting.
- Fever.
- Abdominal pain.
- Thirst (a late symptom).
- Recent eating and drinking habits.
- Others affected?

Examination

- General condition.
- Signs of dehydration:
  - Reduced volume of concentrated urine.
  - Dry mucous membranes.
  - Skin turgor.
  - Sunken eyes.
  - Raised pulse (late sign).
  - BP—including postural drop (very late sign).
- Temperature.

Usually diarrhoeal illnesses will settle. Some will require specific treatments, but the most important factor in minimizing morbidity and mortality rates is hydration. Most patients can maintain their hydration with rest and oral rehydration, although occasionally IV fluids are necessary.

Table 13.3 Common causes of diarrhoea

Condition	Diarrhoea no blood	Diarrhoea with blood
No fever	Food poisoning (bacteria or toxins)	Amoebic dysentery
	Traveller's diarrhoea	
	Viruses	
	Giardia	
Fever	Salmonella	Shigella
		Campylobacter
		Salmonella

General treatment guidelines and rehydration

(See Table 13.4.)
- Rehydration is fundamental.
- Antibiotics are not first-line treatment for diarrhoea. Most episodes are self-limiting and usually settle within 2 days.
- However, a single dose of ciprofloxacin (1 g) at the onset of diarrhoea may shorten the duration and, if symptoms persist, continue ciprofloxacin 500 mg twice a day for 3 days.
- Basic treatment is similar regardless of the cause.
  - Rest.
  - Replace fluids, orally if possible, with oral rehydration fluids (Dioralyte®, Electrolade®, or equivalent)—frequent sips if vomiting.
  - Aim for good volumes (>0.5–1.0 mL/kg body weight/h) of clear urine.
  - Antiemetics may help (suppositories or buccal prochlorperazine (Buccastem®), or IM/IV injection).
  - Paracetamol if febrile or abdominal pain.
  - Avoid dairy products, but don't fast.
  - Avoid loperamide or co-phenotrope (Lomotil®) unless absolutely necessary.
  - Loperamide (4 mg initially, then 2 mg after each loose stool) is useful to limit symptoms if travel is essential or tent-bound by a storm.
  - IV fluids if unable to manage oral fluids (if IV fluids are required the patient should be evacuated). Anecdotally, rectal fluids via a Foley catheter have been used with success.
  - If diarrhoea persists, it could be protozoal; give metronidazole or tinidazole.

When to seek external medical attention:
- Temperature >40°C.
- Significant fever for >48 h.
- Diarrhoea lasting > 4 days.
- Difficulty keeping fluid down.
- Diarrhoea with blood.

Table 13.4 Diagnosis and treatment of diarrhoea and vomiting

Category of diarrhoea	Organisms	Foods	Incubation	Symptoms	Treatment
Diarrhoea— no blood—no fever	Staphylococcus aureus (toxin)	Meat, poultry, dairy produce, particularly, if eaten cold	Usual: 2–4 hRange: 1–7 h	V, AP, (D) short-lived, Abrupt onset	Antibiotics ineffective, as due to toxins
	Bacillus cereus (toxin)	Fried rice, raw or dried foods particularly, if inadequate reheating	Usual: vomiting syndrome 1–6 h Usual: diarrhoea syndrome 6–16 h	V and nausea—lasts <12 h, D (short lived), AP— lasts <24 h	Antibiotics ineffective, as due to toxins
	E.coli (toxin) (known as traveller's diarrhoea)	Faecal contamination of water or food	Usual: 12–48 h	D (watery), AP (cramps) Duration: 2–5 days	Usually self-limiting but single-dose ciprofloxacin 1 g or tetracycline 500 mg may shorten illness
	Clostridium perfringens	Cooked meat, poultry, particularly, if inadequate re-heating	Usual: 8–12 h Range: 4–24 h	D (watery, often violent, AP, V(rarely)	Supportive only
	Cryptosporidium	Faecal contamination of food or water	Usual: 7–10 days Range: 1–28 days	D (watery), AP, bloating	Self-limiting but severe disease in immuno- compromised
	Viral norovirus, rotavirus	Usually person-person or environmental contamination	Usual: 24–72 h Duration: 1–2 days	N—projectile vomiting, mild D, AP R—watery D, V, fever	No antibiotics
	Giardia lamblia protozoal infaction	Contaminated water, often from mountain streams	Incubation: 7–10 days Duration: 2–6 weeks	D (often pale and persistent) AP (cramps), bloating. Flatulence–'eggy burps'	Metronidazole 500 mg three times a day for 5 days or tinidazole single dose 2 g

Diarrhoea—no blood—FEVER	*Salmonella*	Undercooked or raw meat, poultry, dairy produce, eggs	Usual: 12–36 h Range: 6–72 h	D (& blood/mucus) V, AP (cramps), fever Duration: 2–5 days	Usually self-limiting ciprofloxacin 500 mg twice a day if needed
	Cholera	Contaminated water, shellfish or raw food	Incubation: 1–3 days	D (profuse and watery = 'rice water'). Rapid dehydration leading to shock	Fluids +++ (IV). Tetracycline 250–500 mg 6-hrly. Evacuate
Diarrhoea—BLOOD—no fever	Entamoeba (amoebic dysentery; protozoal infection)	Raw or undercooked food Waterborne	Incubation: >7 days Duration: until successfully treated	D (bloody/ gradual onset) AP (cramps), weight loss	Metronidazole 800 mg three times a day for 5 days. Followed by diloxanide 500 mg three times a day for 10 days
	Escherichia coli O157	Meat, poultry, dairy produce Contaminated water	Usual: 3–4 days Range: 1–9 days	D or D with blood, AP (severe) HUS (2–7%)	Antibiotics contra-indicated
Diarrhoea—BLOOD—and FEVER	*Shigella*	Faecal contamination of water or food	Usual: 24–72 h Range: 1–7 days	D (explosive and bloody) AP (cramps), fever, anorexia	Ciprofloxacin 500–750 mg td or trimethoprim 200 mg twice a day
	Campylobacter	Poultry, raw milk, eggs Contaminated water	Usual: 2–5 days Range: 1–10 days	D (often bloody and profuse). AP (severs cramps) 9 fever Duration 2–7 days	Usually self-limiting, Ciprofloxacin 500–750 mg twice daily or erythromycin 500 mg four times a day or 1 g twice daily

Symptom definitions: V, vomiting; D, diarrhoea; AP, abdominal pain. HUS haemolytic uraemic syndrome.
Hawker J, Begg N, Blair I, et al. (2005). *Communicable Disease Control Handbook*. Oxford: Blackwell.

Prevention of diarrhoeal illness

Prevention is better than treatment of diarrhoeal illness on an expedition which, once present, can spread rapidly through the group, disrupting plans, and at worst putting the group at risk. It is possible to prevent it entirely with education and care.

- Meticulous hand hygiene is essential.
- Ensure that there are facilities to wash hands at the latrine, whether soap and water or alcohol gel.
- Hands must be washed before entering a mess tent. A wash basin or alcohol gel at the entrance to the mess tent is a good reminder.
- Boil or sterilize water (➔ Water purification, p. 102) before drinking, brushing teeth, or preparing salads.
- Avoid ice in drinks.
- Check seals on bottled water.
- Take care with salads, unpeelable fruit, shellfish, and avoid raw or undercooked meat (particularly chicken).
- Carefully clean mess tins and other cooking equipment.

Cholera

Infection is through contaminated water. Cholera can reach epidemic proportions where sanitation systems have broken down (natural disasters or in war). Profuse watery diarrhoea and rapid dehydration kill. Incubation is 1–3 days.

Symptoms and signs
- Mild diarrhoea initially.
- Profuse watery diarrhoea ('rice water stools').
- Vomiting.
- Prostration.
- Fever.
- Dehydration.
- Signs of shock.

Treatment
- Rest.
- Fluids +++
- IV fluids.
- Tetracycline 250–500 mg 6-hrly.
- Evacuate.

Typhoid

This is a generalized infection, which later in its course can cause diarrhoea. Initially there may be constipation. Incubation is 7–14 days.

Symptoms and signs
- Fever.
- Headache.
- Abdominal pain.
- Rash (rose spots—2 mm pink papules on torso which fade with pressure).
- After >7 days:

- General deterioration.
- High fever.
- Low pulse (= relative bradycardia).
- After 20 days:
  - Confusion or encephalitis.
  - Gravely ill.
  - 'Pea soup' diarrhoea.
  - Perforation of the terminal ileum.

Treatment
- Rest.
- Fluids—oral or IV.
- Ciprofloxacin 500–750 mg twice a day.
- Evacuate.

Other gastrointestinal problems

These less serious but common problems can, in the wilderness, lead to the sufferer having a miserable time and possibly having to leave the expedition

Constipation

Normal bowel habit varies enormously, from three stools per day to one stool every 3–4 days. Alterations of bowel habit are common on expeditions, with many people developing diarrhoea, but constipation can be equally uncomfortable and inconvenient.

Causes
- Dehydration from exertion.
- High altitude.
- Confinement to a tent during a storm.
- Low-fibre diet.

Symptoms
- Cramping abdominal pains.
- Reduced stool frequency with passage of hard stools.

Examination findings
- Soft abdomen.
- Mild tenderness occasionally.
- May be able to palpate indentable stools in the LIF.

Management
Ensure that expedition food includes adequate dietary fibre. Encourage good hydration, aiming for the regular passing of dilute urine. Simple laxatives (lactulose or senna) may be required if a person is symptomatic, but taking laxatives prophylactically is unwise.

Perianal haematoma

A painful small purple swelling at the anal verge, usually developing after straining at stool. Perianal haematoma usually settle with conservative treatment.

Management
- Anaesthetize the area with a topical local anaesthetic or ice.
- Soften stools.
- If painful or persistent, surgical drainage may produce relief. Make a small stab incision and express the clot.

Perianal abscess

An acute condition of the anus, presenting with pain and swelling in the perianal skin. It develops over a few days and if caught early may resolve with course of antibiotics.

Symptoms
- Perianal pain and swelling.
- Fever.
- Chills and rigors.

Examination findings
- Pyrexia.
- Tender, erythematous perianal swelling.

Management
- Antibiotics (co-amoxiclav or erythromycin + metronidazole).
- Analgesia.
- If very remote some form of drainage will probably be required to enable ambulatory evacuation.
- An abscess generally requires surgical incision and drainage, but some abscesses (such as breast) are now treated with needle aspiration and antibiotics.
- It is reasonable to attempt to drain the abscess with a large needle through the most fluctuant area.
- Local anaesthetic does not work well in inflamed tissue—try oral analgesia, ice packs, and local anaesthetic to the more normal looking skin surrounding the abscess.
- Evacuate for formal drainage.

Pilonidal abscess

An infection most commonly found in the natal cleft, the area over the sacrum between the buttocks. It is caused by an infected ingrown hair and can occur in any hair-bearing area. Most common in males aged 15–35 years old.

Symptoms
- Pain and swelling over the sacrum between the buttocks (there may be a previous history of this or even of previous surgery).
- Discharge (minimal serum to large amounts of pus).

Examination findings
- Swelling in the natal cleft (usually slightly to one side).
- The swelling maybe hot, red, and tender.
- On close inspection of the cleft, tiny black pits maybe visible in the midline (pilonidal pits).

Management
- Antibiotics (penicillin, flucloxacillin, or erythromycin).
- If not settling, drain the abscess under local anaesthetic:
  - Infiltrate a wide area around the abscess with local anaesthetic (preferably non-inflamed tissue; local anaesthesia works better here).
  - Make a longitudinal linear incision off the midline into the most fluctuant part of the abscess.
  - Break down any loculations with a little finger and irrigate with sterile saline.
  - Cover with a dressing.
- If this then fails to settle: *evacuate*.
- If the situation makes draining the abscess inappropriate, evacuate for surgical drainage.

Urological problems

Urinary tract infection

A common problem, particularly among women. Symptoms include urinary frequency, a burning sensation during micturition (dysuria), which is maximal as flow stops (terminal dysuria). Fever is rare unless associated with pyelonephritis. Urethritis is the term given to a collection of symptoms resulting from inflammation of the urethra, most commonly the result of infection, which may sometimes be associated with a sexually transmitted infection (➲ Sexually transmitted infections, p. 506).

Examination
- Often clinically normal.
- Blood, leucocytes, nitrites, and protein on urine dipstick.

Treatment
- Increase oral fluids.
- Co-amoxiclav, trimethoprim, or ciprofloxacin.

Pyelonephritis

An infection of one or both kidneys, usually resulting from an ascending infection from the bladder, but more rarely secondary to ureteric obstruction. Differential diagnosis includes possible retro-caecal appendicitis.

Symptoms
- Sudden onset of fever, sweats, rigors.
- Flank and/or back pain.
- Patient feels 'terrible'.
- Dysuria, urinary frequency, and urgency.

Examination findings
- High fever.
- Loin tenderness.
- Blood, leucocytes, nitrites, and protein on urine dipstick.

Treatment
- Ensure good hydration.
- Ciprofloxacin, co-amoxiclav, or a cephalosporin for 10 days.

Indications for evacuation
- Failure to respond to treatment.
- Systemic sepsis.

Acute urinary retention

An acute, painful inability to void urine despite a desperate need to do so. It almost invariably affects men from middle age onwards. The symptoms are incapacitating and require prompt relief.

Symptoms
- Lower abdominal/suprapubic pain.
- Intense desire to void.
- Dribbling of urine.
- Suprapubic distension.
- History of previous hesitancy, poor stream, and nocturia.

Examination findings
- Distressed patient.
- Distended lower abdomen.
- Palpable bladder, dull to percussion, tender.
- Examination of the prostate may reveal enlargement, but this does not correlate with prostatic symptoms, nor alter management.

Treatment
- Decompress bladder using a Foley urethral catheter if available. Smaller catheters (12–14 F) may be more difficult to pass than larger ones (16–18 F). Do not attempt rigid instrumentation of the urethra in the field.
- If unsuccessful suprapubic needle decompression is required:
  - Aseptic technique.
  - Infiltrate 1% lidocaine two finger breadths above the symphysis.
  - Direct the needle towards the anus whilst aspirating.
  - Aspirate as much urine as possible.
  - May require repeating, but will enable ambulatory evacuation.
- Watch for excessive diuresis, although this situation is more common following chronic urinary obstruction.
- Evacuate.

Renal (ureteric) colic

A collection of symptoms resulting from ureteric obstruction secondary to a kidney stone calculus (calculus).

Symptoms
- Severe unrelieved flank pain that causes patient to writhe around, possibly clutching side of abdomen. Pain radiates around along the course of the ureter into the groin, to the base/tip of the penis or the labia.
- Nausea and vomiting are common.

Examination findings
- Mild loin tenderness.
- Haematuria: on dipstick and occasionally frank.

Treatment
- Pain control:
  - NSAIDs are very effective if no contraindications: diclofenac IM or PR (if vomiting).
  - Additional opiates or tramadol may be required.
- Forced diuresis is of no benefit but maintain adequate hydration.
- Most calculi pass within a few hours, but some become stuck in ureter and require surgical intervention.
- Evacuate if anuric, signs of sepsis, or pain uncontrollable.

Acute scrotal pain

Acute scrotal pain with swelling is a true surgical emergency requiring urgent assessment and treatment. Differential diagnosis includes strangulated hernia (➲ Hernias, p. 393) and testicular torsion, both conditions that must be diagnosed and the patient evacuated.

Testicular torsion

- Any age, commoner near puberty.
- Sudden onset of severe scrotal pain.
- Associated with vomiting.
- Pain on walking.

Examination findings

- Oedematous scrotal skin.
- Discoloured with a blue tinge.
- No relief when elevated (negative Phren's sign).
- Sometimes there are no physical signs other than pain.

Treatment

Scrotal exploration is inappropriate and unrealistic in the wilderness, but it may be worth attempting manual detorsion:

- Lie the patient supine.
- Elevate the testis. Most commonly the testis has rotated medially (inwards or towards the midline). Non-surgical correction or de-rotation has been described and could be attempted if evacuation is difficult. If successful relief is swift.

If unable to untwist:

- Provide strong analgesia and evacuate as quickly as possible.

Epididymitis

An inflammation or pain in the epididymis (which lies on the superior aspect of the testis). In acute epididymitis the pain is often accompanied by inflammation, redness, swelling, and/or warmth.

- More gradual onset than torsion.
- Associated with fever and dysuria.
- Relieved by gentle elevation.
- Careful palpation reveals a tender, swollen epididymis.
- Often caused by an infection. In sexually active men *Chlamydia trachomatous* or *Neisseria gonorrhoeae* are the most common organisms.
- Treatment is with azithromycin or doxycycline.

Prostatitis

An acute infection of the prostate gland by viral or bacterial pathogens. Though uncommon, it can be associated with severe sepsis. Of the bacterial causes, 80% are due to *Escherichia coli*.

Symptoms

- Fever, sweats, rigors.
- Perineal pain.
- Dysuria, frequency, urgency.
- Urinary retention uncommon.

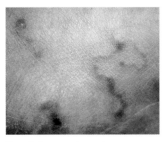

Plate 1 Cutaneous larva migrans.

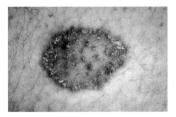

Plate 2 Superficial fungal infection (tinea).

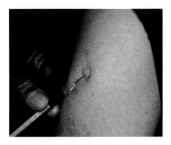

Plate 3 Intradermal injection technique.

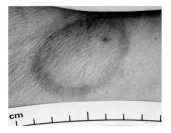

Plate 4 Lyme disease—erythema chronicum migrans.

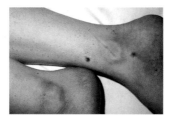

Plate 5 Meningococcal meningitis—early petechial rash.

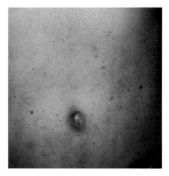

Plate 6 Typhoid rose spots.

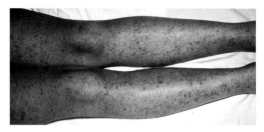

Plate 7 African tick typhus: generalized rash.

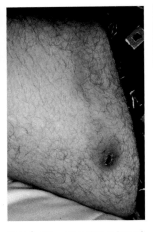

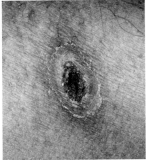

Plate 9 Scrub typhus: eschar.

Plate 8 African tick typhus: eschar and lymphangitic lines.

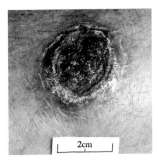

Plate 10 Cutaneous leishmaniasis.

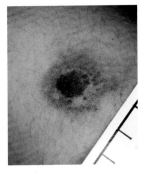

Plate 11 Recluse spider (*Loxosceles*) bite: red-white-and-blue sign 18hr after the bite. Scale in cm.

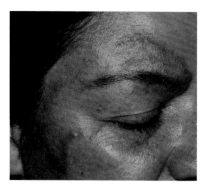

Plate 12 Leprosy misdiagnosed as sarcoid.

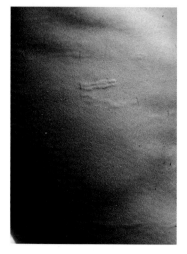

Plate 13 Strongyloidiasis—the rapidly extending linear rash 'larva currens'.

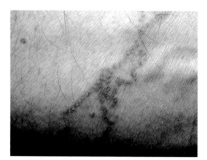

Plate 14 Portuguese Man o' War (*Physalia*) sting.

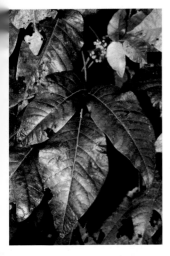

Plate 15 Poison ivy (*Toxicodendron radicans*) trifoliate leaves and berries

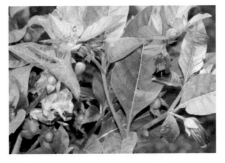

Plate 16 Deadly nightshade (*Atropa belladonna*) flowers and berries.

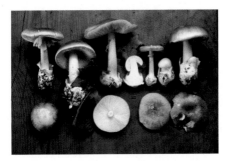

Plate 17 Deathcap mushroom (*Amanita phalloides*). Note white fills and sac at base of stem

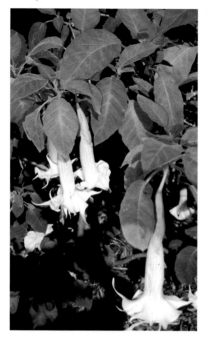

Plate 18 Angel's trumpet (*Brugmansia suaveolans*).

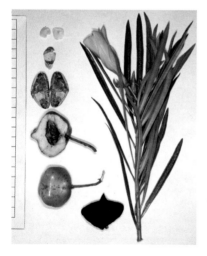

Plate 19 Yellow oleander (*Cascabela thevetia also known as Thevetia peruviana*).

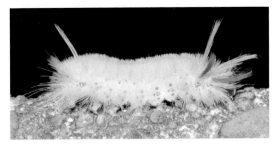

Plate 20 Sycamore tussock moth (Halysidota harrisii).

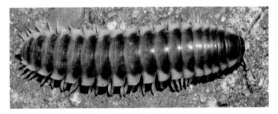

Plate 21 Black and gold flat-backed millipede (*Apheloria virginiensis*).

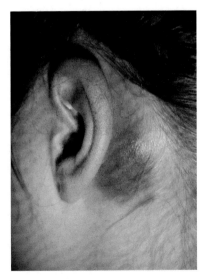

Plate 22 Battle's sign of skull fracture.

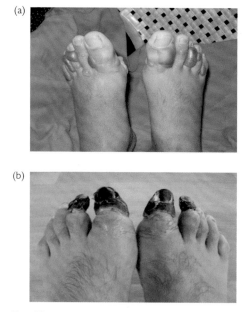

(a)

(b)

Plate 23 a) Frostbite-early b) Frostbite-late.

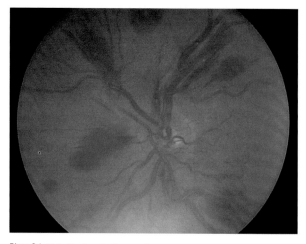

Plate 24 High altitude retinal haemorrhage.

Examination findings
- Pyrexia.
- Tachycardia.
- Boggy tender prostate on rectal examination.

Treatment
In absence of laboratory findings, treat as a bacterial infection. Prolonged courses of ciprofloxacin or co-amoxiclav may be required.

Indications for evacuation
- Systemic sepsis.
- Poor response to treatment.

Gynaecological problems

Gynaecological problems often occur in women who venture into remote regions, even amongst those who have made careful preparations.

Menstrual issues

An 'average' woman loses about 40 mL of blood with each menstrual cycle. Although this amounts to only 8 teaspoonfuls over 4 or 5 days, coping with this can be surprisingly challenging. There may be no privacy to change sanitary protection and no easy access to water. Some medical advisers encourage young women to start the combined oral contraceptive pill to control menstruation, but this is not the solution ➜ Further reading, p. 413, particularly in light of the fact that periods often lighten or even stop during the physical demands of an expedition. Introducing the pill can complicate matters if traveller's diarrhoea interferes with its absorption, thus allowing unpredictable and inconvenient breakthrough bleeding; this is particularly likely in those who have newly started taking the pill but it also occurs in those whose periods are usually regulated by it.

Planning

Ideally, each adventurer will have given some thought to her gynaecological needs long before setting out. One option that is often overlooked is to suppress menstruation by arranging 12-weekly Depo-Provera® injections. This will stop monthly bleeds in most women by the second or third injection. Lack of periods then persist beyond the 3 months between injections, although the woman is, of course, at risk of pregnancy beyond 13 weeks. This contraceptive method has a lot to recommend it amongst travelling women, not least because, being a progesterone-only method, it does not increase the risk of DVT, whereas women taking the combined oral contraceptive pill (or any hormone replacement) have a significantly increased risk; this adds to any risk arising from a long-haul flight, or from ascending to extreme altitude. A progestogen implant (e.g. Nexplanon® has similar advantages, although it can increase menses in some women; to avoid this troublesome side effect, women can be trialled on desogestrel progestogen-only contraceptive pill. Women who bleed on desogestrel are likely to have unwanted bleeding with an implant. Both Depo-Provera® and Nexplanon® need to be organized some time—preferably 6 months—before departure.

Contraceptive types

- *Depo injections* can cause spotting in the first months but thereafter usually suppress menstruation; does not increase DVT risk.
- *Implants* can cause spotting in the first months but thereafter usually suppress menstruation; does not increase DVT risk.
- *Combined pill increases* DVT risk so not good for women ascending to extreme altitude; breakthrough bleeding is often a problem after diarrhoea and in the first 3 months after starting.
- *Progestogen-only* pill can cause spotting, especially in the first month or two; does not increase DVT risk.
- *Intrauterine contraceptive* device tends to increase amount and duration of blood flow; does not increase DVT risk.

- *Intrauterine contraceptive system* can cause spotting in the first months but thereafter usually suppresses menstruation; does not increase DVT risk.
- *Barrier methods* are always worth packing as a backup and for safer sex.

Pain during the first day or two of a menstrual period is often due to blood clots at the neck of the womb and implies a heavier loss than usual. Sometimes, fluid restriction around the first day of bleeding improves symptoms, and so can iron if a woman is anaemic. Those with recurrent and distressing pain on menstruation will be helped by taking a NSAID preparation regularly for a few days starting a day or two before the onset of bleeding. If a woman complains about her periods, ask whether there is any odour or coloured discharge, which suggests a sexually transmitted infection (see ➔ Sexually transmitted infections, p. 506).

Heavy periods in themselves can be quite debilitating but when combined with a poor diet can lead to anaemia. Anaemia then tends to exacerbate heavy menstrual loss and in turn contributes further to anaemia. Iron tablets can often be purchased cheaply overseas.

Logistics

Plenty of sanitary products need to be packed in waterproof containers (zip-lock bags are ideal) and consideration given to responsible disposal. Burying tampons and sanitary towels in desert environments, for example, can allow retrieval by village dogs or exposure by wind. Some sanitary items compost but some towels contain a lot of plastic and do not; washable products are available (e.g. from ℘ http://www.greenbabyco.com). Alternatively, there are devices to collect blood such as the Mooncup® (℘ http://www.mooncup.co.uk). This is a small soft cup with a stalk, which fits in the vagina and collects menstrual blood. It removes the need to carry disposables where they might be difficult to obtain, but clean hands are required to take it out and empty it. The user also needs somewhere to dispose of the still-liquid blood and access to water to clean the Mooncup® before reinserting it. The solution is perhaps to use both reusable and also some conventional disposable supplies.

Vaginal irritation/discharge

Normal vaginal discharge is colourless and its consistency changes with the menstrual cycle. A woman might complain of a change in discharge:

- Yellow or green or foul-smelling discharge implies infection (Table 15.2).
- Vaginal thrush (see Table 15.2); can be treated with miconazole pessaries or oral fluconazole.
- A fishy odour suggests bacterial vaginosis which is cleared with vaginal clindamycin cream inserted for 7 nights or oral metronidazole.
- Foul-smelling black discharge suggests a forgotten tampon; the discharge settles once the tampon is removed.
- Pregnancy also changes the quality of discharge.
- Finally, mid-cycle bleeding might indicate *Chlamydia* infection and must be investigated or treated with doxycycline 100 mg twice a day for 10 days; make diplomatic enquires about possible contacts.

Urinary tract infections

Ascending infections within the female urinary tract are not uncommon in women of all ages; they are more frequent in those who are sexually active. Mild dehydration of the kind experienced in warm climates seems to predispose to UTIs. Sufferers need to continue to drink in quantity, and take 3 days of oral broad-spectrum antibiotic (e.g. co-amoxiclav). If antibiotics are not available, substances which alter urinary pH will help; a teaspoonful of baking soda in a large glass of water is ideal; alternatives are ascorbic acid (vitamin C) or cranberry juice.

Abdominal pain

A woman who complains of significant abdominal pain should be examined especially if the pain is on one side; lateralized lower abdomen pain is often gynaecological in origin but left-sided pain may be caused by GI unease, whilst right-sided pain may be due to appendicitis. A soft abdomen will be reassuring, but vaginal examination is required to exclude problems within the pelvis. An ovarian cyst or fibroid may be palpable during bimanual examination. During vaginal examination, position a finger either side of the cervix so that it can be moved from side to side; if movement of the cervix is painless there is unlikely to be any problem within the pelvis. Equally, pain-free love-making suggests a benign cause for low abdominal pain.

Abdominal pain centred in right or left lower quadrants

Causes of lateralized abdominal pain that usually require evacuation:
- Right-sided pain may be appendicitis (→ Acute appendicitis, p. 390), ectopic pregnancy, or torsion (→ Acute scrotal pain, p. 408): all are serious.
- Ectopic pregnancy—pain on left or right then often erratic menstrual bleeding sometimes described as 'prune juice' appearance; most often 7 weeks (or more) from last period. There may be a tense abdomen (guarding); shock will soon follow and death is a significant risk.
- Twisted ovarian cyst—management depends upon the severity of the pain and size of the cyst; it needs to be assessed in hospital if the cyst is >5 cm in diameter (→ Acute ovarian conditions, p. 394).
- Hernias (→ Hernias, p. 393).

Causes of left- or right-sided abdominal pain that don't usually require evacuation:
- Cystitis—causes malaise and pain on passing urine and sometimes low abdominal pain; blood may be seen in the urine (→ Urinary tract infections, p. 412).
- Ovulation pain—mid-cycle pain located on one side; tender but no guarding; settles in 36–48 h; treat with pain relief. In the longer term the contraceptive pill will stop the pain.
- Gastroenteritis—often left lower abdominal pain associated with passage of stool or flatus; a bland diet reduces symptoms (→ Diarrhoea and vomiting, p. 398).

- Constipation.
- Irritable bowel disease.
- Kidney stones.
- Endometriosis (anti-inflammatory tablets are helpful).
- Salpingitis—pain may be on both sides, but one side is often worse than the other; it may be accompanied by nausea, vomiting, and often fever. Treat with metronidazole 400 mg twice daily and doxycycline 100 mg twice daily for 14 days. Patients should be investigated on reaching home.

Further reading

Sinclair J, Cohen J, Hinton E (1996). Use of the oral contraceptive pill on treks and expeditions. *Br J Fam Plann*, 22, 123–6.
Wilson-Howarth J (2006). *Bugs Bites & Bowels*. London: Cadogan.
Wilson-Howarth J (2006). *How to Shit Around the World*. Palo Alto, CA: Travelers Tales.

Chapter 14

Treatment: limbs and back

Section editor
Jon Dallimore

Contributors
Jules Blackham
Jon Dallimore
Carey M. McClellan
Harvey Pynn
James Calder (1st edition)
James Watson (1st edition)

Limb injuries *416*
Fractures *418*
Dislocations *420*
Shoulder and upper arm injuries *422*
Elbow and forearm injuries *426*
Wrist injuries *428*
Hand injuries *430*
Finger injuries *433*
Nail injuries *434*
Pelvic and hip injuries *436*
Knee injuries *440*
Lower leg injuries *443*
Achilles tendon disorders *444*
Ankle injuries *445*
Foot fractures and dislocations *446*
Spinal injury *448*
Low back pain *450*
Physiotherapy *452*

Limb injuries

Limb injuries may be life-threatening and an initial ABC evaluation should be performed, with respiratory and circulation status regularly re-evaluated (see ➜ Initial response to an incident, p. 180; ➜ Assessment of a casualty, p. 185). Consider the possibility of associated head, spine, chest, abdominal, or pelvic injuries, particularly if the patient is unconscious.

Initial assessment and treatment

- Approach the casualty if safe to do so.
- Ensure that the airway is open, assess the breathing rate, and look for signs of shock (➜ Shock, p. 228). Remember the possibility of cervical spine injury with any significant injury above the collarbones, with multiple injuries, and with head injuries resulting in unconsciousness.
- Control any external bleeding with direct pressure. If the bleeding is catastrophic (traumatic amputation), apply a tourniquet (➜ Control of haemorrhage, p. 196).
- Anticipate and treat shock, particularly with thigh fractures. Where appropriate use a suitable traction splint.
- Remember that painful limb injuries may distract attention from less painful but more significant trunk injuries.
- Expose the affected part and cut off clothing only if absolutely necessary given that in some circumstances clothing, footwear, and waterproofs will be needed to protect the patient from the environment.
- Look for signs of an interrupted blood supply—pale, pulseless, painful, perishingly cold.
- With fractures/dislocations, attempt manipulation early in an attempt to restore distal circulation. Check pulses and sensation before and after any manipulation.
- Look for nerve damage affecting movement and/or sensation.
- Give painkillers.
- Splint fractures using commercially available or improvised materials.
- Transfer to suitable shelter.

Improvised splinting materials on an expedition

- Sleeping mat.
- Paddles.
- Skis or ski poles.
- Slings and karabiners.
- Tree branches.
- Sleeping bags.
- Ropes.

When applying splints, remember that they must be well padded and must immobilize the joints above and below the injury (Fig. 14.1). Where possible, splint with the limb in the anatomical position.

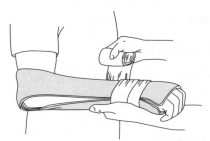

Fig. 14.1 Diagram of a field splint.

Detailed assessment of limb injuries

History
- How did the injury occur? The mechanism is significant; for instance, twisting injuries tend to produce spiral fractures, while a fall onto the heels may produce fractures of the spine or base of skull.
- Did the accident occur in a clean or contaminated environment? Consider IV antibiotics.
- When did the injury happen?
- Was the limb trapped or crushed? (Swelling and compartment syndrome are possible; see also ➲ Crush injuries, p. 277.)
- When was the last tetanus booster? This is very important for open fractures.
- Is the patient allergic to anything?
- Does the patient take any medication?

Examination
- Look for contamination and foreign bodies.
- Check for pulses and capillary refill time.
- Examine carefully for signs of nerve damage: change in sensation, weakness, or paralysis.
- In a wilderness situation, a fracture should be assumed until X-ray studies or clinical examination confirm otherwise.

Capillary refill time
To check for capillary refill press firmly over a fingernail or a bony prominence such as the sternum, forehead, or a malleolus for 5 s to produce blanching. When the pressure is released the colour should begin to return quickly (in <2 s). Slow filling indicates that the patient is extremely cold, shocked, or that the blood supply to the limb is interrupted.

Fractures

Features of a fracture

- Pain/tenderness.
- Loss of function.
- Swelling/bruising.
- Deformity.
- Crepitus.

Fracture classification

A fracture is a soft tissue injury with an underlying break in the bone. Fractures are either open if the skin is broken or closed. They are comminuted if there are more than two fragments. Children's bones may bend, leading to greenstick fractures. Complicated fractures involve damage to blood vessels, nerves, tendons, or organs.

Management of fractures in the field

- Stop bleeding (may require a tourniquet or haemostatic agents).
- Treat shock.
- Monitor pulse, BP, and urine output.
- Give adequate analgesia.
- Take a digital photo of open fractures or significant soft tissue injuries.
- Clean with antiseptic solution and cover exposed bone ends, for example, with saline-soaked gauze, and consider using antibiotics.
- Consider reducing and then immobilize in an appropriate sling/splint.
- Evacuate for X-ray and definitive fracture management.

Dislocations

A dislocation is an injury in which the normal relationships of a joint are disrupted. In some dislocations the bone end may be forced out of a socket (shoulder, hip, and elbow dislocations); in others the joint surfaces may simply be displaced (finger dislocations). Fractures, nerve, and blood vessel injuries may also be present with a dislocation.

Management of dislocations in the field

Correction of dislocations can be technically difficult. Attempts to correct the deformity are justified in certain circumstances, particularly in remote areas. If the blood supply to the distal part of the limb is obstructed by a dislocation, reduction must be attempted. Steady, firm traction along the limb's long axis may correct the deformity or at least relieve the obstruction temporarily. Reduction should be attempted as soon as possible because of increasing muscle spasm. After reduction, splint the limb as for a fracture.

Upper limb supports and slings

Collar and cuff
(See Fig. 14.2.)

In the wilderness this may be improvised by passing a long sock around the patient's neck and wrist of the affected side. This can then be secured using a cable tie or piece of cord. This uses the weight of the arm to apply slight traction to the upper arm and should be used for fractures of the humerus.

High arm sling
(See Fig. 14.3.)

This is mainly used to reduce hand swelling with hand injuries. Avoid excessive flexion of the elbow as this reduces venous drainage of the forearm.

Broad arm sling
(See Fig. 14.4.)

This is commonly used to support the weight of the arm and reduce movement in shoulder and clavicle injuries, dislocations/fractures of the elbow, forearm, and wrist. If used during evacuation of a walking casualty, a swathe around the chest placed on top of the broad arm sling further reduces movement. A broad arm sling may be improvised by pulling the lower edge of a jacket over the arm and then securing with a safety pin.

Arm slings and splints should be worn inside clothing to keep the hand and arm warm.

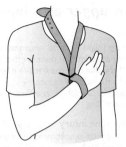

Fig. 14.2 Collar and cuff sling.

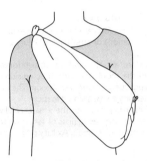

Fig. 14.3 High arm sling.

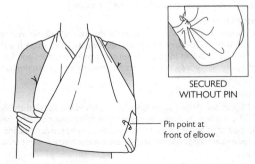

SECURED
WITHOUT PIN

Pin point at
front of elbow

Fig. 14.4 Broad arm sling.

Shoulder and upper arm injuries

Fractured clavicle

This is a common injury following a fall onto the outstretched arm. The clavicle is palpable along its length and there is often obvious deformity and localized tenderness. If the skin over the fracture is tented, then gentle traction with the arm out to the side will reduce the risk of developing an open fracture. Check movement, circulation, and sensation carefully. Treat with analgesia and a broad arm sling.

Acromio-clavicular joint injury

Injury to the acromio-clavicular joint commonly follows a fall onto the point of the shoulder. There is usually a characteristic step together with point tenderness at the joint. Treat with analgesia and a broad arm sling. X-rays will show the grade of injury, and the most severe may require surgical treatment.

Anterior shoulder dislocation

The shoulder joint may be dislocated after violent injury (particularly forced abduction/external rotation) or after minimal injury in those with previous shoulder dislocations.

Most dislocations are anterior and are straightforward to diagnose as there is 'squaring' of the shoulder on the affected side and reduced movement, particularly abduction and forward flexion. The humeral head may be palpated antero-inferiorly to the glenoid fossa.

After any shoulder injury examine the area carefully for complications such as damage to the axillary nerve (loss of sensation over the insertion of deltoid—the 'regimental badge area'). Axillary nerve damage merits expert assessment.

Reduction of shoulder dislocations

On an expedition it is reasonable to attempt reduction in the field, preferably with strong analgesia (± sedation such as midazolam). Reduce using the external rotation method or Spaso method. A clunk is often seen, felt or heard, and the shoulder's normal contour is restored.

External rotation method

Sit the patient as upright as possible. Hold the patient's elbow next to the trunk and, with the forearm mid-prone, slowly externally rotate the shoulder to 90°. The shoulder usually reduces at this point; if it does not, forward flex the upper arm slowly. An assistant may help to manipulate the humeral head into position.

Spaso method

Spaso Miljesic and Anne-Maree Kelly first reported the Spaso technique in 1998.[1] This method is simple, needs minimal force, can be performed by a single operator, and is highly effective even in inexperienced hands. The Spaso technique is relatively atraumatic and countertraction is not required.

---

1 Miljesic S, Kelly AM (1998). Reduction of anterior dislocation of the shoulder. Spaso technique. *Emerg Med*, 10, 173–5.

Lay the patient on their back and give sedation/analgesia as available. Grasp the affected arm around the wrist and slowly lift vertically to 90° shoulder flexion, applying gentle vertical traction as well as external rotation of the shoulder at the elbow. If difficulty is experienced, it may be helpful to use one hand to palpate the head of the humerus and gently push it to assist reduction, while maintaining traction with the other hand.

Stimson's method

Lie the patient prone with the arm hanging down with a 5-kg weight attached to the wrist/hand. This method may take half an hour or more to achieve reduction.

After reduction of any shoulder dislocation

Re-examine for axillary and radial nerve movement/sensation. Check pulses. Rest in a broad arm sling or collar and cuff. Evacuate for X-rays and orthopaedic follow-up/physiotherapy. Recurrent dislocations of the shoulder may not require an X-ray and can be managed with a broad arm sling and early mobilization.

Posterior dislocation of the shoulder

This injury is rare and may follow electric shock or convulsions. It is easy to miss. It results from force applied to the anterior shoulder. The shoulder is internally rotated and there is marked loss of movement. Attempt reduction by applying traction and external rotation with the arm at 90° to the body. Manipulation under anaesthesia may be required.

Inferior dislocation of the shoulder (luxatio erecta)

The patient presents with the arm held above the head. Examine carefully for neurovascular deficits. Attempt reduction by applying traction along the abducted arm, then adduction. If it is not possible to reduce in the field, give strong analgesia, support the arm using padding with sleeping bags or similar, and evacuate for reduction under anaesthesia.

Supraspinatus tendinitis, subacromial bursitis, and rotator cuff injuries

All conditions are caused by acute injury or soft tissue degenerative changes and may be provoked by unaccustomed activity as may occur on wilderness trips. The main symptom is of pain, often following lifting or a fall and onset may be sudden or gradual. Abduction and forward flexion in particular are restricted (unable to upturn a drinks can with arms outstretched in front of patient). There may be a painful arc of movement. Treatment with rest, NSAIDs, and a broad arm sling will usually reduce symptoms. Further assessment will be required if pain and restricted movements persist. Significant loss of ROM in the absence of pain may indicate a complete rotator cuff tear. Avoid prolonged periods of immobilization in a sling.

Fracture-dislocation of the shoulder

If crepitus is felt during manipulation of a shoulder dislocation, suspect an associated fracture and desist from further attempts at reduction in the field until the fracture has been identified or excluded by an X-ray. Support in a broad arm sling, give analgesia, and evacuate.

Fractures of the humerus

These are caused by a fall onto the outstretched arm or onto the elbow. Midshaft fractures can involve the radial nerve as it runs through the spiral groove and result in a wrist-drop.

Treatment for proximal injuries is with a collar and cuff sling. Midshaft injuries may benefit from a splint or broad arm sling and strapping arm against the body. Any involvement of neurovascular structures, particularly the radial nerve or brachial artery, should prompt urgent evacuation for definitive care.

Ruptured long head of biceps

This can be torn during lifting and may not require large forces. It is seen more commonly in elderly males. There is a characteristic bulge of biceps muscle above the elbow but often little pain; bruising may, however, be extensive. Surgical repair may be considered if the arm is not fully functional.

Elbow and forearm injuries

The elbow may be injured by a direct blow or transmitted forces such as a fall onto the outstretched hand. Full extension without pain makes the presence of fracture or serious injury very unlikely.

Elbow dislocation

This requires considerable force and may be associated with fractures. The radius and ulna are usually dislocated posteriorly. Damage to the brachial artery or radial/ulnar/median nerves may occur. Attempted reduction is justified in a wilderness environment, particularly if evacuation to definitive care will take more than a few hours.

Treatment

After suitable analgesia, apply steady traction to the limb by pulling at the wrist. The elbow is usually flexed at around 30°. Countertraction above the elbow with concurrent pushing of the protruding olecranon forwards is essential. Rest in a broad arm sling and evacuate for X-ray and further assessment/rehabilitation. If reduction proves impossible, place in a broad arm sling and give analgesia. Monitor radial pulse and assess for nerve damage.

Epicondylitis—golfer's and tennis elbow

Golfer's elbow refers to inflammation around the common flexor origin at the elbow; tennis elbow involves the same process at the common extensor origin. Both conditions are caused by repetitive hand and wrist movements, particularly rowing and paddling on expeditions. On examination there is tenderness at the medial (golfer's) or lateral (tennis) epicondyles of the humerus and pain on gripping.

Treatment

Rest, anti-inflammatory drugs and, where possible, avoidance of the provoking activity and gentle stretching after 3–4 days.

Olecranon bursitis

The olecranon bursa may become inflamed and painful, sometimes after minor trauma. The lump over the elbow is fluctuant and may be very tender if it becomes infected.

Treatment

This condition may take weeks to resolve but usually only requires rest in a broad arm sling and anti-inflammatory drugs. If there is evidence of spreading infection or fever then give antibiotics. Avoid aspiration in the field because of the danger of introducing infection.

Fractures around the elbow

Displaced fractures around the elbow may be associated with neurovascular injury, particularly the brachial artery. Check distal pulses and seek evidence of neurological deficit. Such fractures usually require orthopaedic assessment and often need internal fixation. With the forearm midprone, splint either in the position found, or with the elbow at 90°. Evacuate for X-rays and further management.

Fractured radial head

This injury can only be diagnosed with the help of radiographs but clinically is suggested by a history of a fall onto the outstretched hand and then pain and tenderness on palpating the radial head. Pronation/supination is often very painful. Support the forearm in a broad arm sling and evacuate for assessment.

Fractures of the forearm

These tend to be unstable fractures and may affect the radius and ulna at the same level, at different levels with spiral fractures, or involve a fracture of one bone with associated dislocation at one of the radio-ulnar joints. Check carefully for neurovascular compromise. Treat with analgesia, splinting, and evacuate for definitive care. If there is evidence of an open fracture, clean and dress the wound and give antibiotics.

Wrist injuries

Fractures of the distal radius

These fractures are commonly caused by a fall onto the outstretched hand. There is often obvious deformity together with pain and swelling. Dorsal displacement of the distal fragment is most common—Colles' fracture. For those familiar with a haematoma block, 6–8 mL lidocaine 2% can be injected into the fracture site before reduction—a haematoma block. All potential wrist fractures on an expedition should be supported in a suitably padded splint and rested in a broad arm sling. Imaging and definitive treatment will be required after evacuation from the field.

Scaphoid fracture

A fall onto the outstretched hand may lead to pain and swelling, together with difficulty gripping. If there is tenderness in the anatomical snuffbox, pain when 'telescoping' the thumb (pushing the straight thumb towards the wrist) or palpating over the scaphoid tubercle, a scaphoid injury must be considered. Avascular necrosis, non-union, and osteoarthritis may complicate scaphoid fractures. On an expedition, immobilize in a below-elbow splint, and evacuate for X-rays and follow up as long-term disability may result from undiagnosed scaphoid injury.

Wrist sprains

If the mechanism of injury makes a fracture unlikely and if findings on examination are non-specific, it is reasonable on an expedition to treat a tender wrist as for a sprain using a support bandage, anti-inflammatories, and early mobilization. If there is any uncertainty or if symptoms are not settling, it is safer to assume that there is a fracture and arrangements should be made to image the wrist in a suitable facility.

Tenosynovitis

Inflammation of tendon sheaths may follow repetitive strain injuries. Characteristically there is pain on moving the wrist or thumb and a 'creaking' or 'buzzing' sensation may be felt over the affected tendons, usually on the dorsum of the wrist. Treatment consists of rest in a suitable splint for up to 3 weeks and anti-inflammatories.

Hand injuries

Initial management of hand injuries

- Stop major bleeding using direct pressure and elevation. Consider the use of a temporary tourniquet (a BP cuff can be used).
- Establish the exact mechanism of injury.
- Remove rings early before swelling develops.
- Hand injuries are very painful and adequate analgesia should be given promptly. After neurological assessment consider early use of local anaesthetic (LA), particularly ring blocks for finger injuries (see Fig. 14.6). Clean hand wounds carefully (the patient may be able to clean the surrounding area first).
- Open fractures should be treated with careful cleaning and antibiotics.
- Punching injuries with a break in the skin (usually at the knuckles) should be considered to be a bite wound (➔ Bites (animal and human), p. 276).
- To avoid later disability, all hand injuries must be carefully assessed and managed.

Examination of the hand

- Record whether the injury affects the patient's dominant hand.
- Compare both hands.
- Look for swelling, deformity, redness, and wounds.
- In the relaxed hand there is increasing flexion from the index to the little finger. A finger which is out of line should raise the possibility of a tendon or nerve injury. Rotation of the digit points to a fracture.
- Ask the patient to make a fist and then fully extend fingers. Look for any obvious motor deficit and crossing of fingers.
- Assess flexor digitorum profundus by holding the proximal interphalangeal joint (PIPJ) extended and asking the patient to flex the finger.
- Assess flexor digitorum superficialis by holding the fingers not being assessed in extension. Ask the patient to flex the finger at the PIPJ.
- Assess the lumbricals by flexing the fingers in turn at the metacarpophalangeal joints (MCPJs).
- Finger extensors can be tested by placing the patient's PIPJs level with a table edge then asking the patient to straighten the finger.
- Test movements at the interphalangeal joints (IPJs), MCPJ, and carpometacarpal joints of the thumb.
- Assess median nerve power by asking the patient to oppose the little finger and the thumb.
- The ulnar nerve may be assessed by abducting or adducting the fingers.
- Check sensation on each side of the digit (digital nerves), in the first web space dorsally (radial nerve), middle finger (median nerve), and little finger (ulnar nerve).

Hand fractures and dislocations

Fractures may be suggested by the mechanism of injury, swelling, bruising, deformity, and loss of normal function. In all cases, check for neurovascular deficit. If suspected, immobilize the hand in a boxing glove dressing (Fig. 14.5) and broad arm sling. Evacuate for imaging and further treatment.

Finger dislocations

Dislocations can occur at the MCPJs or IPJs. After assessing for obvious fractures (small avulsion fractures cannot be diagnosed without imaging), check for any neurovascular damage. It is worth attempting reduction with in-line traction under LA (ring block). If successful, apply buddy strapping or use a boxing glove dressing (Fig. 14.5).

Thumb dislocations

Attempt reduction, then immobilize in a suitable splint or 'boxing glove' (Fig. 14.5). Evacuate for definitive care as internal fixation may be required if there is an associated fracture.

Ligament injuries

These can occur at the metacarpophalangeal or interphalangeal joints. If the joint is grossly unstable when gently stressing the collateral ligaments, surgical treatment may be required. For most ligament injuries, rest with neighbour strapping will allow healing to occur. Warn patients that swelling may take weeks to settle. This occurs in particular with injuries to the volar plate at the PIPJs. If the mechanism of injury involves a forced abduction at the thumb MCPJ (gamekeeper's/skier's thumb), ensure that laxity of the ulnar collateral ligament is tested for. If there is no end point on stressing, surgical repair will be required.

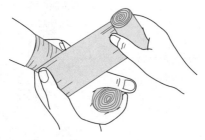

Fig. 14.5 'Boxing glove' dressing.

Tendon injuries

Small cuts or lacerations may damage tendons and these injuries may easily be missed unless hand injuries are carefully assessed. (Beware of any injuries caused by broken glass—evacuation for X-ray is recommended.)

Loss of function is the only reliable sign that a tendon has been damaged, but pain out of proportion to the injury should suggest damage to underlying structures. Ensure that you examine the wound with the fingers moving through their range of movement as tendons move with the finger so the injury may not initially be visible.

Extensor tendon injury

This injury is usually obvious. Partial tendon ruptures are easily overlooked—explore wounds under LA or evacuate for full assessment in a bloodless field.

Flexor tendon injuries

Flexor digitorum superficialis flexes the PIPJ. Flexor digitorum profundus flexes the distal interphalangeal joint (DIPJ).

To test these tendons see ➲ Examination of the hand, p. 430.

Tendon injuries should be repaired in a suitably equipped hospital, not in the field, because of the danger of infection of the flexor sheath that can cause long-term disability.

Finger injuries

On an expedition, fingers can be injured in many ways; they may be crushed in vehicle doors or under heavy weights or during the use of tools/machinery. After release, the digits should be carefully examined (under LA if possible), cleaned, and elevated. Open fractures should be given an antibiotic such as co-amoxiclav and evacuated for X-ray and further management. Always remember to remove rings.

Mallet finger

Rupture of the central slip of the extensor tendon to the distal phalanx results in loss of extension at the DIPJ. This may be associated with an avulsion fracture of the base of the distal phalanx. On an expedition, splint the DIPJ in extension for 6 weeks and arrange for orthopaedic review on return. Do not remove the splint as movement will disrupt the healing tendon.

Finger tip amputation

Provided the bone is not exposed and the area of skin loss is <1 cm^2 it may be possible to treat these injuries in the field. After assessment, clean and dress (using Vaseline® gauze or similar). Re-examine every 2 days. If the wound is not healing, evacuate for imaging and possible terminalization of bone or skin grafting.

Nail injuries

Finger entrapment or crushing injuries may result in partial or complete avulsion of a nail. The finger should be anaesthetized (Fig. 14.6) and cleaned. The patient may be able to help to clean the finger by immersing in warm, clean water. If the nail is displaced it should be removed under LA, any defect should be repaired, the nail should be replaced for protection and the finger dressed and splinted.

Subungual haematoma

Crush injuries to the nail may result in bleeding under the finger nail. The pressure results in throbbing pain which may be relieved by heating a paper clip to red heat and burning a hole in the centre of the nail, using minimal pressure. On an expedition a Leatherman® multi-tool can be used to hold the heated wire paper clip. It may be necessary to reheat the wire on several occasions. Alternatively, a 21 G hypodermic needle can be used to drill a hole in the nail by gentle twisting motion. Once the blood has drained the pain is significantly reduced.

Foreign body under the nail

Splinters of metal or wood under the finger nail are common. A ring block may allow removal with splinter forceps or trimming of part of the nail to allow removal.

Paronychia

See Paronychia, p. 297; Fig. 9.6.

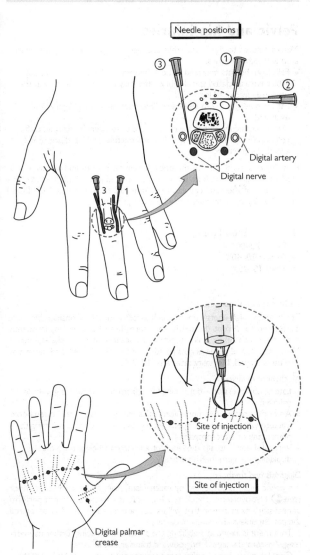

Needle positions

① ② ③

Digital artery

Digital nerve

3 1

Site of injection

Site of injection

Digital palmar crease

Fig. 14.6 Local anaesthesia of hand.

Pelvic and hip injuries

Many fractures to the lower limbs are high-energy injuries and are associated with other injuries:

- Falls from heights may lead to heel, femoral, and pelvic fracture, but 10% have associated spinal injury—this may be masked by pain at the obviously fractured leg.
- Fall from heights >2 m and lower limb fracture = spinal injury until excluded.
- Dashboard injury—knee injury in seated passenger during road traffic collision (RTC) associated with femoral fracture and hip dislocation/acetabular fracture.

Bony injuries to this part of the body are always serious and usually associated with major blood loss. Blood loss for closed lower limb fractures as a proportion of the total circulatory volume are shown in Box 14.1. Blood loss following open fractures may be much greater.

> **Box 14.1 Blood loss**
> - Pelvis: 20–80%.
> - Femur: 20–40%.
> - Tibia: 10–25%.

Pelvic fractures

These follow high-energy trauma such as falls and RTC. Considerable force is required to disrupt the pelvis, therefore these fractures are frequently associated with other major thoracic/spinal/abdominal or skeletal injury. Major vessels and pelvic organs lie adjacent to pelvic bones, and these may also be damaged. Mortality rates are ~10–20%.

Mechanism of injury

- Lateral compression—deforming force from side-to-side, e.g. vehicle rollover.
- Anterior–posterior compression— this may give rise to the 'open book' fracture where the pelvis opens up; e.g. as a result of a rider hitting the petrol tank of a motorcycle.
- Vertical sheer—usually the result of a fall from a height onto one leg, displacing the hemi-pelvis vertically.

Diagnosis and treatment

If a pelvic injury is suspected by mechanism, pain, or hypovolaemic shock (see ➲ Hypovolaemic shock, p. 234), treat as a fracture. Do not perform unnecessary examination that will exacerbate bleeding and do not log roll the patient unless absolutely necessary.

Treatment is aimed at stabilizing the pelvis and reducing further haemorrhage/visceral damage during onward transfer of the patient.

- Control lower limbs—splint legs together at knees and ankles. Flex the knees about 20° and pad any bony prominences.

- Splint pelvis—wrap a folded sheet firmly around the pelvis (upper border of sheet level with anterior superior iliac spines) and tie at the front or use a SAM Pelvic Sling® if available.
- Evacuate urgently and move as little as possible.

Hip fractures

The elderly and those with osteoporotic bones may fracture the neck of the femur with relatively minor trauma; however, the same fracture in younger patients indicates high-energy trauma such as a climbing fall.

Diagnosis and treatment

Often there is a history of a fall onto the lateral aspect of the hip. Pain may radiate to the knee and the affected leg may be shortened and externally rotated. Give analgesia; look for and treat shock. A traction splint may improve comfort during evacuation (see ➜ Femoral fracture, p. 437). If experienced, consider a fascia iliaca nerve block (see ➜ Fascia iliaca block, p. 594).

Hip dislocation

These usually follow a fall from a height or dashboard injury in RTCs. The hip joint usually dislocates posteriorly with or without fracture of the acetabulum. Travellers with hip replacements are at greater risk of dislocation with minimal trauma.

Diagnosis and treatment

There is pain and deformity of the leg, which is shortened and rotated (internally if posterior dislocation). Assess neurological status and distal pulses—hip dislocations may be associated with injury to the femoral or sciatic nerve. If immediate evacuation is possible then splint legs in position and give strong analgesia. If >6 h before evacuation to hospital, then blood supply to the femoral head may become compromised and an attempt at reduction is justified but will require adequate analgesia ± sedation.

Reduction of hip dislocations

In posterior dislocation, the assistant places hands as countertraction on the pelvis (anterior superior iliac spine). Flex the hip to 90° with the knee bent and then apply vertical traction with internal rotation. As the hip relocates externally rotate, extend the hip, and continue longitudinal traction to the lower leg. Wrapping a bandage around the lower leg and foot may allow application of 2.5–5 kg skin traction to be maintained. Check neurovascular status post reduction—relocation may be prevented by entrapment of the sciatic nerve around the femoral neck. The hip may re-dislocate owing to an unstable acetabular fracture. Repeated attempts at reduction are not justified—evacuation is required ASAP for operative intervention.

Femoral fracture

A great deal of force is required to fracture the femur—usually following a fall from a height or RTC. It can be associated with other head, spinal, chest, or abdominal/pelvic trauma.

Diagnosis and treatment

There is pain and deformity of the thigh, together with swelling and fracture crepitus. Assess neurological status and distal pulses. Anticipate and whenever possible treat hypovolaemia (the patient may lose 20% of blood volume rapidly even in closed injury). Splint legs in position (splint to un-injured leg); apply traction through a splint if available to maintain alignment and to reduce bleeding into the thigh compartment. Cover any open wounds with sterile dressings, e.g. saline-soaked gauze.

Strongly consider a fascia iliaca block if suitably experienced (see ➲ Fascia iliaca block, p. 594).

Knee injuries

Knee injuries on expeditions are relatively common. In all cases take a careful history which may give clues to the diagnosis. Ask about previous knee problems such as swelling, clicking, locking, or 'giving way'.

Examination of the injured knee:

- Look for bruising, swelling, redness, deformity, and compare with the uninjured side.
- Feel for an effusion, warmth, or crepitus. Identify any tender areas—joint line or origin/insertion of collateral ligaments.
- Observe straight leg raising (which assesses the extensor mechanism, ➲ Knee extensor mechanism injuries, p. 442).
- Assess movement—extension (0°), flexion (135°).
- Palpate along the medial and lateral joint lines, and over the fibular head for tenderness.
- Test the joint stability—in 30° flexion support the lower leg and apply valgus stress (medial collateral) and in extension a varus stress (lateral collateral) at the knee. With the knee flexed at 90°, place the thumbs on the tibial tubercle and rest index fingers behind the knee. With the hamstrings relaxed, gently draw the lower leg forward, looking for any abnormal shift (anterior draw test).
- McMurray's test for meniscal injury—place thumb and index finger on medial and lateral joint lines, flex the knee, and externally rotate the foot followed by abduction and extension of the knee. Pain and a click suggest a medial meniscal injury. In the acute knee McMurray's test can be difficult and medial or lateral joint line tenderness can be as useful in identifying meniscus injuries.

Haemarthrosis

This is relatively common and refers to bleeding into a joint. Rapid tense swelling develops in 1–2 h. Haemarthrosis may be spontaneous (coagulation disorders and rare vascular tumours) or traumatic (80% after anterior cruciate ligament injury, 10% patella dislocation, 10% meniscal injuries/capsular injuries).

Treatment
RICE, analgesia, and evacuate for further assessment.

Bursitis

There will be good range of movement at the knee. Inflammation of the fluid-filled bursa in front of or below the patella may result from unaccustomed, frequent minor trauma such as kneeling. Rest and NSAIDs usually relieve symptoms. If there are features of spreading cellulitis and a fever, antibiotics should be given (e.g. co-amoxiclav).

Patellar fracture

Sudden knee flexion or a direct blow may result in a fracture of the patella. There is usually pain, swelling (sometimes from a haemarthrosis), and inability to straight leg raise. If suspected, splint the leg almost straight (with 5° of flexion at the knee) and evacuate for imaging and definitive treatment.

Other fractures around the knee

Suspected fractures around the knee should be treated with adequate analgesia and splint, as for patellar fracture. Avoid traction splints if there is a possible fracture in the supracondylar region of the distal femur. Traction may displace the distal part of the fracture posteriorly and damage the popliteal artery.

Patellar dislocation

This is not uncommon and may be a recurrent problem (more common in females). The patella dislocates laterally and, typically, the patient's knee is held flexed with obvious displacement of the patella. Give analgesia and reduce the patella by pressing with the thumbs on the lateral aspect of the patella as the knee is straightened. Once reduced it may be possible to rehabilitate this injury in the field without evacuation.

Dislocation of the knee

This is a rare injury and huge forces are required to produce disruption of the knee ligaments. There is a high likelihood of nerve and blood vessel damage—check distal pulses and sensation carefully. Treat with strong analgesia and immobilize as for patellar fracture before evacuation. Keep monitoring foot pulses, as popliteal artery injury may not be apparent initially. If there are signs of vascular compromise, evacuate urgently for vascular surgery.

Ligament injuries to knee

Medial collateral ligament

The medial collateral ligament runs from the medial epicondyle of the femur to 4 cm distal to the knee joint on the medial aspect of the tibia. An isolated rupture usually results from a direct blow to the lateral aspect of the knee in slight flexion. If there is a rotational component, such as a fall when skiing, there may also be injury to the cruciate ligament.

Diagnosis and treatment

- On examination there is tenderness over the medial collateral ligament ± knee swelling. Test valgus stability with knee flexed 20–30° (in full extension the cruciate ligaments stabilize the knee).
- Mild–moderate (<10 mm opening of joint)—rest, ice, compression, and then early increase range of motion/strengthening with physiotherapy.
- Severe (>10 mm opening of joint)—may require hinged brace for 3–6 weeks after initial management and so will benefit from evacuation for definitive care.

Lateral collateral ligament

The lateral collateral ligament runs from the lateral epicondyle of the femur to the head of the fibula. Isolated injuries are rare but are more usually associated with injury to all the lateral capsular ligamentous structures. This may result in marked instability.

Diagnosis and treatment

- Tenderness ± knee swelling. Test varus stability. An isolated lateral collateral ligament injury may be treated as for medial collateral ligament, but more common complex injury may require evacuation for surgery.

Cruciate ligaments

Anterior cruciate ligament injuries account for 50% of documented knee ligament injuries. Posterior cruciate ligament injury is rare (10% knee ligament injuries). Usually, injuries are caused by non-contact twisting injury, occasionally following hyper-extension. There is pain and difficulty weight-bearing. Swelling usually develops immediately with an ACL rupture. A PCL rupture will have no swelling and a dull posterior knee ache.

Diagnosis and treatment

- There is an acute haemarthrosis following typical history. Examination is often difficult during the acute phase due to pain and swelling. A subjective description of a 'popping' sensation is often noted.
- The Lachman test will usually be positive in an ACL rupture—grip the tibia at 30° flexion and pull it anteriorly over the distal femur. There will be no firm end point. There may also be anterior draw and pivot shift. If suspected, evacuate for X-rays and further imaging (MRI) or arthroscopy. Younger active individuals may have continuing joint instability and may require reconstruction of the cruciate ligament. The PCL will have a positive posterior draw at 90°.

Meniscal injuries

The menisci act as stabilizers for the knee and distribute forces across the articular surfaces. There is usually a history of an axial load with a twisting injury to the knee. 'Degenerative' tears may occur in patients >35 years with very little history of injury.

Diagnosis and treatment

- Patients may complain of the knee 'locking' or 'giving way'. Pain and intermittent swelling may occur. Squatting particularly may aggravate posterior horn tears.
- Acute tears may cause gradual swelling of the knee over 4–6 h and occasionally haemarthrosis. Degenerative tears may settle with physiotherapy.
- Knee arthroscopy is often required if the knee is symptomatic. If the knee is acutely locked, from a loose body, do not attempt to unlock the knee (painful and usually futile). Splint in a comfortable position and evacuate for definitive care.

Knee extensor mechanism injuries

Disruption to any one of these may prevent straight leg raising or active extension of the knee. (NB Tense knee effusion and pain may also prevent straight leg raise without disruption of extensor mechanism.)

Quadriceps tendon rupture

- 80% occur in individuals >40 years. Normally a gap is palpable close to the superior pole of the patella (defect at insertion of vastus medialis).

Patellar tendon rupture

- Usually occurs in those >40 years. Tender inferior pole patella.

Patellar and tibial tuberosity fractures

- Usually occur as result of direct trauma.
- Manage with rest, support, and splinting in extension. Tendons usually require operative repair if the extensor mechanism is disrupted. Fractures often require reduction and fixation if displaced.

Lacerations to sole of foot

These are painful, difficult to manage, and prone to infection. To anaesthetise the area, consider topical LA such as Ametop®, or regional anaesthesia by performing a nerve block of the posterior tibial nerve just posterior to the artery where it runs behind the medial malleolus. This will anaesthetize the majority of the sole of the foot. If the wound is on the lateral sole, consider a nerve block of the sural nerve as it runs behind the lateral malleolus. The tough skin of the sole makes local infiltration of LA painful and ineffective. Remove any foreign bodies and close the wound with glue or Steri-Strips™. There is a significant risk of infection—puncture wounds should be treated with antibiotics prophylactically. Ensure tetanus immunization is up to date.

Plantar fasciitis

This is inflammation of the connective tissue that forms the sole of the foot. There may be pain over the heel, under the arch of the foot forward to the metatarsal heads. It commonly occurs in individuals not accustomed to exercise who suddenly increase exercise intensity. Pain is common for the first few steps of the day or on dorsiflexion of the foot. The condition can be eased with calf stretching exercises and orthotics or cushioned footwear. It can last for up to 2 years.

Spinal injury

(See also Chapter 7 and Chapter 14.)

Spinal cord injuries are relatively rare. However, it is vital that the possibility of spinal injuries is considered in all trauma patients especially:

- High-speed injuries.
- Patients with multiple injuries.
- Falls or those who have been hit by a falling object such as a rock.
- Head-injured and unresponsive patients.

The implications of missing one of these can be life-changing or life-threatening for the patient. Manipulation or inadequate management/immobilization of the spinal-injured patient can cause additional neurological damage and worsen outcome.

Injuries most frequently occur at junctions of mobile and fixed sections of the spine (C6,7/T1, T12/L1). In patients with multiple injuries who have a spinal injury, over half will have a cervical spinal injury. About 10–15% of patients with one spinal fracture will be found to have another.

Management

The aim of spinal management is to prevent any secondary injury to the spinal cord. If a casualty with a spinal injury is moved carefully, they are unlikely to come to further harm but do follow these precautions:

- Ensure that the airway is open. Use the jaw-thrust manoeuvre rather than head tilt and chin lift, which may create further cervical spine injury.
- If necessary, move the head into a neutral alignment (Fig. 14.7). Stabilize the head and neck manually. If available, use a semi-rigid neck collar such as Stifnek select™ together with blocks and tape—in the wilderness socks full of sand or soil can be used.
- Assess breathing and look for and treat any life-threatening chest injury (➔ Breathing, p. 190). Give oxygen if available to keep sats >94%. Adequate oxygenation and tissue perfusion must be maintained as the spinal cord is very sensitive to hypoxia and hypotension.
- Identify any signs of shock and treat cautiously with IV fluids. Ensure an adequate BP (systolic 90 mmHg) and pulse rate. If the pulse rate falls below 45 bpm consider atropine 600 micrograms IV as minimal stimulation may cause asystole owing to unopposed vagal response.
- Rapidly assess the conscious level with AVPU scale or GCS, look at the pupils, and ask the patient if they can move and feel their fingers and toes.
- Only log roll the patient if you suspect a penetrating injury to the back or wounds that require attention. There is little benefit in palpating the spine or performing a rectal examination. Unnecessary log rolling may exacerbate a spinal injury but more importantly an unstable pelvic injury.
- If the patient must be moved, do so with caution but ensure that pressure areas are padded and if there is a spinal injury causing bowel and/or bladder dysfunction, ensure attention is paid to keeping the skin clean and dry.

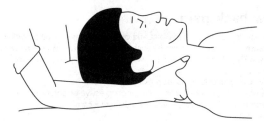

Fig. 14.7 Manual immobilization of the neck.

Clearing the suspected spinal injury

Not all patients who are involved in trauma need to have full spinal precautions maintained. Box 14.2 indicates when a spinal injury can safely be excluded clinically.

If the patient has any of these signs then imaging of the neck is required before cervical spinal immobilization can be removed.

If it is necessary to move the patient, they should be moved carefully, keeping the spine in alignment throughout and should be kept horizontal if at all possible. This is because blood vessels below the level of a spinal cord injury may have lost their spinal reflexes and so cannot contract in response to hypotension. This can cause a precipitous drop in BP and hence further damage to the spinal cord.

Signs of a spinal injury

The patient may complain of:
- Neck or back pain. This may be masked by another more painful injury.
- Loss of movement and/or sensation in the limbs.
- Sensation of burning/electric shock in the trunk or limbs.
- On examination the patient may have swelling or midline tenderness over the spinous processes.

In the unconscious patient a serious spinal injury may be indicated by:
- Hypotension with bradycardia (neurogenic shock).
- The skin may be warm below the level of the lesion.
- Diaphragmatic breathing.
- Flaccid tone.
- Priapism (involuntary erection of the penis).
- Loss of sphincter control.

Box 14.2 Excluding spinal injury ('clearing the spine')
- No midline cervical tenderness.
- No altered level of alertness.
- No evidence of intoxication.
- No neurological abnormality.
- No distracting injury.

Low back pain

Back pain is a common complaint and on expeditions may be provoked by unaccustomed activity or injuries such as lifting awkwardly, falls, or twisting injury. 80% will resolve within 2–8 weeks. Low back pain is very common. Sort into:

- Mechanical back pain (most prevalent).
- Nerve root pain—only concerning if progressive or persistent.
- Serious spinal pathology—will need definitive care.
- Traumatic.
- Infectious.
- Visceral (~2%).
- Suspected cord compression—needs immediate evacuation.

Consider other systemic disease, such as back pain associated with weight loss, fever/rigors, cough/haemoptysis.

History

- Recent back trauma—note the mechanism of any injury.
- Characterize the pain, noting particularly leg symptoms and aggravating and relieving factors.
- Ask if there is any disturbance of bladder/bowel function.
- Ask about previous back injuries or surgery.
- Ask about history of cardiovascular disease, e.g. stroke.
- Presence of red flag signs.

Red flag signs

- Uncontrolled pain, worse at night.
- Fever and/or unexplained weight loss.
- Loss of bladder or bowel control.
- History of carcinoma—particularly thyroid, breast, lung, prostate, kidney.
- Ill health or presence of other medical illness.
- Significant motor weakness or sensory loss.
- Previous osteoporotic fractures.
- Disturbed gait, saddle anaesthesia.
- Age of onset <20 or >55 years.

Examination

'Unwell' patient—immediately assess ABCs and check for presence of pulsatile expansile abdominal mass and presence/absence of femoral pulses (abdominal aortic aneurysm often presents with back pain).

'Well' patient—look for signs of weight loss, scoliosis, and muscle spasm. Watch the patient walk, looking for limping or abnormal posture. Assess spinal movements and note any significant loss. With the patient supine, palpate for tenderness over lumbar spine and sacrum, ribs, and renal angles. Look for muscle wasting in the legs. Perform on both legs:

- Straight leg raise—note angle at which patient detects pain (lumbar nerve root irritation). Normal 70° but compare with other side.
- Check for perineal and perianal sensation. Consider rectal examination to check anal tone.
  See Table 14.1.

Table 14.1 Neurological examination

	Sensation	Motor	Reflex
L3/4	Medial lower leg	Quadriceps	Knee jerk
L5	Lateral lower leg	Extensor hallucis longus	Hamstring jerk
S1	Lateral foot and little toe	Foot plantar flexors	Ankle jerk

Management

- If red flag sign is found, evacuate for specialist investigation of the cause of the back pain.
- In the absence of red flag signs, even with the presence of nerve root pain, conservative treatment should be effective.

Manage symptoms with:
- Reassurance and education that most back pains completely resolve in 2–8 weeks.
- Simple analgesics and NSAIDs, and a short course of a low dose of benzodiazepines (2–5 mg diazepam three times a day for 2 days). Consider opioids for a limited period if needed.
- Use heat not ice.
- Avoid bed rest; encourage gentle, normal movements.
- Consider physiotherapy or manipulation if available.
- Always keep the diagnosis under review if symptoms change.

Physiotherapy

- Most soft tissue injuries will benefit from a short period of rest/
  protection (splinting) followed by early mobilization to prevent stiffness
  and to regain full movements.
- Traditionally RICE forms the basis for simple soft tissue injury
  rehabilitation.
- Rest (for 24–48 h) and ice, if available, applied to the injured part help
  to reduce swelling and pain. Ice should not be applied directly to the
  skin but should be wrapped in a damp cloth and applied intermittently
  for 15 min at a time. If ice is not available, cold packs would be a suitable
  alternative or even placing the injured limb in cold water.
- A crepe or tubigrip bandage may help to support the injury and will
  remind the patient about the injury. If the patient must continue to bear
  weight, compression and ice are beneficial. If complete rest is possible,
  omit compression and instead elevate and use ice.
- Hand and foot injuries benefit from early elevation to reduce discomfort
  and swelling. However, poorly applied elbow or knee compression may
  be harmful if venous return is affected (risk of DVT).

Mobilization

Gentle range of motion exercises should start as soon as possible. Aim for
graded exercises which move joints slightly more each day. Avoid excessive
stretching and try to normalize movement as early as possible within the
limits of pain. Always provide adequate analgesia.

Advice for the patient

- 1–3 days—rest, ice, elevate.
- 3–14 days—perform regular exercises building up activity, avoiding
  excessive discomfort or strain.
- 14 days onwards—injury requires less protection. Concentrate on
  getting the injured part back to full fitness with exercises.
- By 8 weeks all usual activities should have been resumed.

Guide to taping and strapping

Taping or strapping is simply the application of adhesive tape to provide
extrinsic stability and/or to offload weakened structures. Its proprioceptive
qualities play a significant part in protection and rehabilitation. The principal
aim of applying tape is to prevent disability and thus improve otherwise
impaired physical function. Techniques can be used for a multitude of musculoskeletal conditions, either following tissue injury or as a preventative
measure when a history or risk of injury is present. (See Fig 14.8.)

- Because of the incubation period (e.g. fever starting <7 days after entering a malarious area cannot be due to malaria; fever starting >21 days after leaving West Africa cannot be Lassa fever).
- On clinical grounds: e.g. a fever with lymphadenopathy and rash is not compatible with malaria.
- By carrying out a therapeutic trial (e.g. of antimalarial or anti-rickettsial treatment).
- Suspicion of a serious infectious disease such as bacterial meningitis should prompt initiation of blind antimicrobial treatment and urgent evacuation to the nearest base hospital (see ➲ Evacuation, p. 146).
- Confirmation of diagnosis, using a wider range of laboratory and other investigations, may be possible after evacuation to the base hospital identified at the planning stage. Depending on the experience and attitude of local doctors and nurses, the expedition medical officer may still have a role and responsibility at this stage, hence the relevance of some of the information about diagnosis and more advanced treatment given in Box 15.1.

Box 15.1 Some common patterns of infection and pragmatic treatments

- Fever ± headache without other signs—treat for malaria (if exposure was possible):
  - After 48 h still fever but no signs—treat for rickettsia.
  - After 96 h still fever—evacuate.
- Spreading skin inflammation ± pus—treat with flucloxacillin + pus drainage.
- Pain passing urine ± loin pain—urinary tract infection—treat with trimethoprim.
- Coughing up yellow/green phlegm ± pleuritic pain—chest infection—treat with doxycycline or clarithromycin.
- Diarrhoea and vomiting—traveller's diarrhoea—treat with fluids, rehydration salts, and ciprofloxacin or azithromycin.
- Severe abdominal pain with rigid abdomen—peritonitis—treat with fluids and co-amoxiclav and evacuate.
- Headache, stiff neck, photophobia, impaired consciousness, ± rash—meningitis/encephalitis—treat with ceftriaxone and evacuate.

Viral infections

Viral hepatitis

Many different viruses and some bacteria (see ➲ Leptospirosis, p. 471) are capable of producing the clinical and biochemical picture of acute hepatitis. These include some flaviviruses (see ➲ Viral encephalitides, p. 460), herpes viruses, such as Epstein–Barr virus (EBV) and Cytomegalovirus (CMV) and the 'hepatitis viruses' (A to G) that specifically target the liver (see Fig. 2.2 and Fig. 2.3). Of the specific hepatitis viruses, A and B are of particular concern to the traveller who should have received appropriate vaccination. Hepatitis C is only a concern to those who inject drugs or who receive medical care overseas.

Transmission and incubation period
- *HAV* is transmitted faecal–orally and rarely by blood transfusion, needle stick, and sexually. Incubation is 4–6 weeks.
- *HBV*, sometimes associated with HDV ('delta agent') is transmitted by transfusion, needle stick, from mother to baby at birth, or sexually. Incubation is 4–24 weeks.
- *HCV* is transmitted by needle stick, transfusion, rarely from mother to baby at birth, and sexually. Incubation is 2–26 weeks.
- *HEV* is transmitted faecal–orally and zoonotically via pork and other animal products. Incubation is about 6 weeks. Many epidemics attributed to HAV are thought to have been due to HEV. Pregnant women are susceptible to severe disease.

Clinical
Many infections are anicteric and some asymptomatic. In the rest, cholestatic jaundice appears after a few days of general malaise, anorexia, nausea, vomiting, fever with chills, weakness, fatigue, headache, aches and pains, and upper abdominal discomfort. Dark urine, pale stools, and pruritis are common. Signs include right upper quadrant tenderness, tender hepatomegaly, spider naevi, and vasculitic or urticarial rashes. Splenomegaly is common with CMV and EBV but not with the specific hepatitis viruses. Fulminant, potentially-fatal, hepatic failure may occur with HBV, rarely with HAV, presenting with hepatic encephalopathy. The acute illness, which may relapse, lasts days or weeks and in severe cases is complicated by persistent nausea, vomiting, ascites, oedema, or liver failure. Chronic viral carriage, chronic hepatitis, cirrhosis, and hepatoma are complications of HBV (HDV) and HCV infection.

Diagnosis
Urine dipstick testing reveals urobilinogen (early) and bilirubin (later). If laboratory services are available, rapidly rising serum aminotransferase concentrations (to thousands of units) suggest hepatitis and the diagnosis is confirmed by serology or antigen detection. High alkaline phosphatase suggests 'surgical' obstructive jaundice (e.g. gallstones).

Treatment

There is no specific treatment for acute viral hepatitis. Hepatotoxic drugs and alcohol must be avoided. Rest and low-fat diet improve comfort. Corticosteroids and low-protein diet have no proven benefit. It is essential that the patient attends an infectious diseases unit on return, to screen for other blood-borne viruses and to exclude chronic HBV, HDV and HCV infection, any of which may require specific treatment.

Prevention

(See also ➲ Hepatitis A, p. 33; ➲ Hepatitis B, p. 34.)

Effective vaccines are available against HAV and HBV (and HDV) and are strongly recommended to all travellers to developing countries. HBV vaccine is mandatory for medical personnel. Avoidance of HAV and HEV involves food and water hygiene, especially in hyperendemic third world countries. For the parenterally/sexually transmitted viruses such as HBV and HBC, extreme caution is necessary with blood and blood products unless they have been properly screened. Surgical and dental procedures, ear piercing, tattooing, acupuncture and injections in or out of hospital, unprotected sex, and intimate contact that risks inoculation of blood or tissue fluids, even sharing a tooth brush, are potentially hazardous.

Websites
- ℰ http://www.cdc.gov/ncidod/diseases/hepatitis
- ℰ http://www.who.int/topics/hepatitis/factsheets/en

Poliomyelitis

Poliomyelitis, caused by the polioviruses (enteroviruses), has been eliminated from the Western hemisphere but wild poliovirus (WPV) infections still occur in a few African and Asian countries (Fig. 15.1). In 2013, WPV cases were confirmed in Pakistan, Afghanistan, Syria, Nigeria, Chad, Niger, Kenya, and Ethiopia with a major resurgence in Somalia. WPV1 was found in sewage in Israel. In March 2012, India was officially removed from the WHO's list of countries with active transmission of endemic polio. This status will be monitored for 3 years before the country can be classed as 'polio-free'.

Transmission: is faecal–oral.

Clinical

Most infections are asymptomatic or cause only mild upper respiratory tract symptoms, but in about 1% of cases, there is aseptic meningitis or flaccid paralysis of one limb or more extensive quadriplegia or bulbar and respiratory paralysis due to infection of spinal anterior horn cells. Other viruses such as enterovirus 71, adenoviruses, and Japanese encephalitis virus can also cause polio-like flaccid paralysis.

Prevention

Everyone must be vaccinated or boosted if visiting an endemic area >10 years after their previous vaccination. Inactivated (Salk) vaccine is used increasingly. In the UK, it is combined with tetanus and diphtheria vaccine (DPT) (see Table 2.1). Oral (Sabin) vaccine (live, attenuated virus) can cause vaccine-related poliomyelitis (0.5–3.4 cases/1 million vaccines).

Website

ℰ http://www.who.int/topics/poliomyelitis/en

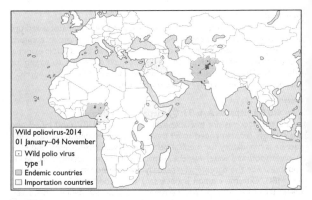

Fig. 15.1 Distribution of wild poliovirus 2014 (January to November).

Viral encephalitides

Japanese encephalitis

This is a common, dangerous, vaccine-preventable, mosquito-borne flavivirus encephalitis of Asia and parts of Oceania (see Fig. 2.4). There are 30,000–50,000 cases reported annually with 10,000–15,000 deaths. Forty clinical cases in travellers have been reported over 30 years.

Prevention: a new Vero cell vaccine ('IXIARO') is recommended (two doses 4 weeks apart followed by a booster after 1 year. Children over 2 months but less than 3 years old receive half the adult dose).

Tick-borne encephalitis (TBE)

Tick-borne encephalitis, caused by a flavivirus, occurs throughout a vast area from Germany and the whole of Scandinavia in the west, through eastern Europe, Baltic countries and central Asia to the far west of the Russian Federation (Russian spring—summer encephalitis; see Fig. 2.6). Each year, 3000 clinical cases are reported in Europe and >10,000 in Russia. The incidence is increasing in all countries except Austria where an aggressive vaccination policy has proved effective.

Transmission: hard ticks (*Ixodes ricinus, I. persulcatus*) transmit three subtypes of TBE flaviviruses. Infection can also be acquired by drinking unpasteurized dairy products, especially goats' milk.

Clinical: a feverish illness (myalgia, headache and fatigue) may appear 4–28 days after the tick bite; 1–33 days later about 1/3 will develop meningitis, meningoencephalomyelitis, myelitis, or meningoradiculitis.

Diagnosis (at the base hospital): can be confirmed by detecting viraemia (early) or serologically.

Treatment is symptomatic.

Prevention: (see ➋ Tick-borne encephalitis, p. 37) vaccination (two doses 4–6 weeks apart followed by a booster at 1 year) is effective for those walking and camping in tick-infested coniferous forests of endemic areas, especially during the tick season (May–October and 'Russian spring–summer encephalitis'). In Austria, everyone is vaccinated. Avoid tick infestation (➋ Ticks, p. 288) and unpasteurized (goats') milk products.

West Nile fever

West Nile fever, caused by a flavivirus, occurs in Africa, Europe, Asia, Australia and the Americas. Kunjin virus is the Australian subtype.

Transmission is by *Culex* mosquitoes, primarily among migratory birds but sometimes to humans, horses, and other mammals and also by blood transfusion.

Clinical: after an incubation period of 3–15 days, about 20% of infected people develop a dengue-like feverish illness. Fewer than 1% have meningitis or encephalitis, although these may prove fatal in elderly patients. Rashes and lymphadenopathy are uncommon.

Diagnosis: confirmation is serological.

Prevention: there is no vaccine. Avoid mosquito bites (see Box 15.3), especially from dusk to dawn. Wear gloves when handling bird carcasses.

Website

• ♫ http://www.cdc.gov/ncidod/dvbid/westnile/index.htm

Rabies

Rabies ('hydrophobia') is a zoonotic encephalomyelitis caused by several different rabies viruses (lyssaviruses) of mammals (e.g. classic rabies virus, Australian and European bat lyssaviruses, Duvenhage, etc.) that can be transmitted to humans by bites. Most of the world is endemic for rabies (see Fig. 2.5). Domestic dogs are by far the most important source of human rabies worldwide. Other vectors include cats, wolves, foxes, jackals, skunks, mongooses, raccoons, vampire bats (Caribbean and Latin America only), flying foxes (fruit bats), and insectivorous bats. Bites by rodents pose negligible risk. Monkey bites are common among visitors to S/SE Asian temples, but the risk of rabies is exceedingly low. However, all mammal bites and scratches should be taken seriously because rabies is such a fatal disease.

Rabies is especially common in parts of Africa, the Indian subcontinent, South-East Asia, China causing >60,000 human deaths each year and untold fear and suffering.

Transmission

Virus-laden saliva is inoculated through the skin by a bite or scratch and the virus can also penetrate intact mucosae. Transmission between humans has been proved only via infected corneal and solid organ grafts from unsuspected rabies-infected donors.

Clinical

The virus spreads from the wound along nerves to reach the CNS, caus-ing fatal encephalomyelitis. The incubation period is usually a few months but can vary from 4 days to many years. Often, the first symptom is itching at the site of the healed bite wound. Within a few days, headache, fever, confusion, hallucinations and hydrophobia develop. Attempts to drink water induce spasm of inspiratory muscles and an indescribable terror. Ascending flaccid paralysis is another type of presentation. Except for a few bat-associated cases in USA, rabies encephalomyelitis is inevitably fatal, usu-ally after a few days. However, rabies is readily preventable.

Prevention

Avoid all unnecessary and close contact with domestic, wild or pet mam-mals, especially carnivores and bats. Beware of wild animals that appear unusually tame or aggressive: they may be rabid!

In case of mammal bites licks or scratches

Irrespective of the risk of rabies, mammal bites, scratches, and licks on mucous membranes or broken skin should be thoroughly cleaned immediately.

> Pre-exposure rabies vaccination (3 doses, days 0, 7, and 28) (➲ Rabies, p. 36) is strongly recommended for all travellers to rabies-endemic regions because optimal post-exposure prophylaxis may not be readily available and this is a deadly disease! Cost can be reduced if a group of two or more travellers are vaccinated together, using 0.1 mL by the intra-dermal (ID) route.

- Scrub wound with soap and water, ideally under a running tap.
- Rinse and apply povidone–iodine or strong (40–70%) alcohol (gin and whisky contain more than 40% alcohol).
- Give tetanus toxoid.
- Consider other mammal bite pathogens (e.g. *Pasteurella multocida*), but prophylactic antibiotics (tetracycline, amoxicillin, or co-amoxiclav) are not justified except for severe/deep bites and those on the hands.
- In a rabies-endemic country, if the skin has been broken by the bite or scratch, or if a mucosal membrane or open wound, including a scratch, has been contaminated with the animal's saliva, start post-exposure prophylaxis (see Box 15.2). The decision should be made as soon as possible by a doctor working in the area where the bite has occurred. On no account should it be delayed until the traveller's return to their own country. If in doubt, start prophylaxis!

Websites

- ℱ http://www.cdc.gov/ncidod/dvrd/rabies
- ℱ http://www.who.int/rabies/en

Box 15.2 Post-exposure prophylaxis of rabies

Modern tissue/cell culture vaccines, such as human diploid cell vaccine (Sanofi-Pasteur), vero cell vaccine (Sanofi-Pasteur Verorab®) and purified chick embryo cell vaccine (Novartis-Chiron Rabipur® and RabAvert®), are potent and safe. Consider including at least one dose of rabies vaccine in your medical kit as emergency ID post-exposure booster treatment.

For those who *have* received three doses of pre-exposure immunization in the past:
- *Either* two IM post-exposure booster injections of vaccine should be given on days 0 and 3 but no rabies immune globulin (RIG) is necessary.
- *Or* give 0.1 mL of vaccine ID at each of four sites (deltoids, lateral thighs or suprascapulars) on one occasion only.

For those who *have not* previously received a course of rabies vaccine:
- RIG is infiltrated around the bite wound and any remaining is given IM (lateral thigh). Human RIG 20 units/kg body weight; equine RIG 40 units/kg.

And:

Rabies tissue culture vaccine (detailed in ⊅ Rabies, p. 36):
- *Either* IM (deltoid) injections of one vial, 1 mL (0.5 mL for Verorab®) of reconstituted vaccine on days 0, 3, 7, 14 and 28.
- *Or* ID four-site injections (so that a small papule is produced—see Plate 3, just like with BCG vaccination).
  - On day 0: divide one ampoule of vaccine between *four* sites (both deltoids and both thighs or suprascapular regions).
  - On day 7: 0.2 mL (in the case of 1 mL vials) or 0.1 mL (in the case of 0.5 mL vials) at each of *two* sites (both deltoids).
  - On day 28: single site 0.2/0.1 mL.

Early, vigorous cleaning of the bite wound (see ⊅ Wounds, p. 268; ⊅ In case of mammal bites licks or scratches, p. 462) combined with vaccination and use of RIG has proved very effective in preventing rabies. If no suitable vaccine is available where and when the exposure occurs, the traveller should be repatriated immediately to start post-exposure prophylaxis as a matter of urgency.

No case of rabies has been reported in anyone who was exposed to rabies after receiving pre-exposure prophylaxis and in whom post-exposure booster shots of vaccine were given.

Viral haemorrhagic fevers

Yellow fever

Yellow fever (YF) is the classic flavivirus haemorrhagic fever. It occurs only in Africa and South America (see Fig. 2.7). Ninety per cent of cases are reported from Africa. In 2013, it was confirmed in Sudan (Darfur), Ghana, Cameroon, Ethiopia, Niger, and Congo DR. There have been as many as 200,000 cases of YF each year, with 30,000 deaths. Deaths of six unvaccinated travellers have been reported in the past 10 years.

Transmission: is by *Aedes* mosquitoes. Jungle (sylvatic) YF is transmitted between monkeys and occasionally humans by tree hole breeding mosquitoes in South America and Africa, while urban epidemics are transmitted between humans by peri-domestic *Aedes aegypti*.

Clinical: after an incubation period of 3–6 days, around 5% of those infected become feverish with chills, headache, photophobia, myalgia, back ache, pain in limbs and knees, nausea, vomiting, epigastric pain, and prostration. Heart rate may be slow relative to the temperature. After a temporary remission, jaundice, generalized bleeding (black vomit, melaena), acute kidney injury, shock, and coma may supervene.

Diagnosis: at the base hospital): leucopenia and thrombocytopenia are typical. Confirmation is by detecting virus in blood or liver tissue (post mortem) or serological.

Treatment: supportive.

Prevention: (see ➔ Yellow fever, p. 38) vaccination is recommended for all visitors to the endemic area and is a statutory requirement in many countries. For example, you will not be allowed to fly from Ecuador to Brazil without a valid vaccination certificate. The live, attenuated 17D vaccine is contraindicated before the age of 9 months, in pregnant women, and in the immunosuppressed. There have been problems with vaccine supply (India), safety, fake vaccine and fake certificates (India, West Africa). YF-associated neurological disease (YEL-AND) is an abnormal allergic response to the vaccine, as with other vaccines (e.g. flu) causing postvaccinal encephalitis, Guillain–Barré syndrome, etc. It occurs in 1.0/100,000 doses in people aged 60–69 years and 2.3/100,000 doses in people aged ≥70 years. YF-associated visceral disease (YEL-AVD) is a severe infection (case-fatality >60%) caused by massive replication of the vaccine virus with multiple organ failure occurring only after primary vaccination in 0.4/100,000 doses. In those >60 years old and YF vaccine naïve, the combined incidence of YEL-AND and YEL-AVD increases to around 1/50,000, the highest risk for any vaccine currently in use.

Websites
- ℘ http://www.nathnac.org/pro/factsheets/yellow.htm
- ℘ http://www.nhs.uk/Conditions/Yellow-fever/Pages/Prevention. aspx
- ℘ http://wwwnc.cdc.gov/travel/yellowbook/2014/chapter-3-infectio us-diseases-related-to-travel/yellow-fever

Dengue fever ('break bone' fever)

Dengue viruses are flaviviruses, responsible for 50–100 million cases of dengue each year throughout the tropics, notably in South-East Asia, South America, and the Caribbean, and increasingly in urban areas (Fig. 15.2). There are four serotypes, DEN-1 to -4.

Transmission

Day-biting, peri-domestic mosquitoes such as *Aedes aegypti* and *Ae. albopictus* transmit the four types of dengue virus between humans.

Clinical

In most foreign travellers, dengue causes an acute fever associated with headache, backache, pains in the muscles and joints ('break bone' fever), and a rash. A reddish blotchy rash that may blanch on pressure often appears after a temporary lull in the fever. Petechial haemorrhages may be found in the skin and conjunctivae.

Severe dengue

200,000–500,000 cases of severe, life-threatening dengue occur each year, with 5% case fatality, usually in children born and being brought up in endemic areas who are suffering their second infection with a dengue virus type different from that causing their first attack. However, severe and even fatal, apparently primary, dengue infections have been seen in adults, including travellers. After 2–7 days of fever, spontaneous bleeding (nose, gums, GI) and increased capillary permeability leads to shock, haemoconcentration, and thrombocytopenia.

Diagnosis (at the base hospital)

Diagnosis is supported if the blood count shows leucopenia with relative lymphocytosis and thrombocytopenia often with raised liver enzymes and may be confirmed serologically.

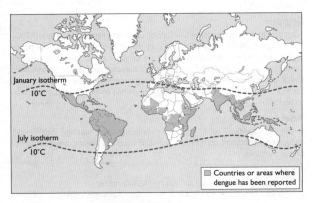

Fig. 15.2 Global distribution of dengue 2011.

Treatment

For primary dengue only symptomatic treatment is needed (bed rest, control of fever and pain with paracetamol). Suspected severe dengue warrants immediate evacuation and correction of hypovolaemia, hypoglycaemia, and electrolyte and acid–base homeostasis but avoidance of corticosteroids, heparin, NSAIDs, and aspirin. Supportive treatment reduces case fatality to <1%.

Prevention

Wear sensible clothing (see Box 15.3 and ➲ Insect protection and repellents, p. 771) during the daytime biting period and apply DEET-containing repellents to exposed skin surfaces. A vaccine is long awaited.

Websites
- ℘ http://www.cdc.gov/Dengue
- ℘ http://www.who.int/topics/dengue/en

Arenaviruses: Lassa fever (West Africa) and Bolivian, Argentine, and Venezuelan haemorrhagic fevers

These *Arenavirus* zoonoses are acquired through contact with urine of peri-domestic or feral rodents. In West Africa there are thought to be 300,000–500,000 cases of Lassa fever, with 5000 deaths each year. In parts of Liberia and Sierra Leone, the prevalence of Lassa fever among hospital admissions is 10–16%. The overall case fatality rate is 1%, up to 15% among hospitalized patients. Pregnant women and their fetuses are at very high risk. Worldwide, >30 cases of imported Lassa fever have been described, the most recent from Liberia to USA.

Transmission

By contact with urine of multimammate rat (*Mastomys natalensis*) and between humans by contamination with infected blood, needle sticks, and sexual contact.

Symptoms

After an incubation period of 6–21 days, Lassa fever presents with insidious fever, malaise, headache, and painful sore throat with visible exudative pharyngitis, conjunctivitis, backache, chest pain, cough, nausea, vomiting and diarrhoea, but no jaundice (despite hepatitis), bleeding or rash. Hypovolaemic shock (associated with facial oedema) may supervene after about 1 week. Early antiviral treatment with ribavirin (tribavirin) reduces case fatality five- to tenfold.

Prevention

Avoid all contact with rodents (including not eating them) and rodent-contaminated accommodation and food in endemic areas. No vaccine is available.

Websites
- ℘ http://www.who.int/csr/disease/lassafever/en
- ℘ http://www.cdc.gov/ncidod/dvrd/spb/mnpages/dispages/vhf.htm

Filoviruses: Marburg and Ebola viruses

In 2013–2014, these filoviruses caused epidemics of highly fatal haemorrhagic fever in Congo DR and Uganda. The first West African epidemic of Ebola virus disease broke out in Guinea in early February 2014, spreading to Sierra Leone and Liberia, with a few cases in adjoining countries. By December 2014, 19,065 cases and 7,388 deaths had been recorded (case-fatality 39%). The natural reservoir is probably fruit bats, while other mammals, including higher primates, can be infected. Epidemics probably start when infected wild mammals ('bush meat') are killed and eaten.

Transmission
Contact with organs, blood, secretions, or other body fluids of infected patients.

Symptoms
After an incubation period of 2–21 days there is sudden fever, fatigue, headache, vomiting, diarrhoea, loss of appetite, weakness, myalgias, and a generalized non-prutitic, papular, desquamating, erythematous rash without jaundice (despite hepatitis). In West African patients, hypovolaemia from severe vomiting and diarrhoea is a prominent feature, while bleeding, usually manifest as blood in the stools, is relatively uncommon. Case fatality ranges from 30% to 90%.

Prevention
By avoiding epidemic areas, especially bat caves and contact with patients' blood, vomitus, stool, sputum, and other body fluids and secretions, and risk of parenteral infection by needles and sharps.

Website
- ⅊ http://www.cdc.gov/vhf/ebola
- ⅊ http://www.who.int/mediacentre/factsheets/fs103/en

Bunyaviruses: Crimean–Congo, Hantavirus, and Rift Valley fevers

Crimean–Congo haemorrhagic fever (CCHF)

This occurs in Eastern Europe, the Middle East, Africa, and Asia, in 2013 in Russia, Kosovo, India, Bulgaria and South Africa. In 2012 a man, infected in rural Afghanistan, died in UK. It is transmitted by ticks or in infected animal blood (abattoirs, ritual sacrifice). After 3–7 days' incubation period, there is sudden fever, headache, photophobia, nausea, vomiting, generalized body pains, thrombocytopenia, leucopenia, and severe bleeding with a case fatality of 15–80%. Treatment with ribavirin may be helpful. No vaccine is available. Avoid tick bites (➲ Prevention of tick-transmitted infections, p. 288) and parenteral exposure.

Hantavirus haemorrhagic fever with renal syndrome (HHFRS or Korean haemorrhagic fever)

This occurs in Europe, especially Scandinavia, Germany and the Balkans, and Asia. Hantavirus pulmonary syndrome (HPS) occurs in the Americas. In 2012, deer mice (*Peromys cusmaniculatus*) transmitted hantavirus to ten campers in Yosemite National Park, USA, three of whom died.

HHFRS is spread by aerosol from rodent urine or bites. After a long incubation period (12–16 days, up to 2 months), fever, facial flushing, and subconjunctival haemorrhages develop, followed by shock, pulmonary oedema, and acute kidney injury. The case fatality is up to 15% (50% in HPS). Avoid rodent contact and human-to-human spread in HPS. No vaccines are generally available.

Rift valley fever (RVF)

In Africa and the Middle East, RVF is spread from camels and domestic ruminants by mosquitoes and contamination by infected blood in abattoirs. In 1997–98 and 2006–07, there were epizootics in Kenya, Tanzania, Burundi, and Somalia. 684 cases with 155 deaths were reported in Kenya (case fatality 23%), 264 with 109 deaths in Tanzania (41%) and 114 with 51 deaths in Somalia (45%). After 3–6 days' incubation, there is acute fever, mucocutaneous haemorrhages, conjunctivitis, photophobia, eye pains, blinding retinitis, and lymphadenopathy, with occasional progression to disseminated intravascular coagulation (DIC), severe bleeding, encephalopathy, hepatorenal failure, and death. Veterinary vaccines are marketed. Avoid mosquito bites and contact with infected animal blood.

Website

• ℘ http://www.cdc.gov/hantavirus

Chikungunya fever

Chikungunya is a dengue-like Aedes mosquito-transmitted alphavirus infection that has caused massive epidemics in Indian Ocean islands, Comoros, Mauritius, Seychelles, Madagascar, Mayotte, and Réunion, Africa, Latin America, and Caribbean and Pacific islands (>1.3 million cases) since 2006. Hundreds of cases were imported into France and other European countries from Réunion and the other islands popular with tourists. Local (autochthonous) transmission of Chikungunya by indigenous *Aedes albopictus* mosquitoes was established around Ravenna, Italy, causing thousands of cases. More than 200 imported cases have been identified in the UK, mainly from the Caribbean and Latin America.

Clinical

After 2–4 days' incubation there is sudden fever, headache, malaise, conjunctivitis, arthralgia, arthritis (ankles and small joints), myalgia, and low back pain with rash in half the cases. Rashes are very variable: erythematous (blanching), vesicular, bullous, dyshydrotic, keratolytic, purpuric, and hyperpigmented, associated with facial oedema, erythema nodosum, and aphthous ulcers. Joints may be severely and persistently involved with effusions and bursitis. A useful sign is pain on pressure in the anatomical snuff box. Severe and occasionally fatal features are meningoencephalitis, Guillain–Barré polyradiculopathy, myocarditis, hepatic dysfunction, and acute kidney injury.

Prevention
An effective vaccine has been developed in the USA but is not generally available. Antimosquito measures are the only protection.

Website
• ⌕ http://www.who.int/mediacentre/factsheets/fs327/en

Bacterial infections

Brucellosis

This globally prevalent zoonosis of goats, sheep and camels (*Brucella melitensis*), cattle (*B. abortus*), and dogs (*B. canis*) has been eliminated from <20 countries. More than 500,000 new cases of *B. melitensis* infection are reported each year.

Transmission

The main risk of infection, except for farmers, is ingestion of milk products, especially soft white goats' cheeses, and raw meat.

Clinical

After an incubation period of 1 week to several months, every system can be involved and so the range of symptoms is enormous. Commonly there is acute or insidious persistent fever with chills, arthralgias, septic arthritis, back ache, spinal tenderness signifying osteomyelitis, granulomatous hepatitis, meningoencephalitis, endocarditis, and epididymo-orchitis and other genitourinary infections.

Diagnosis

At the base hospital or after return home in the case of long incubation periods, blood, marrow, and other cultures (prolonged, using special media) and serology (IgG agglutinins difficult to interpret) may prove diagnostic.

Treatment

Doxycycline (oral 100 mg twice a day) and rifampicin (oral 600–900 mg/day) for 45 days or doxycycline for 45 days and streptomycin (0.5–1.0 g/day IM) for 2 weeks are the most effective regimens.

Prevention

Avoid all unpasteurized milk and milk products, especially cheeses and undercooked meat products in parts of the world where brucellosis is prevalent, such as Africa, the Middle East and Latin America.

Diphtheria

Diphtheria (*Corynebacterium diphtheriae*) usually infects the upper respiratory tract or skin and its toxin can affect the heart, nerves, and kidneys. Although largely eliminated by childhood vaccination, diphtheria still occurs in developing countries and has increased in the former Soviet Union.

Transmission

From human-to-human by aerosol or contact with respiratory tract secretions.

Clinical

After an incubation period of 2–5 days there is inflammation of mucosae, usually of the fauces, nasal cavity, trachea, larynx or bronchi, development of the classic greyish-yellow pseudomembrane, local lymphadenopathy, and swelling of the neck ('bull neck'). Diphtheria can cause skin ulcers apparently indistinguishable from simple bacterial ulcers, but they have an area of anaesthesia round them which can be detected by testing pinprick sensation (see ● Tropical ulcers, p. 292).

Treatment

High-dose benzyl penicillin (12 g each day in six divided doses) or erythromycin will eliminate the infection but antitoxin is needed for severe toxic effects, and emergency tracheostomy or needle cricothyroidotomy (➜ Surgical airways, p. 188) may be needed to relieve airway obstruction. Suspected diphtheria warrants immediate evacuation.

Prevention

(See also Table 2.1.)

Childhood immunization in combination with tetanus and pertussis is routine in most countries. For boosting immunity in adult travellers, adsorbed diphtheria (low dose) and tetanus vaccine (formol toxoids) is recommended for adults and adolescents.

Leptospirosis

Leptospirosis is a zoonotic infection by *Leptospira icterohaemorrhagiae* and related strains or serovars, affecting rats, dogs, pigs, sheep, cattle, other mammals including humans, and reptiles and amphibians throughout most parts of the world. Increasing numbers of cases are being detected in South Asia. Leptospirosis is an occupational disease of farmers and sewer workers. Those involved in fresh water sports (canoeing, sailing, water skiing) and exposure to watery, flooded environments are also at risk. During the 10-day Eco-Challenge-Sabah 2000 multisport endurance race, 26% of 304 athletes caught leptospirosis. Andy Holmes, a British Olympic gold medal oarsman died of leptospirosis in 2010.

Transmission

Infection is acquired when broken skin or intact mucosae are in contact with fresh water contaminated by infected mammals' urine.

Clinical

The incubation period is 2–26 (mean 10) days. Most infections are subclinical or mild but in about 10% severe features, including jaundice, hepatorenal failure, pulmonary haemorrhage, and shock may develop. Symptoms include fever, rigors, headache, myalgia, backache, painful tender calves, meningism, and gastrointestinal and pulmonary haemorrhages. Jaundice and subconjunctival haemorrhages are common signs.

Treatment

Early treatment with oral doxycycline (100 mg twice daily for 1 week) for suspected mild disease and high-dose parenteral benzylpenicillin may be effective.

Prevention

Avoid contact with fresh water likely to be contaminated by rats and other mammals especially if you have skin abrasions. Doxycycline in the dose taken for malaria prophylaxis (100 mg each day) or 200 mg once each week is protective. Post-exposure prophylaxis after immersion in a river or lake might be appropriate in some circumstances.

Lyme disease

Lyme disease, named after Lyme, Connecticut, USA, is the most common vector-borne disease in North America, where there are about 20,000 new cases reported each year. It is common in north-eastern, mid-Atlantic, and north-central states in people aged 5–14 years and 45–54 years. It occurs in Europe, especially Estonia, Latvia, Lithuania, Russia, and in northern Asia. It is caused by *Borrelia burgdorferi* in North America and by *B. garinii* (Lyme neuroborreliosis or Bannwarth syndrome) and *B. afzelii* in Europe.

Transmission

From mice, deer, and other mammals to humans is by bites of hard (*Ixodes*) ticks.

Clinical

After an incubation of 7–10 days, a red macule/papule and later an expanding red ring (erythema migrans) usually appears around the tick bite site (Plate 4) and is associated with local lymphadenopathy, fever, chills, headache, myalgia, arthralgia, and meningism. The classic erythema migrans does not always appear. Unilateral facial nerve palsy, radiculopathy, carditis with heart block, arthritis, and other rashes may occur.

Diagnosis

Confirmed by serology at the base hospital.

Treatment

Early treatment with oral doxycycline 100 mg twice daily for 14–21 days is curative. About 15% of patients show a mild exacerbation of symptoms (Jarisch–Herxheimer reaction) within 24 h of starting treatment.

Prevention

Anti-tick measures (see ➲ Prevention of tick-transmitted infections, p. 288) are important. Chemoprophylaxis before tick attachment is not justified and afterwards only within strict criteria.

Website

• ℛ http://www.cdc.gov/lyme

Melioidosis

Melioidosis, a dangerous infection caused by soil-dwelling *Burkholderia pseudomallei,* is increasingly recognized in South East Asia, Northern Australia, the tropical Americas, and as an imported travellers' disease. Infection is usually through exposure of skin lesions to wet fields and floods, rarely by ingestion of infected fresh water and inhalation. Severe cases are usually immunosuppressed by diabetes mellitus, chronic renal failure, urinary lithiasis, alcoholic cirrhosis, malignancy, corticosteroid or other immunosuppressant treatment. Infection may be latent for many decades (e.g. in US veterans of the Vietnam war).

Clinical features

Local infections and abscesses may involve cutaneous/subcutaneous tissues, lungs, parotidis, lymph nodes, bones, joints, liver, spleen, genital tract and brain. A septicaemic illness is the commonest presentation, often associated with a primary pneumonia but chronic fever and weight loss also occur. Case fatality varies from >40% in north-east to 14% in Australia.

Diagnosis
Can be confirmed only where there are good bacteriological facilities.

Treatment
Involves supportive care, drainage of collections of pus and prolonged antimicrobial therapy, first with parenteral ceftazidime or a carbapenem, then with oral trimethoprim-sulfamethoxazole for 12–20 weeks.

Prevention
Vulnerable people should avoid exposure to wet or inundated areas in endemic areas, especially if they have open wounds

Meningitis

Bacterial (pyogenic) meningitis is an acute infection involving the meninges and CSF. Common causes in younger people are the meningococcus (*Neisseria meningitidis*), pneumococcus (*Streptococcus pneumoniae*), and *Haemophilus influenzae* b (Hib) although all they are increasingly controlled by routine childhood vaccination. Meningococcal meningitis is common across the sub-Sahelian zone of Africa, extending from Senegal to the Sudan ('meningitis belt'; see Fig. 2.1), where there are annual cold season epidemics of group A or C disease. Outbreaks may also occur where there are gatherings of people from all over the world, such as in Mecca for the Hajj (check ℰ http://www.promedmail.org for news of current epidemics).

Other causes of acute meningitis include viruses (e.g. *Herpes simplex*, enteroviruses, mumps, etc.); causes of more insidious meningitis/encephalitis are tuberculosis, fungi (e.g. *Cryptococcus*), free-living amoebae (*Naegleria*, *Acanthamoeba*, and *Balamuthia*) and even worms (e.g. *Parastrongylus*).

Transmission
By aerosol from infected carriers or cases.

Symptoms
- Sudden fever.
- Severe headache.
- Photophobia.
- Nausea.
- Vomiting.
- Diarrhoea.
- Myalgia.

Meningococcal meningitis

A petechial/purpuric rash is characteristic. It is initially macular, often starts on the forearms or shins, and may be visible on the conjunctivae (Plate 5). It spreads over the trunk and face, and may become vasculitic with geometrical areas of skin necrosis. Stiff neck (meningism) is the diagnostic sign of meningitis. Ability to flex the neck so that the chin touches the chest or shake the head from side to side virtually excludes meningism. Impairment of consciousness and seizures (children) are ominous developments. Very rapid evolution to classic meningococcal septicaemia (profuse rash, shock, bleeding, peripheral gangrene, multiple system failure) occurs in a minority of cases. Meningococcal septicaemia may also occur in the absence of meningitis.

Pneumococcal meningitis

There may be an obvious source of infection (e.g. pneumonia, otitis media).

Diagnosis

Unless the diagnosis can be rapidly confirmed by lumbar puncture and CSF examination (unlikely in most expeditions), suspicion of bacterial meningitis warrants immediate, parenteral, preferably intravenous, antibiotic treatment, and urgent evacuation to the base hospital.

Treatment

Ceftriaxone or cefotaxime (2 g IV or IM 12-hrly) are the antibiotics of choice, covering all causes of bacterial meningitis except *Listeria monocytogenes* (special risk in pregnant women and some immunosuppressed patients; add ampicillin). Benzylpenicillin 2.4g IV or IM 4-hrly is effective for meningococcal infection. If parenteral treatment is impossible, amoxicillin 2g 4-hrly, or chloramphenicol 100 mg/kg each day in four divided doses can be given by mouth.

Prevention

(Also see ➔ Meningococal menigitis, p. 32.)

Hib vaccine (since 1992), meningococcal group C vaccine (since 1999) and conjugated pneumococcal vaccine since 2006 have been routinely offered to children in Britain. Travel to the African meningitis belt (see Fig. 2.1) or other areas of current epidemic meningococcal meningitis, justifies group A,C,W135,Y vaccine ('ACWY Vax'). Recombinant protein multicomponent Meningococcal Group B Vaccine now available. Contacts are treated with ciprofloxacin (500 mg single dose) or rifampicin (600 mg twice daily for 2 days).

Plague

About 2700 cases and 200 deaths from plague are reported each year (case fatality 7%), mainly from Madagascar and other African countries, and southern Asia, but a few are from the western USA (Fig. 15.3). Plague is flea-borne from rodents to humans. Warning of an impending epidemic is a die-off of rats, mice, marmots, etc.

Prevention

If your expedition is going to a notorious plague area (see ℘ http://www.cdc.gov/plague) and an epidemic is in progress, consider going elsewhere or taking preventive measures such as avoiding rodents and their parasites, and taking chemoprophylaxis (doxycycline, ciprofloxacin, or co-trimoxazole). No vaccines are currently available.

Website

- ℘ http://www.cdc.gov/plague

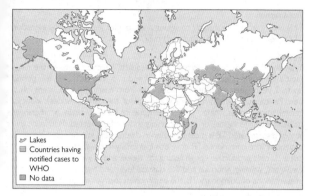

Fig. 15.3 World distribution of plague.

Tetanus

Tetanus remains endemic in developing countries and still carries a high case fatality but all visitors from western countries should be fully protected by vaccination from childhood although a booster of tetanus toxoid may be necessary (see Table 2.1).

Tuberculosis

Tuberculosis is the world's most prevalent bacterial infection, infecting 2 billion people, 1/3 of the world's population. The incidence is 8.8 million new cases of active disease and 1.1 million deaths each year, 23% of which are in India and 17% in China. Throughout most of Africa, Eastern Europe, Asia, and Latin America the incidence exceeds 50/100,000 of the population/year. All these figures are increasing as a result of the HIV pandemic. The causative organism, *Mycobacterium tuberculosis,* shares the genus with other species of mycobacteria, environmental or non tuberculous mycobacteria (NTM) that are not usually pathogenic to humans. They are more commonly found in the environment, sometimes causing disease in immune compromised patients (such as *M. avium* complex in HIV-immunosuppressed patients) but only rarely causing problems in the immunocompetent. All mycobacteria have the characteristic staining property that the Ziehl Neelsen (ZN) stain taken up by their cell walls is not decolorized by acid or alcohol, hence 'acid and alcohol fast bacteria' (AAFB or AFB). Many people are infected as children, sometimes leading to serious clinical disease such as disseminated ('miliary') TB. In most cases, infection is controlled by a normal immune response and held dormant as latent TB infection (LTBI). LTBI may be reactivated at any time to produce clinical TB disease. It is more likely to occur in someone who becomes immune suppressed due to cancer, HIV infection or immune suppressive drugs such as steroids and the new biologic agents such as infliximab.

Transmission

This is by aerosol created by coughing and, to a far less extent, by ingestion of *M. bovis*-infected (unpasteurized) milk.

Clinical

Typically, if the immune response is inadequate, infection involves the lungs (apical cavitating pneumonia), mediastinal nodes or pleura during the period up to 2 years after exposure or much later from reactivation of latent infection. Pericardium, lymph nodes (e.g. scrofula of the cervical nodes), kidneys, genital tract, bones, joints, gut or peritoneum, spleen, brain or meninges (tuberculous meningitis) or any organ may be affected. Fulminant miliary or disseminated TB is most common in children and immunocompromised patients. More commonly, TB develops insidiously. No symptom is diagnostic, but a chronic productive cough lasting for weeks and associated with malaise, weakness, wasting, anorexia and the classical fever and night sweats are typical presentations of pulmonary TB, the commonest form of the infection.

Diagnosis (at the base hospital)

Confirmed by staining or culturing *Mycobacteria* in sputum or elsewhere or detecting characteristic histopathology in biopsies. A strongly positive Mantoux test suggests active infection but a negative result is uninterpretable.

Mantoux test: inject 0.1 mL of solution, containing two Tuberculin Units of Statens Serum Institute (SSI) tuberculin RT23, ID into the volar surface of the forearm. After 48–72 h, measure the diameter of palpable induration (*not* of the red weal!). A diameter of >15 mm suggests active infection; 6–15 mm may be caused by previous BCG immunization (℘ http://www.immunisation.nhs. uk/files/mantouxtest.pdf). For detecting latent TB, consider interferon-gamma testing for those with a +ve Mantoux test, or those who have had BCG.

Treatment

Quadruple therapy with isoniazid, rifampicin, pyrazinamide, and ethambutol or streptomycin is usually effective, but drug resistance is emerging. Multidrug resistant (MDR-TB), extensively drug-resistant (XDR-TB) and totally drug-resistant (TDR-TB) infections have been reported. Other antibiotics to which these strains may respond include capreomycin, amikacin, and kanamycin.

Prevention

(Also see ➋ Tuberculosis, p. 37.)

ID BCG vaccination (Plate 3) provides variable but potentially valuable protection against TB (especially miliary TB and tuberculous meningitis in children) and leprosy. Those born in hyperendemic countries should have been given BCG at birth (look for the scar). BCG vaccination of Mantoux/ interferon-gamma negative expedition members is recommended if the destination is in a hyperendemic area and if the programme involves mixing with local people in crowded high-risk environments such as hostels, prisons, refugee camps, hospitals or clinics. HIV-immunocompromised people should consider taking prophylactic isoniazid (300 mg each day with pyridoxine 50 mg/kg each day) or isoniazid with rifampicin. However, there are potentially serious drug interactions with antiretrovirals and so expert advice should be sought.

Website

- ℘ http://guidance.nice.org.uk/CG117

Atypical *Mycobacteria*

These *Mycobacteria* usually cause chronic skin and soft tissue infection. Transmission is by direct inoculation or inhalation. They may need to be considered in chronic non-healing wounds in travellers on return from the expedition and require specialist diagnosis and treatment in a referral centre in the home country.

They include:

- *M. leprae*—causes leprosy, a skin disease of historic and global importance which is unlikely to infect short-term travellers. It has, however, affected expatriates who have lived for long periods in socially deprived conditions (e.g. missionaries in Papua New Guinea). It affects the skin and peripheral nerves (Plate 12). Diagnosis is confirmed by skin biopsy and demonstration of acid-fast-bacilli at specialist centres. Treatment is with dapsone, clofazimine, and rifampicin.
- *M. marinum* (➲ Marine wound infections, p. 294): soft tissue granulomas spreading up the limb lymphatic drainage in fish handlers and tropical fish enthusiasts.
- *M. chelonae* and *M. fortuitum*: similar presentation to *M. marinum*, but derived from soil inoculation.
- *M. avium/intracellulare*: causes painless mycobacterial lymphadenitis usually of the cervical or submental glands in children, *or* disseminated disease with fever in HIV/AIDS patients.
- *M.ulcerans*—causes Buruli or Daintree ulcer, an infection of subcutaneous fat leading to expanding ulcers.

Typhoid and paratyphoid (enteric fevers)

Infections by *Salmonella typhi* and *S. paratyphi* A, B, and C are still common in the Indian subcontinent, Vietnam, and Indonesia (100–1000 cases/100,000 population/year). Worldwide, there are an estimated 15–30 million cases and 500,000 deaths each year.

Transmission

By faecal–oral spread from water and food infected by human carriers (up to 1% of the population in some communities).

Clinical

After an incubation period of 3–60 (usually 7–14) days, the illness starts insidiously with fever, headache, malaise, abdominal discomfort, some bowel disturbance (often constipation but sometimes diarrhoea), cough, sore throat, and epistaxis. Signs include a slow pulse rate in relation to the fever, hepatosplenomegaly, a blanching macular rash on the abdomen (rose spots (Plate 6)), rhonchi in the chest, and abdominal tenderness (especially right iliac fossa). Untreated patients may develop severe complications in the second to fourth weeks of illness: perforation, intestinal haemorrhage, shock, and coma.

Diagnosis

By blood, stool, urine, or bone marrow culture.

Treatment

Fluoroquinolones, such as ciprofloxacin 0.5–1.0 g each day in two divided doses for 7–14 days, are usually effective, but resistance is now common in Asia and is emerging elsewhere. Parenteral ceftriaxone (50–60 mg/kg/day for 7–14 days) or oral cefixime (20 mg/kg/day for 7–14 days) or oral azithromycin for non-severe cases (10–20 mg/kg/day for 7 days) can be used in areas of high fluoroquinolone resistance.

Prevention

Strict food and water hygiene (Chapter 3) are crucial. Effective inject-able and oral vaccines, covering typhoid but not paratyphoid, are available and strongly recommended for all expeditions to developing countries (see Table 2.1).

Typhus

Rickettsial bacteria cause a large variety of arthropod-borne acute febrile diseases in most parts of the world, usually with a distinctive rash. Louse-borne epidemic typhus (*Rickettsia prowazeckii*) remains an epidemic threat in poorer countries, mite-borne scrub typhus (*Orientia tsutsuga-mushi*) is prevalent throughout South-East Asia (Fig. 15.4), tick-borne Rocky Mountain spotted fever (RMSF) (*R. rickettsii*) is one of the most dreaded infections in North America, and tick-borne African tick fever (*R. africae*) is commonly acquired by safari travellers in Southern Africa.

Transmission

By tick or mite saliva during their blood meal, by louse or flea faeces inocu-lated through skin or mucosae by scratching.

Clinical

After an incubation period of 4–14 (average 7) days, fever, chills, head-ache, photophobia, nausea, vomiting, abdominal pain and cough may develop. This is followed 3–5 days later by a generalized maculopapular and eventually petechial rash (Plate 7). A papule appears at the site of the infected bite in spotted fevers such as African tick fever (Plate 8), RMSF and Mediterranean boutonneuse fever and in scrub typhus (Plate 9). This evolves into a black-scabbed eschar with lymphangitis and local lymphad-enopathy. Severe multisystem complications may ensue.

Diagnosis

Confirmation is serological.

Treatment

Early treatment with oral doxycycline 200 mg or chloramphenicol 2 g in four divided doses each day for 2–3 days is appropriate for clinically suspected rick-ettsial infections. The therapeutic response is often dramatic and diagnostic.

Prevention

Vaccines are not generally available. Doxycycline in the dose taken for malaria prophylaxis (100 mg each day) or 200 mg once each week is pro-tective. Scrub typhus is suppressed rather than eradicated and so it may appear after cessation of chemoprophylaxis. Prevention of tick, louse, flea, and mite infestation is crucial (➔ Prevention of tick-transmitted infections, p. 288).

Website
- ℘ http://www.cdc.gov/ncidod/dvrd/rmsf/index.htm

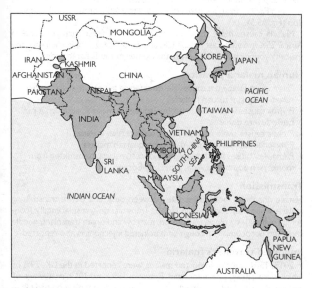

Fig. 15.4 Distribution of scrub typhus.

Further reading

Wormser GP, Dattwyler RJ, Shapiro ED, Halperin JJ, Steere AC, Klempner MS, *et al*. (2006). The clinical assessment, treatment, and prevention of lyme disease, human granulocytic anaplasmosis, and babesiosis: clinical practice guidelines by the Infectious Diseases Society of America. Clin Infect Dis, 43(9), 1089–134. Erratum in: Clin Infect Dis, 2007, 45(7), 941.

Malaria

Malaria occurs throughout the tropics: north to Kyrgyzstan, south to north-eastern South Africa, west to Mexico, and east to Vanuatu in the western Pacific, an area inhabited by more than 40% of the world's population (Fig. 15.5).

Malaria causes more than 500 million cases of fever each year, 75% in Africa, 25% in South-East Asia. It kills at least 600,000 people each year, the majority young children and pregnant women in sub-Saharan Africa.

Human malaria parasites

- *Plasmodium falciparum* causes life-threatening falciparum malaria, also called 'malignant tertian malaria'.
- *P. vivax* causes vivax malaria or 'benign tertian malaria', although it can cause severe disease.
- *P. ovale* causes ovale malaria, also 'benign tertian malaria'.
- *P. malariae* causes malariae malaria or 'quartan malaria'.
- *P. knowlesi* causes life-threatening knowlesi malaria, transmitted from monkeys in South-East Asia, especially Borneo.

Transmission

Female *Anopheles* mosquitoes bite between dusk and dawn, transmitting malaria while they suck human blood. Transmission transplacentally (congenital malaria), via blood transfusion, marrow and organ transplant, needle stick, and nosocomially through contaminated injections is also reported.

Imported traveller's malaria

In 2013, 1501 cases of imported malaria were reported in the UK, 79% of which were caused by *P. falciparum*. Between 1993 and 2012, an average of nine deaths have been reported each year, mostly in people who had taken no prophylaxis. In 2012, 1691 cases of imported malaria were reported in the USA, 58% caused by *P. falciparum* with nine deaths. Most of the deaths could have been prevented if travellers had been better educated about mosquito protection and correct chemoprophylaxis and if they had sought prompt medical attention when they fell ill during the first few weeks or months after returning home.

Incubation

The minimum interval between an infective mosquito bite and the first symptom (incubation period) is about 7 days, but most travellers with falciparum malaria become ill within a month of returning home; exceptionally, there may be a delay of more than a year. More than 1% of vivax infections present more than a year after leaving the tropics.

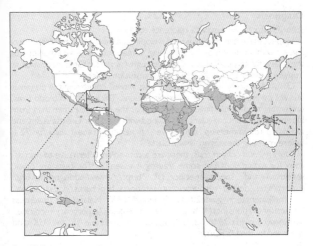

Fig. 15.5 Distribution map for malaria.

Symptoms

- Acute severe fluctuating fever with rigors.
- Severe headache.
- Pain in muscles and back.
- Nausea.
- Diarrhoea.
- Loss of appetite.
- Postural hypotension.
- Prostration.
- *Absence* of sore throat, rash, lymphadenopathy.

Classic periodicity of fever (every day—quotidian—in knowlesi malaria; every other day—tertian—in falciparum, vivax, and ovale malarias; every third day—quartan—in malariae malaria) is uncommon but the fever often recurs at the same time every day.

Signs

- There may be none and the patient may be afebrile.
- Petechiae, tender enlarged liver and spleen, pale conjunctivae, and jaundice are worth looking for.
- *Falciparum* malaria in non-immunes (those who have not acquired temporary immunity to malaria through repeated infections) can be a rapidly evolving and potentially life-threatening disease (exceptionally, first symptom to death in 24 h). Worrying features are severe prostration, impaired consciousness (cerebral malaria), seizures, profound anaemia, deep jaundice, hypoglycaemia, shock, renal failure, spontaneous systemic bleeding (suggesting DIC), and respiratory distress.

Diagnosis

(See ℘ http://www.malaria-reference.co.uk)

Suspect malaria in anyone who develops acute fever >7 days after entering, or within a few months of leaving, a malarious area whether or not they have taken prophylaxis. Consider unusual risks of infection, such as 'runway', 'airport', 'needle stick', and transfusion malarias.

Classic microscopy: this remains the best way of confirming the diagnosis but will be impracticable for most expeditions. Thick and thin blood films, preferably made from finger prick blood at the bedside rather than from blood stored in anticoagulant, are stained with Field's or Giemsa stains and examined (oil immersion, high power). If negative, repeat daily for 72 h before rejecting the diagnosis of malaria.

Rapid malaria antigen tests: these are a convenient alternative to microscopy for expeditions but some training is essential. The tests are quick, sensitive, and species-specific (℘ http://www.finddiagnostics.org/export/sites/default/resource-centre/reports_brochures/docs/malaria_rdt_implementation_guide2013.pdf). BinaxNOW® Malaria test (Inverness Medical Innovations Inc) (℘http://www.alere.co.uk/emergency-medicine/binaxnowr-malaria-26/product-listing.htm) is available in the UK and approved by the US FDA.

Differential diagnosis

At the base hospital, malaria must be distinguished from other tropical fevers (typhoid, typhus, relapsing fevers, leptospirosis, dengue, and other viral haemorrhagic fevers), less exotic infections such as glandular fever (EBV), pyogenic bacterial infections, meningitis, viral hepatitis, viral encephalitis, HIV seroconversion illness, and heatstroke.

Treatment

Suspected malaria warrants immediate evacuation.

Falciparum malaria

- Wherever *P. falciparum* infection may have been acquired assume it is chloroquine-resistant.
- For adults who can swallow tablets and keep them down:
  - Artemether-with-lumefantrine (Riamet®, Co-artem®, or Co-artemether®): adult and children >12 years and >35 kg in weight dose four tablets at 0, 24, 36, 48, and 60 h *or*
  - Proguanil hydrochloride-with-atovaquone (Malarone®): adult dose four tablets (children 11–20 kg 1; 21–30 kg 2; 31–40 kg 3 tablets) daily for 3 days *or*
  - Quinine sulfate: adult dose 600 mg (three tablets) (children 10 mg/kg) 8-hrly for 5–7 days followed by either doxycycline 200 mg for 7 days or (pregnant women or children) clindamycin 450 mg three times daily (children 20–40 mg/kg in three divided doses) for 5 days.

Severe falciparum malaria

For adults who are vomiting and unable to swallow and retain tablets or who have severe prostration, impaired consciousness, jaundice, profound anaemia, hypoglycaemia, renal failure, spontaneous systemic bleeding/DIC, black urine or respiratory distress:

- Sodium artesunate is the drug of choice despite emerging resistance in south-east Asia (⌨ http://www.cdc.gov/malaria/diagnosis_treatment/artesunate.html): loading dose 2.4 mg/kg by IV injection followed by 1.2 mg/kg by IV injection daily for a minimum of 3 days, followed by oral antimalarial (e.g. artemether-with-lumefantrine).
- Quinine dihydrochloride; loading dose 20 mg/kg by IV infusion over 4 h (or IM), then, after 8 h, maintenance dose 10 mg/kg by IV infusion over 4 h (or IM) 8-hrly until able to swallow tablets. Complete the course with quinine sulfate followed by either doxycycline 200 mg for 7 days (*not* for children or pregnant women) or clindamycin 450 mg three times daily (children 20–40 mg/kg in three divided doses) for 5 days. *Quinine may cause hypoglycaemia!*
- Artemether: loading dose 3.2 mg/kg by IM injection followed by 1.6 mg/kg by IM injection for a minimum of 3 days followed by oral antimalarial (e.g. artemether-with-lumefantrine).

'Benign' malarias

For adults, chloroquine (BASE!) 600 mg (usually four tablets) (children 10 mg BASE/kg) followed by 300 mg after 6–8 h (children 5 mg BASE/kg) followed by 300 mg daily for 2 days (children 5 mg BASE/kg) (total dose ~25 mg BASE/kg body weight). Eradicate liver cycle with primaquine (see ➲ Prevention of the 'benign' malarias (*P. vivax, P. ovale,* and *P. malariae*), p. 488) (beware of G6PD-deficiency!). In New Guinea and adjacent areas of Indonesia (for example, Lombok), *P. vivax* has become resistant to chloroquine. A double dose of chloroquine or the standard dose of mefloquine, followed by a 4-week course of primaquine, can be used to treat such resistant infections.

Prevention of malaria

Assessing the risk

Within malarious countries, the areas of malaria transmission may be patchy, depending on environmental factors such as temperature, altitude, vegetation, and season. Thus there is no malaria transmission in some African capital cities that are at a comparatively high altitude, such as Addis Ababa and Nairobi, and in other areas malaria transmission occurs only during a brief rainy season. Seek reliable local advice about malaria transmission at the places and times when the expedition will be there. Even within a transmission area, the risk of being bitten by an infected mosquito can vary from less than once per year to more than once per night. The risk of catching malaria during a 2-week visit without any protection has been estimated as about 0.2% in Kenya and 1% in West Africa.

People who are especially vulnerable to malaria, including pregnant women (see Box 15.3), should seriously reconsider whether they really need to enter a malarious area.

Box 15.3 Principles of personal protection against malaria

- Awareness of risk: vulnerable individuals, such as pregnant women, infants, splenectomized or otherwise immunocompromised people, should avoid entering a malarious area.
- Antimosquito measures: kill, exclude, repel, and avoid mosquitoes.
- Sensible clothing: long sleeves and long trousers between dusk and dawn.
- Diethyl toluamide (DEET)-containing insect repellent applied to exposed skin.
- Insecticide (pyrethroid)-impregnated mosquito bed net or screened (air-conditioned) accommodation sprayed with insecticide each evening.
- Vaporizing insecticide in the sleeping quarters (burning mosquito coil, electrical, knock-down insecticide).
- Chemoprophylaxis: Malarone®, doxycycline or mefloquine (Lariam®) or other drugs, depending on the particular geographical area (see ➲ Antimalarial chemoprophylaxis: two strategies, p. 485). (*Remember that there have been NO deaths in UK travellers who have complied with an appropriate chemoprophylaxis regimen.*)
- Standby treatment: artemether-with-lumefantrine quinine or Malarone®.
- In case of feverish illness within a few months of return: see a doctor and mention malaria specifically!
- Avoid all alternative/homeopathic remedies for prevention or treatment of malaria (🔗 https://www.gov.uk/government/publications/malaria-homeopathic-remedies).

Anti-mosquito measures

- *Sleeping quarters:* malaria-transmitting mosquitoes bite in or near human dwellings during the hours of darkness and so the risk of infection can be reduced by insect-proofing sleeping quarters or by sleeping under a mosquito net. Individual, lightweight, self-supporting mosquito nets are available. Protection against mosquitoes and other biting invertebrates (sandflies, lice, fleas, bed bugs, ticks) is greatly enhanced by sleeping under insecticide-treated nets (ITNs). The net is soaked in a pyrethroid insecticide such as 10% permethrin (75 ml or 200–500 mg per m² of material every 6 months). Even better, long-lasting insecticidal nets (LLINs) are factory-treated to retain their activity for at least 20 washes and 3 years of use. Screens and curtains can also be impregnated with insecticide. In addition, bedrooms should be sprayed in the evening with a knock-down aerosol insecticide (e.g. Etofenprox®, Malathion®, Deltamethrin®) to kill any mosquitoes that may have entered the room during the day. Mosquitoes may also be killed or repelled by vaporizing synthetic pyrethroids (D-allethrin, S-bioallethrin, transfluthrin) on an electrical vaporizing mat (such as No Bite® and Buzz Off®) where electricity is available, or over a methylated spirit burner (Travel Accessories UK Ltd, PO Box 10, Lutterworth, Leicester LE17 4FB, UK). Burning cones or coils of mosquito-repellent 'incense' may also be effective.

- *Protective clothing:* to avoid bites by any flying insect, high-necked, light-coloured, long-sleeved shirts and long trousers afford better protection than vests and shorts. To avoid malaria-transmitting mosquito bites, this sensible clothing should be worn, particularly after dark, even on the beach. Cotton clothes and ankle bands can be impregnated with DEET and other materials can be impregnated with permethrin insecticide.
- *Repellents:* exposed areas of skin should be rubbed or sprayed with repellents containing NN-diethyl-m-toluamide (DEET) or p-methane-diol ('Mosiguard Natural'). Insecticide-containing soaps ('Mosbar', Simmons Pty Ltd, Box 107, Chadstone, Victoria 3148, Australia) and suntan oil are available.

Antimalarial chemoprophylaxis: two strategies

Two different strategies have been proposed for antimalarial chemoprophylaxis. In areas of high incidence (more than 10 cases of malaria per 1000 of the local population per year) such as West Africa, the risk of infection outweighs the risk of side effects of taking antimalarial drugs and so chemoprophylaxis is justified. However, in areas of low incidence (less than ten cases of malaria per 1000 of the local population per year), such as Central America and Southeast Asia, the risk of taking antimalarial drugs outweighs the risk of infection and so reliance is placed on full anti-mosquito measures and carrying a course of standby emergency treatment (SBET) to be taken if the traveller develops symptoms suggestive of malaria while out of reach of medical care (see Table 15.1)

Compliance: the failure of travellers to take their antimalarial tablets regularly, and in particular to continue taking them for long enough after leaving the malarious area (4 weeks for all but Malarone® which need only be taken for 7 days), also reduces the effectiveness of chemoprophylaxis. During bouts of vomiting and diarrhoea (traveller's diarrhoea), these drugs may not be adequately absorbed.

Choice of drug: risk of contracting malaria should be balanced against the relative efficacy and risk of side effects of a particular prophylactic drug.

Chemoprophylactic drugs and combinations

Mefloquine (Lariam®)

Mefloquine is effective against some multiresistant *P. falciparum* strains but has some unpleasant side effects: nausea, stomach ache, and diarrhoea in 10–15% of people who take it; insomnia and nightmares; giddiness and ataxia (unsteadiness and incoordination) in some; and a rare 'acute brain syndrome' (psychosis and even seizures).

Contraindications include: a history of previous adverse reactions to this drug, hypersensitivity to quinine, depression, any type of neuropsychiatric disease, and epilepsy. Airline pilots, scuba divers, those who have suffered a traumatic brain injury, and those whose work demands manual dexterity should choose another drug unless they have already proved tolerant of mefloquine.

Adult dose is 250 mg once a week.

Start weekly mefloquine 4 weeks before leaving for the malarious area in case side effects demand a change in treatment. All antimalarial drugs that kill parasites in the bloodstream must be continued for 4 weeks after return so that late-emerging parasites (hepatic merozoites), protected as long as they remain in the liver, are eliminated when they enter the circulation.

Atovaquone–proguanil (Malarone®)

This is a safe, effective, but expensive drug. Malarone® acts on liver stage parasites and so need be taken for only 7 days after leaving the malarious region. The dose is one tablet each day for adults. It is best avoided in pregnancy.

Doxycycline (Vibramycin®)

No antimalarial drug offers absolute protection. Much depends on compliance. Travellers who become feverish and ill, especially in the early months after their return, should consult a doctor and mention the possibility of malaria. If there is any doubt, referral to an infectious/ tropical disease unit for exclusion of malaria is an urgent necessity. Antimalarial prophylactic drugs should be stopped until the diagnosis is confirmed or rejected.

This tetracycline antibiotic has proved useful for prophylaxis in areas where mefloquine resistance is prevalent, such as the Thai–Cambodian border region. It gives some protection against other travellers' diseases such as typhus, leptospirosis, and some types of traveller's diarrhoea. One 100 mg tablet should be taken every day. Side effects include oesophagitis, photosensitive rashes, skin irritation, diarrhoea, and oral/oesophageal or vaginal thrush. It should be taken while standing up on a full stomach with plenty of fluid to reduce the risk of its becoming stuck in the oesophagus and causing irritation/ulceration. It is best avoided in pregnant women and is contraindicated in children under 12.

Proguanil (Paludrine®) and chloroquine (Avloclor®, Nivaquine®, Malarivon®)

Proguanil—adult dose two tablets (each of 100 mg) every day—and chloroquine—two tablets (each of 150 mg BASE) once a week—is no longer recommended for Africa, the Amazon region, South-East Asia, Assam, and Oceania but remains effective prophylaxis elsewhere. It is safe in pregnancy and (in a lower dose) in children. The only side effects are rare mouth ulcers, mild indigestion, and hair loss. The combination is available in the UK as Paludrine®/Avloclor® (AstraZeneca).

Chloroquine taken for up to 5–6 years continuously in the dose recommended for prophylaxis against malaria does not cause damage to the eyes, but those who have taken it for >6 years continuously (total cumulative dose approaching 100 g) should have their vision checked.

Table 15.1 Choice of prophylactic strategy in different geographical areas: chemoprophylaxis or standby emergency treatment (SBET)

Country	Strategy	Drug
Central America + Hispaniola	SBET	Chloroquine
South America: Brazil—Rondônia, Roraima, Acre; Guyana, Suriname, French Guiana—interior	Chemoprophylaxis	Malarone®, mefloquine or doxycycline
South America: other malarious areas	SBET	Riamet® or Malarone®
Africa (including Madagascar): malarious areas	Chemoprophylaxis	Malarone®, mefloquine or doxycycline
Middle East: malarious areas	SBET	Riamet® or Malarone®
Central India, Assam, SE Bangladesh[a]	Chemoprophylaxis	Chloroquine-proguanil/Malarone®, mefloquine or doxycycline[a]
Some parts of Burma, Laos, Cambodia, Vietnam[a]	Chemoprophylaxis	Malarone® or doxycycline
Rest of Indian subcontinent and Southeast Asia + China: malarious areas[a]	SBET	Riamet® or Malarone®
Lombok, Eastern Indonesia, New Guinea, Solomon Islands	Chemoprophylaxis	Malarone®, mefloquine or doxycycline
Vanuatu	SBET	Riamet® or Malarone®

[a] For more details see:
🔗 http://www.hpa.org.uk/webc/HPAwebFile/HPAweb_C/1203496943523

Schlagenhauf P, Petersen E. (2013). Current challenges in travelers' malaria. Curr Infect Dis Rep, 15(4), 307–15.
🔗 http://www.dtg.org/uploads/media/Malariakarte_2011_02.pdf

Pregnant women

Pregnant women should avoid entering a malarious area because of the risks to them and their fetus. If exposure is absolutely unavoidable, full anti-mosquito precautions and chemoprophylaxis are essential. The hazards of getting malaria, particularly *P. falciparum* malaria, during pregnancy exceed the small but finite hazard of adverse effects to the baby of the antimalarial drugs. Proguanil and chloroquine are safe. Mefloquine may be an acceptable alternative where there is a high risk of infection and this combination is ineffective. Doxycycline and Malarone® should be used only if there is no alternative.

Standby emergency treatment (SBET)

SBET is appropriate for two categories of travellers:
1. Those visiting areas of low malaria risk (see Table 15.1) who are not taking antimalarial chemoprophylaxis.
2. Those visiting remote areas with a high risk of malaria who are taking appropriate chemoprophylaxis (in case of infection breaking through their prophylaxis).

Both groups should carry a course of standby treatment to be taken if they develop a malaria-like fever but do not have ready access to hospitals and diagnostic laboratories. This must not delay their seeking medical treatment at the base hospital as soon as possible. Appropriate drugs for standby treatment are:
• Artemether-with-lumefantrine (Riamet®, Co-artem®, or Co-artemether®): adult dose four tablets at 0, 24, 36, 48, and 60 h *or*
• Quinine sulfate: adult dose 600 mg 8-hrly for 5–7 days followed by either doxycycline 200 mg for 7 days or clindamycin 450 mg three times daily for 5 days *or*
• Proguanil hydrochloride-with-atovaquone (Malarone®) four tablets daily for 3 days (unless in category 2 this drug is being taken for prophylaxis).

Prevention of the 'benign' malarias (*P. vivax*, *P. ovale*, and *P. malariae*)

Weekly chloroquine or mefloquine prevent *P. vivax*, *P. ovale*, and *P. malariae* malarias. However, *P. vivax* and *P. ovale* can establish themselves in the liver despite chloroquine prophylaxis, and may re-emerge to cause relapsing infections months or years later. Primaquine, adult dose 15 mg a day for 2 weeks, eradicates latent liver infection (hypnozoites) and should be given to travellers who have spent more than a few months in areas where these species are endemic (beware of G6PD-deficiency!). In parts of Indonesia, particularly Irian Jaya, and in Papua New Guinea, Thailand, the Philippines, and the Solomon Islands, Chesson-type strains of primaquine-resistant *P. vivax* require a 4-week course of primaquine.

Resources

Websites
- ✍ http://www.who.int/malaria/docs/TreatmentGuidelines2006.pdf
- ✍ http://www.hpa.org.uk/infections/topics_az/malaria/Treat_guidelines.htm
- ✍ http://www.cdc.gov/malaria

Other information
Advice about malaria can be obtained from the following tropical medicine units:
- Malaria Reference Laboratory (Health Protection Agency) London, UK:
  - Tel: +44 (0) 20 7636 3924 (advice on prophylaxis only).
  - Tel: +44 (0) 20 7927 2427 (advice on laboratory diagnosis).
  - Fax: +44 (0) 20 7637 0248.
  - Tel: +44 (0) 9065 508908 (24-h 100 p/min).
  - ✍ http://www.nathnac.org
- Hospital for Tropical Diseases, London, UK:
  - Emergency Admission Tel: +44 (0)20 7387 9300 and ask for the Duty Doctor on Bleep 5845.
  - Tel: +44 (0)845 155 5000 and ask for Duty Tropical Diseases Doctor.
  - Fax: +44 (0)20 7388 7645.
  - ✍ http://www.thehtd.org
- Liverpool School of Tropical Medicine, Liverpool, UK:
  - Tel: (0900–1700 h) +44 (0) 151 708 9393.
  - Tel: (24 h; ask for tropical/ID physician on call) +44 (0) 151 706 2000.
  - Fax: +44 (0) 151 708 8733 or +44 (0) 151 705 3368.
  - ✍ http://www.liv.ac.uk/lstm/travel_health_services/travel_clinic/index.htm
- Oxford Centre for Clinical Vaccinology and Tropical Medicine, John Warin Ward, Churchill Hospital, Oxford, UK:
  - Tel: (24 h; ask for I D consultant on call) +44 (0)1865 741 841.

Other protozoal infections

Leishmaniasis

Leishmania can cause a spectrum of skin, mucosal membrane, and visceral infections in humans and animals in the Mediterranean, Middle East, Africa, Asia, and in North, Central and South America (Fig. 15.6). An estimated 1.5–2 million cases of cutaneous leishmaniasis and 500,000 cases of visceral leishmaniasis (kala-azar) occur each year.

Transmission

Leishmania are transmitted from infected humans or animals by the bite of tiny sandflies (*Phlebotomus, Lutzomyia*).

Clinical

Cutaneous leishmaniasis—days to months after the infected sandfly bite, a nodule appears that grows, crusts, and ulcerates over weeks to months. The classic 'oriental sore' is 1–5 cm in diameter, painless with raised edges and granulating apple jelly base, and small satellite lesions on an exposed area (Plate 10). Lesions may slowly heal or persist, recur, and spread. Mucocutaneous leishmaniasis—infection with some Latin American *Leishmania* presents with a cutaneous ulcer but (sometimes years) later destructive lesions develop in the nasopharyngeal mucosa. Visceral leishmaniasis (kala-azar)—there is fever, massive splenomegaly, hepatomegaly, wasting, hypersplenism, and secondary bacterial infection. Post-kala-azar dermal leishmaniasis may develop, after apparent recovery. HIV-immunosuppressed patients are especially vulnerable.

Diagnosis

Scrapings from the nodular edge of the sore are stained with Giemsa and examined microscopically. Mucosal lesions are biopsied. Kala-azar can be confirmed serologically (direct agglutination test or rK39 dipstick test) (⅊ http://bmj.com/cgi/doi/10.1136/bmj.38917.503056.7C) and in hospital, Leishman–Donovan bodies are sought in splenic or bone marrow aspirate, liver or lymph node biopsy or buffy coat.

Treatment for cutaneous leishmaniasis

Small sores can be excised, larger ones can be injected with sodium stibogluconate (Pentostam®) twice weekly for 2–3 weeks or the lesions can be left to heal. Oral fluconazole 200 mg/day for 6 weeks is proving effective for cutaneous Old World leishmaniasis caused by *L. major* and *L. tropica*. For infections acquired in Latin America; unless *L. brasiliensis, L. panamensis,* and *L. guyanensis,* which carry the risk of mucosal involvement, can be excluded; prolonged courses of IV treatment with drugs such as Pentostam®, pentamidine, paromomycin (*L. aethiopica*), ketoconazole, or fluconazole (*L. major, L. mexicana*) are needed. For kala-azar, oral miltefosine or prolonged courses of IV treatment with drugs such as Pentostam® or amphotericin are needed.

Prevention

Avoid bites by nocturnally active sandflies tiny enough to penetrate ordinary mosquito nets but deterred by pyrethroid-impregnated bed and face nets, wear sensibly ample clothing and apply DEET-containing repellent to skin, cotton clothing, and ankle bands.

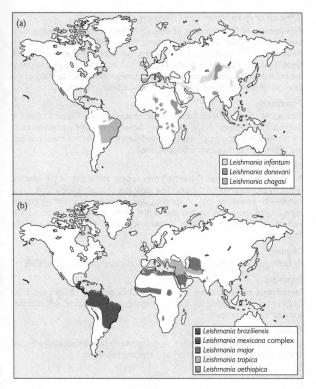

Fig. 15.6 Leishmaniasis distribution

African trypanosomiasis (sleeping sickness)

An estimated 40 000 new cases of sleeping sickness occur each year in a number of smallish areas scattered throughout West, Central, East, and southern Africa (Fig. 15.7). There is currently a resurgence of the disease in Angola, Central African Republic, Uganda, Nigeria, and adjacent countries following the breakdown of control measures. A few foreign travellers, especially to the game parks of eastern and southern Africa, have been infected.

Transmission

Tsetse flies (*Glossina*) transmit the trypanosomes causing Gambian sleeping sickness (*Trypanosoma brucei gambiense*) between humans and those causing Rhodesian sleeping sickness (*T. b. rhodesiense*) between humans and animal reservoir hosts (game, antelopes, etc.).

Clinical

A small ulcer with a scab ('chancre') may appear at the site of the infected tsetse fly bite and, within the next few days, intermittent fever begins, associated with headache, loss of appetite, and enlargement of lymph glands, especially in the posterior triangle of the neck. Eventually, there is invasion of the CNS, and patients become apathetic, sleepy, and eventually comatose.

Diagnosis

By finding motile trypanosomes in lymph node aspirates, blood, or CSF.

Treatment

Pentamidine or suramin are used before CNS invasion. Drugs used after CNS invasion (detected by CSF examination), melarsoprol, eflornithine, and nifurtimox are toxic.

Prevention

Chemoprophylaxis is not feasible. Avoid tsetse fly bites by wearing sensible clothing (light-coloured, not blue) and applying repellents.

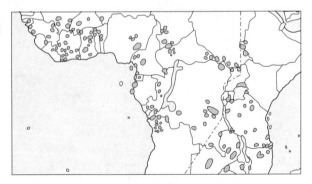

Fig. **15.7** Distribution of African trypanosomiasis.

Whip worm (Trichuris)

Whip worm infection (30–50 mm long, greyish-white or pink) is acquired by ingesting eggs. Massive infections cause anaemia, colitis with blood and mucus in the stools, and sometimes appendicitis and rectal prolapse. Visible worms may be passed.

Pin worms (Enterobius vermicularis)

(2.5–13 mm long, white) lay their eggs around the anal verge, causing intense nocturnal pruritus ani, scratching and excoriation of perianal skin, and insomnia. Eggs contaminate the microenvironment and are spread among the family by ingestion or inhalation. The host is reinfected by licking contaminated fingers. Diagnosis is confirmed by microscopic detection of eggs stuck to strips of sellotape applied to the anal margin on waking.

Treatment

All these round worm infections can be treated with albendazole 400 mg single dose or mebendazole 100 mg twice each day for 3 days. However, those with hookworm infection may need haematinics for iron deficiency, and treatment of pin worm infection should include the whole household and must be repeated after 1 week.

Flukes

Schistosomiasis (bilharzia)

This fluke infection occurs in Africa, the Middle East, eastern South America, China, and South-East Asia (Fig. 15.10). Infection is acquired through contact with fresh water from lakes and sluggish rivers, usually by bathing or washing with water taken from these sources. Infected humans contaminate the lake by defecating or urinating into it and infect, in turn, the intermediate snail hosts. Snails release tiny cercariae into the water which burrow through the skin of bathers.

Clinical

The earliest symptom of possible infection is 'swimmer's itch', experienced soon, sometimes minutes, after contact with infected water. Some people develop an acute feverish illness associated with an urticarial rash and blood eosinophilia a few weeks after infection ('Katayama fever'). Later symptoms include passing cloudy or frankly blood-stained urine or dysentery and, rarely, ascending paralysis and loss of sensation in the lower limbs. Travellers usually get worried about bilharzia when they get back from their trip and remember bathing in forbidden lakes or hear that schistosomiasis has been diagnosed in another member of the party.

Diagnosis

Search for characteristic ova in stool, urine (midday, centrifuged, end-stream sample is optimal) or rectal biopsy, or by a blood test.

Treatment

Treatment is fairly simple with one to two doses of praziquantel (Biltricide®).

Prevention

Avoid bathing in sluggish fresh water sources in endemic areas. Local advice may be misleading. Lake Malawi, officially declared free of bilharzia, has been the source of many imported cases of bilharzia in the UK over the last few years.

Screening of returned travellers

Although routine screening is not indicated, groups of people travelling with and presumed to have shared the same exposure as a confirmed case deserve to be tested, as do those who were at particularly high risk. Ova can be detected as soon as 3–4 weeks after exposure. If asymptomatic travellers are screened, wait 3 months after exposure before doing a blood test. Many travellers who have swum in Lake Malawi have purchased praziquantel locally to take immediately. However, what they buy may not contain any praziquantel, and taking it immediately post-exposure (swim) is far too early in the life cycle for it to be effective.

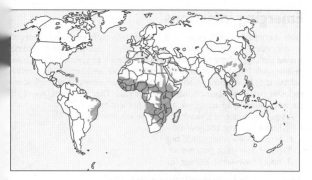

Fig. 15.10 Geographic distribution of schistosomiasis.

Liver flukes

Liver fluke (*Clonorchis, Opisthorchis*) (7–25 × 3–5 mm) infections acquired by eating fresh water fish are very common in South-East Asia and China. Liver fluke *Fasciola hepatica* (20–30 × 8–13 mm) and intestinal fluke *Fasciolopsis buski* (20–75 × 8–20 mm) infections result from ingestion of metacercariae attached to water cress, water chestnuts and other fresh water plants. Anorexia, right upper quadrant abdominal pain, tenderness and hepatomegaly, and episodes of cholangitis are typical of liver fluke infection, while nausea, anorexia, abdominal discomfort, lienteric diarrhoea (passing undigested food) are typical of heavy *F. buski* infections.

Treatment

Praziquantel 25 mg/kg three times daily after meals for 2 days is effective.

Tape worms (cestodes)

Beef (*Taenia sagginata*) (4–12 m long, 5–7 mm thick whitish, semi-transparent) or pork (*T. solium*) (3–8 m long, 5–7 mm thick, yellowish) tape worms are acquired by eating inadequately cooked meat containing viable cysticerci (e.g. 'measly' pork). Passing a long tape worm through the anus or seeing the elongating and contracting whitish reproductive segments (proglottids) (18–30 × 5–7 mm) in the stool or vomitus are the commonest symptoms, but nausea, abdominal pain relieved by eating, pruritus ani, and weight loss are common. (Cerebral) cyticercosis, a complication of *T. solium* infection, presents with seizures.

Treatment

Niclosamide 2 g as a single morning dose or praziquantel 10–20 mg/kg as a single dose after breakfast is effective.

Emerging infections

Over the past decade, a number of entirely new pathogens have emerged as important causes of (sometimes epidemic) human disease; some known pathogens have mutated into drug-resistant strains and others have re-emerged. Members of expeditions to remote areas might, like 'sentinel animals', be exposed to some of these known emerging and unknown reclusive pathogens enzoonotic in wild animals. They should be aware of current epidemics to assess risk and plan prevention.

A free online journal is devoted to these infections:

- ℗ http://wwwnc.cdc.gov/eid
- ℗ http://www.promedmail.org
- ℗ http://www.cdc.gov/mmwr
- ℗ http://www.who.int/wer/en

Severe acute respiratory syndrome (SARS)

Infections caused by the SARS corona virus emerged in China in November 2002. The last case was reported in China in April 2004, but SARS could re-emerge at any time. The epidemic affected >8000 patients in 37 countries in five continents, with a case fatality of 9%. The origin of human cases was palm civets and other carnivores but ultimately bats. Several new human coronaviruses have been discovered since the SARS epidemic, including HCoV-NL63, HCoV-HK and MERS-CoV (see ➲ Middle East respiratory syndrome coronavirus (MERS-CoV), p. 501).

Transmission

By droplets and close human-to-human contact, especially in hospitals.

Clinical

After an incubation period of 1–14 (average 4) days, fever (>38°C), myalgia, lethargy, malaise, chills, non-productive cough, sore throat, breathlessness, pleurisy, and watery diarrhoea may develop. There were chronic sequelae in survivors. The diagnosis can only be suspected in a patient who fails to respond to antibiotic treatment and has an epidemic or contact history.

Diagnosis

Confirmed by serology after about 10 days of illness. No effective specific treatment or prophylaxis is known.

Prevention

By avoiding epidemic areas and especially hospitals and by wearing face masks. Markets in which wild mammals are sold for food in China pose a hypothetical risk of infection. No safe vaccine has yet been developed.

Websites

- ℗ http://www.who.int/csr/sars/guidelines/en
- ℗ http://www.cdc.gov/ncidod/sars
- ℗ http://www.hpa.org.uk/infections/topics_az/SARS/menu.htm

Middle East respiratory syndrome coronavirus (MERS-CoV)

This new coronavirus disease emerged from Saudi Arabia in September 2012. More than 818 cases including 352 deaths have been reported (case-fatality 43%). Deaths were mainly in people with chronic co-morbidities. Although currently confined to the Arabian Peninsula including Madinah, site of the annual Hajj in KSA and adjacent countries (Iran, Jordan, etc.), it has been exported to several Western countries in travellers. Possible mammalian reservoirs include camels, cats, and various species of bats. The infection presents as a severe acute pneumonia with respiratory distress and acute kidney injury. It can spread between humans (e.g. to hospital staff). The virus is thought to have pandemic potential. Recent travellers returning from the Middle East who develop severe acute respiratory infections (SARI) should be tested for MERS-CoV.

Avian influenza H5N1

Avian flu is caused by H5N1 influenza virus which naturally infects wild birds and has caused large outbreaks in domestic poultry. The first human cases were identified in Hong Kong in 1997 and it re-emerged in 2003, by 2013 causing 633 infections with 377 deaths (case fatality 60%) in Asia, Europe, the Near East, and Africa, the most in Indonesia and Vietnam. Over 90% of cases have been <40 years old.

Transmission

By close contact (aerosol) with infected birds (usually poultry) and eating their uncooked blood or meat. Suspected human-to-human spread is very rare.

Clinical

Typical 'flu-like' symptoms such as fever, cough, sore throat, myalgia, conjunctivitis, and pneumonia with acute respiratory distress requiring mechanical ventilation.

Treatment

Oseltamivir and zanamivir may be effective for treatment and prevention of H5N1 viruses, but resistant strains have already evolved.

Prevention

Candidate vaccines have been approved. Watch the epidemic news (see following websites) and avoid contact with poultry and wild birds as far as possible, especially commercial or backyard poultry farms and live poultry markets. Do not eat uncooked or undercooked poultry or poultry products, including dishes made with uncooked poultry blood. H5N1 vaccines are being developed. If there is an epidemic, prophylactic/therapeutic oseltamivir will be distributed by the WHO and perhaps by some embassies in affected countries. Face mask (preferably N-95) are recommended for high-risk environments by some authorities.

Websites

- ℅ https://www.gov.uk/government/publications/
  avian-influenza-guidance-and-algorithms-for-managing-human-cases
- ℅ http://www.who.int/csr/disease/avian_influenza/en
- ℅ http://www.cdc.gov/flu/avian

Avian influenza H7N9

This strain of avian influenza emerged from China in April 2013 causing >140 confirmed cases with a case-fatality of >30%. New cases were reported in Hong Kong in late 2013. Exposure is to poultry in contaminated environments, especially live-poultry markets (chickens, ducks, pigeons; not migratory birds). Compared to H5N1 victims the patients are older and more likely to be males. It causes rapidly progressive pneumonia, respiratory failure, ARDS, and death. Patients had been exposed to poultry and contaminated environments, especially live-poultry markets, where H7N9 was found in chickens, ducks and pigeons. Migratory birds do not seem to be affected.

H1N1 pandemic swine flu

This new H1N1 'triple reassortant' swine virus, with avian and human flu virus components, arose in Mexico, spreading worldwide via air-travel routes. Between April 2009 and August 2010, it caused 284,500–570,000 estimated deaths (18,500 lab confirmed). Seasonal flu vaccines were ineffective, but those born before the 1950s were protected. The disease was usually mild, sometimes with diarrhoea and vomiting. Case-fatality 0.03%. Severe cases (ARDS) were associated with pregnancy, asthma, pulmonary, cardiovascular, neurological and autoimmune diseases, diabetes and obesity. Chemotherapy and the WHO's vaccine tender process proved highly contentious.

Other emerging viruses

Australian bat lyssavirus, closely related to classic rabies virus, was discovered in 1996 in flying foxes (fruit bats) and other bats. It has caused three known human deaths in people who handled bats.

New paramyxoviruses (Henipaviruses) are a group of viruses associated with flying foxes and other bats in South Asia and Australia. They include the Nipah virus that caused an epidemic of encephalitis, mainly among pig farmers in Malaysia and Singapore in 1999. In total, 258 cases were reported with a case fatality of 40%.

Human bocavirus is a newly recognized parvovirus associated with lower respiratory tract infection in children in Europe, Thailand, China, Japan, and Australia.

Monkey pox virus, previously known as a rare cause of a febrile smallpox-like disease in children in equatorial Africa, caused a multistate outbreak of >70 human cases in USA in 2003. Pet prairie ('dogs') marmots had apparently been infected by rodents imported from West Africa.

Emerging bacteria

New antibiotic-resistant strains of bacteria are constantly emerging (℞ http://www.cdc.gov/drugresistance).

Drug-resistant strains are increasingly important globally causing infections which may not respond to conventional antibiotics.

Emerging antibiotic-resistant strains: some examples are:
- Penicillin-resistant pneumococci which cause pneumonia or meningitis. These are usually sensitive to ceftriaxone.

- Methicillin- and vancomycin-resistant *Staphylococcus aureus*, which may be community-acquired, and Panton–Valentine Leucocidin (PVL)-positive strains of *S. aureus*. The majority of strains of *Staph. aureus* causing skin and soft tissue infection in the USA and several other countries are resistant to flucloxacillin which is the mainstay of staphylococcal treatment. Strains that produce the toxin PVL may cause more severe systemic and recurrent infection. Group A streptococci (GAS), *Strep. pyogenes*, although not antibiotic resistant, can cause very severe septic shock by toxin mediated immune modulation. The focus is usually soft tissue, although it can be the throat or genital tract. The recognition and management of impending sepsis is crucial. In the absence of a hospital, fluid resuscitation and oral linezolid (600mg 12-hrly), expensive and probably difficult to acquire, may be an effective holding measure for severe MRSA and invasive GAS.
- Extended spectrum beta-lactamase (ESBL)-producing *E. coli*, carbapenemase producing *Klebsiella pneumoniae* (with New Delhi Metallo-beta-lactamase-1 (NDM-1)) and other Gram-negative organisms have become highly resistant to many if not all antibiotics. These multi-resistant organisms pose a major global health hazard. They cause the same infections as sensitive Gram-negative organisms, i.e. urinary, biliary, and intra-abdominal sepsis, but fail to respond to conventional antibiotics. In many countries such organisms have entered the food chain through water and food and are selected out as the predominant bowel organisms by antibiotic treatment. They are usually carried harmlessly, but should be considered when infections fail to respond to treatment. Microbiology investigations may be essential to establish sensitivity.
- *Stenotrophomonas maltophilia* and other environmental pseudomonads are may become important in critically ill patients, particularly those with intravascular lines, ventilation, and who have also received broad spectrum antibiotics. These organisms are also multiply resistant, although co-trimoxazole is the treatment of choice for *Stenotrophomonas*.
- Vancomycin- and teicoplanin-resistant *Enterococcus faecium* are important in certain hospital units. Linezolid is active against these organisms.
- Multiply resistant gonococci; fluoroquinolone-resistant typhoid bacilli (*Salmonella typhi*) and tetracycline-resistant scrub typhus (*Orientia tsutsugamushi*) all require expert management.
- *Acinetobacter baumannii* is an intrinsically multiresistant bacterium associated with some recent blast victims from Afghanistan and Iraq. It has caused some nosocomial outbreaks.
- *Rhodococcus equi* can cause severe lung disease in HIV-immunocompromised people, and *Arcanobacterium haemolyticum* causes bacterial pharyngitis. Both are diphtheria-like bacteria.
- Emerging rickettsia-like organisms include *Ehrlichia chaffeensis* which causes human monocytic ehrlichiosis, *Anaplasma phagocytophilum* (human granulocytic anaplasmosis), and *Ehrlichia ewingii* (human granulocytic ehrlichiosis) are rare pathogens. Diagnosis is available by PCR at the Rare and Imported Pathogens laboratory, Public Health England.

Other emerging pathogens

- *Cyclosporiasis*: since 1996, the coccidian protozoan, *Cyclospora cayetanesis*, has been increasingly recognized as a cause of giardiasis/cryptosporidiosis-like GI symptoms in travellers. There have been some epidemics related to imported berries, herbs, and salads.
- *Balamuthia mandrillaris* is a free-living amoeba of tropical fresh water environments that can cause devastating cutaneous, nasal, and intracerebral disease.
- *Microsporidiasis*: many species of protozoan *Microsporidia* (e.g. *Encephalitozoon* spp.) are now recognized as causes of keratoconjunctivitis and GI, biliary, urinary, and respiratory tract, and muscle infections in severely immunocompromised people.

Sexually transmitted infections

Definition
Any disease transmitted by sexual contact.

Epidemiology
Sexually transmitted infections (STIs), although mostly curable, are often asymptomatic, are easily transmissible, can cause serious complications, and can affect anybody.

Incidence
The exact data for infections worldwide is unknown, although the WHO estimated 499 million new cases of curable STIs globally in 2011, with the largest numbers in South/South-East Asia, sub-Saharan Africa, Latin America, and the Caribbean.

Causes
Of the eight main infections transmitted sexually, four are curable; bacterial STIs *Chlamydia trachomatis, Neisseria gonorrhoeae,* and syphilis (*Treponema pallidum*), and *Trichomonas vaginalis* (a parasitic flagellate protozoan). The remaining four are incurable though preventable and treatable viral STIs; human immunodeficiency virus (HIV), herpes simplex virus (HSV), human papilloma virus (HPV or warts), and hepatitis B. Hepatitis types A and C can also be transmitted sexually.

Risk factors
Any unprotected sexual contact, including skin-to-skin contact (for HSV and HPV), and fluid-to-fluid contact.

Prevention
Must be considered prior to travel:
- Hepatitis A vaccination (usually two injections 6 months apart) (➔ Hepatitis A, p. 33).
- Hepatitis B vaccination (usually four injections over 6 months) (➔ Hepatitis B, p. 34).
- Abstinence if possible.
- Avoid sexual contact with higher risk groups (e.g. sex workers).
- Barrier contraception/condoms—take them with you. Condoms purchased abroad may not conform to British safety standards and are often smaller and so may break.
- Protected oral sex: some infections (e.g. chlamydia and gonorrhoea) can also be carried in the throat and can be transmitted this way. Hepatitis A can be transmitted through oral–anal routes. Use flavoured condoms and dental dams (squares of latex for oral–vaginal/oral–anal contact).

Treatment
For up-to-date STI treatment guidelines see the website of the British Association for Sexual Health and HIV (BASHH): ℘ http://www.bashh.org

Sexual assault
See ◗ Sexual assault, p. 165.

Urethral discharge

Definition
Pus/fluid coming from the urethral orifice in the glans penis.

Causes
Most common causes are chlamydia, gonorrhoea, and non-specific urethritis (NSU). HSV can also cause urethral discharge, but would usually be accompanied by painful genital sores/blisters.

Organisms
Chlamydia
- Caused by bacterium *Chlamydia trachomatis.*
- Transmitted via oral/vaginal/anal contact, or direct inoculation of infected secretions from one mucous membrane to another.
- 50% of men asymptomatic.
- Typically clear/white urethral discharge ± dysuria.

Gonorrhoea
- Caused by bacterium *Neisseria gonorrhoeae.*
- Transmitted via oral/vaginal/anal contact, or direct inoculation of infected secretions from one mucous membrane to another.
- 10% of men asymptomatic.
- Typically yellow/green urethral discharge ± dysuria.

Non-specific urethritis (NSU)
(Assuming chlamydia and gonorrhoea are not the cause).
- Up to 30% have no bacterial pathogen.
- Possible causes are *Trichomonas vaginalis* (1–17%), *Mycoplasma genitalium* (20%), urinary tract infection, candida, foreign bodies, chemical irritation (e.g. soaps, washing powders).
- Typically clear/white discharge may only be present on urethral massage ± dysuria.

Investigations
These depend on the equipment available. Ideally, a Gram-stained urethral smear to confirm diagnosis of gonorrhoea and NSU, leucocyte esterase diptick for NSU on first catch urine, nucleic acid amplification test (NAAT) test on a first catch urine for *Chlamydia* and gonorrhoea, and culture on urethral swab for gonorrhoea.

Management
- Avoid sexual contact to prevent further transmission.
- Ensure partner(s) are informed and treated prophylactically.
- Ideally, test the patient as soon as possible to avoid STI complications.
- Consider treating if investigations are not possible and there is uncomplicated infection (no testicular pain, no eye symptoms).
- If patient is treated, suggest full STI screen when returns home.

Treatment

BASHH guidelines suggest:

- *Chlamydia*: doxycycline 100 mg twice a day for 1 week (beware photosensitivity) *or* azithromycin 1 g stat *or* erythromycin 500 mg four times a day for 7 days (less efficacious than doxycycline and more likely to cause side effects).
- Gonorrhoea: ceftriaxone 500mg IM (or other 3rd-generation cephalosporin) *plus* treatment for chlamydia is current global recommendation. Other regimens include cefixime 400mg PO stat *or* ciprofloxacin 500 mg PO stat *plus* treatment for chlamydia *but* high resistance worldwide.
- NSU: treat as for chlamydia. Avoid soaps etc. to genital area.
- If treating blind, consider drug regimen that could treat chlamydia and gonorrhoea plus UTI such as ofloxacin 200 mg twice daily for 1 week.

Complications

- Epididymo-orchitis—inflammation of one or both testes (presentation usually with unilateral testicular pain).
- Sexually acquired reactive arthritis (SARA)—immune response in the joints to a bacterial STI, causing pain ± swelling and stiffness at one or more joints.
- Conjunctivitis.
- (Uncommon) gonococcal metastatic septicaemic arthritis and skin lesions.

Vaginal discharge

Definition: fluid coming from the vagina. A 'normal' vaginal discharge is usually clear/milky, does not smell, may change during a woman's cycle, and keeps the vagina healthy. Changes in vaginal discharge that may indicate a problem are:

- Increase in amount.
- Change in colour or smell.
- Irritation, itchiness, soreness, or burning.

Causes and symptoms

See Table 15.2.

Investigations

Microscopy of Gram-stained vaginal smears may allow diagnosis of gonorrhoea, *Candida*, and bacterial vaginosis. Direct observation by a wet smear for *Trichomonas*. Ideally more complicated lab tests are employed if they are available, i.e. nucleic acid amplification tests (NAAT) for chlamydia and gonorrhoea.

Management

- Avoid sexual contact to prevent further transmission.
- Ensure partner(s) are informed and treated prophylactically.
- Ideally, test the patient as soon as possible to avoid STI complications.
- Suggest testing rather than treating blind if possible.
- Consider treating blind if confident of diagnosis (e.g. patient has had same previously) and suitable medication available.
- If patient treated, suggest full STI screen when returns home.

Table 15.2 Vaginal discharge causes and symptoms

Infection	Typical symptoms
Chlamydia	70% asymptomatic
	Purulent vaginal discharge, dysuria, intermenstrual/ post-coital bleeding, low abdominal pain
Gonorrhoea	50% asymptomatic
	Increased/change in discharge (especially colour and smell), low abdominal pain
Trichomonas vaginalis	10–50% asymptomatic
	Change in vaginal discharge (varying thickness, sometimes frothy, often yellow/green), vulval irritation, dysuria, offensive odour
Bacterial vaginosis	Thin/watery, white/grey, homogeneous, offensive, fishy-smelling discharge. Not STI
Candidiasis (thrush)	Thick, white, curdy 'cottage cheese' discharge, vulval itching, soreness, and erythema. Vulval fissures, external dysuria. Not STI

Treatment

BASHH guidelines suggest:
- *Chlamydia*: doxycycline 100 mg twice a day for 1 week (beware photosensitivity) *or* azithromycin 1 g stat.
- Gonorrhoea: ceftriaxone 500 mg IM (or other 3rd-generation cephalosporin) *plus* treatment for chlamydia is current global recommendation. Other regimens include cefixime 400 mg PO stat *or* ciprofloxacin 500 mg PO stat *plus* treatment for chlamydia *but* high resistance worldwide.
- *Trichomonas*: metronidazole 2 g orally stat.
- Bacterial vaginosis: only treat if symptomatic—metronidazole 400 mg twice a day for 5 days.
- Avoid soaps/shower gels/scented products to genital area.
- *Candida*: clotrimazole pessary (varying dosages), clotrimazole cream *or* fluconazole 150 mg stat capsule. Avoid soaps/shower gels/scented products to genital area, avoid tight-fitting clothes. Oral treatments and cream are preferable on expedition.

Complications

Untreated *Chlamydia*/gonorrhoea can lead to:
- Pelvic inflammatory disease (PID) (➜ Pelvic inflammatory disease, p. 395)—upper genital tract inflammation, causes low abdominal pain, pyrexia, systemic illness.
- Possible infertility owing to scarring/blocking of fallopian tubes.
- SARA—immune response in the joints due to a bacterial STI, causing pain ± swelling and stiffness at one or more joints.
- Conjunctivitis.
- (Uncommon) gonococcal metastatic septicaemic arthritis and skin lesions.

Genital sores and ulcers

Open wounds of skin or mucous membrane in genital area. If lesion originates from sexual contact causative organisms are likely to be syphilis or genital herpes (Table 15.3).

Syphilis

Caused by bacterium *Treponema pallidum*, it is currently increasing in Western countries.

There are three stages:

- Early (primary, secondary, and early latent <2 years).
- Late (late latent >2 years).
- Tertiary (with neurological and cardiovascular involvement).

Syphilis is transmitted via oral/vaginal/anal contact, blood-to-blood contact, or mother-to-baby contact (vertical transmission).

The incubation period is 9–90 days for primary symptoms.

Genital herpes

- Caused by herpes simplex virus type 1 or 2.
- Transmitted via skin-to-skin contact (oral/vaginal/anal).
- Incubation period is typically 2–10 days but can be years.

Investigations/diagnosis

For experienced medical practitioners, visual diagnosis is possible. Dark ground microscopy from lesions in early syphilis can confirm infection, otherwise serological test for *Treponema pallidum* is performed. Early false negatives are possible, so repeat if there is high clinical suspicion. HSV viral culture from swab from genital lesions is ideal.

Management

- Avoid sexual contact to prevent further transmission.
- Test patient as soon as possible to avoid complications if STI present.
- Suspected syphilis needs infection confirmation, specialized medical attention, and supervised treatment.
- Consider self-treating herpes if the patient gives a history of HSV, and there appears to be uncomplicated infection (no urinary retention).
- Avoid sharing towels/flannels as there is a very slight risk of transmission.

Treatment

BASHH guidelines suggest:

- *Early syphilis:* benzathine benzylpenicillin 2.4 MU IM *or* (if penicillin allergy) doxycycline 100 mg PO twice a day for 14 days. Treatment differs in pregnancy, if neurological/ophthalmic involvement in early syphilis and in late latent syphilis.
- *Herpes:* treatment needs to be started within 5 days of the first symptoms. Aciclovir 200 mg five times per day for 5 days *or* famciclovir 250 mg three times per day for 5 days *or* valaciclovir 500 mg twice per day for 5 days *and* saline bathing, topical anaesthetic agents, analgesia.

Table 15.3 Genital sores and ulcers

Infection	Typical symptoms
Syphilis	Primary: single, painless, indurated ulcer (chancre) with a clean base discharging clear serum. Regional lymphadenopathy
	Secondary: multisystemic involvement, generalized polymorphic rash, often affecting palms and soles
Genital herpes	Painful blisters/sores and ulceration of genital/perianal area. May be accompanied by burning, tingling, itching, dysuria, and urethral/vaginal discharge. Systemic symptoms of fever are common in primary infection. Chronic condition, symptoms can recur

Complications
- Syphilis—reactions to treatment (Jarisch–Herxheimer/anaphylaxis).
- Herpes—urinary retention, secondary bacterial infection.

Differential diagnoses
- Behçet's disease (chronic immune condition. Symptoms of mouth ulcers ± genital ulcers, skin lesions, eye and joint inflammation).
- Chancroid (caused by bacteria *Haemophilus ducreyi*, mainly found in developing third world countries).
- Trauma—possible cause if patient recalls specific incident.

Genital lumps and other sexually transmitted infections
See Table 15.4.

Table 15.4 Genital lumps and other sexually transmitted infections: causes and symptoms

Infection	Typical symptoms
Genital warts	Small, pink/white lumps, sometimes 'cauliflower-shaped', itchy, usually painless. Visually same as warts elsewhere
Molluscum contagiosum	Small, round, 'spots', often have white head or small dimple in centre
Folliculitis	Infected hair follicle causing painful pus-filled swellings in genital area, erythema; may have yellow head

Genital warts
- Caused by human papilloma virus (HPV).
- Transmitted through sexual contact (including skin-to-skin contact).
- Treated with cryotherapy, podophyllotoxin 'paint', or imiquimod.
- Psychological distress is the main difficulty; treatment can wait until repatriation as complications are unlikely.

Molluscum contagiosum
- Caused by species of molluscipoxvirus.
- Transmitted through sexual contact (including skin-to-skin contact).
- Avoid sharing towels/flannels/clothing.
- Treatment (if required) with cryotherapy.
- Psychological distress is the main difficulty; treatment can wait until repatriation as complications are unlikely (but can get secondary bacterial infection).

Folliculitis
- Often bacterial cause.
- Common in areas that rub, e.g. buttocks and groin.
- May burst by itself; keep area clean, saline bathing.
- Treat with antibiotics considered if no improvement.

Human immunodeficiency virus and prevention

Definition

HIV is a retrovirus that suppresses the body's immune response, and is responsible for acquired immune deficiency syndrome (AIDS), a collection of specific opportunistic infections.

Incidence

HIV disproportionately affects sex workers, men who have sex with men, and people who inject drugs. There were an estimated 34 million living with HIV at the end of 2011, 50% unknowingly, with 2.5 million new infections that year. The areas with the highest prevalence of HIV are sub-Saharan Africa, South-East Asia, Russia, the Caribbean, and South America. See UNAIDS for excellent incidence data.

Transmission

HIV is present in blood (including menstrual blood), semen, and vaginal fluids. Transmission can occur if infected fluids pass between people. There are three main routes of transmission:
- Unprotected sexual contact (including oral sex).
- Blood-to-blood contact.
- Mother-to-baby.

Risk factors
- Unprotected sexual contact.
- Injecting drug use/sharing injecting equipment.
- Needlestick injuries/contaminated sharps.
- Contaminated blood products.
- Mucous membrane exposure (e.g. splash of blood/semen/vaginal fluid into the eye).

HIV prevention
- Abstinence from sexual activity.
- Safe sex—condom use for all sexual activity (see ➲ Prevention, p. 506).
- Avoid sexual contact with higher risk groups (e.g. sex workers, high-incidence countries).
- Ensure safe injecting equipment/sharps—take your own with you.

Post-exposure prophylaxis
Consider as a last measure where all other methods of HIV prevention have failed. This comprises a 4-week course of antiretroviral (anti-HIV) medication, started up to 72 h (but ideally ASAP) after possible exposure to attempt to abort HIV infection. It is not guaranteed to work, and medication usually has significant side effects. It was previously used for healthcare workers following needlestick injuries from HIV-positive patients, but is now also considered after sexual exposure (PEPSE; see Table 15.5).

Table 15.5 Situations in which PEPSE would be considered[1]

Sexual activity	Source status			
	HIV-positive viral load detectable	HIV positive viral load undetectable	Unknown, high prevalence group/area	Unknown, low prevalence group/area
Receptive anal sex	Recommended	Recommended	Recommended	Not recommended
Insertive anal sex	Recommended	Not recommended	Consider	Not recommended
Receptive Vaginal sex	Recommended	Not recommended	Consider	Not recommended
Insertive vaginal sex	Recommended	Not recommended	Consider	Not recommended
Fellatio with ejaculation	Consider	Not recommended	Not recommended	Not recommended
Fellatio without ejaculation	Not recommended	Not recommended	Not recommended	Not recommended
Splash of semen into eye	Consider	Not recommended	Not recommended	Not recommended
Cunnilingus	Not recommended	Not recommended	Not recommended	Not recommended

1 Clinical Effectiveness Group (BASHH) (2006). UK Guideline for the use of post-exposure prophylaxis for HIV following sexual exposure. *Int J STD AIDS*, 17, 81–92.

The currently recommended drug regime is Truvada® one tablet once daily plus Kaletra® two tablets twice daily or four tablets once daily for 28 days (for latest updates refer to ℘ http://www.bashh.org.uk). Treatment is very expensive (approximately £1000 for 28 days), so 'starter packs' of 3–5 days could be taken on expedition with immediate repatriation to continue treatment. If the expedition does not have PEPSE, some countries may have the recommended drugs available to buy—seek advice in the local area.

Common side effects are diarrhoea, nausea, and vomiting, so antiemetics (domperidone 10–20 mg three times a day when required) and anti-diarrhoeals (loperamide 4 mg stat followed by 2 mg after each loose motion to maximum of 12 mg in 24 h) may be needed.

Risk-benefit analysis should be undertaken and decisions made in each case. Consider whether the person might already be infected with HIV and their ability to adhere to (vital) and tolerate the drug regimen, especially in remote areas. (See Table 15.6.)

Table 15.6 Risk of HIV transmission following an unprotected sexual exposure from a known HIV positive individual (℘ http://www.bashh. org/documents/4076.pdf)

Type of exposure	Estimated median (range) risk of HIV transmission per exposure
Receptive anal intercourse	1.11% (0.042–3.0%)
Insertive anal intercourse	0.06% (0.06–0.065%)
Receptive vaginal intercourse	0.1% (0.004–0.32%)
Insertive vaginal intercourse	0.082% (0–0.004%)
Receptive oral sex (fellatio)	0.02% (0–0.004%)
Insertive oral sex (receiving fellatio)	0%

Chapter 16

Psychological and psychiatric problems

Section editor
James Moore

Contributors
Claire Davies
Karen Forbes
Debbie Hawker
James Moore
Marc Shaw
Jon Dallimore (1st edition)
Michael E. Jones (1st edition)
Ian Palmer (1st edition)

Introduction: psychological and psychiatric problems *516*
Stressors in the wilderness *517*
Considerations before departure *518*
Psychiatric conditions *522*
Psychological reactions to traumatic events *526*
Post-traumatic stress disorder *530*
Serious psychological threats *534*
Recreational drugs and alcohol *538*
After the expedition *540*

Introduction: psychological and psychiatric problems

Expeditions by definition involve travel, usually into remote areas, and include activities unlikely to form part of a normal working week. Any change from the normal pattern of life can be stressful, and participants must adapt to a multitude of novel experiences, enjoyable and otherwise. Most fit, healthy, and well-prepared individuals should adapt readily to the physical and psychological effects of stress, but occasionally travellers encounter circumstances that result in long-term psychological issues.

Small groups are likely to consist of companions who are previously acquainted in other settings, and an informal process of selection may have occurred. Those in larger groups may have had little or no contact with other participants prior to the journey, especially if the group has been organized as a charity trek, adventure race, or commercial expedition. The longer the expedition, the more stressful or arduous the activity, the greater is the likelihood that psychological problems will surface.

Stressors in the wilderness

The physical demands of the expedition

The physical demands of the expedition are likely to cause a lowered reserve for dealing with other stressors, including making new relationships within the group.

If participants have joined their first expedition they may be unprepared for the intensity of contact involved in sharing tents or cramped sleeping accommodation. Experienced members may be intolerant of the difficulties experienced by those unused to, e.g. close quarter living, jungle style sanitation, the reduced opportunity for keeping clean, and the absence of home comforts. In polar extremes 24-h daylight or darkness are well-recognized causes of stress, leading to illnesses such as 'seasonal affective disorder' (SAD)—a problem documented by early explorers. If possible, plan a team-building exercise before the expedition that introduces some of these stressors to observe how people may adapt to the physical demands of the expedition.

Cultural adjustment

During an expedition, contact with indigenous peoples may be limited or very intense. The opportunity for developing understanding of different cultural values may be limited by language barriers unless fluently bilingual interpreters are present.

Factors which may reduce cultural transitional stress include:
• Previous exposure to that culture and knowledge of local languages.
• Understanding cultural adaptation and local values and customs.
• A flexible, resourceful temperament, and the ability to tolerate ambiguity with a good sense of humour.

All these factors should be borne in mind when screening potential expedition team members.

Pre-existing problems

Increasing numbers of individuals with a prior medical history of mental health problems are undertaking expeditions, and this can result in problems during the expedition and possibly a need for repatriation. Problems are most likely if members have a pre-existing psychological morbidity that was either not declared, or considered unimportant, during the selection process (see this chapter; ➔ Creating expedition teams, p. 26; ➔ Medical screening, p. 46).

Considerations before departure

Assessing vulnerability

Some form of psychological health screening of potential expedition members is highly desirable and becomes increasingly important for longer expeditions. An acute psychosis, although rare, may cripple the progress of an expedition until repatriation can be organized. Losing a member of the team because of illness may affect the overall skills of the group.

No screening process will ever distinguish perfectly between those who will thrive on an expedition and those who will develop problems; however the risks of serious adverse events can be reduced with some simple measures. Information should be sought from several sources.

Application forms

These should be constructed carefully so that all questions have to be answered (see ➋ Advising those with common pre-existing conditions, p. 50). GPs completing medical forms should be informed that any prior psychological history is fundamentally important, and that non-disclosure could be detrimental to the safety of both the applicant, and the rest of the team. Non-disclosure may invalidate medical insurance. However, it is also important to stress that disclosure of mental health issues is primarily to enable individuals to prepare for the rigours of expedition life and not necessarily to prevent them from participating.

Work references

Work references are particularly important because they are provided by people in regular contact with the candidate who see them when they are not trying to create a specific impression.

Interviews

Interviews should be at the core of any selection process. Panel members must include those involved in the expedition, individuals who have previous experience in the field in similar situations, and are aware of small group dynamics and their influence on morale and psychology of the group. The interview can include:

- *Employment history*: relationships at work and the reasons for job changes should be explored. Candidates who give up easily may not be the best team members for a physically and psychologically demanding expedition.
- *Personal and family mental health history:* the assessor should ask about any consultations with the GP for any form of emotional ill health and any previous referrals for psychiatric help or counselling, as well as any untreated episodes.
- *Substance abuse:* any abuse of alcohol or drugs should be noted. Insight into any past difficulties, and healthy strategies for dealing with any future problems would balance concerns about previous substance abuse.
- *Adaptability and resilience to deal with stressful events:* it can be helpful to ask the candidate to describe how they have been affected by stress in the past. What sort of things do they find stressful? What are their

vulnerability points and their coping mechanisms? How adaptable are they to change?

- *Personal relationships*: individuals have many different motivations for embarking on an expedition. Recent relationship failures are often cited as motivation for adventure. Although individuals may feel mentally stable, their coping mechanisms for the rigours of an expedition may be weakened.

Unsuitability due to mental health history

Each expedition will be different, and the ability to help those with complex psychological needs will depend on the location, purpose, duration, staffing levels, and medical competence of the team.

- *Serious mental illness*: includes schizophrenia, bipolar disorder, hypomania, severe depression or anxiety. People with schizophrenia are more prone to psychotic breakdown when their environment is altered; bipolar and manic disorders often require potent medication for control, and failure to take medication may lead to relapse. Those on lithium need access to laboratory monitoring and are at risk of lithium toxicity in the event of dehydration. Expeditions tend to be stressful, and are not suitable for most people with serious mental illness.
- *Untreated psychological disorder*: any current psychological disorders should have been treated and followed by a symptom-free period where the individual has been able to cope with other stressful situations.
- *Anxiety*, depression or panic attacks: repeated episodes of anxiety and depression will raise concern.
- *Recent loss*: following recent bereavement, divorce, or broken relationship, it is wise to delay before making a potentially stressful trip.
- *Eating disorders* (➔ Pre-expedition preparation, p. 519): previous anorexia nervosa or bulimia nervosa must have been controlled for a year or two such that the applicant has healthy eating routines, does not engage in self-induced vomiting or laxative abuse, and is maintaining a satisfactory BMI.
- *Deliberate self-harm and previous suicide attempts*: a recent psychiatrist's report may be required to ensure that the individual is safe to travel to a remote area, has resolved any outstanding issues, and will not be a risk to themselves.
- *Drug or alcohol abuse*: a period of abstinence and recovery of 1 year is suggested following a rehabilitation programme.

Pre-expedition preparation

As with any other pre-existing medical condition, individuals with a mental illness should have coping mechanisms and appropriate treatment planned prior to departure. In some instances it might be prudent to create a contract between the individual, the team leader and a medical professional detailing:

- What is considered acceptable behaviour whilst on expedition.
- What individuals should do if they feel they are struggling to cope.
- The consequences of crossing any pre-determined boundaries.

For example, for a person with anorexia nervosa:
- Agree a pre-arranged acceptable calorie intake.
- Agree that if unable to maintain the pre-arranged food input, the individual will discuss this issue with a named individual.
- Agree treatment strategies and a plan of action: e.g. communication with relative/counsellor via satellite phone, dietary changes, or change in level of activity.
- Agree that failure to respond to pre-agreed strategies will result in curtailing of expedition activities, followed by repatriation.

All parties involved should sign this agreement. It will also be necessary to review insurance policies and ensure individuals have appropriate repatriation cover.

Stresses on an expedition

Human resilience increases when basic needs are attended to: food and water, shelter, rest, and time for recreation. Poor living conditions and excessive tiredness result in poor decision-making. Common causes of stress include relationship problems, poor leadership, lack of control, poor understanding of roles and a lack of support. Such stressors should be explored before departure to try to match expectations to organization. Appropriate pressure leads to excitement and improves performance; although excessive pressure can cause team members to feel overwhelmed and exhausted. Strategies that can boost resilience include:
- Ensuring basic needs are met as far as possible.
- Reviewing expectations—are they realistic?
- Clarifying areas of uncertainty.
- Talking things through.
- Taking time out where possible—including for leaders.

Psychiatric conditions

Psychopathology in people working overseas, even after rigorous selection, is common, and those engaged in expeditions and other prolonged visits into wilderness locations are at risk.

Anxiety disorders

Anxiety may be generalized or focused on particular concerns such as snakebite or flying. Features are as for panic disorder (see ➲ Anxiety disorders, p. 522).

Anxiety about health is normal when travelling internationally, but can be a problem if it becomes extreme or remains, despite reassurance. It may be made worse on expeditions which are isolated from competent medical help.

Aviophobia (fear of flying) is experienced by up to 20% of air passengers. Behavioural therapy and, in particular, systematic desensitization, is a very effective treatment, and medication such as beta blockers or one-off doses of benzodiazepines can complement physical techniques and cognitive strategies to overcome the fear. There are several UK-based courses such as ℘ http://www.virtualjetcentre.co.uk/fear-of-flying (South west) or ℘ http://www.gatwick-airport-uk.info/fear-of-flying.htm

Panic disorder is the presence of recurrent panic attacks; a discrete period of intense fear or discomfort, involving at least four of the following symptoms:
• Palpitations.
• Sweating, shaking.
• Shortness of breath or feeling of choking.
• Chest pain.
• Nausea/abdominal symptoms.
• Dizziness.
• Feelings of unreality or being detached from oneself.
• Fear of losing control or going crazy.
• Fear of dying.
• Numbness or tingling sensations.
• Chills or hot flushes.

Management of anxiety or panic consists of calm reassurance and, in the case of rapid breathing, breathing in-and-out of a paper bag, cupped hands or abdominal breathing (all intended to help slow breathing down). If symptoms persist, an expert opinion should be sought. Anxiolytic drugs, psychological therapies, or both may be advised.

Depression

It is important to distinguish clinical depression from the low mood which all people experience from time to time. Homesickness, concerns about how one may cope, environmental stressors, and fatigue may all produce similar symptoms during an expedition. Depression may follow a clear trigger such as bereavement but it may have no obvious precipitant. Characteristic features of clinical depression include:
• Low mood (particularly in the morning).
• Lack of motivation and low energy levels.

- Poor sleep, particularly early morning wakening.
- Persistent weepiness.
- Preoccupation with worries or feelings of guilt.
- Excessive alcohol consumption.
- Possible suicidal thoughts. Those with active plans for suicide are at high risk. Asking about suicidal plans does not increase the risk of the person harming themselves.

Management of depressed people is likely to require expert help in the form of psychological therapy and/or medication, particularly if there are suicidal features. Repatriation may be required.

Psychosis and acute confusional states

Psychoses are severe mental illnesses and are rare, but they can develop while travelling and may be provoked by medication such as mefloquine (Lariam®) or illicit drugs such as marihuana, amphetamines, and cocaine. However, it is important to remember that physical illness may be the cause for abnormal behaviour: see ➲ Delirium/confusion, p. 252.

- Protozoal tropical infections—cerebral malaria, African trypanosomiasis (sleeping sickness), and amoebic dysentery.
- Bacterial infections—typhoid and meningitis.
- Other causes—hypoglycaemia, head injury, viral encephalitis, hypo/ hyperthemia

Features of psychosis/acute confusion include:
- Bizarre behaviour.
- Paranoia.
- Disinhibition.
- Hallucinations, delusions.
- Thought disorder.
- Pressure of speech.
- Disorientation in time, place, or person.
- Lack of insight.
- In practice it may be difficult to distinguish between physical and psychiatric illness. Absence of fever, orientation in time and place, and auditory hallucinations tend to point towards a psychiatric problem. Visual hallucinations tend to indicate physical illness.

A psychotic or confused patient may not be cooperative with treatment or safety procedures. Approaches to increase engagement include:
- Maintaining a calm environment.
- Repeated gentle persuasion.
- Explaining what is happening.
- Acknowledging that the situation may be frightening for them.
- Treating them as normally as possible.
- Avoiding restraint unless vital for their own safety.

Someone with an acute psychotic illness should be evacuated for expert assessment and treatment, usually with a psychotropic medication. Consider sedation with olanzapine 5–10 mg PO (available in orodispersible form). Haloperidol 0.5–3 mg two or three times daily is an alternative and can be used in delirium; it must be given with an anticholinergic such as benzhexol or procyclidine. Mental health laws differ between countries, or may be absent.

Eating disorders

Approximately 2% of adult females and occasionally males have been diagnosed with an eating disorder. The main eating disorders are:

- *Anorexia nervosa:* a conscious reduction in calorific input stemming from low self-esteem and other varied stressors. Symptoms include severe weight loss, dizziness, abdominal pain, growth of soft, fine hair (lanugo) all over the body, amenorrhoea, withdrawal—particularly at meal times, perfectionist behaviour, excessive exercising (including micro-exercising during mealtimes).
- *Bulimia nervosa:* individuals become caught in a cycle of over-eating large quantities of food, then purposefully vomit, omit food, or take laxatives as a method of 'purging'. Symptoms include halitosis, abdominal pains, irregular periods, constipation, puffy cheeks, sore throat, kidney and bowel problems.
- *Binge eating disorder (BED):* individuals consume large amounts of food in relatively short periods of time. Unlike patients with bulimia nervosa they do not purge.
- *Eating disorders not otherwise specified:* individuals who display partial signs and symptoms of the previous three eating disorders.

Eating disorders are both complex and chronic in nature. It is unlikely that issues causing these illnesses will be resolved on expedition. Successful management will hinge on the individual's concordance with either pre-arranged management plans, or those formulated whilst away. It is not unusual for the care of an individual suffering from an eating disorder to become stressful, particularly around meal times, as they seek increasingly more covert ways of reducing their calorific intake. Mealtime behaviour might include:

- Delaying eating.
- Dissecting or tearing food into tiny pieces.
- Playing with or hiding food.
- Offering food to other members of the team.

Strategies for managing mealtimes may include:

- Acknowledging the eating difficulty but reinforcing the need to start/ continue eating.
- Firm but supportive prompting.
- Ensuring others around the table act as role models.
- Maintaining contact after mealtimes, allowing food to digest, preventing opportunities for purging and an opportunity to offer support feedback.

It is important to avoid the emotional game of dietary chess, where success or failure rides on an individual's ability to hide food or make someone complete a meal. Firm but supportive care, where there is clarity of boundaries and consequent repercussions, must be paramount.

Learning and intellectual disorders

Increasing numbers of adolescents embark on youth expeditions. Between 2% and 8% of this age group have been diagnosed with a learning or intellectual disorder, so it is not uncommon to encounter these issues whilst away. Such disorders can have multiple physiological, social, and environmental components, the most common conditions being:

- *Conduct disorders (CDs):* persistent aggressive and disobedient behaviour that cannot be attributed to ordinary childhood mischief or poor behaviour. Symptoms include aggression or violence, inability to adhere to social boundaries, or a disregard for safe behaviour.
- *Attention deficit hyperactivity disorders (ADHD):* a term used to describe 2–5% of hyperactive children and adolescents who have difficulty concentrating. Symptoms include appearing constantly distracted, an inability to sit still, and poor social skills. Problems such as autism, conduct disorders, and neurological conditions are found to coexist in children with ADHD.
- *Autism spectrum conditions (ASD):* a group of conditions caused by abnormal brain development and function. Characteristics include inappropriate behaviour, poor social skills, and communication. Characteristics vary according to age and level of development. Asperger's syndrome is a common ASD, often associated with high-functioning individuals.

Preparation is the key to the effective management of learning or intellectual disabilities, but relies on individuals disclosing sensitive and often stigmatized conditions prior to departure. As with some psychological conditions, contracts detailing acceptable behaviour, boundaries and repercussions are important. Whilst away, management strategies should include:

- Encouragement, positive support, and plenty of praise.
- Consistency, fairness, and appropriate discipline.
- Breaking tasks into smaller, simpler components.
- Providing simple instructions for tasks or responsibilities.
- Avoiding food additives.

Individuals with learning or intellectual disorders are often misunderstood, feel stigmatized, and become marginalized. These issues become a barrier to effective communication and support. Fostering an atmosphere of mutual respect will maximize effective management.

See ℅ http://www.rcpsych.ac.uk/healthadvice/problemsdisorders.aspx for useful information and further reading about these conditions.

Nocturnal enuresis

1–2% of adolescents over the age of 15 suffer from bed-wetting. Although the causes can be physiological, the effects are psychological, affecting self-esteem and confidence. Whilst on an expedition individuals may attempt to control the volume of urine created by drinking less which can, in the expedition setting, lead to potentially hazardous dehydration.

Desmopressin (1-deamino-8-D-arginine vasopressin or DDAVP®) is a potent antidiuretic used in the management of nocturnal enuresis, causing increased water reabsorption in the renal tubules. If taken too often (something a nervous or embarrassed expedition member might do), or taken alongside the increased fluids often required in hot or humid climates, it can result in a significant and hazardous risk of hyponatraemia (see also → Fluid-induced hyponatraemia, p. 762).

Hyponatraemia may also be induced with the concomitant use of NSAIDs.

Psychological reactions to traumatic events

(See also ➲ Death on an expedition, p. 166; and ➲ Sexual assault, p. 165.)

Most expeditions will be completed with only minor untoward events. However, anyone taking a group into the field, particularly those responsible for young people, must be aware of how to care for the group's psychological welfare should illness, accident or, at worst, death occur. These events might occur within the group whilst on expedition, but it is also possible that leaders might be responsible for informing an expeditioner of events that have occurred at home. Possible traumatic events include:

• Death on the expedition.
• Grave illness or injury.
• A member of the team going missing.
• A hostage situation.
• Death or serious illness of a relative or close friend at home.

In some situations the whole group will have witnessed what has happened. In others, the leader may have to inform the members of the group about the traumatic event or its repercussions. Box 16.1 on 'Breaking bad news' gives some guidance on how to do this (See Box 16.1). Further details are available at: ✎ http://dartcenter.org/files/breaking_bad_news_0.pdf

When a traumatic event occurs, leaders should assume that some people may be stunned and bewildered, or react with incapacitating anxiety or hysteria. The leader and/or medic needs to identify quickly how people are reacting and use them appropriately. Those reacting effectively may be needed to help in rescue efforts or to ensure the safety of the others.

What should the leader and medic do?

In the event of a disaster, care of the victim is the first priority; however, other group members, the leader, rescuers, family and friends, and expedition organizers will all experience different psychological reactions. The psychological care of the victim and the rest of the group and self-care are the leader and medic's responsibility. They should provide accurate information in a timely fashion for the rest of the group.

Care of the victim

Whilst an ill or injured group member is awaiting evacuation, their physical comfort, security, and dignity must be maintained; e.g. ensuring they are covered and have privacy. If the person is conscious they should be kept informed of what is happening. They may be very distressed or bewildered. It is important to be patient, honest, to allow them time to talk, and to accept what may be muddled and rapidly changing thoughts and emotions, and reassure them these are normal.

If the victim is unconscious, their right to privacy and dignity must still be respected. It should also be assumed they can hear; they should have company, be kept informed, and be spared pessimistic conversations happening around them.

Psychological first aid

Psychological first aid (PFA) should be offered to the rest of the group. This includes:

- Ensuring safety (including from unhelpful rumours or media).
- Practical help, e.g. food and shelter.
- Providing information.
- Offering comfort and reassurance; calming people down.
- Discussing communications with people outside the group. Relatives and friends of everyone involved ought to receive information in an appropriately supportive manner, not through uncontrolled use of social media.
- Facilitating contact with family members.
- Listening.

An important aim is to reduce arousal levels as this will reduce the risk of post-traumatic stress disorder developing (➔ Post-traumatic stress disorder, p. 530). A free manual on PFA is available at: ☌ http://www.ptsd.va.gov/professional/manuals/psych-first-aid.asp

Care of the group

Having ensured the initial safety of the group, the leader is responsible for ensuring their needs for food, water, and shelter are met, and then for providing a supportive environment. In a small, functional group this may be relatively simple and possible on a one-to-one basis.

In a larger group, particularly if fault or blame might be apportioned around the cause of the traumatic event, the task will be more difficult and the leader might choose to arrange a debriefing meeting 24–72 h after the event, after the practicalities of medical care, evacuation, and informing relatives have been completed. The primary aim of this meeting would be to facilitate a supportive emotional environment and get a functional team home. In most instances it is inappropriate to attempt to establish causality of an event, or attribute blame, immediately after it has occurred. Many facts surrounding critical incidents only become visible after proper investigation and without the added complications of acute emotional attachment.

An operational debriefing concentrates on evaluating procedures and tasks, and dealing with practical matters. The team may also agree on the next steps (e.g. whether to continue the expedition or return home).

A critical incident debriefing provides an opportunity for the group to talk about the facts of what has happened, and their thoughts and feelings. The process is non-judgemental. Common responses to trauma are normalized, and people are taught that these usually disappear naturally with time. Information is provided about helpful coping mechanisms. Group support is encouraged, future plans are discussed, and people are told how to obtain further help if it is needed. Critical incident debriefing should not take place too soon (within 24 h of a traumatic event), and sufficient time should be allocated for the process (at least 2 h). It can occur remotely (e.g. over the Internet).

Debriefing should be facilitated by an individual with sufficient skills or experience as, done incorrectly, it can cause significant short or long-term distress.

Reactions to traumatic events or bad news

Group members witnessing or being involved in a traumatic event and an expeditioner given bad news from home may react in similar ways.

To be bereaved is to be deprived of someone or something of value. We may grieve for a person, but we may also grieve for other losses, such as friendship, hope, or our perceptions of safety and immortality. People who are grieving may have feelings of numbness, sadness, anxiety, anger, guilt, or yearning; they may experience physical sensations of a 'flight or fright' reaction, with dry mouth, hollow stomach, breathlessness, or tachycardia; they may be confused, bewildered, disbelieving, and disorientated. In close relationships they may even have auditory or visual hallucinations of the person who has died. Their behaviour may be altered, with crying, restlessness, loss of appetite, sleep disturbance, and absent-mindedness, which could compromise the individual's safety on an expedition.

The vast majority of people who are bereaved of someone close to them, or who experience a traumatic event, recover with time and the support of family and friends. Bereavement and loss are a normal part of life. In the aftermath of such an event, individuals should be reassured that the jumble of emotions, sensations, thoughts, and behaviours they are experiencing are normal and does not mean there is something wrong with them or they are 'going mad'. Expeditioners who are so distressed by grief they might compromise their own or the group's safety might have to be evacuated, but there may be good arguments for keeping a supportive group together. Evacuation may also be necessary to facilitate attendance at a funeral, which is an important part of the grieving process.

It is important to stress that difficulty with grieving or PTSD may occur even with good leadership, because of the person's pre-existing personality or mental health, or because of the nature of the event. The leader's job is to provide a supportive environment so that recovery is encouraged, where possible, and to get the team home safely.

Post-traumatic stress disorder

Symptoms of PTSD may develop after experiencing 'a stressful event of an exceptionally threatening or catastrophic nature'. Sufferers involuntarily re-experience the event or aspects of it and these 're-experiencing symptoms' may feel very real, frightening, and distressing. Victims often have recurrent flashbacks or nightmares and may avoid triggers reminding them of the event, or return continuously to why it happened or how it could have been avoided. They may have emotional numbing or be in a constant state of alertness, being fearful, irritable, easily startled, and having difficulties with concentration and sleeping. Such symptoms are normal up to 6 weeks after an incident. Persistent problems indicate the need for psychiatric or psychological input.

Who develops post-traumatic stress disorder?

The chances of developing PTSD are higher in women than men and differ according to the traumatic event. The risk of developing PTSD is highest after rape (about 20% in women), other sexual attack, being threatened with a weapon, and kidnapped or taken hostage. About 10% of people seeing accidents, death or injury, and natural disasters will go on to develop PTSD.

Psychological reactions to a crisis or tragedy

When the tragedy becomes known to the expedition, team members may go through a variety of reactions: grief, guilt, acceptance and then resolution:

- 'This can't have happened.'
- 'I don't believe it.'
- 'This is ridiculous—he was only here in this camp an hour ago.'
- 'Tell me that again!'

Psychological debriefing is the generic term for immediate interventions following trauma (usually within 3 days) that seek to relieve stress with the intent of mitigating or preventing long-term pathology. In the first days after the death of a colleague, expeditioners are advised to:

- Talk about the dead colleague, talk about the death, talk about their positive and negative feelings for their colleague. Talk about the nightmares that may result, and what these nightmares are and how they were handled.
- In the first 8 weeks expeditioners should not try to push flashbacks, intrusive images, or nightmares away. These are all ways the psyche is trying to work through and make sense of an abnormal situation.
- Advice should be given *not* to drink or indulge in recreational drugs 'more than normal', as both impede the brain's processing of the trauma.
- All within the group need to remind themselves that they are not going crazy (a common feeling) but that they are reacting normally to an abnormal situation.

- Avoidance of discussion of the incident is the single best predictor of PTSD, a condition that leads to nearly one in five sufferers committing suicide. The whole group must slowly confront the situations that they are avoiding. In the early stages after the tragedy this involves talking about the event and about the dead colleague. Such discussion may include the need or desire either to continue with the mission or to return home, and may predispose to feelings of selfishness (that turn into guilt), selflessness, remorse, blame, and whether there is willpower to go on. Collectively the expedition survivors should talk in terms of:
  - 'We were shocked.'
  - 'We thought we'd have to quit.'
  - 'We decided to continue to honour our fallen friend.'
  - 'This is what he/she would have wanted us to do.'
- Initial counselling needs to occur within the group. Symptoms of PTSD may develop several weeks after the event, and team members should then seek help through their GP or healthcare professional. The value of formal counselling in these circumstances is highly controversial; some experts feel it is essential, while others suggest it may make PTSD worse rather than better.

People are most likely to recover after a traumatic event if they experience positive and supportive responses from those around them. Blaming and negative thoughts about the event are unhelpful. Ensure basic needs are met and facilitate an open environment where the survivor can talk if needed. Forcing people to talk when they are not ready can be detrimental.

Box 16.1 Breaking bad news

S—setting up the interview

- Prepare yourself.
- Have as much information as possible.
- Think about the questions the person will ask.
- Ensure privacy, avoid interruptions.
- Involve significant others.
- Sit down.
- Make eye contact.

P—assess perception

- What do they already know?
- What do they think has happened?

I—obtain the person's invitation

- Gain permission to give more information, e.g. 'Can I tell you what happened this afternoon?' or 'I need to tell you what happened this afternoon.'

K—give knowledge and information

- Give a warning: 'I'm afraid I have some bad news for you.'
- Avoid blurting it all out—give information in small chunks.
- Avoid excessive bluntness, but be clear and avoid euphemisms.
- Check for understanding periodically.
- Respect the level of knowledge the person wants, e.g. some will just want to know the person has died while some will want to know how and why.

E—address emotions with empathic responses

- Observe for emotional responses.
- Identify the emotion and the reason for it to yourself.
- Empathize: e.g. 'I can see you are really upset.' 'This must be very difficult for you.' 'I'm so sorry this has happened.'
- Avoid 'I know how you feel': you don't.
- Give time and respect silence.
- Use touch if appropriate.

S—strategy and summary

- Summarize what has been said.
- Agree what should happen next for expedition members, e.g. does the person wish to stay on the expedition, or do they want to go home, or who would they like to 'buddy' them?

Adapted from a protocol for breaking bad news to patients with cancer. Baile WF, Buckman R, Kudelka AP, et al. (2000). SPIKES—a six-step protocol for delivering bad news. *Oncologist*, 5, 302–11.

Serious psychological threats

The most extreme psychological threats of an expedition relate to death, serious accident or illness, RTCs, mugging/assault/carjacking, or kidnapping/hostage-taking.

Unfortunately, kidnapping and hostage-taking remain prevalent in many areas of the world. They probably represent the most extreme and sustained form of psychological (and sometimes physical) abuse.

It is important to be aware of any such risks in the locations to be explored (see ℘ https://www.gov.uk/foreign-travel-advice). Clear contingency plans are advisable. A reputable 'survival in hostile region' course may help in learning how to avoid becoming captured (℘ http://www.akegroup.com). The course should include training in how to cope if kidnapping does occur.

Surviving kidnapping

All kidnappings are undertaken for gain, usually after careful surveillance. Captors are criminal and/or political; whilst of perceived value, captives of criminals are relatively safe. The fate of political hostages is less certain. Kidnappers' previous behaviour is the best predictor of outcome. Kidnapping is not personal; most victims are a pawn in another's game. The aim of those kidnapped is to survive.

Kidnapping may be conceptualized in three phases:
- Capture.
- Incarceration.
- Release.

Capture

Kidnappers obtain compliance through extreme violence, dominance, and uncertainty. Capture and release are the most dangerous times of kidnapping. If escape is unlikely, heroics should be avoided. Weapons should not be used, unless the captive is skilled in their use. Sensory deprivation may be used to isolate the captive and is disorientating, by design. After the initial shock of abduction, there may be a short-lived euphoria at having survived, followed by a pattern of enforced sensory deprivation, threats, abuse, and hardships.

On abduction:
- Be calm, composed, patient, polite, and cooperative.
- Obey all orders.
- Keep quiet unless spoken to.
- Move slowly and deliberately—ask first.
- Listen closely to what is going on.
- Keep clothes and belongings if possible.
- Rest/sleep/eat/drink whenever possible/offered.
- Inform captors of any medical requirements.

Incarceration

Immediately establish a routine that focuses on maintaining physical and mental hygiene, health, and fitness. Physical health requires eating the food and drink offered. Physical fitness improves resistance to infection, raises mood, and may allow for a successful escape attempt. Mental fitness requires awareness of uncontrollable (external) and controllable (internal, self-induced) stressors. A positive frame of mind is important. Release is the most likely outcome; someone will be working for release of hostages.

A primitive existence will develop, centred upon bodily functions, sleeping, and eating in an atmosphere of intimidation and ruthlessness. Self-questioning and blame are destructive to self-esteem and self-worth, and lead to inertia, depression, and despair. Emotional lability is common. Any pre-existing psychological or psychiatric predispositions may be triggered. Physical activity is the best counter to this.

Compassion is required for those who are not coping well. Captors' attempts to 'split' the group will severely worsen the situation for all captives. Maintaining clear lines of communication and interest in each other's welfare is protective. The intimacy engendered by enforced proximity and shared adversity may lead to deep personal attachments/ antipathies. A group leader should be appointed if taken as a group.

Captors vary in their abilities to mistreat their charges. Dehumanization promotes maltreatment. Trying to understand captors and developing rapport by active listening and drawing attention to your human needs, e.g. hunger, thirst, and bodily functions may be beneficial.

To prevent dehumanization:
- Remain calm and courteous.
- Develop rapport and negotiate (with care) for basic needs.
- Act to maintain self-respect and dignity.
- Avoid whining, begging, or arguing.
- Prepare for a long captivity.
- Seek information on captors, time, place, deadlines.
- Look for humour in all things and help each other.
- Keep the mind active: chess, writing/reciting poems, plots of plays, films, novels.
- Focus on previous good experiences.
- What to do if/when.
- Monitor body language.
- Do not believe all given information.
- Maintain religious or spiritual beliefs—without irritating others.

Release

Maintain belief in rescue, and be patient. Peaceful resolution is the default option, as violent conclusion may involve killings. Deadlines are dangerous for all parties. Any escalation of violence by kidnappers will increase the likelihood of an armed solution. Thus always assume there are plans for a forceful solution. Think ahead; obtain as much information as possible about deadlines. Armed forces are most likely to enter through windows or doors, thus stay away from portals, locate a safe place, and wait.

On hearing gunfire or explosion:
- Go to ground.
- Keep your hands visible at all times.
- Make *no* attempt to help.
- Make *no* sudden movements.

- Follow all instructions immediately.
- Rescuers will assume you are a kidnapper—expect extremely firm handling.
- Never exchange clothing with captors.

There is a natural euphoria on release. This may be tempered if locally employed individuals remain behind or were killed. Relationships formed during captivity may influence the healing process. Problems present before capture will remain unresolved. Depending on the event, consideration should be given to the competing physical, psychological, and social variables, and the variety of interested parties involved, e.g. family, friends, colleagues, employers, pressure groups, politicians, doctors, and media.[1]

Resource

See ℜ http://www.hostageuk.org for further information, including guidelines to help families cope, and advice on handling the media.

---

1 Palmer I (2004). What to do if you are taken hostage. *BMJ Career Focus*, 329, 157–8.

Recreational drugs and alcohol

Worldwide, levels of drug abuse are rising, with evidence suggesting illegal drug use in up to 1/3 of some groups of travellers. Drug use on expeditions is rare, although do not assume that expedition members are immune to inquisitive behaviour, especially if the expedition finds itself located amongst bushes of wild plants such as marihuana.

The consequences of drug misuse on expedition are considerable, ranging from life-threatening illness to life-threatening judicial sentencing. In addition, the consequences might not be confined to the individuals participating, but also to other non-participants on the expedition. Have policies on drug use and make them known before the expedition.

When managing drug abuse on expedition, consider the implications of involving local authorities, especially the police. Advice should be sought carefully and involve the expedition leadership team. However, decisions such as these should not prevent the patient from receiving life-saving hospital treatment.

General approach

The average expedition medical kit is unlikely to contain the appropriate medicines for managing an individual who is under the influence of drugs.

Immediate management

- Rapid assessment of the patient (ABCDE (see ➜ Rapid primary assessment and resuscitation, p. 214), Measure P, BP, RR, temperature, glucose level).
- Resuscitation where appropriate.
- Medical and nursing care, including:
  - Rule out organic, psychiatric, and medicinal reactions as cause of signs and symptoms of drug misuse.
  - Removal and safe storage or destruction of drugs.
  - Consider further expedition participation and repatriation of individual.

Considerations

- Drugs are not always taken alone—always consider alcohol.
- The patient's condition might change abruptly: don't get caught out.

Basic drug categories and field management

Stimulants

Field management
- Reduce hyperpyrexia.
- Consider diazepam 0.1–0.3 mg/kg PO for anxiety/agitation.

Opioids

Field management
- Airway and respiratory support.
- If RR <10: naloxone at a dose of 0.8 mg IV repeated every 2–3 min until RR ≥10.

Hallucinogenics

Management
- Mainly supportive—quiet reassurance, calm, and quiet environment.
- In severe agitation, consider sedative agents (IM lorazepam 1–2 mg and/or IM haloperidol 5–10 mg).

Hypnotics
- Nitrazepam, temazepam, flunitrazepam.

Management
- Airway and respiratory support.
- In hospital, effects antagonized by flumazenil.

Alcohol
- Alcohol misuse is a leading cause of preventable death/illness either via excessive ingestion or as a co-factor in accidents. Be aware that alcohol is illegal in some countries with strict penalties for possession. Excessive alcohol consumption may also be culturally unacceptable in some areas.
- Alcohol is a problem when an individual's consumption has a recurrent adverse effect on day-to-day activities including those of others. Even small amounts of alcohol can adversely affect perception, reaction time, and decision-making. Traditional/home-made alcohol may be of unpredictable potency and purity posing additional risks.
- Policies on alcohol should be made clear at the outset of the expedition including what code of conduct is expected of participants.
- Individuals with alcohol dependence are unlikely to have declared this during the medical screening process. Sudden alcohol withdrawal symptoms are a real possibility on expeditions where access to alcohol is limited or not possible.

Management of alcohol withdrawal
- Consider offering a benzodiazepine or carbamazepine.
- If these are unavailable and the patient is becoming increasingly agitated, one could consider providing small quantities of an alcoholic drink to prevent acute withdrawal symptoms.
- Lorazepam can be used for the treatment of delirium tremens.
- Beware of the risk of acute alcohol withdrawal seizures.

After the expedition

For the majority, expeditions are positive experiences that enhance self-esteem and, in young people, contribute to maturity. Expeditions will change all those involved; the individual and those they interact with at work, socially, and at home. It takes time for the 'system' to readjust to the returnee and vice versa. Readjustment requires acceptance, adjustment, and accommodation. Prepare people that a period of 'reverse culture shock' is normal and this may include a period of mourning. Reconnection with enjoyable activities at home and contact with other expedition members is helpful. Accept that change is irrevocable and inevitable but not necessarily negative.

Severe problems persisting for >3 months or those interfering with day to day function merit the following:

- Full physical and mental state examination and appropriate treatment. Persistent physical symptoms for which there is no demonstrable organic cause occur regularly amongst expatriates, including those who have been on expeditions. It is vital that physical causes are thoroughly excluded with a detailed medical history and physical examination and appropriate investigations. Once this process is complete, other factors which may be generating symptoms can be explored.
- Where appropriate, referral to general practitioner and/or counsellor with experience in psychiatric problems associated with travel and/or traumatic illness and injury. For example: ℘ https://www.interhealthworldwide.org

Resource

A WHO web-based guide to the management of stress disorders can be found at: ℘ http://www.ncbi.nlm.nih.gov/books/NBK159725

Chapter 17

Risks from animals

Contributor
David A. Warrell

Animals that can cause severe trauma 542
Treatment of trauma caused by animals 548
Venomous land animals 550
Venomous marine animals 566
Poisonous fish and shellfish 574

Animals that can cause severe trauma

Animals, wild and domesticated, especially large ones, should always be treated with great respect and not approached unnecessarily. Popular TV wildlife programmes have tended to diminish our perception of the risk posed to travellers by giant pachyderms and apex predators. Tigers, lions, leopards, and other big cats, hyenas, domestic dogs, jackals, wolves, bears, elephants, rhinos, hippopotamuses, buffaloes, bison, wild and domestic cattle, moose, elk, other large deer and antelopes, domestic and wild pigs, rams, tapirs, chimpanzees, baboons, ostriches, cassowaries, and even ferrets have killed people.

Learn about the likely hazards by asking the local residents. Be vigilant at all times. Beware of wandering alone and unprotected, especially between dusk and dawn when most attacks by large mammals occur. Travel in groups, do not stray from vehicles, and do not take dogs with you; they attract large predators. A competent look-out armed with a large-calibre rifle (0.375 or more) is essential if you are working in the open where big game animals roam. However, firearms can become a danger and a liability unless they are in the hands of an experienced warden, ranger, or hunter.

Bears

All bears, even giant pandas, are potentially dangerous carnivores. Mothers with cubs are responsible for 80% of attacks on people. In North America, where backpackers and campers in national parks are victims of daytime/evening attacks, black bears (*Ursus americanus*) were responsible for about 5.8 attacks and 0.3 deaths/year, while brown bears (*U. arctos*), including grizzlies and Kodiak bears, were responsible for about 1.65 attacks and 0.6 deaths/year in the 1990s. Brown bears also kill and injure people in Romania, Scandinavia, and other parts of Europe. Asian sloth bears (*Melursus ursinus*) killed 48 people and injured 687 in Madya Pradesh, India (1989–94).

Prevention

In bear country, hikers should travel in groups, making plenty of noise so that bears are not taken by surprise. Never go too close (e.g. to photograph them), especially when there are cubs about and keep away from carrion and garbage tips that attract scavenging bears. Warning signs that the bear is irritated include standing up, hissing or growling, yawning, and head swinging. If a bear approaches or charges you, avoid eye contact and do not attempt to hide, run away, or climb a tree. When it is within a distance of 30 feet, it may be repelled by discharging a pepper spray (10% capsicum oleoresin) towards its eyes. If this fails and the attacker is a grizzly bear, roll into a ball, interlocking your hands behind your neck, protecting your face with your elbows, and your back with your backpack. Stay in this position for long enough to ensure that the bear has gone away. If the attacker is a black bear, growl, shout, and fight back with any available weapon. Do not store food in camp but hang it in a tree >100 yards/m away, >14 ft (4 m) from the ground and >4 ft (1.25 m) away from the tree trunk.

Polar bear

Polar bears (*U. maritimus*) are the most predatory, aggressive, and dangerous of all bears, killing six people in Canada (1965–85), and attacking 50 people in Svalbard (Spitzbergen, Norway) (1973–86) (➲ Wildlife in cold regions, p. 610). In Arctic regions, keep a look out for these increasingly hungry animals. Travel in groups, carry a firearm (calibre 0.308 or 12-bore shot gun) and flares, and know how to use them. If you see a bear, make a lot of noise, keep as far away as possible, and remain up wind so that it senses your presence and will not be startled by your sudden appearance. If the bear approaches, fire a flare or warning shot, but at 25 m shoot to kill if it continues to advance. Protect camps with bear fences with trip wires, take it in turn to be on bear watch and use guard dogs. At close quarters, use pepper spray, hit the bear on its nose or shoot it.

Websites

℘ http://www.canadianrockies.net/backpack.html#bear
℘ http://kho.unis.no/doc/Polar_bears_Svalbard.pdf

Big cats

Attacks by lions, tigers, leopards, American mountain lions (cougar, puma), jaguars, and other large felines are increasing in many areas.

Lion

In Kenya and Tanzania there were historical epidemics of fatal attacks by man-eaters. Between 1990 and 2005, 563 human deaths and 308 injuries were reported in south-east Tanzania. Lions are attracted to farms by marauding bush-pigs but end up killing farmers sleeping in shelters in their fields.

Mountain lion (puma, cougar)

In North America, there are an average of 5.6 mountain lion attacks and 0.8 deaths each year.

Tiger

India is famous for its man-eaters. In the Sundarbans (India–Bangladesh border), tigers kill up to 100 people every year during daylight attacks.

Leopard

In India and Pakistan, individual man-eating leopards have claimed hundreds of lives. As human population and farmlands expand, leopards increasingly coexist, even in suburban areas, and the incidence of attacks is rising. Leopards usually attack at night and may enter dwellings.

Big cats usually attack humans from behind, seizing the head or throat and shaking the victim to break the cervical spine or biting at the base of the skull. Severe scratches are inflicted.

Prevention

Big cats are best observed from a vehicle, hide, or from the back of an elephant. Females with cubs and solitary males are the most aggressive. Firearm protection is necessary for walking safaris in dangerous areas. Long-term camps should be protected by high fencing and campfires. In the Sundarbans, wearing face-like masks on the back of the head reduced tiger attacks on villagers. If you are attacked, fight for your life, using any available weapon and making as much noise as possible.

Camels and horses

Domesticated and wild beasts of burden can lethally kick, bite, crush, and bolt! Treat them with great respect and stand well clear of the head or tail ends unless you are an expert.

Dogs and wolves

Bites by domestic and feral dogs are common worldwide. More than 200,000 patients bitten by dogs attend hospital in England and Wales each year. In the USA, each year, dogs bite 4.5 million people: 885 000 require medical attention (reconstructive surgery in 31,000) and 12 are killed. Children are especially vulnerable. Walkers and joggers in both urban and rural areas frequently encounter aggressive dogs guarding their owners' properties and strays.

Unless they are rabid, wolves usually keep away from humans and rarely attack, but there have been fatalities, especially in children, in Europe (Estonia, Poland, Spain, Russia, Belarus), Iran, India, and North America.

Prevention

Avoid dogs' territories as far as possible and do not disturb bitches with puppies or dogs that are eating or sleeping. Carry a heavy stick or club and fill your pockets with stones. If attacked, avoid eye contact and do not run away, but shout, protect yourself with your backpack, and fight back with sticks and stones.

Website

⅋ http://www.cdc.gov/ncipc/duip/biteprevention.htm

Elephants

Elephants (maximum height 4 m, weight 7000 kg) are the largest land animals and are highly dangerous. Each year, they kill about 300 people in India and 50 in Sri Lanka and Kenya. Humans may be grasped by the trunk, thrown high in the air, trampled, and then gored. A high proportion of attacks prove fatal. Elephants attack because they are guarding calves or territory, are sick, injured, frightened or, in the case of bulls, are in 'musth', episodes of increased testosterone production indicated by black oily discharge from temporal glands (between the eye and ear), urinary incontinence, priapism, green algal staining of the penis, and extreme aggression. Early warning signs of irritation before a charge are trumpeting, raised head and trunk, spread ears, swaying body, and lashing tail. 'Mock' charges and attacking charges, with lowered head and curled trunk, may be indistinguishable.

Prevention

Always treat elephants with extreme respect and caution even if they are working or performing animals. Walking safaris in elephant country are dangerous. Experienced rangers with firearms of appropriate calibre are essential. If you sight elephants, travel downwind of them, avoiding, in particular, cows with calves, and solitary bulls. If charged by an elephant, it is futile to run or try to climb a tree. The only hope is to face the animal, shout, and wave your arms. Vehicles may not provide adequate protection.

Hippopotamuses

These massive (maximum height 1.65 m, weight 4500 kg) and irritable African herbivores wallow on the beds or banks of rivers and lakes by day, remaining submerged for periods of up to 6 min. They come ashore to graze at night. Especially in Kenya, Tanzania, Niger, and Botswana, they are notorious for capsizing canoes and drowning their occupants (usually fishermen), for trampling people under foot, and, in water or on land, inflicting terrible bite wounds with their 50-cm long canines. However, they kill fewer people than elephants, lions or crocodiles.

Prevention

Avoid swimming, diving, and canoeing in hippo-infested waters. Look out for ripples suggesting a submerged animal and, when it emerges, for warning yawn and grunting. If you are in a boat, escape into deeper water. On land, never block a grazing hippo's trail or its retreat to the water and beware of cows with calves. You cannot outrun a hippo. If charged, hide behind or climb a tree.

Hyenas

Campers resting by day or sleeping in the open at night in Africa have been seized by the head and severely mauled by hyenas causing horrific head and facial injuries. Attacks and deaths are reported from Malawi, Mozambique, Ethiopia, Kenya, and elsewhere.

Pigs and peccaries

Wild, domesticated, and feral pigs are armed with sharp tusks and can attack swiftly and unexpectedly, especially in Melanesia. Penetrating abdominal injuries with prolapse and strangulation of the intestine, pneumothorax, open fractures, laceration of tendons, and artery and nerve injuries have been described.

Prevention

For protection against these lethal animals in Papua New Guinea, an expert's considered advice was: 'carry two spears'.

Crocodiles and alligators

Between 1928 and 2009, 567 encounters with alligators (*Alligator mississippiensis*) (maximum length 4.6 m, weight 453 kg) were reported in the USA, 139 provoked by handling, and 24 fatalities. Florida is worst affected. The black caiman (*Melanosuchus niger*) (maximum length 6 m, weight 1100 kg) is the most dangerous crocodilian of the Amazon region. Nile crocodiles (*Crocodylus niloticus*) (6.1 m, 900 kg) kill about 1000 people each year in Africa. A famous American infectious diseases physician was seized by a crocodile from a canoe on the Limpopo River, Botswana in March 2006, and an experienced South African tour guide was taken from a kayak on the Lukuga River, DR Congo in December 2010. In northern Australia, 27 deaths from 60 attacks by the salt water crocodile (*C. porosus*) (7 m, 2000 kg) have been reported since 1876. This species is responsible for many attacks and killings in the Purari-Kikori delta region in the Gulf of Papua New Guinea. Mass killings by crocodiles have been described in the Nile at the time of Alexander the Great, in the Second World War

(Japanese army off Ramree Island, Burma), and recently after flooding in Ethiopia. Many victims are killed outright and eaten, their bodies never recovered. Victims reaching hospital usually survive but most will require debridement, amputations, and skin grafting. Forty per cent are left with permanent deformities. Fatalities are increasing in Ethiopia, Tanzania, Malawi, and PNG. *Pseudomonas, Enterococcus, Aeromonas, Clostridium, Serratia, Citrobacter, Bacteroides, Burkholderia*, and *Vibrio*, including *V. vulnificus*, have been implicated in crocodile/alligator bite infections (see ➋ Marine wound infections, p. 294).

Prevention

Take advice from local people. Walkers should keep well away from the water's edge. Avoid footpaths by lakes, rivers, and waterfalls. Do not pitch camp too close to water, do not attract crocs by throwing in waste food, and keep children and dogs under control. Never bathe between dusk and dawn. Canoeing is hazardous in croc-infested waters. Do not trail extremities in the water. If attacked on land, run. If attacked in the water, fight back, hitting the animal on the nose and eyes with any available weapon.

Sharks

Between 2000 and 2012, 885 unprovoked attacks by sharks and 77 fatalities were reported (averages of 68 attacks and 6 deaths each year). Most attacks are in Florida, Australia, and South Africa. Surfers and wind surfers are most at risk, followed by swimmers, snorkelers, divers and waders. Great white (*Carcharodon carcharias*) (length 716 m, weight 2250 kg), tiger (*Galeocerdo cuvier*) (5.5 m, 900 kg), and bull (*Carcharhinus leucas*) (3.5 m, 360 kg) sharks are the most dangerous, but more than 70 species that grow longer than about 2 m are potentially lethal. Sharks can inflict truly appalling wounds, resulting in devastating blood loss from severed arteries, causing shock, and the risk of drowning. Common targets are buttocks, thighs, or shoulders. The rough placoid scales can cause abrasions.

Prevention

Avoid bathing in shark-infested waters, between sand bars and the deep ocean, where dead fish have been thrown into the water, where many sea birds are feeding, and where there is sewage effluent. Reduce risk by bathing in groups, close to the shore, only in daylight, and not if you are injured or menstruating. Do not wear jewellery or brightly coloured or patterned clothing. Spear fishermen should not carry their catch. Avoid looking like a seal, a major prey species of dangerous sharks, when you are lying on a surf board. Neither splash excessively nor swim with pet dogs. If attacked by a shark, fight back, hitting it on the nose and clawing at its eyes and gills. Get out of the water as soon as possible. Surface swimmers and surfers are usually targeted rather than divers. Scuba divers who encounter sharks can avoid attacks by descending to the ocean floor, hiding beneath rocks or reefs, and staying in groups. Various chemical and electrical-field repellents, chain mail protective suits and 'bang sticks' (firearms) have been developed but none is of proven benefit.

Website

꧂ http://www.flmnh.ufl.edu/fish/sharks/isaf/2012summary.html

Other fish

Most fish can inflict a painful and damaging bite if handled carelessly on a line or in a net, with a high risk of infection (see ➋ Marine wound infections, p. 294). Barracudas, marlin, sailfish, titan trigger fish and rays can be aggressive. In the great river systems of South America, piranhas are capable, at the very least, of biting a chunk out of a foot or hand trailed over the side of the boat. Tiny catfish (Portuguese 'candirú', Spanish 'canero'), their tropism for the gills of the large fish that they parasitize confused by the smell of urine, may, like aquatic leeches, penetrate the urethra, vagina, or anus of bathers, especially women who are menstruating. At Hospital Santa Rosa, Puerto Maldonado, Peru, some half a dozen cases are seen at the local hospital every year. Indo-Pacific marine gar fish or needle fish (*Tylosurus*) can leap out the water at night, attracted by a light, and fatally impale the fisherman.

Prevention

Prevention of all these unusual hazards is to take local advice and to take sensible precautions (e.g. don't bathe in the nude!).

Treatment of trauma caused by animals

First aid of severe injuries

- Secure the victim out of danger and out of the water.
- Control bleeding by direct pressure or tourniquet.
- Close perforating injuries with pressure dressings.
- Start IV fluid volume repletion.
- Evacuate to the base hospital.
- Assume that all injuries are infected. Clean wounds urgently and thoroughly with soap and water, and apply iodine and alcohol solutions. For multiple/severe dog- and cat-bite wounds and bites of face and hands, start prophylactic co-amoxiclav, doxycycline, or erythromycin. For other bites, use penicillin, an aminoglycoside (e.g. gentamicin for 48 h) and metronidazole; for marine wounds see ➔ Marine wound infections, p. 294.
- Cover risk of tetanus and rabies.

Emergency treatment at the base hospital

- Replace blood loss.
- Attend to local mechanical complications such as fractures, tension pneumothorax, damage to large blood vessels, perforation of the bowel, and lacerations of other abdominal viscera.
- Debride or amputate dead tissue, removing animals' teeth, etc.
- Irrigate with saline and betadine and drain.
- Delay primary suturing for 48–72 h, except for head and neck wounds which should be sutured immediately.

Further reading

Packer C, Ikanda D, Kissui B, Kushnir H (2005). Lion attacks on humans in Tanzania. *Nature*, 436, 927–8.

Packer C, Swanson A, Ikanda D, Kushnir H (2011). Fear of darkness, the full moon and the nocturnal ecology of African lions. *PLoS One*, 6(7), e22285.

Woodroffe R, Thirgood S, Rabinowitz A (eds) (2005). *People and Wildlife. Conflict or Coexistence?* Cambridge: Cambridge University Press.

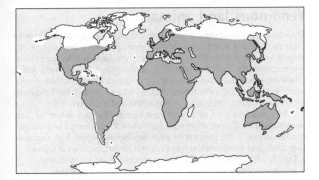

Fig. 17.1 Map of venomous land snake distribution.

Venomous land animals

Travellers' fears about venomous animals are usually exaggerated. Although most parts of the world, especially the tropical regions, are inhabited by animals with potentially lethal venoms, it is the local people (agricultural workers, hunters, and their children) rather than travellers who suffer. However, venomous bites and stings have caused a few fatalities in travellers, explorers, and researchers. Risk is reduced by sensible behaviour, protective clothing, and training in prevention and treatment.

Before embarking on an adventurous journey, find out about the local venomous fauna of your wilderness destination. If it is infested with dangerous animals or if the purpose of your expedition involves high exposure (e.g. zoological or botanical surveys in a rain forest), proceed as follows:

- Decide whether to take your own supply of antivenom (antivenin, antivenene or antisnake-bite serum); this is justified only if the expedition is at high risk of venomous bites and stings, the area is more than a few hours' evacuation time from medical care, and your party includes someone capable of injecting the antivenom and dealing with an anaphylactic reaction.
- Check the availability of antivenom at the nearest (base) hospital.
- Identify a national centre for antivenom production, supply, and treatment (see ➲ Resources, p. 575 for addresses and websites of foreign manufacturers). Antivenoms for bites by foreign snakes cannot be ordered in UK.
- Acquire the necessary knowledge about preventing and treating envenoming. Educate the expedition members at an early stage about prevention and first aid, and rehearse treatment and evacuation of bite/sting victims.

Snake-bite

Snake-bite is an important cause of death in agricultural communities in some parts of West Africa, Burma, the Indian subcontinent, New Guinea, and among indigenous Amerindians of the Amazonian region. In India alone, there were 46,000 snake-bite deaths in 2005. Most parts of the world are inhabited by venomous snakes (Fig. 17.1). The medically important groups are elapids, vipers, pit vipers, back-fanged (colubrid) snakes and burrowing asps (Figs 17.2, 17.3, and 17.4).

Europe
- Vipers only, e.g. adder *Vipera berus*.

Africa and the Middle East
- Elapids (Fig. 17.2), e.g. cobras and spitting cobras (*Naja*), mambas (*Dendroaspis*).
- Vipers (Fig. 17.3), e.g. saw-scaled vipers (*Echis*), puff adders (*Bitis*), desert horned-vipers (*Cerastes*).
- Colubrids (Fig. 17.4), e.g. boomslang (*Dispholidus*), twig snake (*Thelotornis*), keel-backs (*Rhabdophis*).
- Burrowing asps (*Atractaspis*) (Fig. 17.4).

sia
- Elapids, e.g. cobras (*Naja*) and kraits (*Bungarus*).
- Vipers, e.g. Russell's vipers (*Daboia*), saw-scaled vipers (*Echis*).
- Pit vipers, e.g. Malayan pit viper (*Calloselasma rhodostoma*), green tree vipers, habus, and mamushis (*Cryptelytrops*, *Trimeresurus*, *Gloydius*, etc.).
- Colubrids, e.g. keel-backs (*Rhabdophis*).

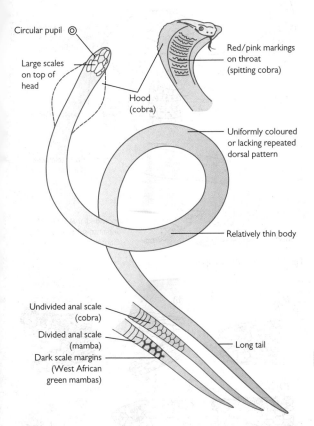

Circular pupil

Large scales on top of head

Hood (cobra)

Red/pink markings on throat (spitting cobra)

Uniformly coloured or lacking repeated dorsal pattern

Relatively thin body

Undivided anal scale (cobra)

Divided anal scale (mamba)

Dark scale margins (West African green mambas)

Long tail

Fig. 17.2 Typical African elapid snake.

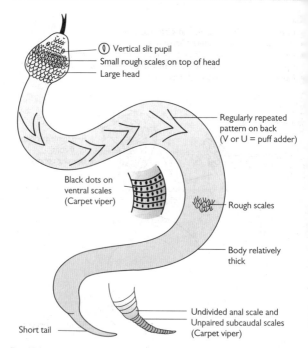

- Vertical slit pupil
- Small rough scales on top of head
- Large head

Regularly repeated pattern on back (V or U = puff adder)

Black dots on ventral scales (Carpet viper)

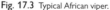

Rough scales

Body relatively thick

Undivided anal scale and Unpaired subcaudal scales (Carpet viper)

Short tail

Fig. 17.3 Typical African viper.

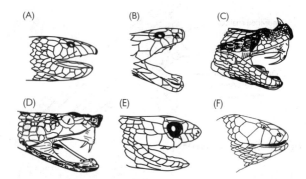

Fig. 17.4 Snake fangs: (A) Sea snake. (B) Cobra. (C) Viper. (D) Pit viper. (E) back-fanged snake (boomslang). (F) Burrowing asp.

Australasia
- Elapids only, e.g. taipans (*Oxyuranus*), black snakes (*Pseudechis*), brown snakes (*Pseudonaja*), tiger snakes (*Notechis*), death adders (*Acanthophis*).

The Americas
- Elapids, e.g. coral snakes (*Micrurus*).
- Pit vipers, e.g. lance-heads (*Bothrops*), moccasins (*Agkistrodon*), bushmasters (*Lachesis*), rattlesnakes (*Crotalus*).

The Indian and Pacific Oceans
- Elapids, sea snakes.

Clinical features

The following are the main groups of clinical features [and the snakes that cause them]:

- Local pain, swelling, bruising, blistering, regional lymph node enlargement, and tissue damage (necrosis) [vipers, pit vipers, burrowing asps, some cobras].
- Incoagulable blood (20-min whole blood clotting test—see ➲ Indications for antivenom treatment, p. 556) and spontaneous systemic bleeding (from gums, nose, skin, gut, genitourinary tract) [vipers, pit vipers, Australasian elapids, colubrids].
- Shock (hypotension) [vipers, pit vipers, burrowing asps].
- Descending paralysis progressing from ptosis and external ophthalmoplegia to bulbar and respiratory muscle paralysis [elapids, a few vipers and pit vipers].
- Generalized skeletal muscle breakdown (rhabdomyolysis) (generalized myalgia, muscle tenderness, and myoglobinuria-black/'Coca-Cola-coloured' urine positive for blood on stix testing) [sea snakes and a few other elapids, vipers, pit vipers].
- Acute kidney injury (oliguria/anuria, ECG changes of hyperkalaemia) [sea snakes, a few vipers, pit vipers and colubrids].

Treatment of snake-bite

First-aid treatment of snake-bite must be applied immediately by the victim or other people who are on the spot.

> ### First-aid treatment of snake-bite
> - Reassure the bitten person.
> - Do not interfere with the bite site in any way.
> - Immobilize the victim, especially their bitten limb, using pressure-immobilization or pressure-pad (see ➲ Pressure-immobilization, p. 554; ➲ Pressure-pad, p. 555).
> - Arrange urgent evacuation to medical care.
> - Treat pain.
> - *Do not* attempt to catch or kill the snake.
> - Avoid all traditional, herbal and 'quack' remedies.

- *Reassure* the patient, who may be terrified by the thought of sudden death: only a minority of snake species are dangerous; even the most notorious species may bite without injecting enough venom to be harmful ('dry bites'); the risk and rapidity of death from snake-bite have been greatly exaggerated—lethal doses of venom usually take hours (cobras, mambas, sea-snakes) or days (vipers, rattlesnakes, and other pit vipers) to kill a human, not seconds or minutes as is commonly believed; *correct treatment is very effective.*

- *Remove* tight rings, bracelets, and clothing from the bitten extremity before it becomes swollen.
- *Immobilize* the whole patient, especially their bitten limb, with a splint or sling to delay spread of venom from the bite site. Pressure-immobilization or pressure-pad are effective but training is necessary.
- *Evacuate* the victim to medical care (e.g. to the expedition doctor, clinic, or base hospital), as quickly, safely, passively, and comfortably as possible: vehicle, motorbike, bicycle, boat, stretcher or even fireman's lift are suitable. Ideally, the patient should lie in the recovery position to minimize the risk of aspirating vomit (a common early symptom of systemic envenoming) and should keep as still as possible to avoid exercising any part of the body, especially their bitten limb. Don't waste time before starting the journey; get going!
- Give analgesia as snake-bite can be very painful: paracetamol or codeine are suitable but avoid aspirin or non-steroidal anti-inflammatory agents as they increase the risk of bleeding.
- Do not attempt to catch or kill the snake: if it has been killed already, take it along as useful clinical evidence. But never handle a dead snake with bare hands; even a severed head may strike!
- Do not use traditional methods: incisions, suction, tourniquets, electric shock, ice packs, instillation of potassium permanganate crystals, herbs, black/snake stone, etc. are useless and potentially harmful.

Pressure-immobilization (PI) and pressure-pad (PP)

These first-aid treatments are important for elapid bites that can cause rapidly evolving paralysis. However, in the field, snake identification is usually uncertain. Immediate application of PI or PP is therefore recommended for all cases of snake-bite except where an elapid can be confidently ruled out (e.g. Europe and north of latitude 43°). Pressure can be released later if an elapid bite can be confidently excluded. The aim is to empty and compress lymphatics and veins draining the bitten limb (in the case of PI) or draining the bite site (in the case of PP), to prevent systemic spread of venom neurotoxins into the systemic circulation where they may cause life-threatening paralysis. This can be achieved with an external pressure of 50–70 mmHg (roughly equivalent to the firm binding of a sprained ankle).

Pressure-immobilization

The whole bitten limb is bound, using several robust elastic bandages (10 cm wide, 4.5 m long)[1] and incorporating a splint (e.g. SAM® splint), starting around the fingers or toes and finishing at the axilla or groin (Fig. 17.5A). Don't bind too loosely! If it is too tight, it will become an arterial tourniquet, the limb will become ischaemic, cyanosed, and painful, and peripheral pulses at the wrist or ankle will be impalpable.

---

1 Mölnlycke Setopress PEC high compression bandage Type 3c, 10 cm x 3.5 m, applied at more than 40 mmHg using visual pressure guide, is recommended ℘ http://csc.uk@molnlycke.com

Pressure-pad
A firm pad approximately 8 × 8 × 3 cm thick, made, for example, by folding a bandage or piece of cloth, or using foam rubber, is applied directly over the bite site, using a broad non-elastic circumferential bandage around the bitten limb (Fig. 17.5B).

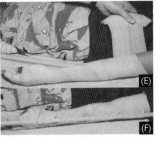
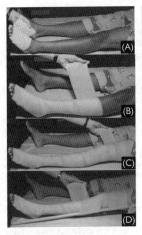

Fig. 17.5A Pressure-immobilization methods. Applying pressure-immobilization bandages a–c: firm binding of the bitten limb with a wide elasticated bandage, starting beyond the bite site, extending up to the groin; d: incorporating a splint; e–f: same for upper limb with elbow extended. Images courtesy of Dr David Williams, Papua New Guinea.

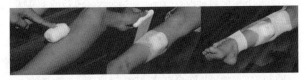

Fig. 17.5B Pressure-immobilization methods. Application of pressure-pad directly over the bite wound, bound in place and the bitten limb immobilized with a splint. Images courtesy of Dr David Williams, Papua New Guinea.

Indications for antivenom treatment

Any of the following:

- Spontaneous systemic bleeding.
- Incoagulable blood: failure of the patient's blood to clot solid when placed in a new, clean, dry, glass vessel and left undisturbed for 20 min *or* persistent bleeding (>30 min) from the fang punctures or other wounds, including venepuncture sites.
- Shock: low or falling BP or cardiac arrhythmia.
- Paralysis.
- Black/dark red-brown/'Coca Cola-coloured' urine (indicating rhabdomyolysis or massive haemolysis).
- Local swelling: involving more than half the bitten limb *or* swelling after bites on the fingers and toes *or* swelling after bites by snakes whose bites have a high risk of causing necrosis.
- Mild local swelling alone is not an indication for antivenom. Never give antivenom unless you have adrenaline (epinephrine) available to treat early anaphylactic reactions to the antivenom.

Choice of appropriate antivenom

Before giving antivenom make sure that its range of specificity includes the snake likely to have bitten your patient.

Most antivenoms are polyvalent and are able to neutralize venoms of all the medically important venomous species of the region for which it is intended. For example, in India, all antivenoms cover the 'big four' venomous species: cobra, common krait, Russell's viper, and saw-scaled viper; in Latin America some antivenoms cover the local lanceheads, rattlesnakes, and bushmaster (*Lachesis*). Monovalent antivenoms can be used if only one dangerous species occurs in the area (e.g. adder *V. berus* in UK, Netherlands, Belgium, Luxemburg, Poland and Scandinavia), if the snake has been reliably identified, or if a diagnostic clinical syndrome of envenoming appears. For example, in the savanna region of northern third of Africa, incoagulable blood is virtually diagnostic of saw-scaled viper (*Echis*) bite.

Administration of antivenom

- Give prophylactic adrenaline/epinephrine, adult dose 0.25 mg of 0.1% SC before starting antivenom to reduce the risk of a severe reactions.
- For optimal effect, administer antivenom by slow IV injection* (2 mL/min) or IV infusion diluted in 250–500 mL isotonic fluid over 30–60 min.

- NB Only in an extreme emergency should untrained people administer antivenom; for example, when the victim is many hours away from medical care, develops severe envenoming (see Fig. 17.6), and is deteriorating. Only in this unusual situation, give antivenom by multiple deep IM injections into the thighs (not the buttocks). Massage injection sites to increase absorption and apply firm pressure bandages to prevent bleeding.

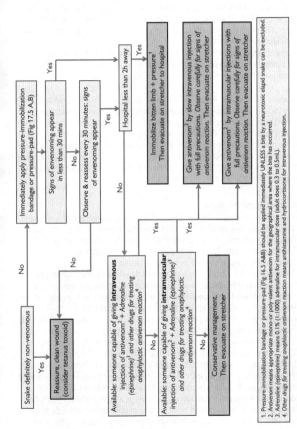

Fig. 17.6 Algorithm to guide use of antivenom in remote wilderness situations.

1. Pressure-immobilization bandage or pressure-pad (Fig 16.5 A&B) should be applied immediately UNLESS a bite by a neurotoxic elapid snake can be excluded.
2. Antivenom means appropriate mono- or poly-valent antivenom for the geographical area where the bite has occurred.
3. Adrenaline (epinephrine) means 0.1% (1:1000) adrenaline for intramuscular dose (adult dose 0.3 to 0.5mL).
4. Other drugs for treating anaphylactic antivenom reaction means antihistamine and hydrocortisone for intravenous injection.

Elements within the algorithm:

Snake definitely non-venomous
— No → Immediately apply pressure-immobilization bandage or pressure-pad (Fig 17.5 A,B)
— Yes → Reassure, clean wound (consider tetanus toxoid)

Signs of envenoming appear in less than 30 mins
— No → Observe & reassess every 30 minutes: signs of envenoming appear
— Yes →

Observe & reassess every 30 minutes: signs of envenoming appear
— No →
— Yes →

Hospital less than 2h away
— Yes → Immobilize bitten limb + pressure[1]. Then evacuate on stretcher to hospital
— No → Available: someone capable of giving **intravenous** injection of antivenom[2] + Adrenaline (epinephrine)[3] and other drugs for treating anaphylactic antivenom reaction[4]
  — Yes → Give antivenom[2] by slow intravenous injection with full precautions. Observe carefully for signs of antivenom reaction. Then evacuate on stretcher
  — No → Available: someone capable of giving **intramuscular** injection of antivenom[2] + Adrenaline (epinephrine)[3] and other drugs for treating anaphylactic antivenom reaction[4]
    — Yes → Give antivenom[2] by intramuscular injections with full precautions. Observe carefully for signs of antivenom reaction. Then evacuate on stretcher
    — No → Conservative management. Then evacuate on stretcher

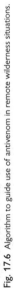

- Initial dose depends on the type of antivenom, species of snake, and severity of symptoms: often four to five 10 mL ampoules.
- Watch the patient closely for at least 2 h after starting antivenom for signs of anaphylaxis: restlessness, fever, itching, urticarial rash, angioedema, vomiting, breathlessness and wheezing, tachycardia, and fall in BP.
- Treat anaphylaxis immediately with adrenaline (epinephrine), adult dose 0.5 mL of 1 in 1000 solution IM (lateral thigh); this can be repeated after 10 min if it is not effective. Asthmatic reactions require additional inhaled bronchodilator.
- Repeat initial dose after 6 h if the blood remains incoagulable when re tested, or after a few hours if life-threatening bleeding, shock, or paralysis are undiminished.

Paralysis caused by Asian cobras and Australasian death adders may respond to anticholinesterases such as edrophonium, neostigmine, or physostigmine. Atropine 0.6 mg is given IV followed by 10 mg edrophonium (Tensilon®) by slow IV injection or 0.02 mg/kg neostigmine bromide/metilsulfate (Prostigmin®) by IM injection (all adult doses). If there is an improvement in muscle power within the next 20–30 min, treatment can be continued with SC neostigmine metilsulfate, 0.5–2.5 mg every 1–3 h up to 10 mg/24 h maximum (adult dose).

Treatment of complications
- *Hypovolaemic shock:* massive external bleeding or leakage of blood and tissue fluid into a swollen limb may leave the patient with an inadequate circulating volume so that the BP falls (check for postural drop from lying to sitting up). Transfusion with plasma expanders such as 0.9% saline or Hartmann's solution may be needed.
- *Respiratory failure:* from respiratory muscle paralysis must be treated with assisted ventilation; mouth-to-mouth or Ambu bag connected to a tight-fitting face mask, endotracheal tube, laryngeal mask airway, or i-gel, whatever is available and effective in the circumstances.
- *Acute kidney injury:* some patients become anuric or oliguric soon after bites by Russell's vipers, some pit vipers, Australasian elapids, and sea snakes. They must be managed conservatively until they reach the base hospital. Correct hypovolaemia by giving IV fluid until the jugular venous pulse becomes visible when the patient is propped up at 45°, then restrict fluids.
- *Wound infection* may be introduced by the snake's fangs or by ill-advised tampering at the bite site producing local inflammation (difficult to distinguish from envenoming) or an obvious abscess which should be aspirated. A tetanus toxoid booster is appropriate immediately after the bite. In cases of obviously infected or necrotic wounds, treat with antibiotics such as co-amoxiclav or chloramphenicol.
- *Surgical complications:* at the base hospital, necrotic tissue should be debrided and the skin defect covered with split skin grafts. Fasciotomy to relieve suspected compartment syndrome (e.g. anterior tibial compartment) is very rarely indicated and should be considered only after normal haemostasis has been restored with adequate antivenom treatment and raised intracompartmental pressure confirmed by direct measurement (e.g. using a Stryker pressure monitor).

Spitting cobra-induced eye injuries

Spitting cobras occur in Africa and parts of south-east Asia. They can spray venom defensively for a metre or more towards the glinting eyes of a perceived aggressor. Venom falling on the conjunctivae causes agonizing chemical conjunctivitis with profuse tearing, leucorrhoea, and blepharospasm. Corneal ulceration, infection, and permanent blindness may result.

Emergency treatment

Irrigate the eye(s) immediately with large volumes of any available bland fluid, ideally water under the tap (but milk or even urine is better than nothing: 'Please urinate into my eye!'). Single (only!) instillation of 1% adrenaline or local anaesthetic (e.g. tetracaine) eye drops with oral paracetamol relieves pain. Exclude corneal abrasions by fluorescein staining or slit lamp examination and apply prophylactic topical antibiotic (e.g. tetracycline, chloramphenicol). Prevent posterior synechiae, ciliary spasm and discomfort with topical cycloplegics (e.g. 2% atropine). Give topical antihistamine (e.g. 'Antistin') for allergic kerato-conjunctivitis. Topical or intravenous antivenom and topical corticosteroids are contraindicated.

Prevention of snake-bites

Do

- Avoid all snakes and snake charmers.
- Open and shake out sleeping bags and clothing before use.
- Tap boots before wearing to dislodge any unwanted inhabitants.
- Check ground before sitting at the base of trees.
- Wear boots, socks, and long trousers when walking in undergrowth or deep sand.
- Wear boots and use a torch when walking off or on the track at night, especially after heavy rain and also when relieving yourself at night (many snakes are most active at night).
- Be cautious and wear gloves when collecting fire wood.
- Remember that banks and streams are common snake haunts.
- Travel with a local guide who is much more likely to see camouflaged snakes.
- Sleep off the ground (hammock or camp bed) or use a sewn-in ground sheet and mosquito-proof tent or sleep under a mosquito net that is a well-tucked-in under your sleeping bag. This will protect against night-prowling kraits (Asia) or spitting cobras (Africa) which often bite people while they are asleep on the ground.

Do not

- Put hands blindly down inside rucksacks—empty out contents.
- Put hands or poke sticks into burrows or holes.
- Put hands up onto branches or ledges that can't be seen.
- Swim in rivers matted with vegetation in which snakes may be hiding or in muddy estuaries where there are likely to be sea snakes.
- Straddle logs—better to step up onto them then over.
- Disturb, corner, provoke, or attack snakes. Never handle them, even if they are said to be harmless or appear to be dead (some snakes sham death!).
- Move, if you do corner a snake by mistake. Snakes strike only at moving objects so keep absolutely still until it has slithered away although this demands almost inhuman sangfroid!

Lizard bite (parts of Middle and Central America only)

Gila monster (*Heloderma suspectum*) (up to 55 cm long) of south-western USA and adjacent Mexico and the Mexican beaded lizard or escorpión (*H. horridum*) (up to 80 cm) of western Mexico south to Guatemala are the only dangerously venomous lizards. However, some monitors (*Varanidae*) (notably the Komodo dragon (*Varanus komodoensis*)) and other lizards have now been shown to secrete venomous saliva. Helodermids' venom glands and grooved fangs are in their lower jaws. They only bite people who attack/handle them, hanging on like bulldogs, making it very difficult to disengage and increasing the exposure to envenoming. Lever its jaws apart with a screw driver, put it under the tap, place its four feet on the ground or introduce some alcohol into its mouth.

There is immediate severe local pain, spreading tender swelling, erythema and regional lymphadenopathy, weakness, dizziness, tachycardia, hypotension, syncope, angioedema, sweating, rigors, tinnitus, nausea, and vomiting. No fatal cases are confirmed.

Treatment

Antivenom is not available. A powerful analgesic may be required. Hypotension should be treated with plasma expanders and perhaps adrenaline or noradrenaline depending upon response.

Arthropods

Bee, wasp, hornet, yellow jacket, and ant sting hypersensitivity (Hymenoptera)

Stings by these insects are a common nuisance in many countries. Bees (*Apidae*) and wasp-like insects including yellow jackets and hornets (*Vespidae*), occur world-wide. Fire ants (*Solenopsis*) inhabit the Americas and jumper ants (*Myrmecia*) are found in Australia (especially Tasmania). Stings by all these hymenoptera can cause rapidly developing, potentially-lethal, systemic anaphylaxis in approximately 2–4% of the population who have become sensitized to their venoms. Other people may develop delayed, massive and persistent local swelling and inflammation which is unpleasant but not life-threatening.

Clinical

Symptoms of anaphylaxis can evolve in seconds. They include urticaria, angio-oedema, shock, unconsciousness, bronchoconstriction, GI symptoms (nausea, vomiting, diarrhoea), double incontinence, and, in women, uterine contractions. Venom-specific IgE is detected by radioallergosorbent test (RAST) or prick skin/patch testing, confirming hypersensitivity (see Fig. 8.8).

Prevention

People who have had anaphylaxis must carry self-injectable adrenaline (e.g. EpiPen®, Emerade®) with them at all times, but most have little idea how to use them in an emergency (Fig. 17.7). The technique should be practised with an EpiPen® Trainer. Allergic subjects should wear an identifying tag (e.g. MedicAlert™ or MediTag™) to indicate their problem (e.g. 'allergic to wasp stings—give adrenaline') in case they are found incoherent or unconscious.

1. Pull off the grey safety cap, as shown in diagram (a).

2. Hold the auto-injection as shown in diagram (b) and place the black tip on your thigh, at right angles to your leg. Always apply to the thigh.

3. Press hard into your thigh until the auto-injection mechanism works and hold the device in place for 10 seconds. The EpiPen® unit can then be removed. Massage the injection site for 10 seconds

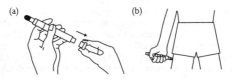

(a)   (b)

Fig. 17.7 Epipen® technique.

Desensitization: those with a history of systemic anaphylaxis to a sting who are RAST or skin test-positive for the appropriate venom can be effectively desensitized before the expedition. Control of the hypersensitivity takes about 8 weeks, while cure takes 3–5 years.

Mass attacks

In tropical countries, rock climbers and other travellers have been attacked by large swarms of aggressive bees, resulting in fatal falls. In Zimbabwe, a man survived 2000 bee stings despite terrible symptoms of massive histamine release. Some accidents could have been prevented by seeking local advice. Thundery weather is known to upset bees but a perceived threat to their nest is the commonest provocation.

In the face of an attack, run away very fast, ideally into undergrowth, or immerse yourself under water. For climbers, a fall is the greatest danger. First, secure yourself, then use anorak, rucksack, or tent for protection. South Asia has aggressive giant honey bees 3 cm long and in South America there have been many deaths from mass attacks by furious swarms of Africanized ('killer') honey bees. Multiple stings can cause haemolysis, rhabdomyolysis, bronchospasm, pneumonitis, and acute kidney injury. No antivenom is commercially available.

Blister beetles ('Spanish fly', 'Nairobi eye')

These beetles exude vesicating fluid containing cantharidin when inadvertently touched or trapped (e.g. in antecubital fossa when elbow is flexed), causing erythema, itching, and formation of large, painless, thin-walled blisters. 'Spanish fly' (*Cantharis vesicatoria*, family Meloidae) is iridescent green. 'Nairobi eye' and similar blistering conditions in Australia and South East Asia are caused by pederin-containing secretions of rove beetles (*Paederus*, family Staphylinidae; Fig. 17.8). Toxin from crushed beetles or blister fluid is easily spread to other sites such as the eye by fingers. Treatment is palliative.

Moth and caterpillar sting ('lepidopterism', 'erucism')

These insects, in particular brightly coloured, hairy caterpillars, such as the sycamore tussock moth (*Halysidota harrisii*) (see Plate 20) can cause severe problems: local pain, inflammation, nettle rash, blistering, and arthritis on contact and, in northern South America, systemic bleeding and incoagulable blood. Treatment is non-specific (anti-histamines, corticosteroids, analgesics) except in the case of the most dangerous genus of moth caterpillars (*Lonomia*), for which a specific antivenom is manufactured in Brazil.

Spider bite

The most dangerous genera of spiders are:

• *Latrodectus*—black/brown widow spiders (Americas, southern Europe, Southern Africa, Australia, New Caledonia; Fig. 17.9).
• *Phoneutria*—wandering, armed or banana spiders (Latin America; Fig. 17.10).
• *Atrax* and *Hadronyche*—(Sydney) funnel web spiders (Australia).
• *Loxosceles*—brown recluse spiders (Americas, southern Africa, and Mediterranean).

Many completely innocent (hobo, wolf, white-tailed, sac) spiders have been vilified as causes of 'necrotic arachnidism', attributable to other ulcerative conditions.

Clinical

Bites usually happen when the victim brushes against a spider that has crept into curtains, clothes, or bedding. *Latrodectus*, *Phoneutria*, and *Atrax* are neurotoxic, causing local puncture marks and surrounding erythema, severe pain spreading from the bite site, cramping abdominal or chest pains simulating an acute abdomen or myocardial infarction, muscle spasms, weakness, profuse sweating, salivation, goose flesh, fever, nausea, vomiting, priapism, anxiety, feelings of doom and alterations in pulse rate and BP. Local pain, sweating, and gooseflesh at the site of bite are useful signs. Some genera of Old World tarantulas (Theraphosidae) can cause severe muscle spasms. *Loxosceles* venom is necrotic, causing evolution, over a few hours at the site of bite, of pain and a circumscribed lesion ('red-white-and-blue sign') (Plate 11). Rarely, there are systemic effects: fever, scarlatiniform rash, haemoglobinuria, coagulopathy, and acute kidney injury.

Deaths are unusual except among children. Antivenoms are manufactured in countries such as South Africa, Australia, Mexico, and Brazil, where severe spider bites are common.

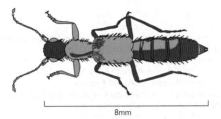

8mm

Fig. 17.8 Nairobi eye beetle (*Paederus eximius* or *P. sabaeus* Staphylinidae).

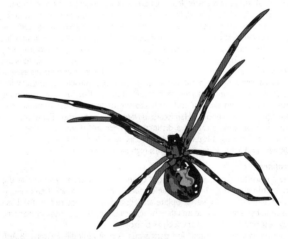

Fig. 17.9 Brown widow spider *Latrodectus geometricus*.

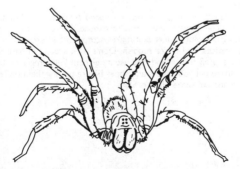

Fig. 17.10 Brazilian wandering spider *Phoneutria*.

Scorpion sting

The most dangerous scorpions are:

- *Leiurus quinquestriatus*, *Androctonus* spp., *Hemiscorpius lepturus*, and *Buthus* spp. in North Africa and the Middle East.
- *Parabuthus* spp. in South and North-East Africa.
- *Centuroides* spp. in North America (15,000 stings by *C. exilicauda* per year reported in Arizona, USA) and Mexico.
- *Tityus* spp. in Latin America and the Caribbean (Fig. 17.11).
- *Hottentotta tamulus* in the Indian subcontinent.
- All are found in dry desert or hot dusty terrains.

Clinical

Almost all stings (except *H. lepturus*) are excruciatingly painful and fatalities do occur, especially in children. Systemic symptoms reflect release of autonomic neurotransmitters, initially acetylcholine (causing vomiting, abdominal pain, pancreatic secretion, sphincter of Oddi constriction, bradycardia, salivation, nasolacrimal secretion, generalized sweating, priapism etc.) then catecholamines (causing piloerection, palmar sweating, hypertension, tachycardia, pulmonary oedema, ECG abnormalities). *Centuroides* envenoming causes erratic eye movements, fasciculations, muscle spasms simulating tonic–clonic seizures, and respiratory distress. *Parabuthus* envenoming causes ptosis and skeletal and respiratory muscle paralysis; some species can squirt their venom. *Hemiscorpius lepturus* (Iran, Iraq, Pakistan, and Yemen) envenoming causes a distinctive syndrome of painless sting, local erythema, bruising, blistering and necrosis, bleeding tendency, myocardial damage, and acute kidney injury with high case fatality.

Treatment

The severe local pain is best treated by infiltrating local anaesthetic at the site of the sting (e.g. 1–2% lidocaine), ideally by digital block if the sting is on a finger or toe. Powerful opiate analgesia may be required. In the base hospital, hypertension, acute left ventricular failure, and pulmonary oedema may respond to vasodilators such as prazosin.

Antivenoms are available for dangerous African/Middle Eastern, South African, American, and Australian species.

Prevention

When establishing camp in scorpion-infested country, first clear the area of rocks, undergrowth, and debris to expose the scorpions. By night, a UV lamp is a useful adjunct as it makes scorpions fluoresce. They hide in cracks, crevices, and under rubbish. Don't walk around in bare feet, be sure to sleep off the ground, and use a permethrin-impregnated bed net. Always shake out your boots and shoes before putting them on (see also ➲ Prevention of snake-bites, p. 559).

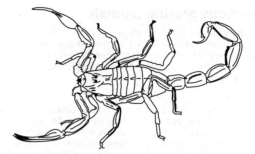

Fig. 17.11 Brazilian scorpion *Tityus serrulatus*.

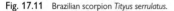

Other venomous invertebrates

Bites by some tropical centipedes can be dangerous as well as painful. Millipedes such as *Apheloria virginiensis* (see Plate 21) can squirt highly irritant defensive secretions, causing blistering and staining of skin and mucosae. No specific treatment is available. Giant freshwater water bugs (beetles) (Belostomidae) can inflict painful bites. Some ticks in North America (e.g. *Dermacentor* spp.), eastern Australia (*Ixodes holocyclus*), and Europe can inject a neurotoxin while sucking blood. If one of your team develops an ascending flaccid paralysis while in these countries, search hairy areas and the external auditory meatus, and detach any ticks as soon as possible using the correct technique (see ➋ Removing ticks, p. 288). Paralytic symptoms should then subside.

Venomous marine animals

Although venomous bites and stings can occur in temperate waters, the risk is much greater in tropical seas (Indo-Pacific, Red Sea, Eastern Mediterranean and Caribbean). Often, the animal is not seen or identified, but the circumstances and symptoms may be helpful in establishing the likely cause (see Fig. 17.17).

Sea-snake-bite

Sea-snakes occur in colossal numbers in warmer oceans, estuaries, rivers and a few inland lakes, but not in the Atlantic or the Red Sea (Fig. 17.12). They are encountered mainly by fishermen in the Indo-Pacific region but bite only if handled (e.g. while being picked out of hand nets or off fishing lines). Heads and tails may be difficult to distinguish. Bites are usually painless leaving small puncture marks, often multiple and containing broken-off teeth. The principal symptoms of envenoming are progressive myalgia and muscle tenderness with trismus, passing dark (Coca-Cola coloured) urine (myoglobinuria), ptosis, descending paralysis threatening respiratory failure, and acute kidney injury. Rhabdomyolysis can be so severe that potassium released from damaged muscles causes cardiac arrest. Hyperkalaemia may be controlled with IV calcium chloride, sodium bicarbonate or insulin and dextrose. Treatment is the same as for other snake-bites (see ➜ Treatment of snake-bite, p. 553). Wet suits are protective against the bites of all but the longest-fanged and most aggressive of sea snakes.

Fish sting

More than 1200 species of fresh water and especially marine fish are venomous, but only about 200 species can cause dangerous stings. They inhabit both tropical and temperate waters. Important species include stingrays, mantas, catfish, weevers, toadfish, stargazers, stone lifters, scorpion fish, stone fish, sharks, and dogfish. Their venomous spines are in the gills, fins, or tail. Beautiful lion, zebra, tiger, turkey, or red fire fish (*Pterois, Dendrochirus*; Fig. 17.13) are popular aquarium pets. Stingrays are common in the oceans and in rivers of South America and Equatorial Africa. If trodden upon they lash their tails, impaling the ankle with a venomous spine (Fig. 17.14).

Stings occur when fish are:

- Handled by fishermen or tropical aquarium keepers.
- Trodden on or touched by bathers and waders on beaches or by people fording rivers in the Amazon region, especially in the dry season.
- Irritated by swimmers and scuba divers around coral reefs.

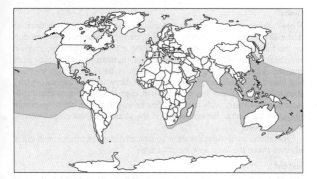

Fig. 17.12 Distribution of sea snakes.

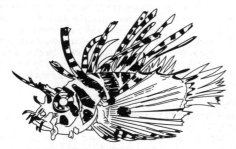

Fig. 17.13 Lion fish *Dendrochirus*.

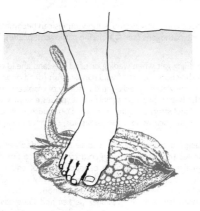

Fig. 17.14 Stinging action of stingray.

Clinical

There is immediate excruciating pain followed by swelling and inflammation at the site of the sting. Rarely, severe systemic effects may develop during the following minutes or hours: vomiting, diarrhoea, sweating, irregular heartbeat, fall in BP, spasm or paralysis of muscles, including respiratory muscles, and fits. Stingrays' barbed spines may be large enough to cause fatal trauma (pneumothorax, penetration of thoracic or abdominal organs), as in the case of Steve Irwin who swam over a large stingray that fatally punctured his heart with its spine. Spines invested with their venomous integument are often left embedded in the wound and will cause infection unless removed.

Expeditions involving activities in aquatic environments should find out in advance about the local venomous hazards.

First aid

The agonizing local pain is dramatically relieved by immersing the stung part in hot but not scalding water. Test the temperature with your own elbow. If you have a thermometer, check that the temperature does not exceed 45°C. Hotter water will cause a full thickness scald. Ad hoc methods of local heating have been described: a lighted cigarette, cigar or lighter advanced to within inches of the wound, or a damp towel wrapped round a hot engine block. Alternatively, 1% lidocaine or some other local anaesthetic can be injected, ideally as a digital block (see Fig. 19.1). The venomous spines of stingrays and catfish are often barbed but must be removed as soon as possible.

Antivenom

CSL Australia produces an antivenom for stonefish (genus *Synanceja*) that covers stings by some other scorpion fish. Exceptionally, a stung patient might need mouth-to-mouth respiration and external cardiac massage. Atropine (0.6 mg IV for adults) should be given if there is hypotension attributed to bradycardia.

Infection

Both venomous and non-venomous fish wounds can become infected with unusual marine pathogens (see ⊃ Marine pathogens, p. 294).

Prevention

Employ a shuffling gait when wading or prod the sand ahead of you with a stick to disturb venomous fish. Avoid handling fish (dead or alive) and keep clear of fish in the water, especially in the vicinity of tropical reefs. Footwear, the thicker the better, protects against most species except stingrays.

Cnidarian (coelenterate) sting: jellyfish, Portuguese man o' war ('blue bottle'), sea nettle, sea wasp, cubomedusoids, sea anemones, stinging corals, etc.

The tentacles of these marine animals are studded with millions of stinging capsules (nematocysts) triggered by contact to fire their venomous stinging hairs into the skin. This produces lines of painful blisters and inflammation in distinctive patterns. Hypersensitivity may lead to recurrent urticarial rashes over many months. The venom of some species, such as the notorious box jellyfish (*Chironex fleckeri* and *Chiropsalmus* spp.) of

Northern Australian and Indo-Pacific waters, has caused >70 deaths since 1883. Severe systemic effects can result in cardiorespiratory arrest within minutes of the stings. 'Irukandji' syndrome is caused by *Carukia barnesi* and other tiny transparent cubomedusoids. There is severe musculoskel-etal pain, anxiety, trembling, headache, piloerection, sweating, tachycardia, hypertension, and pulmonary oedema starting within about 30 min of the sting and persisting for hours. Other medically important jellyfish include Portuguese men o' war (*Physalia*) which are worldwide in distribution, and have caused a few fatalities and local gangrene owing to arterial spasm (Plate 14); *Stomalophis nomurai* of the north-west Pacific, China, and Japan which can cause fatal pulmonary oedema; the sea nettle (*Chrysaora quinquecirrha*) which is very widely distributed but is most common in Chesapeake Bay, USA, and the mauve stinger (*Pelagia noctileuca*), which can swarm in enor-mous numbers causing stinging epidemics in the Adriatic and other parts of the Mediterranean.

Coral cuts are common injuries inflicted by coelenterates in tropical waters. Painful superficial grazes and cuts result when tender areas of the body are inadvertently brushed against coral outcrops. Mechanical injury from the spiky calcified crust is combined with envenoming and the risk of a marine bacterial infection (see ➔ Marine pathogens, p. 294).

Treatment
- Remove the victim from the water to prevent drowning.
- Prevent further discharge of nematocysts on fragments of tentacles stuck to the skin:
  - For *Chironex* spp. and other cubozoans, including Irukandji (Indo-Pacific region, perhaps Caribbean), apply commercial vinegar or 3–10% aqueous acetic acid solution. This is not recommended for stings by other jellyfish.
  - For *Chrysaora* spp. apply a slurry of baking soda and water (50% w/v).
  - Tentacles should be washed off, removed by hand or with a shaving razor.
  - *Do not use* alcoholic solutions such as methylated spirits and suntan lotion as they cause massive discharge of nematocysts.
- Relieve agonizing pain:
  - *Chironex* spp. and *Physalia*—hot water treatment (as for fish stings; see ➔ First aid, p. 568) has proved more effective than ice.
  - Pressure immobilization is no longer recommended.
- Treat severe envenoming:
  - Cardiopulmonary resuscitation on the beach has saved lives.
  - Antivenom for box jellyfish, 'Sea wasp' (*C. fleckeri*), is manufactured in Australia. Ideally, give IV, but it has been given on the beach by surf lifesavers by IM injection.
  - Coral cuts: should be cleaned and debrided as far as possible, irrigated, cleaned with antiseptic and dressed. Infection should be treated promptly (see ➔ Marine pathogens, p. 294).

Sea urchin and starfish injuries (echinoderms)

The sharp venomous spines and grapples of some sea urchins may become deeply embedded in the skin, usually of the sole of the foot when the animal has been trodden upon. Wounds may be stained blue-black. Soften the skin with salicylic acid ointment and then pare down the epidermis to a depth at which the spines can be removed with forceps. If the spines are visible, it is tempting to try to remove them immediately, but this may be difficult or impossible. They are absorbed over several days provided they are broken into small pieces in the skin. If they penetrate a joint or cause infection, surgical removal is necessary.

Molluscs: octopus bite and cone shell sting

The blue-ringed octopuses of the Indo-Australasian region rarely exceed 20 cm in diameter but have caused fatal envenoming after unnoticed, painless bites (Fig. 17.15). Cone shells (Fig. 17.16) are beautiful collectors' items but they can envenom by harpooning and implanting a venom-charged arrowhead. Stings may be unnoticed, causing spreading numbness and paralysis. Beware of picking up these attractive animals bare-handed. Their stings can be fatal. No antivenom is available. Treatment of mollusc bites and stings is purely supportive, based on the knowledge that their venoms (tetrodotoxin in the case of the blue-ringed octopus) are ion-channel agonists/ antagonists that may cause paraesthesiae, paralysis, and cardiac arrest.

Annelids: bristle worm bites and stings

Most species of these polychaete annelid marine worms (e.g. lugworms, sandworms) are <10 cm long but one species grows to 3 m. Their paddle-like parapodia are armed with sharp setae that can become embedded, causing pain and irritation while bites can also be painful. Some species may inject toxins by stinging and biting.

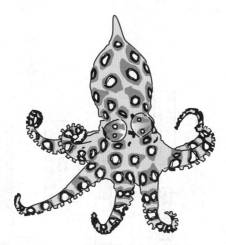

Fig. 17.15 Blue-ringed octopus (*Hapalochlaena maculosa*).

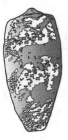
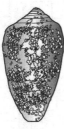
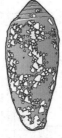
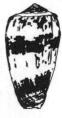

Conus geographus   *Conus textile*   *Conus aulicus*   *Conus striatus*

Conus tessulatus   *Conus abbas*   *Conus tulipus*   *Conus lividus*

Fig. 17.16 Cone shells.

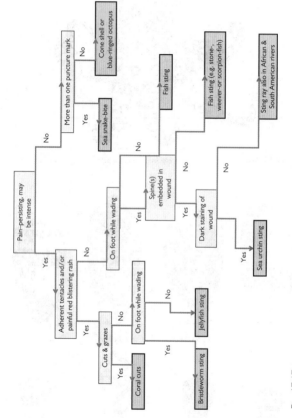

Fig. 17.17 Diagnosis of envenoming of unknown cause in a tropical sea.

Poisonous fish and shellfish

Everywhere, but especially in the tropics, the flesh of many species of fish, shellfish, and other marine animals is dangerously poisonous, always or seasonally, when ingested by humans and other animals.

Ciguatera poisoning

Symptoms develop 1–6 h after eating warm-water shore or reef fish (groupers, snappers, parrot fish, mackerel, moray eels, barracudas, and jacks). There are >50,000 cases each year and, in some Pacific Islands, up to 1% of the population is affected each year, with a case fatality of 0.1%. GI symptoms resolve within a few hours, but paraesthesiae and myalgia may persist for a week or even months.

Tetrodotoxin poisoning

Scaleless porcupine, file, trigger, puffer, and sun fish (order: Tetraodontiformes) become poisonous at certain seasons. Puffer fish ('fugu') is popular in Japan. Neurotoxic symptoms develop 10–45 min after eating the fish and death from respiratory paralysis may follow 2–6 h later. There may be no GI symptoms. Skin changes include erythema, petechiae, blistering, and desquamation. 'Zombification' in Haitian 'ju-ju' has been attributed to the use of this toxin. Tetrodotoxin, ultimately derived from bacteria, accumulates in parrotfish (*Scaridae*), Californian newts (*Taricha*), toads (*Atelopus*), blue-ringed octopuses (see Fig. 17.15), starfish, the eggs of horseshoe crabs (*Limulidae*) and in certain species of angelfish, polyclad flatworm, *Chaetognatha* (arrow worm), nemertean (ribbonworm), and xanthid crab.

Scombroid poisoning (histamine-like syndrome)

Bacterial contamination and decomposition of dark-red-fleshed fish (tuna, mackerel, bonito, skipjack), and canned sardines and pilchards generates histamine. *An early warning is immediate tingling or smarting of the lips and tongue at the first mouthful!* A few minutes to a few hours later, there is flushing, burning, sweating, urticaria, pruritus, headache, abdominal colic, nausea, vomiting, diarrhoea, bronchial asthma, giddiness, hypotension, and collapse.

Paralytic shellfish poisoning

Bivalve mollusks (mussels, clams, oysters, cockles, and scallops) become toxic when there is a 'red tide' of algal blooms. Many fish, sea birds, and mammals perish. Within 30 min of ingestion, paralysis begins and may progress to fatal respiratory paralysis within 12 h in 8% of cases. Milder gastrointestinal and neurotoxic symptoms (neurotoxic shellfish poisoning) without paralysis may occur.

Treatment

- In all cases, attempt to eliminate the toxic materials from the gut by gentle gastric lavage and purgatives, and give repeated doses of activated charcoal which is of unproven benefit but is unlikely to do harm.
- Scombroid poisoning responds to antihistamines and bronchodilators.
- Severe cases of paralytic poisoning require assisted ventilation.
- Victims of tetrodotoxin poisoning have recovered despite fulfilling the criteria for brain death.

Prevention
Note! Marine poisons are not destroyed by cooking or boiling.

Do
- Take local advice about what it is safe to eat.

Don't eat
- Seafood if there is an obvious 'die off' of marine life (rows of dead fish and sea birds on the shore).
- Shellfish if there is a 'red tide'.
- Very large reef fish (ciguatera poisoning) and any parts of any fish other than muscle (i.e. no skin, viscera, gonads, roe, etc.).
- Notorious poisonous species such as Moray eels (ciguatera), parrotfish (saxitoxin and others), large sharks (ciguatera, carchatoxin, trimethylamine), marine and fresh water puffer fish (tetrodotoxin/ saxitoxin) and, especially, horseshoe crabs' eggs, a delicacy in Thailand (*Carcinoscorpius rotundicauda*—Thai 'mengda talai' and *Tachypleus gigas*—Thai 'mengda chaan') (tetrodotoxin).
- Livers of any carnivorous polar mammal (polar bear, seals, cetaceans, huskies, etc.) because of the risk of fatal vitamin A toxicity.

Resources

Advice on venomous bites and stings
United Kingdom:
- TOXBASE® Administered by National Poisons Information Service (Edinburgh) website (registered users) http://www.toxbase.org
- 24/7 poisons information in the UK: 0844 892 0111.
- Phone: +44 (0)131 242 1383 (office).
- FAX: +44 (0)131 242 1387.
- mail@toxbase.org

United States:
- American Association of Poison Control Centers 24/7 help line: 1-800-222-1222.
- Oklahoma City Anti-venin Index: 1-405-271-5454.
- Poisondex central office, Denver, Colorado: 1-800-332-3073.
- Miami-Dade Fire Rescue Anti-Venin Bank: 1-786-336-6600.

Useful websites
Snake-bite in South and South-East Asia:
- ℘ http://www.searo.who.int/entity/emergencies/ documents/9789290223774/en

Snake-bite in Africa:
- ℘ http://www.afro.who.int/en/clusters-a-programmes/hss/ essential-medicines/highlights/2731-guidelines-for-the-prevention-and-c linical-management-of-snakebite-in-africa.html

Envenoming worldwide:
- ℘ http://www.toxinology.com
- ℘ http://www.vapaguide.info

Antivenoms: general
- ℘ http://globalcrisis.info/latestantivenom.htm
- ℘ http://www.who.int/bloodproducts/snake_antivenoms/en
- ℘ http://www.toxinfo.org/antivenoms/Index_Product.html
- Australian antivenoms:
- ℘ http://www.csl.com.au/docs/1022/475/A%20Clinician%27s%20 Guide%20to%20Venomous%20Bites%20&%20Stings%202013%20-%20 FINAL%20Web-S2,0.pdf
- ℘ http://www.toxinology.com/generic_static_files/cslavh_antivenom. html

South African antivenoms:
- ℘ http://www.savp.co.za

Venomous snake taxonomy updates:
- ℘ http://pages.bangor.ac.uk/~bss166/update.htm

Marine: Australia
- ℘ http://www.marine-medic.com.au
- ℘ http://www.anaesthesia.med.usyd.edu.au/resources/venom/ marine_enven.html

Plants and fungi

Contributor
David A. Warrell

Dangers of living off the land 578
Effects of contact with skin 579
Effects of ingestion 580
Fungal poisoning 582
Treating plant and fungal ingestion 584

Dangers of living off the land

'I wanted to eat of the fruit of all the trees in the garden of the world.'
(Oscar Wilde)

Please don't do it!

The abundance of appetizing, fragrant, and diverse fruits, leaves, and fungi offered by the wilderness environment may tempt the expeditioner to 'live off the land'. This ideal is enthusiastically encouraged in some military survival exercises and by certain heroic TV personalities! However, without expert guidance such attempts may prove lethal. In Europe, especially in France, Scandinavia, and Russia, enthusiastic amateur mushroom hunters seek novel gustatory experiences, but every year thousands are poisoned and hundreds die. Toxic plants and fungi are easily confused with edible ones and it is salutary that even expert botanists and mycologists are occasionally poisoned. You should not be reassured by seeing wild animals and birds feeding with apparent impunity. They have adapted to avoid poisoning in many clever and evolutionary ways. For example, Zanzibar's red colobus monkeys (*Piliocolobus kirkii*) eat charcoal to prevent poisoning by phenolic compounds in the Indian almond (*Terminalia catappa*) and mango (*Mangifera indica*) leaves that are their staple diet. Sometimes poisoning results from rash experimentation in quest of psychedelic experiences, using fungal psilocybin or tropane-containing plants. In South India and Sri Lanka, toxic plants are commonly employed as a means of self-harm (e.g. yellow oleander—*Cascabela thevetia* and Kerala suicide nut—*Cerbera manghas* or *C. odollam*).

Since recognizing danger is the secret of survival, an essential adjunct to this chapter is a profusely illustrated guide, CDRom (e.g. ✍ http://www. kew.org/data/poisplts.html), or website covering the poisonous (and edible) plants and fungi of the expedition's location.

Prevention of plant and fungal poisoning

Do

- Educate expedition members about the local toxic flora.
- Rely on your own food supplies.
- Confine collection of food from the environment to what you can identify with certainty as being safely edible or what is confidently recommended by local indigenous people.
- *Remember!* Cooking does not destroy fungal toxins!

Don't

- Experiment.
- Eat 'forbidden fruits': those resembling familiar cultivated fruits may be highly poisonous. To a non-expert, the death cap toadstool looks very like an edible mushroom (see ➡ Fungal poisoning, p. 582).
- Eat wild fungi and certainly none with white gills (see Fig. 18.1).
- Accept invitations to inhale, 'snort', or ingest the local psychedelic brew: a splitting headache, nausea, vomiting, and terrifying hallucinations are more likely than any pleasurable trance or 'out of body' experience.

Effects of contact with skin

Contact dermatitis is by far the commonest risk posed by plants. Examples include stinging nettles, euphorbias, and 'dumb cane' (*Dieffenbachia*).

Allergic dermatitis may be caused by a large variety of plants, notably poison ivy (*Toxicodendron (Rhus) radicans*) (see Plate 15) whose leaves have a trifoliate pattern ('leaves of three, leave them be'), poison oak (*Toxicodendron diversilobum*), primula (*Primula obconica*), and citrous fruits. Some plant saps are photosensitizing, resulting in erythema, papules, vesicles, bullae, and persistent hyperpigmentation confined to exposed areas.

Treatment

Treatment is based on immediate decontamination by washing with water, followed by symptomatic use of systemic antihistamines and topical corticosteroids.

Prevention

To avoid further contact, try to identify the cause. Since photosensitization is a common sequel, try to reduce solar exposure. In general, avoid unnecessary contact of bare skin with plants, especially those that have stinging hairs or are exuding latex or sap. If your expedition is botanical, learn to recognize some of the most notoriously irritant plants in advance and wear gloves when necessary.

Effects of ingestion

When to suspect plant poisoning
Within minutes to hours (exceptionally 24 h) after ingesting any part of a wild fruit, plant, or fungus (mushroom or toadstool):
- Nausea, vomiting, abdominal colic, diarrhoea.
- Confusion, hallucinations, or convulsions.
- Atropinic, nicotinic, or muscarinic symptoms.
- Cardiac arrhythmias.
- Flushing in response to alcohol ingestion.
- Oliguria/anuria.

Effects on gut
Many of the plants that cause contact dermatitis also irritate the gut. Cuckoo pint/arum lily, dumb cane, and many other plants have an irritant sap containing oxalate crystals. Ingestion causes immediate soreness, reddening, and blistering of buccal mucosa, salivation, and dysphagia. Most poisonous plants cause rapidly evolving nausea, abdominal cramps, vomiting, and diarrhoea (e.g. laburnum, anemone, hellebore, horse chestnut, ivy, privet, pokeweed, and snowberry). Some even more toxic plants cause severe GI symptoms after a delay of several hours up to 2 days (e.g. autumn crocus (*Colchicum autumnale*), glory lily (*Gloriosa superba*), jequirity bean (*Abrus precatorius*), and castor oil bean (*Ricinus communis*).

Effects on cardiovascular system
Bradycardia, heart block, other arrhythmias, ECG changes ('digoxin effect'), and GI irritation are caused by foxglove (*Digitalis purpurea*), white/pink oleander (*Nerium oleander*), yellow oleander (*Cascabela thevetia*, also known as *Thevetia peruviana*) (see Plate 19), monkshood (*Aconitum napellus*), yew (*Taxus baccata*), and death camas (*Zigadenus*).

Effects on nervous system
- Hallucinogenic: e.g. cannabis (*Cannabis sativa*), khat (*Catha edulis*), morning glory (*Ipomoea*), and peyote (*Lophophora williamsii*).
- Convulsant: e.g. cowbane (*Cicuta virosa*), ackee (*Blighia sapida*), and nux vomica (*Strychnos nux-vomica*). Cowbane poisoning causes gastroenteritis, increased secretions, and long-lasting intense episodes of generalized tonic–clonic convulsions, resulting in severe metabolic acidosis and multiple organ failure. Consumption of unripe ackee fruit is responsible for 'Jamaican vomiting sickness' associated with hypoglycaemia and fatal encephalopathy.
- Atropine-like: e.g. deadly nightshade (*Atropa belladonna*) (see Plate 16), angels' trumpets (*Brugmansia suaveolens*) (see Plate 18), and thorn apple or Jimson weed (USA) (*Datura stramonium*) and related species such as devil's trumpet (*D. metel*). Clinical effects are: 'red as a beet, dry as a bone' (flushed, hot, red, dry face), tachycardia, and dilated pupils (mydriasis), and, in serious poisoning, arrhythmias, urinary retention, psychosis, convulsions, coma, and fatal respiratory failure. Some of these plants are hallucinogenic and therefore desirable to some people.

- *Nicotine-like*: e.g. spotted hemlock (*Conium maculatum*), responsible for killing Soctrates and Hamlet's father, first stimulates and then paralyses autonomic ganglia, and can cause convulsions and respiratory arrest.

Effects on liver

Pyrrolizidine alkaloid-containing plants such as comfrey (*Symphytum offici-nale*) can cause hepatic veno-occlusive disease, which has occurred mainly in Jamaica, India, and Afghanistan. Nausea, abdominal pain and distension, hepatomegaly, and sometimes fever and vomiting develop a few days after ingestion.

Effects on kidneys

Oxalate-rich plants such as rhubarb (*Rheum rhabarbarum*), dock, and sorrel (*Rumex*), and plants containing other nephrotoxins may damage the kidneys.

Poisonous food plants

Staple food plants in many tropical countries can be poisonous if inade-quately soaked, dried, fermented, or cooked:

- Cassava (*Manihot esculenta*), sweet potato, yam, some fruit kernels, pips, and cherry laurel (*Prunus laurocerasus*) can cause acute or chronic cyanide poisoning.
- In Africa, tropical ataxic neuropathy and spastic paraparesis ('konzo') are attributed to cassava poisoning.
- Inadequately cooked beans and pulses (Leguminosae) can cause diarrhoea, while long-term exposure can lead to retarded growth and may even be fatal:
  - Lathyrism is an epidemic paralytic disease (e.g. in the Denbia depression of Ethiopia) caused by a neurotoxic amino acid in chick peas (*Lathyrus sativus*).
  - Favism occurs in some Mediterranean and Middle Eastern countries. Those with congenital glucose-6-phosphate dehydrogenase deficiency may develop intravascular haemolysis after eating broad (fava) beans (*Vicia faba*).

Fungal poisoning

Fungal poisoning is usually sporadic and accidental but occasionally may be homicidal, suicidal, or epidemic. In Europe (especially France, Scandinavia, and Russia), where there are many enthusiastic collectors and connoisseurs of wild mushrooms, poisoning is more common than elsewhere in the world. In 1999, 357 people were poisoned and 39 died from death cap mushroom (*Amanita phalloides*) poisoning in Voronezh in central Russia. Toxicity of fungi varies with location and season, from year to year, and with individual susceptibility.

The death cap, the world's deadliest mushroom or toadstool (see Plate 17), looks superficially like an edible mushroom (*Agaricus*) but it has white gills (radiating linear structures under the mushroom's cap) and a sac or volva at its base, whereas the edible mushroom has dark brown or black gills and no volva at the base of its stem (Fig. 18.1).

Poisoning with early symptoms (within a few hours)

- *GI symptoms*: vomiting, diarrhoea, and abdominal pain are usually transient but sometimes more intense, resulting in fluid and electrolyte disturbances. They may be caused by many species of common fungi, including honey agaric (*Armillaria mellea*) and *Boletus luridus*.
- *Cholinergic effects (muscarinic poisoning)*: abdominal pain and diarrhoea, sweating, lacrimation, salivation, miosis, bronchorrhoea, and sometimes bronchospasm, bradycardia, and hypotension may develop 5–120 min after ingesting *Inocybe* and *Clitocybe* spp.
- *Confusion (ibotenic poisoning)*: nausea, vomiting, confusion, disorientation, anxiety, euphoria, hallucinations, visual disturbances, ataxia, muscle cramps, and coma may develop 20–120 min after ingestion of panther cap (*Amanita pantherina*), fly agaric (*Amanita muscaria*), and *Amanita strobiliformis*.
- *Hallucinations (psilocybin poisoning)*: LSD-like, mainly visual hallucinations are induced by eating 'magic mushrooms' (*Psilocybe, Conocybe, Gymnopilus, Panaeolina, Panaeolus, Pluteus,* and *Stropharia* spp.). Within 30 min, there is mydriasis, tachycardia, euphoria, confusion, dizziness, and vomiting.
- *Antabuse-like reactions (Coprine poisoning)*: eating ink cap (*Coprinus atramentarius*) or club foot (*Clitocybe clavipes*) may produce a reaction similar to that induced by disulfiram (Antabuse®). If alcohol is drunk within 72 h of eating the fungi, there is flushing of the skin, metallic taste, sweating, mydriasis, nausea, vomiting, anxiety, confusion, dyspnoea, severe headache, tachycardia, chest pain, and hypotension.

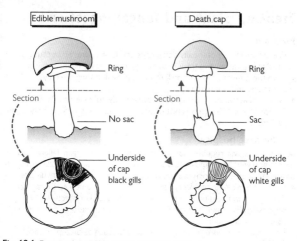

Fig. 18.1 Distinguishing edible mushrooms from death cap.

Poisoning with delayed symptoms (6 h to several days)

- Gastroenteritis *with hepatotoxicity and nephrotoxicity (Amatoxin poisoning)*: may result from eating the death cap (*Amanita phalloides*; Fig. 18.1), destroying angel (*Amanita virosa*), fool's mushroom (*Amanita verna*), *Conocybe filaris*, and some *Galerina* and *Lepiota* spp. Abdominal pain and vomiting, but in particularly severe cases, watery or bloody diarrhoea, starts 6–24 h (usually 12 h) after ingestion, leading to dehydration. After a period of apparent recovery, lasting up to 72 h, fatal hepatorenal failure may supervene.
- *Gastroenteritis with neurological symptoms (gyromitrin poisoning)*: there is gastroenteritis with a feeling of bloating, severe headache, vertigo, pyrexia, sweating, diplopia, nystagmus, ataxia, cramps, delirium, and sometimes coma, lethargy, hypoglycaemia, hepatic damage, haemolysis, and renal damage starting 2–24 h after ingesting false Morel (*Gyromitra esculenta*) or inhaling fumes while it is being cooked.
- *Renal damage (orellanine poisoning)* may develop 2–17 days after eating *Cortinarius* species. There is fatigue, intense thirst, headache, chills, paraesthesiae, tinnitus, and abdominal, lumbar, and flank pain. After a transient polyuric phase, oliguria and anuria may ensue.
- *Ergotism ('St Anthony's fire')* results from eating cereal crops whose seed heads are infected with the hard, purplish-black fruiting bodies of *Claviceps purpurea*. Symptoms include vasoconstriction, leading to peripheral gangrene and muscular tremors, convulsions, and hallucinations.

Treating plant and fungal ingestion

First aid

- Gastric lavage is potentially dangerous and is discouraged because of the risks of aspiration and trauma to pharynx and oesophagus.
- Give the patient a glass of milk to drink provided they are fully conscious and not vomiting.
- Give oral activated charcoal 50 g immediately, followed by 25 g every 2 h for at least 48 h (this is not evidence based but is very unlikely to be harmful).

At the base hospital

Severe cases will require supportive treatments for organ failure such as mechanical ventilation and renal dialysis, with therapy for hypovolaemia, acid–base disturbances, hypoglycaemia, cardiac arrhythmias, and convulsions.

- For *cholinergic (muscarinic) symptoms*—atropine (adult 0.6–1.8 mg IV).
- For *central and peripheral anticholinergic (atropine-like) effects*—physostigmine (adult 1–2 mg IV) to control hallucinations, delirium, and psychotic behaviour.
- For *confusion or hallucinations*—tranquillizers such as diazepam (adults 5–10 mg).
- For *psychotic behaviour*—chlorpromazine or haloperidol may be required.

Specific antidotes:

- For poisoning by yellow oleander, other *Apocynaceae,* and any plant containing cardiac glycosides: digoxin-specific antibodies (ovine Fab fragments such as Digibind™ or DigiTab™).
- For severe autumn crocus (*Colchicum autumnale*) poisoning: colchicine-specific Fab antibodies.
- For amatoxic fungal poisoning: infuse silibinin (silybin, silymarin) 5 mg/kg IV over 1 h, followed by 20 mg/kg/24 h (available in Germany but not in the UK or USA) or large doses (300,000–1,000,000 U/kg/day by continuous IV infusion) of benzylpenicillin. N-acetyl cysteine might reduce liver damage. In severe cases, liver transplantation is life-saving.
- For gyromitrin fungal poisoning: pyridoxine 25 mg/kg over 30 min, glucose IV, and promote diuresis.

Resource

Poisonous Plants and Fungi in Britain and Ireland. ISBN 1 900347 92 X. Interactive CDRom from Publications Sales, Royal Botanic Gardens, Kew, Richmond, Surrey TW9 3AE, UK. ℘ http://www.kew.org/data/poisplts.html

Advice about plant and fungal poisoning

United Kingdom

TOXBASE® Administered by National Poisons Information Service (Edinburgh) website (registered users): ℘ http://www.toxbase.org
24/7 poisons information in the UK: 0844 892 0111.
Phone: +44 (0)131 242 1383 (office). FAX: +44 (0)131 242 1387.
Email: mail@toxbase.org
Plants and fungi identification: telephone advice service for urgent poisoning case enquiries—Kew Gardens. Phone: +44(0)020 8332 5000.

Chapter 19

Anaesthesia in remote locations

Contributors

Rachael Craven

Joe Silsby (1st edition)

Introduction to field anaesthesia 586

When to give an anaesthetic 587

Know your limits 588

Local infiltration anaesthesia 590

Peripheral nerve blocks 594

Spinal anaesthesia 596

Ketamine anaesthesia 600

Sedation 602

Suggested minimum equipment and drugs for field
   anaesthesia 604

NB While local anaesthetic (LA) infiltration using recommended doses is safe, other forms of sedation and anaesthesia described in this chapter normally demand extensive specialist training. Untrained or inexperienced personnel should attempt these techniques only in circumstances where life or limb is threatened and help unavailable.

Introduction to field anaesthesia

The basic principles that govern field anaesthesia are similar to those governing conventional hospital anaesthesia, but the practical aspects of working safely in remote locations and the adverse conditions under which the operations may be performed can be a formidable challenge even to experienced specialists.

Anaesthesia must be:
- Simple.
- Safe for the patient.
- Adaptable to the constraints of the situation.
- Essential for life or limb preservation.

Four types of field anaesthesia can be differentiated:
- *Military*: armed forces may provide highly sophisticated retrieval, resuscitation, surgery and intensive care facilities in the field, and the logistics to evacuate casualties to secondary care facilities within 72 h. Such arrangements are inapplicable to the majority of expeditions.
- *Mass casualties*: non-combatants during conflicts and casualties of major disasters may present in large numbers to healthcare facilities run by non-governmental organizations (NGOs) such as Médecins Sans Frontières or the International Red Cross. There are often shortages of personnel, equipment, drugs, and disposables and backup facilities are rare. The principle of the 'best for most' is paramount. Trauma, general surgery, and obstetric emergencies may all require treatment.
- *Surgical camps*: several NGOs now provide planned surgical treatment for people living in areas of developing countries where such care is not usually possible. They establish short-term surgical camps with the objective of taking reasonable standards of care and follow-up to places where these services are not usually available. Examples include surgical camps for cataract removal, and facial cleft repairs.
- *Expeditions*: polar expeditions, ships' crews, and exploration groups may spend prolonged periods in isolation where accidents and acute surgical conditions can occur. Individuals may require treatment necessitating sedation or anaesthesia prior to, or whilst awaiting, evacuation. Minor ailments might also require treatment using LA during such expeditions.

When to give an anaesthetic

Avoid anaesthesia if possible

Some conditions usually treated by surgery are more safely dealt with in the field by IV fluid resuscitation, analgesia and antibiotics. Examples include acute surgical conditions such as suspected appendicitis, where conservative management should allow sufficient time for evacuation of the patient (➲ Acute appendicitis, p. 390).

Life- or limb-saving situations

Sedation or anaesthesia may be essential to save life or limb before evacuation. Examples include:

- Lower limb fracture-dislocation with occlusion of the blood supply requiring rapid reduction to restore the blood supply and save the leg before evacuation.
- Entrapment of a casualty by rockfall requiring amputation of a limb for extraction.

Effective sedation or anaesthesia may be a necessary adjunct to fluid resuscitation and analgesia.

Treatment to prevent complications

Other situations may not require evacuation but do need treatment to prevent further complications. Examples include removal of foreign bodies from tissues, incision of abscesses, cleansing and suturing of superficial lacerations and wounds. Often LA techniques provide a safe and effective way of anaesthetizing for these procedures.

> Use general anaesthesia in the field only as a last resort when there is no other option.

Know your limits

All anaesthetics are potentially dangerous; an anaesthetic given by inexperienced hands can cause more harm than good. When selecting a technique consider:

- The risks and benefits to the patient—both of operating and of doing nothing.
- The physiological state of the patient. If they have lost blood or are dehydrated due to illness, pre-anaesthetic resuscitation is vital.
- The drugs and equipment available.
- The effects and side effects of the chosen anaesthetic technique.
- What help is available; simultaneously trying to operate and look after the patient is very difficult.
- The capabilities of the anaesthetic administrator and of the surgeon.
- Local or regional anaesthesia is usually safer than general anaesthesia.
- Airway management requires considerable expertise—ventilating using a bag and mask can be technically difficult, and unskilled attempts may result in inadequate ventilation or distention of the stomach.
- Mal-placement of a tracheal tube or laryngeal mask airway will obstruct breathing and can kill. Airway adjuncts should be used only after appropriate training and knowledge of how to identify correct placement.
- The side effects of potent drugs and complications of anaesthesia or surgery can be difficult or even impossible to deal with in remote locations.

Local infiltration anaesthesia

When to use it

Minor surface surgery such as:
- Wound suturing.
- Small superficial abscesses—although LAs are less effective in the presence of infection.
- Digital blocks.
- Dental work (see Chapter 11).
- Pain relief—following some animal bites and stings.
- Topically on the surface of the eye or other mucus membranes.

Advantages
- Safe.
- Easy to learn.
- Minimal equipment required.
- Additional monitoring unnecessary.

Disadvantages
- Not appropriate for large or multiple areas if maximum safe dose will be exceeded.
- LA toxicity, whilst rare, is a challenge to treat in remote situations.
- Not always effective, especially if affected area is inflamed or infected.
- Inadvertent intravascular injection may cause systemic toxicity even without using the 'maximum' dose.

Local anaesthetic agents

Lidocaine
Most widely available LA.
- Dose: 3 mg/kg plain lidocaine to a maximum of 300 mg; or 7 mg/kg with adrenaline (epinephrine) 1:200,000 up to a maximum of 500 mg.

Prilocaine
Good if large volumes will be required and is fairly safe but relatively short acting.
- Dose: 5 mg/kg plain or 8 mg/kg with adrenaline (epinephrine) to a maximum of 400 mg.

Bupivacaine
Slower onset but long duration of action, which can be useful. Never inject intravascularly as can cause irreversible cardiac arrest.
- Dose: 2 mg/kg with or without adrenaline, to maximum of 150 mg.

To calculate a drug dose
- Drugs in solution are quoted as percentage concentrations.
- 1% means 1 g of drug has been dissolved in 100 mL of solvent.
- So:
  - 1% solution = 10 mg/mL; 0.25% solution = 2.5 mg/ mL.
- If your casualty weighs 70 kg and you are using lidocaine the maximum safe dose for lidocaine is 3 mg/kg, which for this patient is $3 \times 70 = 210$ mg
- Therefore the maximum volume of lignocaine you can infiltrate is:
  - 210/10= 21 mL of the 1% solution or 210/20 = 10.5 mL of the 2%.

Symptoms and signs of overdose
Mild
- Perioral paraesthesia.
- Tinnitus.
- Metallic taste.
- Blurred vision.

Moderate
- Restlessness.
- Slurred speech.
- Nystagmus.
- Tremor.

Severe
- Fits.
- Coma.
- Hypotension.
- Dysrhythmias.
- Cardiac arrest.

Treatment
- Stop injection.
- Resuscitate using ABC approach.
- Diazepam 10 mg or other benzodiazepine for fits.
- If available give 20% lipid emulsion 1.5 mL/kg to a maximum of 3 boluses and start an infusion at 15 mL/kg/h, continue until stable or maximum dose of lipid of 12 mL/kg has been given.

Local infiltration techniques
First calculate the maximum safe dose for your casualty.

If you think a large volume may be required consider using a LA solution containing adrenaline (epinephrine) 1:200,000 unless it as an area supplied by end arteries such as fingers, toes, penis, or tip of ear.

Wound infiltration
- Wearing sterile gloves, clean the skin with antiseptic solution.
- Draw up calculated volume of LA into syringe.
- Using a 23 or 25 G needle, inject subcutaneously along both sides of the wound. Aspirate prior to injection to avoid intravascular injection.
- Alternatively inject in a diamond shape around the wound or abscess with a single entry point at either side of the area to be anaesthetized.

Digital nerve block
See also Fig. 14.6.
- Used for surgery distal to the base of the proximal phalanx of fingers or toes.
- Never use adrenaline-containing solutions.
- If available, choose a 25 mm 25 G needle.
- Infiltrate LA on either side of the base of the proximal phalanx, in a vertical plane from the dorsal surface until the needle almost reaches the palmar surface (Fig. 19.1). Inject 2–3 mL of 1% lidocaine or prilocaine, or the same dose of 0.25% bupivacaine on each side of the digit, then add a small additional dose over the dorsum of the digit.

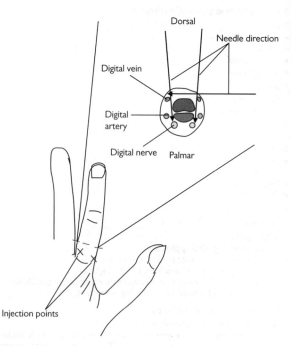

Fig. 19.1 Digital nerve block.

Haematoma block
- Used to reduce fractures of the distal radius and ulna or occasionally also distal tibia and fibula.
- Not suitable for use on open fractures.
- Wear sterile gloves and clean the skin with antiseptic solution.
- Palpate the fracture line and introduce the needle into the fracture site aspirating as you go to identify fresh blood from the fracture haematoma. (Fig. 19.2).
- Once in the haematoma inject 6–8 mL of 2% lignocaine (for a 70 kg adult). Plus a further 2–3 mL in ulna styloid area.
- Onset of anaesthesia takes about 10 min.

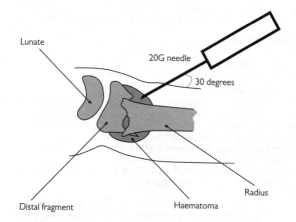

Lunate

20G needle

30 degrees

Radius

Distal fragment

Haematoma

Fig. 19.2 Haematoma block showing injection into haematoma at fracture site.

Peripheral nerve blocks

What they are

Injection of LA around a nerve or nerve plexus to provide anaesthesia and analgesia in its area of distribution.

When to use them

- Longer-lasting analgesia for limb fractures during evacuation.
- When infiltration techniques would require more than the maximum safe dose.

Advantages

- Longer-lasting anaesthesia than with infiltration.
- Larger area of anaesthesia than can be provided with infiltration.

Disadvantages

- Technically more difficult.
- Potential for damage to nerve.
- Potential for intravascular injection and LA toxicity.

Fascia iliaca block

This block has been identified by the Association of Anaesthetists of Great Britain and Ireland as a block suitable for non-medical practitioners since its injection point when performed correctly is away from both nerves and major blood vessels, and is therefore relatively safe.[1]

- *Indication:* analgesia for femoral shaft and neck of femur fractures, anterior thigh, and above-knee amputation.
- *Equipment:* blunted needle, 1–2 mL 1% lignocaine for skin infiltration, 30–40 mL of a suitable percentage LA.
- *Method:*
  - Calculate maximum safe dose of LA (see ⟳ To calculate a drug dose, p. 591), this is a volume-dependent block so you need to choose a percentage that will allow you to inject a large volume, e.g. 30 mL 0.25% bupivacaine.
  - Ensure you have IV access.
  - Identify your landmarks: a line connecting the anterior superior iliac spine and the pubic tubercle divided into thirds. Mark the injection point 1 cm caudal to the junction of the lateral and middle third (Fig. 19.3).
  - Clean the skin with antiseptic.
  - Infiltrate skin at injection point with 1% lignocaine.
  - Using a blunted needle pierce the skin at the injection point at right angles to the skin.
  - Advance the needle cranially at an angle of 60° until you have felt two 'pops' of fascia lata and fascia iliaca.
  - Aspirate before injecting and every 5 mL during injection to ensure no intravascular placement.

1 ⟳ http://www.aagbi.org/sites/default/files/Fascia%20Iliaica%20statement%2022JAN2013.pdf

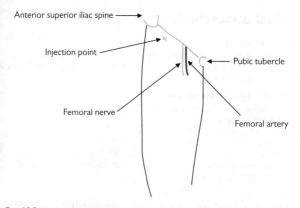

Anterior superior iliac spine ⟶

Injection point ⟶

⟵ Pubic tubercle

Femoral nerve

Femoral artery

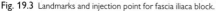

Fig. 19.3 Landmarks and injection point for fascia iliaca block.

Axillary nerve block
This block is technically more demanding than the fascia iliaca block, and since the injection point is by a major nerve plexus and large blood vessels it has a higher risk of both nerve damage and intravascular injection. However, in experienced hands it is an excellent block to use in the field for both anaesthesia and analgesia of the upper limb.

Spinal anaesthesia

When to use it

Spinal anaesthesia is an excellent technique to use in the field, but is not a technique for the inexperienced. It is very suitable for surgery below the umbilicus, such as lower limb surgery.

Contraindications and cautions

- Hypovolaemia and uncorrected dehydration.
- Generalized sepsis.
- Suspected or known clotting problems.
- Infection at site of injection.
- Spinal anaesthesia is associated with falls in BP: a cannula, IV fluids, and vasopressor drugs are essential to counteract this effect. Resuscitation equipment must be available.

Equipment

- Antiseptic solution, sterile gloves, syringes, and disposable spinal needles are required.
- Vasopressor, e.g. ephedrine 30 mg ampoules—dilute into 10 mL.

Preparation

- Explanation to patient.
- Obtain IV access, ideally with 14 or 16 G cannula.
- Fluid pre-load: 500–1000 mL of crystalloid.
- Vasopressor available, e.g. 30 mg ephedrine in 10 mL saline.
- Check BP.

Procedure

- Same as for a diagnostic lumbar puncture.
- Sit the patient with their feet supported, back arched forwards, vertebrae pushed backwards, and chin tucked towards chest. Useful to have helper.
- Tuffier's line joins the iliac crests crossing the dorsal spine at the fourth lumbar vertebra. Above this line is the L3/4 interspace, and below is the L4/5 interspace. *Do not go above L3 as the needle may injure the spinal cord* (Fig. 19.4).
- Using sterile gloves, clean a large area around the planned insertion site with antiseptic.
- Raise a subcutaneous wheal of LA (e.g. 1% lidocaine) at L3/4 or L4/5.
- Using a 22–29 G disposable spinal needle (preferably 25–29 G as there is less risk of postdural puncture headache), insert the spinal needle at the chosen interspace in the midline. Advance with 15° cephalad (towards the head) angulation until a click or pop is felt at an approximate depth of 4–6 cm (dura punctured) (Fig. 19.5).
- If bone is hit first, withdraw the needle to just below skin and re-insert, usually with more cephalad angulation, checking that you are in the midline.
- Withdraw stylet and check free flow of CSF. If blood flows, withdraw the spinal needle completely and try again. If the patient complains of shooting pain on insertion, withdraw needle immediately, check pain settles, and try again.
- Inject the local, ensuring that the spinal needle is not moved inadvertently.
- Following injection, lie patient on back with legs flexed for 10 min.

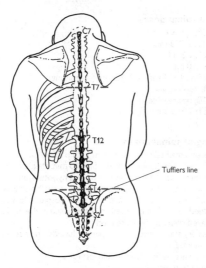

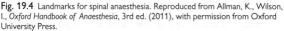

Fig. 19.4 Landmarks for spinal anaesthesia. Reproduced from Allman, K., Wilson, I., *Oxford Handbook of Anaesthesia*, 3rd ed. (2011), with permission from Oxford University Press.

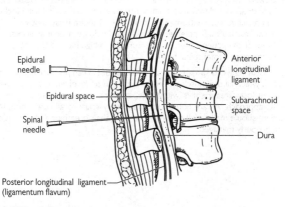

Fig. 19.5 Position for spinal anaesthesia injections. Reproduced from Allman, K., Wilson, I., *Oxford Handbook of Anaesthesia*, 3rd ed. (2011), with permission from Oxford University Press

Suggested spinal doses
- Heavy 0.5% bupivacaine:
  - T6–T10: 2.5–3 mL.
  - T11–L1: 2.5 mL.
  - L2–L5: 2.0 mL.
  - S1–S5 (saddle block): 1.0–1.5 mL (stay sitting).
- Plain 0.5% bupivacaine:
  - T6–T10: not reliable.
  - T11–L1: 2.5–3.0 mL.
  - L2–L5: 2.5 mL.

Monitoring of spinal anaesthesia
- After injection maintain verbal contact with patient.
- Check BP every few minutes for the first 10 min, then every 5 min.
- Nausea is quite common—it often indicates hypotension. Treat with fluids and a vasopressor such as ephedrine 3–6 mg boluses IV.
- Opioids, often included in spinal injections in hospital practice, should not be added to spinal anaesthetic mixtures used in the field as they may cause delayed respiratory depression.
- Before surgery starts, test that the patient has lost their sense of pain in the relevant area.
- A spinal bupivacaine injection should last for 2–4 h.
- Urinary retention may occur.
- Patients can mobilize after the block has completely worn off.
- The spread of blocks is more variable if plain, as opposed to heavy or hyperbaric solution, is used.
- Beware of 'high blocks'. The patient will notice numbness or weakness in their arms and may find it difficult to take a deep breath. High blocks can result in more extreme falls in BP, which require treatment with vasoconstrictors. Supplementary oxygen should be given if available. Monitor the patient carefully to ensure that a high block does not progress to a total spinal block.

Excessive cephalad spread of a large volume of LA can produce a 'total spinal' in which all the muscles of respiration can be involved. Consciousness can be lost. Treatment is with fluids, ephedrine, and resuscitation on an ABC approach. A rare complication and very scary to all concerned, the patient should make a full recovery providing their breathing and circulation are properly managed.

Ketamine anaesthesia

Ketamine is widely used in field and developing world anaesthesia. Its ease of administration should not tempt the inexperienced to use it except in desperate circumstances.

When to use it
- For general anaesthesia, if local and regional anaesthetic techniques are not possible.
- At sedative/analgesic doses for fracture reduction, abscess drainage, and burns dressings, etc.

Advantages
- Sole agent required for induction and maintenance of anaesthesia.
- Increases sympathetic tone so BP well maintained even in shocked patients.
- Respiration is not depressed (especially useful at altitude).
- Airway is normally well maintained.
- Strong analgesic.
- Doses can be given as IV boluses, IV infusions, or IM.
- Can be used in low 'sedative-analgesic' doses for reduction of fractures, splint application, small abscess drainage, and burns dressings.

Disadvantages
- Drug ampoules dispensed in a variety of strengths, check which you have.
- Anaesthetized patients often have involuntary movements; their eyes may remain disconcertingly open.
- Salivation increases. Consider atropine (0.6 mg IV) at induction.
- Aspiration and respiratory arrest are still possible, so full resuscitation equipment must be available.
- Some patients get unpleasant hallucinations following ketamine anaesthesia.

Monitoring
Clinical and, if available, BP and pulse oximetry.

Technique
- Obtain IV access.
- Apply monitoring and oxygen if available.

Induction
- IV dose for anaesthesia: 1–2 mg/kg. Onset 1–2 min, lasts 10–15 min.
- IM dose for anaesthesia: 8–10 mg/kg IM. Onset 5 min, duration 20–30 min.

It is safer to give a smaller dose and titrate to effect than to give the full dose straight off. You can always give more but you can't take it out!

Maintenance
- Give intermittent bolus 0.5–1 mg/kg IV every 15–20 min.
  Or
- Continuous infusion for longer cases:
  - Add 500 mg of ketamine to a 500 mL bag of crystalloid fluid (= 1 mg/mL), run at 2–4 mg/kg/h.
  - Stop infusion 30 min before expected end of procedure.

To set up an infusion
- Most drip sets are 20 drops per mL (but check packaging).
- If you use an infusion concentration of 1mg ketamine/mL then a rate of:

  (Patients wt in kg) drops/min = 4 mg/kg/h
- I.e. if the patient weighs 70 kg, then 70 drops/min equates to approximately 4 mg/kg/h.
- In the absence of more sophisticated equipment, set drops/min rate by timing against watch, and then ask an assistant to regularly check that the rate does not vary.

Emergence
- 'Emergence phenomenon' can be unpleasant.
- Try to permit patient to wake naturally in a quiet and calm environment.
- Consider IV benzodiazepine, such as diazepam or midazolam 0.1 mg/kg with induction.

Sedation

Definition
A state of reduced consciousness where verbal contact with the patient is maintained.

When to use it
For short, uncomfortable procedures to provide anxiolysis and amnesia.

Advantages
- May avoid need for general anaesthesia.
- Ketamine and methoxyflurane provide analgesia as well.

Disadvantages
- Risk of cardiorespiratory depression with benzodiazepines and ketamine, therefore must have resuscitation equipment available.
- Benzodiazepines have no analgesic effects.
- Caution if using opiates with sedatives as easier to over-sedate.

Techniques
Ideally the same level of monitoring and oxygen as for general anaesthesia.

Benzodiazepines
- Midazolam 0.07–0.1 mg/kg IV or diazepam 0.05–0.1 mg/kg IV.
- Titrate to response, give 1–2 mg doses and allow at least 3 min between each dose for effect.
- Anxiolysis and amnesia but no analgesia.
- Flumazenil 0.1–1 mg can be used to reverse the effects of benzodiazepines.

Ketamine
- Dose 0.3–0.8 mg/kg IV or 2–4 mg IM.
- Titrate to effect using a divided dose.
- Allow 5–10 min for IM effect.
- Provides anxiolysis, amnesia, and analgesia.

Methoxyflurane (penthrox/green whistle)
- An inhaled potent analgesic with some amnesia and anxiolysis.
- Only available in Australia and New Zealand, withdrawn elsewhere due to nephrotoxicity.
- When used at analgesic doses no nephrotoxic effects seen.
- Comes as a green plastic inhaler (the green whistle) with 3 mL ampoules of methoxyflurane.
- Patients self-administer and should inhale intermittently as required.
- One dose of 3 mL lasts ~30 min.
- A second and final dose of 3 mL can be given if required.
- A maximum weekly dose of 15 mL should not be exceeded or nephrotoxic effects may occur.

Suggested minimum equipment and drugs for field anaesthesia

Airway
- Self-inflating bag and selection of face masks.
- Oral (Guedel) airways and nasal airways.
- Portable, e.g. hand- or foot-powered, suction unit. Suction catheters.
- Laryngoscope and blades plus spare bulbs and batteries.
- Oral endotracheal tubes with 15 mm connectors.
- Airway bougie.

Intravenous
- Selection of cannulae, needles, and syringes.
- Tourniquet, securing tape, or dressings for cannulae.
- Crystalloid, e.g. Hartmann's solution or 0.9% sodium chloride.
- Giving sets.

Resuscitation
- Adrenaline (epinephrine), atropine.
- Ephedrine.

Local anaesthetic
- Lidocaine/bupivacaine for LA.
- Preservative-free 'heavy' bupivacaine 0.5% for spinal anaesthetic.

Anaesthetic/sedation drugs
- Ketamine.
- Benzodiazepine such as midazolam.
- Opioid such as morphine, or other analgesic such as tramadol.
- Naloxone and flumazenil to reverse above.
- If intubation a possibility, muscle relaxant and neostigmine.

Spinal
- Spinal needles: 22, 25, or 27 G needles.

Monitoring
- Portable battery-powered pulse oximeter, stethoscope, sphygmomanometer.

Miscellaneous
- Antiseptic cleaning solution, sterile and non-sterile gloves, sterile swabs.
- Nasogastric tubes, scissors.
- Torch/headlight.

Local facilities
- Will possibly have use of local hospital facilities.
- Likely to be basic, especially in developing countries.
- If possible, rely on own equipment and drugs.

Oxygen sources
- Compressed oxygen cylinders may have faulty pressure gauges, making estimation of remaining supply unreliable.
- Cylinders may come in a variety of colours, and may not have consistent or reliable labelling.
- Oxygen concentrators are reliable if serviced and power supply guaranteed; these yield ~90% oxygen at flows <4 L. With age the concentration may decrease.
- Ideally use techniques not dependent on oxygen availability.

Drugs
- Quality assurance of drugs sourced in developing countries may be poor.
- Store drugs appropriately, especially muscle relaxants such as suxamethonium and atracurium, which should be kept cool, especially in the tropics.
- Be vigilant of 'use by' dates.

Anaesthetic delivery equipment
- Carefully check any anaesthetic equipment if you plan to use it. Is it safe/complete?
- Draw-over vaporizers and Oxford inflating bellows are reliable if well serviced.
- Halothane vaporizers can be cleaned with trilene or ether.
- The use of unfamiliar equipment by the inexperienced is dangerous.

Monitoring
- Equipment sourced locally may be poorly maintained, incomplete, or faulty.
- Pulse oximeters are often available, ECG and automated BP usually absent.
- Clinical observation—mucous membrane colour, capillary refill, central pulses, and precordial stethoscope are all useful.
- Ideally utilize a conscious anaesthetic technique, e.g. spinal or regional/ local.

Further reading
Allman KG, Wilson IH (2011). *Oxford Handbook of Anaesthesia*, 3rd ed. Oxford: Oxford University Press.

Craven R (2007). Ketamine. *Anaesthesia*, 62(suppl.1), 48–53.

Dobson MB (2000). *Anaesthesia at the District Hospital*. Geneva: World Health Organization.

Vreede E (2001). *Field Anaesthesia—Basic Practice*. Médecins Sans Frontières. Available via e-mail: guide.anaesthesia@msf.org

Cold climates

Section editor
Chris Imray

Contributors
Ian Davis
Chris Johnson
Clive Johnson
Howard Oakley
Barry Roberts

The polar environment 608
Travel in cold climates 612
Whiteout 613
Humans in polar areas 614
Preparations for a polar trip 618
Infectious diseases in polar areas 620
Hypothermia 622
Freezing cold injuries 626
Non-freezing cold injury 632
Snow blindness (photokeratitis) 634
Skin problems 636
Problems of prolonged polar travel 636

The polar environment

Wilderness medicine in a cold or polar environment involves all the challenges of remote medicine but with additional climatic stresses that impact on all aspects of living, travelling, and surviving. In addition to being cold and windy, these regions are often extremely remote and may include dramatic high-altitude mountains and glaciers—hostile, yet beautiful environments under threat from global warming.

Weather

The characteristic feature of cold climates is that the temperature remains below freezing for lengthy periods of the year, resulting in accumulations of snow and ice. Polar environments surround both poles and extend to lower latitudes during winter, similar conditions are found at high altitude anywhere on earth. The predominance of snow in a polar climate disguises the fact that many polar environments have very little precipitation; Antarctica is one of the driest places on earth, but winds move the snow around, regularly generating blizzard conditions. Sub-Arctic continental environments such as the Yukon, Alaska, and Siberia have bitterly cold winters, but their summers can be mild or even hot, with a rich diversity of wildlife, flowers, insects, and even a significant risk of huge forest fires.

The dominant factors in polar and cold climates are air temperature, wind speed, and sunlight. Around freezing point, high humidity (freezing fog) can make conditions feel bitterly cold, but humidity falls at lower temperatures and ceases to be a significant influence.

The windchill index combines temperature and windspeed to estimate the hazards to humans of the environment. Formulated by Siple and Passal in 1945, the original calculations were based upon the rate at which plastic bags of water froze. North American studies in 2003 instead studied the rate of cooling of exposed human faces, and derived a complex mathematical formula[1] to calculate the cooling effect of the climate. In practice it is easier to use online calculators[2] or one of the numerous downloadable weather apps to judge the hazard of the environment. For those without communication links, Fig. 20.1 and Fig. 20.2 provide equivalent information.

Prevailing meteorological conditions may be modified by local circumstances; for instance, wind speed and therefore windchill are reduced by contour features, trees, and clothing, but increased by skiing or travelling on a skidoo. Temperatures may be lower in sheltered valleys, but travel that is safe in the valley can become dangerous when crossing an exposed and windy pass. Bright sunshine raises the apparent temperature considerably. Careless behaviour can lead to frostbite in conditions that should pose a low physical risk. (See Table 20.1.)

---

1 http://www.nws.noaa.gov/om/winter/windchill.shtml

2 http://www.onlineconversion.com/windchill.htm

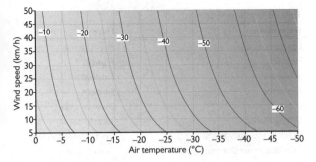

Fig. 20.1 Windchill index. Reproduced with the permission of the Minister of Public Works and Government Services Canada, 2007.

The following are approximate values

Temperature (°C) Wind (km/h)	−15	−20	−25	−30	−35	−40	−45	−50
10	*	*	22	15	10	8	7	2
20	*	30	14	10	5	4	3	2
30	*	18	11	8	5	2	2	1
40	42	14	9	5	5	2	2	1
50	27	12	8	5	2	2	2	1
60	22	10	7	5	2	2	2	1
70	18	9	5	4	2	2	2	1
80	16	8	5	4	2	2	2	1

*Frostbite unlikely.
The wind speed, in km/h, is at the standard anemometer height of 10 m (as reported in weather observations).

Frostbite possible in 2 min or less	2
Frostbite possible in 3–5 min	5
Frostbite possible in 6–10 min	10

Fig. 20.2 Windchill—minutes to frostbite. Reproduced with the permission of the Minister of Public Works and Government Services Canada, 2007.

Table 20.1 Polar environment

Environmental	Medical
Low temperatures	Hypothermia
High winds	Frostnip
Whiteout	Frostbite
Avalanche	Sunburn
Crevasse	Snow blindness
Shifting sea ice	Trench foot
Wildlife (especially bears)	Contaminated water
Thin lake, stream, or marsh ice	Dehydration
Transport (ski and skidoo)	Slips and falls
Insects in summer season	Recreational hazards

Risk analysis

(See also ➲ Avalanches, p. 642.)

Novice travellers in cold environments may encounter many hazards—most of them unfamiliar:

- Visitors to snowy areas want to enjoy the recreational opportunities, but the environment is not always accorded the respect it deserves. Icy areas around living accommodation are a common place for injuries—spread grit or ash to improve grip.
- Skiing, snowboarding, and sledging are hazardous, and an expedition with scientific goals and limited medical backup must minimize the risk that team members injure themselves during their leisure time.
- Rocks may be frost-fractured and unstable, while ice climbing is a high-risk pastime.
- Steep snow slopes will present avalanche risks and glaciated terrain will often be crevassed.
- Tracked vehicles have small turning circles and unprotected machinery. Noise and limited visibility prevents their drivers from being fully aware of their surrounding—skiers and pedestrians must stay well away. Skidoos range from slow load haulers to racing vehicles; keep your legs and arms inboard, follow trail rules, and beware of wire fences.
- Cold weather and alcohol don't mix. Drunkenness leads to injuries and the risk of hypothermia. Many circumpolar peoples have exceptionally low alcohol tolerance and should not be encouraged to drink alcohol, particularly when they are in the field.

Wildlife in cold regions

(See also Chapter 17.)

Animal life at the two poles differs considerably. In the south, hazards are rare and can be avoided by watching animals from a sensible distance and keeping away from the sea ice edge. Research scientists are at greater risk.

Killer whales and leopard seals are potential threats in or on the water and ice edge. Fur seals bite intruders in their colonies, while bull elephant seals will aggressively guard their territory. At both poles, birds, particularly terns, will attack intruders on nesting sites by flying at their heads; an umbrella or walking pole may prevent collisions.

In northern areas, bears, wolves, elk, and moose pose substantial threats. By far the commonest problem occurs on roads at night. Moose use roads as convenient thoroughfares and as salt licks, as a result are frequently hit by cars, sadly often with fatal results to both animal and humans. In Newfoundland there are about 700 moose/vehicle collisions each year, and elk create serious problems for Scandinavian drivers. Away from roads, these large animals can also be a threat. Avoid approaching male moose during the autumn rutting season, and do not stray between a mother and her calf. At other times, the animals are generally placid and can be safely observed from a distance.

Bears are a danger. In North American tourist areas national park rangers monitor bear activity and offer advice about travel, closing campsites and trails if aggressive bears have been reported. Advice on dealing with a bear encounter is widely available.[3]

Most bears prefer to keep away from humans and will move on if parties make noisy progress through the wilderness. Brown and grizzly bears usually hibernate in winter and are the greatest threat if early autumn snow forces them down from the mountains into tourist areas. Do not leave food where it is accessible to bears. They become accustomed to this easy source of food, threaten humans, and then have to be culled or transported to very remote areas. Travellers on back-country trails should carry pepper sprays.

Polar bears are a very serious danger, particularly in areas such as Northern Canada and Svalbard (Spitzbergen), which are increasingly popular adventure tourism destinations. Campsites can be protected by a perimeter alarm system of ropes, bells, or empty cans; sledge dog teams can be spanned around the periphery, and it may be essential to carry firearms, and clearly appropriate training is crucial (➔ Polar bear, p. 543). The risk of polar bear attack can reduced if visitors stay in cabins instead of tents, use trip wires that detonate explosives, use guard-dogs, and deploy someone on polar bear watch who is armed.

During the summer huge numbers of biting insects breed in the ponds and marshes of low Arctic regions; clothing with ankle and wrist elastics, and midge hoods will make life bearable.

3 ℘ http://esrd.alberta.ca/recreation-public-use/alberta-bear-smart/default.aspx

Travel in cold climates

Improvements in transport, navigation, equipment, and communications have made access to remote polar areas much easier. Using a combination of fixed and rotary winged aircraft and coastal craft, logistic companies can supply and support polar expeditions, but travel remains costly and weather restricted, sometimes making casualty evacuation very difficult.

Once at the destination, travel may involve traditional technologies such as by walking, snowshoes, dog sleds, or skis, or more modern solutions such skidoos, superjeeps, ski cats, or kite skis. Environmental hazards such as crevasses and avalanches, and meteorological variations such as diurnal temperature change or whiteout may affect route timing and choice. Navigation may utilize maps, compasses, sextants, or GPS. Modern technology greatly enhances an explorer's ability to navigate in difficult weather and terrain, but only while the batteries last.

Whiteout

Whiteout is a meteorological condition where there is lack of contrast, visibility may be excellent, or masked by fog. With no visual points of reference it is easy to walk or ski over a cornice, travel in circles, or even fall over while standing still. Though sometimes necessary, travel in whiteout is undesirable and may be very hazardous.

Search and rescue

Avalanche transceivers are essential in mountainous areas and familiarity with their expeditious use is vital if buried victims are to have a chance of being extricated alive.

Mobile phone coverage extends to fairly remote areas of Scandinavia; satellite phones are valuable, though expensive, when beyond the range of terrestrial equipment and essential if you have arranged a 24-h 'doctor on call' emergency service. In 2013, only the Iridium system guarantees polar coverage. Checking the adequacy of coverage of any system prior to departure is essential. Short wave radio communications can be disrupted by auroral activity. Satellite beacons (emergency position-indicating beacons; EPIRBs) are becoming increasingly useful particularly if there is a satellite phone failure (battery, damaged, or lost), but require sophisticated SAR services in the area.

Environmental impact of humans

Polar and cold environments are threatened by global warming, their habitats fragile and vulnerable to the increasing numbers of visitors. The concept of sustainable ecotourism needs to be championed. All visitors to these precious areas need to be aware of the impact of their visit and try to minimize the effects (⊃ Assessing an expedition's environmental footprint, p. 125).

Humans in polar areas

Humans have little physiological ability to acclimatize to cold environments. The only proven response to chronic cold exposure is the Lewis 'hunting response'. Fit, experienced workers who regularly expose their hands to temperatures below 5°C can develop a cyclical vasodilatation of the skin vessels that enables them to maintain higher mean hand temperatures than new arrivals in a cold environment. At a time when hunting and fishing required hand agility at low temperatures, this mechanism had survival benefit. However, most modern polar travellers will not regularly expose their hands to such low temperatures, and those who do run the risk of suffering recurrent minor cold injury instead of acclimatizing. Native peoples in circumpolar areas have a short, stocky build, suggesting that an endomorphic body shape has survival benefits in very cold climates.

Travellers in cold dry climates encounter few problems if the temperature is above −10°C. As temperatures fall further:

- The need to humidify dry air causes the nose to drip.
- Facial and anorak hood encrustation with icicles develops.
- Lips become dry and cracked—a good moisturizing sunscreen is essential. During prolonged arctic journeys travellers can have serious problems with lip ulceration and bleeding.
- Bright sunlight can cause snow blindness, but sunglasses or goggles can be difficult to use in very cold conditions as condensation from forehead or eyes freezes on their surface.
- Strong sunlight and UV light reflecting off a bright reflective snow or ice surface greatly increases the risk of sunburn on any exposed skin. Protect skin with high SPA creams, including the undersides of chin, ears, and nose.
- Strenuous exercise in very low temperatures, below −40°C, can result in chest pain, possibly caused by very cold air reaching the bronchi. Asthma is commoner amongst cross country skiers than in the general population.

Chronic conditions that may be exacerbated by cold dry air include:

- Cold-induced asthma.
- Peripheral circulatory problems, including Raynaud's syndrome, and the presence of cold agglutinins in the blood.
- Angina.
- Sufferers from these conditions should consider whether they will be able to travel and work safely—if in doubt test the effects of the cold by persuading your local butcher to let you into the cold store.

Children in cold weather

Children can be safely taken into cold climates, but must be properly dressed and closely supervised as they can lose body heat rapidly. Early signs of chilling include grumpiness and a reluctance to move. Young children should not be carried in backpacks in the cold; the parent may slip and fall, while the youngster's legs can become constricted by the base of the pack, resulting in poor circulation and cold injury to the legs. Ski pulks— sledges for towing youngsters in the snow—are popular in Scandinavia; legislation bans their use if the air temperature is below −10°C. Parents or guides should regularly check to ensure that their charges' hands and feet have not become numb. An exercising adult may be unaware of how cold the resting youngster has become.

Accommodation, heat, light, and fuel

Polar expeditions will usually choose a permanent building as a base camp for their work. When the camp involves several buildings, doorways should be linked by hand-lines, as it is easy to become disorientated in darkness or a blizzard. This particularly applies to latrines sited some distance from the base. Fire is a serious threat in areas where water is not available to extinguish flames. Store fuel away from the main base building, there should also be an emergency dump of clothing and food in case of a serious conflagration.

In extreme cold and at high altitude, cooking gas cylinders should be warmed (body warmth or sunlight) before use. Consider keeping the cylinder in a sleeping bag at night. When in use, raise the cylinder off the cold ground using a thin insulating board. Consider the mix of fuels being used. Pure propane has a boiling point of −42°C, but requires a heavy steel canister to safely contain it. Butane has a boiling point of −1°C, but does not vaporize well when the temperature drops well below freezing. In cold weather an appropriate cold weather blend is the best solution and usually a mix of 80–85% iso-butane and 15–20% propane is optimal (e.g. MSR IsoPro® fuel, Snow Peak GigaPower® fuel, or Jetboil JetPower® fuel).

Snow holes are warmer than tents in extreme conditions, but more laborious to construct. Tents and snow holes must be positioned away from avalanche runs and trails; both should be well marked so that vehicles and skiers do not accidentally cross them, and they can be re-located in poor weather.

When camping on glaciated terrain, camps need to be carefully assessed by a roped climber using an avalanche probe to rule out hidden crevasses and mark the safe perimeter using bamboo canes or 'wands'. Only then should the team unrope and once unroped, they should remain inside the designated safe area at all times.[4]

Carbon monoxide poisoning

Carbon monoxide poisoning and dangerously low oxygen levels are both serious risks in closed areas if candles or cooking stoves are used. If a candle flame burns low or goes out, oxygen levels are dangerously low. Carbon monoxide from cooking stoves is odourless and causes insidious poisoning. Headache and nausea usually precede unconsciousness, but the cause may not be apparent to fatigued travellers, or at altitude where such symptoms are common. Tents designed for extreme conditions are very windproof, particularly if they become partially buried in drifting snow; ventilators may block with condensation and must be checked regularly. Cooking with the tent door partially open in all but the most extreme weather is strongly recommended. Deaths have occurred. Supplementary oxygen should be given to a survivor and the victim evacuated. If facilities exist in the area, hyperbaric oxygen is an effective treatment.

4 Imray C, Tipton M, Dhillon S, Montgomery H (2013). Surviving in a crevasse. *Lancet*, 381(9881), 1903–4.

Water

Fresh water can usually be obtained by melting snow, and is safe to drink unless it comes from an area frequented by animals or birds. Clear and separate designation of the latrine area and water source has to be established from the outset. Using a small volume of water at the base of a pan of snow greatly increases the speed at which the snow (mainly air) will melt. Large amounts of fuel[5] are needed to melt snow, particularly at very low temperatures, so whenever practical dig or drill through overlying snow to obtain stream water running below. The upper layers of sea ice usually contain little salt and are potable. In the Northern hemisphere, deer and beaver may live close to apparently pristine melt streams and can contaminate the water with *Giardia*. Glacier outwash streams contain fine, highly abrasive rock dust in suspension; this is a powerful laxative. If in doubt, filter water and then boil or sterilize it (➋ Water purification, p. 102).

Because polar air is very dry, sweat evaporates quickly and fluid losses may be underestimated. Dehydration is a risk during the first days of an expedition; even if people do not feel thirsty, they should drink sufficiently to ensure that they urinate dilute, pale urine. A combination of malaise, headache, and raised body temperature is common when groups first arrive in the cold; this may be a mild form of heat exhaustion. Bathing in cold climates is a masochistic pastime. On shorter expeditions and when facilities permit, people and clothes should be washed whenever possible to prevent fungal skin infections and boils. In the field, 'wet wipes' can provide a practical way of maintaining hygiene. However, without washing, the Inuit and members of prolonged field expeditions develop a natural balance with their body oils and the risk of infection reduces. To avoid offence, it is wise to shower shortly after returning to heated accommodation!

Food

Around base camp, or travelling using motorized transport, energy requirements will be similar to those of an outdoor worker in the UK (3000 kcal/ 12000 kJ per day), but man-hauling sledges and cross country skiing are extremely energetic pastimes requiring two to four times this energy intake, and eating enough is challenging. Typically a 5–10 min rest every hour to snack and rehydrate is the only way of adequately fueling during a strenuous climb. A greater proportion of the diet is likely to be made up of fatty foods, and a wide selection of high calorie snacks and foods should be available. In the past, polar expeditions have lived off the land, but nowadays most Arctic species are protected and licences are required before they are hunted. The internal organs of some polar animals contain toxic amounts of vitamin A and should never be eaten. When travelling in areas where big mammals hunt, you should ensure that food is stored appropriately. Airtight containers in rucksacks and animal-proof food dumps reduce the risk of unwanted visitors.

---

5 At least double the fuel requirements for your stove if temperature is −40°C.

Sanitation

Polar environments are extremely fragile ecosystems in which organic matter degrades very slowly. Removing waste is your gift to future generations. In Antarctica, expeditions are required to ship out all their waste, including faeces and sanitary materials. National Parks in North America, Canada, and Greenland also have specific requirements about waste disposal, which is a 'pack in—pack out' policy.

Supplies

Cold will affect many items, including batteries, contact lens fluids, and drugs. Aqueous drugs freeze, crystallize, and may degrade in the cold; therefore powdered preparations and plastic containers should be selected whenever possible. Critical items can be kept warm by body heat or heat packs used to maintain temperature.

Detailed advanced planning is required to accurately predict food and fuel consumption. Contingency plans and adequate reserves are required. Stoves are lifesavers in the hostile polar environment and spare parts or spare stove is essential. Optimal choice of fuel will depend upon a number of factors including the number travelling, the destination, the duration and ease of re-supply.

Preparations for a polar trip

- Dental check-up, as problems may be exacerbated by the cold.
- If you take regular medication, make sure you take enough to last the entire trip plus extra in case of delays. Inform other team members, so they are aware of the dose and where the medication is kept.
- If you wear spectacles, take a spare pair and have prescription sun glasses made. Make sure ski goggles are the type that fit easily over glasses.
- Make sure that boots fit well and are 'broken-in' before starting out. Physical and mental endurance are essential on multi-day trips. Middle-aged participants in 'adventure' holidays that involve long distances skiing, snow-shoeing, or pulling sledges must have prepared properly.
- Consider rabies vaccination if the disease is endemic amongst local sledge dogs.
- Appropriate insurance is essential; it remains difficult, dangerous, and very expensive to evacuate casualties from remote polar areas.
- Tents, skis, and other equipment must be appropriate to the area visited and capable of surviving extreme conditions.

Just having the appropriate equipment is not enough. Familiarity with when and how to use it is often overlooked and is just as important. The 'week-end warrior' or the affluent but inexperienced polar traveller is a potential danger to both himself and his companions.

Clothing

Careful consideration needs to be given to the range and choice of clothing taken to cold and polar regions. Active individuals will typically use a flexible layering system, with a wicking non-absorbable base-layer building up through a series of insulating layers to an outer wind/waterproof shell. Those riding on sledges or skidoos may prefer a heavily insulated over-garment, though these can restrict movement. The final choice will vary between individuals and will reflect the ambient temperature, the wind chill, the altitude, their susceptibility to cold, and the activity undertaken. Synthetic and natural fibres and fabrics have different advantages and disadvantages; these need to be understood if the benefits are to be fully utilized.

Clothing should be adequate to prevent body cooling, but excessive clothing results in a build-up of body heat and sweating, which is undesirable as perspiration condenses in clothes, reducing their insulation. Although modern breathable synthetic fabrics function adequately in cold dry climates, many experts prefer cotton 'ventile' shell garments. After prolonged use without washing, woollen base layers such as merino are less malodorous than synthetics. Energetic cross-country skiers often wear thin garments, but must carry windproofs in case conditions change; the groin area can become painfully cold and requires effective thermal protection, e.g. using thermal windproof underpants. If such 'wind-pants' are not worn, the penis is alarmingly vulnerable to frostbite. At any rest or meal break, conserve heat by putting on a belay jacket or zipping up anorak vents, and by putting on scarf, hats, and gloves.

Mittens are superior to gloves at retaining peripheral heat in very cold climates and should be used with wrist or 'idiot loops'. Chemical hand warmers are useful when hands or feet become uncomfortably cold, and are a great morale booster for children in the snow, but should be used with caution if peripheries have become numb, as there is the risk of thermal heat injury. Loose fitting, well-insulated footwear, with gaiters to prevent snow getting onto socks, are desirable. Battery-powered heated insoles are available if feet are to be exposed to the cold for lengthy periods at low exercise levels; for instance, when travelling by skidoo, or making scientific observations. However the practicality of using any electrical or chemical technique over sustained periods is unrealistic. Whenever possible, boots should be warmed and dried; over a period of days they accumulate moisture and can freeze if taken off in a tent overnight.

Eyes

Eyes must be protected from UV glare by appropriate sunglasses or goggles (see ➲ Snow blindness (photokeratitis), p. 634). For those with visual defects, contact lenses, prescription sunglasses or spectacles with photochromic lenses all work reasonably well. Wearing ordinary spectacles under goggles is cumbersome. Anyone whose vision is so poor that they always need to wear glasses or contact lenses must plan to avoid the difficulties that would arise from loss or breakage: as a minimum, a spare pair of spectacles should be taken. Below −20°C, glasses invariably mist over, and contact lenses may be preferable. However, contact lenses can adhere or even freeze to the eye. Forced or clumsy removal can then result in corneal abrasion, requiring topical treatment with antibiotics and local anaesthetic (➲ Contact lenses, p. 325).

Metal spectacle frames can become very cold and cause cold injury if in direct contact with the skin; opticians sell silicone sheaths that cover the side arms. Plastic-framed glasses or snow goggles are preferable, but become brittle at low temperatures. Carry spare filters for goggles as these too can crack after prolonged exposure to the cold.

Infectious diseases in polar areas

In the past, imported infectious diseases such as diphtheria, measles, and TB tragically decimated circumpolar native populations, but infectious diseases are nowadays uncommon in polar areas. Some sledge dogs carry rabies, and inoculation is advisable if the expedition is visiting an endemic area. Sexually transmitted infections have a worldwide distribution. After prolonged residence in a cold climate—e.g. over-wintering on a polar base—travellers will be particularly susceptible to upper respiratory tract infections.

An increasing number of visitors are being airlifted onto the Antarctic plateau (2500 m/8000 ft+) to compete in races or personal challenges. The combination of cold and altitude with pre-existing upper respiratory tract infections has resulting in several incidents where previously fit individuals have developed severe pulmonary symptoms, possibly as a result of a combination of infection and altitude sickness.

Hypothermia

In the field, diagnosis can be difficult, but anyone whose torso feels 'as cold as marble' should be treated as a cold casualty. Diagnosis can be confirmed by measuring body temperature using a low reading rectal thermometer, preferably a calibrated electronic device with the sensor inserted to 15 cm beyond the anal sphincter. Conventional oral thermometers do not measure low body temperatures, and infrared tympanic membrane thermometers can be inaccurate by several degrees, particularly when the ear has been exposed to cold, heat, or water.

Hypothermia is a drop in the victim's core body temperature to an extent that their ability to function normally is impaired. Normal core temperature is 36.5–37°C. Temperatures below 35°C cause progressive symptoms similar to drunkenness and known as the 'umbles': the victim stumbles, grumbles, mumbles, & fumbles. They may shiver uncontrollably, but do not always do so and—rejecting help—may vehemently deny that anything is wrong. Untreated, they will eventually become comatose and die. (See Table 20.2.).

Swiss field staging system[6,7]

Stage 1: mild hypothermia
Core temperature, 35–37°C (95–98.6°F) associated with shivering and poor fine motor coordination.

Stage 2: moderate hypothermia
Core temperature, 32–34.9°C (89.6–94.8°F) associated with violent shivering, stumbling and confusion despite alertness and finally collapse.

Stage 3: severe hypothermia
Core temperature, <32°C (<89.6°F) with cessation of shivering, reduced level of consciousness progressing to stupor, paradoxical behaviors such as burrowing and undressing, bradycardia and tachyarrhythmias, reduced respiration cold diuresis, organ failures, and death.

6 Brugger H, Durrer B, Adler-Kastner L, Falk M, Tschirky F (2001). Field management of avalanche victims. *Resuscitation*, 51, 7–15 (figure 3, p. 11).

7 State of Alaska Cold Injuries Guidelines. Available at: ℔ http://dhss.alaska.gov/dph/Emergency/Documents/ems/assets/Downloads/AKColdInj2005.pdf

Prevention

Hypothermia is uncommon in a properly clothed fit person, but develops if someone is injured, lost, short of food and/or water, or if their clothing is inadequate or wet, especially in windy conditions. Typically it develops insidiously over several hours, but death (usually from 'cold shock' or drowning when disabled by hypothermia) can occur within minutes if someone is immersed in cold water.

Table 20.2 Approximate core body temperatures at which serious malfunction develops

Body core temperature (°C)	Associated symptoms
37	Normal body temperature
36	
35	Judgement may be affected: poor decision-making. Feels cold, looks cold, shivering
34	Change of personality, usually withdrawn—'switches off/doesn't care'. Inappropriate behaviour—may shed clothing. Stumbling, falling, confused
33	Consciousness clouded, incoherent. Shivering stops
32	Serious risk of cardiac arrest. Body cannot restore temperature without help. Limbs stiffen
31	Unconscious
30	Pulse and breathing undetectable
29	
28	Pupils become fixed and dilated
27	
26	
25	
24	Few victims recover from this temperature
23	
22	
21	
20	
19	
18	
17	
16	
15	
14	Lowest recorded temperature of survival[8]

8 Gilbert M, Busund R, Skagseth A, Nilsen PA, Solbø JP (2000). Resuscitation from accidental hypothermia of 13.7 degrees C with circulatory arrest. *Lancet*, 355, 375–6.

Field management

Experts disagree about the best treatment for severe hypothermia and this has led to conflicting advice in textbooks. However, the controversies are irrelevant to most expeditions as they are unlikely to carry the advanced resuscitation equipment now available to mountain rescue groups. The aim of treatment is to restore the body heat of the victim:

- Seek shelter—building, tent, snow hole, survival bag, or group shelter.
- Remove damp outer clothing. Wrap casualty in additional dry insulation such as a sleeping bag. If this is impossible, place inside a heavy plastic bag and seal around the neck to eliminate evaporative heat loss. Do not bother using inefficient 'space blankets'.
- Lie down and insulate from the ground using, for instance, rucksacks.
- If conscious:
  - Restore body heat by providing warm drinks, warming the air with a stove, and sharing the body heat of unaffected rescuers.
  - Chemical heat pads can be helpful if they are available, but ensure that they do not cause burns.
  - Do not give alcohol.
  - Ensure casualty rests and is kept under close supervision for at least 24 h.
- If unconscious or body temperature very low:
  - Ensure breathing does not obstruct, try to prevent further heat loss, arrange urgent evacuation if feasible.
  - Rewarm using any method that can be improvised.
  - Support circulation with warmed IV fluids if available.

It may be very difficult to tell whether a hypothermic casualty is dead or alive. Breathing will be slow and shallow, while the pulse may be slow, thready, and palpable only in the neck and groin. If unsure, assume that the casualty is alive. In an isolated base camp, the best that can be done is to keep the victim as warm as possible, ensure that their breathing does not obstruct and, if possible, infuse some warmed IV fluid to maintain hydration. The patient needs to be turned regularly to ensure that they are not lying in one position for a prolonged period. Advanced life support measures such as intubation or the insertion of a laryngeal mask airway can precipitate intractable ventricular fibrillation, but may sometimes be a necessary risk. Similarly, starting external cardiac massage may tip the hypothermic heart into ventricular fibrillation. Once started, cardiac massage should be maintained until the patient has been rewarmed or delivered to a hospital: in very remote areas this makes it inadvisable to start massage because evacuation will be impractical.

If you do start CPR, it is clearly difficult to give evidence-based advice on how long to continue. Following immersion in very cold water, there have been cases of full recovery following several hours of external cardiac massage. The most effective form of rewarming from severe hypothermia is extracorporeal circulatory rewarming, but this will require rapid evacuation to a tertiary care hospital. Declaring a victim dead is more confidently done if they are warm, but the difficulty here lies in warming up someone in the wilderness enough to be able to do this.

The Scottish Mountain Safety Forum in 1997 produced guidelines to assist with decision-making (Table 20.3).

Table 20.3 Recommendations for evacuation of cold-injured people

	Criteria	Action
Definitely alive	Conscious	Insulate from heat loss Rewarm Monitor regularly Evacuate
Definitely alive	Unconscious Respiration and/or pulse present	Insulate from heat loss Rewarm only after arrival at hospital Maintain airway Evacuate in recovery position
May be alive	No respiration No circulation (1 min) Clear airway No obvious fatal injury Temperature below 32°C	Radio/phone for medical advice with evacuation plan Rewarm only after arrival at hospital
Definitely dead	No respiration No circulation (1 min) Airway blocked Obvious fatal injury Temperature below 32°C	Evacuate as dead

Sequelae

Recovery from mild hypothermia is usually uneventful, although the victim may feel exhausted for hours or a few days. Although rare, fulminating acute pancreatitis can cause rapid deterioration during or after rewarming.

Severe hypothermia, especially if the patient has been unconscious for some time, requires careful monitoring in hospital. Extracorporeal warming with warm air (e.g. Bair Hugger) is important, and whilst peritoneal lavage and bladder irrigation can be used, cardiopulmonary bypass is necessary to rewarm the profoundly hypothermic casualty. Arrhythmias, muscle damage, and kidney failure can develop. Maintaining the patient at 33°C for 48 h before fully rewarming may reduce complications.

Freezing cold injuries

See Fig. 20.3.

Frostnip

Frostnip is a superficial reversible freezing of the skin surface, which resolves completely within 30 min of starting to rewarm the frozen part. In the field, it looks as though pale wax has been dropped on the skin. Typically affecting parts of the body that are exposed to prevailing cold and wind, such as chin, cheeks, and earlobes, frostnip is rare if the environmental temperature is above −10°C, but common in conditions below −25°C. Strong winds, either natural, or generated by travel (running, skiing, or skidooing), increase the risk. Some experienced cold-weather travellers believe they can feel the onset of frostnip as a sudden burning 'ping' sensation. Once established, the lesions are numb and painless.

Pathophysiology

There is vasoconstriction of the cutaneous blood vessels endothelial cell damage, and freezing of the outermost layers of the skin. Deeper tissues are unaffected.

Prevention

Novice visitors to very cold climates must be constantly aware of the dangers of the environment. Using a system of 'buddy' pairs is sensible if travelling in adverse conditions, with the buddies checking each other regularly for cold injuries. Simple measures to prevent cold injuries include:
- Protective clothing (multiple loose layers are ideal).
- Avoid clothing that constricts blood flow to any part of the body.
- Stay dry, and avoid prolonged cold exposure.
- Try to protect your face from high winds using a facemask or the hood of an anorak.
- Use shelter as much as possible to reduce force of wind.
- Wear an insulated hat that covers the ears.
- Wear gloves to protect your fingers, and in extreme cold, insulated mitts with 'idiot loops'.
- Wear appropriately insulated boots, socks should not cramp feet.
- Maintain adequate nutrition and hydration.
- Avoid alcohol and smoking.
- Supplemental oxygen above 7500 m.
- Chemical and/or electrical hand and foot warmers for short severe exposure (such as a summit bid).
- Metal in contact with the skin, e.g. metal-framed spectacles, earrings, or other facial piercings, increases risk of cold injury.

For men, the protective value of beards is a hotly debated topic. In some Scandinavian countries, ointments are sold that are claimed to reduce the risk of cold injury. Evidence suggests that these are not effective and some may actually increase the risk of injury.

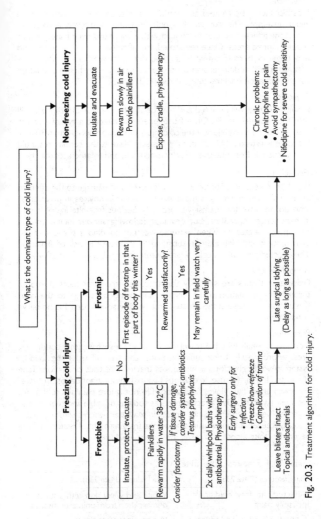

Fig. 20.3 Treatment algorithm for cold injury.

What is the dominant type of cold injury?

Non-freezing cold injury
- Insulate and evacuate
- Rewarm slowly in air. Provide painkillers
- Expose, cradle, physiotherapy

Freezing cold injury

Frostnip
- First episode of frostnip in that part of body this winter? — Yes
- Rewarmed satisfactorily? — Yes
- May remain in field but watch very carefully

Frostbite — No
- Insulate, protect, evacuate
- Painkillers. Rewarm rapidly in water 38–42°C
- *Consider fasciotomy* If tissue damage, consider systemic antibiotics. Tetanus prophylaxis
- 2x daily whirlpool baths with antibacterial, Physiotherapy
- *Early surgery only for* · Infection · Freeze-thaw-refreeze · Complication of trauma
- Leave blisters intact. Topical antibacterials
- Late surgical tidying (Delay as long as possible)

Chronic problems:
- Amitriptyline for pain
- Avoid sympathectomy
- Nifedipine for severe cold sensitivity

Treatment

Frostnip should be treated as soon as possible, before permanent tissue injury develops. The skin can be gently warmed by blowing exhaled air across the affected skin, or by contact with a warm ungloved hand. Do not rubbed nipped areas. Once rewarmed, the affected area will look red and may tingle or burn. Frostnip is an indication that weather conditions are hazardous and additional skin protection is required or shelter should be sought. No additional treatment is required.

Sequelae

Initially the area will look red and may be slightly swollen, but the skin will return to normal rapidly. Once frostnipped, the affected areas of skin are susceptible to repeat injury. If the cold injury does not resolve within 30 min, if a zone is repeatedly injured, or if the skin blisters, the condition should be regarded as frostbite, the casualty evacuated, and treated accordingly.

Frostbite

Frostbite is freezing of body tissues, with extensive damage to the affected areas. This type of injury is most likely to occur in novices in polar areas who do not care for themselves properly. Serious frostbite injury is rare in experienced travellers, but develops following serious injury, immersion in cold water, or when extreme weather conditions prevent travel. Dehydration and high altitude substantially increase the risk of frostbite. The affected part will be cold, white, numb, and rigid. (See Table 20.4.)

Pathophysiology

Frostbitten tissues are seriously damaged, cell structures being disrupted through the formation of ice crystals and osmotic damage to the cells. Circulation will cease in the affected area with muscles frozen and no nerve conduction.

Prevention

Consider carefully whether travel is necessary in severe weather conditions, dress appropriately, drink sufficient fluids, and pair off using the 'buddy' system. Avoid tight clothing and boots that may restrict circulation. Tape gloves to clothing (or use 'idiot loops') so that they cannot be lost in a gale, and carry spare hat, gloves, and socks. Do not ignore painfully cold hands and feet; try to rewarm affected parts as soon as possible and seek shelter urgently. Never immerse hands or feet in seawater near freezing: seawater typically freezes at temperatures below the freezing point of tissues, making severe frostbite a common result. Beware of cold fuels.

Table 20.4 Features of frostbite

Early features (Plate 23a)	Late features (Plate 23b)
Affected part feels cold and possibly painful	White and waxy skin with distinct demarcation from uninjured tissues
Continued freezing produces paraesthesia and/or numbness	Woody, insensate tissues
Areas of blanching blending into areas of apparently uninjured skin	Progression to bruising and blister formation (usually upon thawing)

Predisposing factors
- *General:* unusually cold weather, prolonged exposure to cold, inadequate clothing, inadequate use of appropriate clothing, homelessness, smoking, dehydration, old age, ethnicity, high altitude.
- *Systemic disease:* peripheral vascular disease, diabetes mellitus, Raynaud's disease, sepsis, previous cold injury.
- *Psychiatric illness.*
- *Pharmaceutical:* beta blockers, sedatives, neuroleptics, smoking.
- *Trauma:* any immobilizing injury but especially head and spinal injuries, and proximal limb trauma compromising distal circulation.
- *Intoxication:* alcohol and illicit drug use.

Field management
Frostbite injuries are usually serious and the casualty will usually need to be evacuated. Although undesirable, a victim can continue to travel with a frozen limb, but, once the affected area has been thawed, they will be incapacitated. Try to protect the numb area from further damage until shelter is reached.

Initial base management
- Once shelter and safety are reached the limb can be thawed.
- Give the victim painkillers; the rewarming process will be very painful.
- Place the affected part in clean water and warm the water quickly and carefully to 40°C. Ensure that the water never becomes hot enough to cause additional thermal damage. Stir the water constantly to ensure good heat transfer.
- Once warmed, protect the damaged areas from pressure and do not allow them to re-freeze.
- Cover raw areas with sterile dressings and change regularly.
- Wherever possible leave blisters intact. Although some experts suggest removing the tops from white, but not blood blisters, discuss before following this treatment pathway.
- Treat with a simple antibiotic (penicillin, erythromycin); a non-steroidal painkiller such as ibuprofen provides both pain relief and may improve healing.

Severe limb frostbite

The only reason for delaying rapid rewarming is if an arm or leg is very badly frozen. In such cases, the cellular structure of the deep tissues can be seriously damaged and the patient requires urgent transfer to hospital. As the tissues thaw, they swell, and pressures in the deep fascial compartments may exceed arterial pressure, leading to complete ischaemia of the limb. Fasciotomy prior to rewarming can prevent this disaster, but requires full investigation prior to surgery. (See ➲ Crush injuries, p. 277; Fig. 20.4.)

Thrombolysis or iloprost
In individuals who have sustained a severe frostbite injury and where they can be evacuated to a major vascular or plastics unit within 24 h of the injury (this may be possible in Alaska, European Alps, Scotland, etc) it may be possible to reduce final tissue loss by the use of intra-arterial tissue-plasminogen activator or iloprost[9]. Contraindications to thrombolysis (associated major trauma, recent stroke, GI bleed, etc.) need to be ruled out.

9 Handford C, Buxton P, Russell K, Imray CE, McIntosh SE, Freer L, et al. (2014). Frostbite: a practical approach to hospital management. *Extrem Physiol Med*, 3, 7.

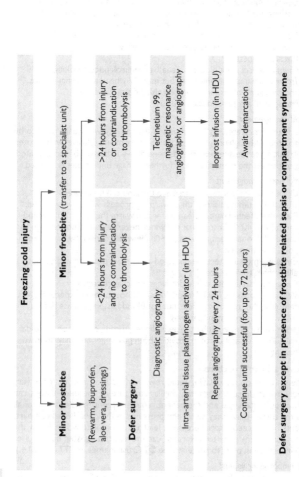

Fig. 20.4 Algorithm for the management of acute frosbite. Reproduced from Hallam M et al. BMJ, Nov 19 2010; 341:bmj.c5864, with permission from BMJ.

Sequelae

In the early phase after rewarming, the affected area will look red, blistered, and severely swollen. Raw areas leak copious amounts of serous fluid. Later, peripheral parts of affected limbs will turn black and mummify. Systemic antibiotics and tetanus prophylaxis should be given to anyone who has significant amounts of dead or dying tissue.

The mainstay of continuing treatment is the whirlpool bath into which affected parts are placed for 30 min twice daily. An appropriate antibacterial should be added to the water. Exposure in a warm environment and early mobilization should be encouraged; smoking should be forbidden.

In temperate climates, where frostbite is very rare, vascular surgeons are familiar only with dry gangrene caused by vascular insufficiency. Such patients have deep-seated, often painful, gangrene, and require amputations. Frostbite injuries can look very similar but the damage is usually more superficial and, unless infection develops, surgical interventions should be avoided until a natural demarcation line becomes obvious between dead and healthy tissue. Better scanning techniques and anti-prostaglandin drugs are improving the outlook for patients with serious frostbite injuries.[10,11,12]

Internet and satellite phones frostbite advice

A recent development that allows access to expert advice in difficult situations is the use of the Internet and satellite phones. A virtual opinion or more specialized advice can be sought from anywhere in the world using a combination of digital images and phone advice.[13]

10 Hallam MJ, Cubison T, Dheansa B, Imray C (2010). Managing frostbite. *BMJ*, 341, c5864. Available at: 🔗 http://www.researchgate.net/publication/49628759_Managing_frostbite?ev=prf_pub

11 Wilderness Medical Society *Practice Guidelines for the Prevention and Treatment of Frostbite*: 🔗 http://www.wemjournal.org/article/S1080-6032%2811%2900077-9/fulltext

12 Russell KW, Imray CH, McIntosh SE, Anderson R, Galbraith D, Hudson ST, *et al.* (2013). Kite skier's toe: an unusual case of frostbite. *Wilderness Environ Med*, 24(2), 136–40.

13 🔗 https://www.thebmc.co.uk/how-to-get-expert-frostbite-advice

Non-freezing cold injury

Non-freezing cold injury is a protean condition that occurs in cold, wet conditions ('trench foot'), shipwreck survivors ('immersion foot'), wet jungle ('paddy foot'), even those with dependent and immobile legs ('shelter limb'). Common to these is a period of relative ischaemia in the feet or hands, during which there is impairment or loss of sensation, followed by hyperaemia when they are rewarmed, often accompanied by lasting and severe pain. Predisposing factors are similar to those of frostbite, but tissues do not freeze. Cold exposure is longer in duration, typically hours or days, although non-freezing cold injury can occur in less than an hour. Individuals of African ethnicity are particularly susceptible to developing the condition.

Pathophysiology

Although less understood than frostbite, current evidence suggests that cold and ischaemia damage nerves and the vascular endothelium in local tissues. Rewarming then results in further damage from free radicals and inflammation.

Prevention

High standards of foot care are essential, with frequent regular replacement of wet socks with dry ones, and wiggling of toes to try to maintain blood flow. Even assiduous care can only postpone the onset of injury, so periodic removal from cold, wet conditions is also necessary. Footwear that relies on eliminating evaporative heat loss ('vapour barrier') or surrounding the feet with impermeable materials leads to accumulation of sweat next to the skin, resulting in non-freezing cold injury. Foot care routines and drying are even more important when rubberized or impermeable boots are worn.

Management

Cases that present before rewarming must be allowed to rewarm slowly, and thus non-freezing cold injury must be distinguished from frostbite, which should be rapidly rewarmed. Sometimes the only clue is that socks remained wet and did not freeze. Many cases present after rewarming, with florid redness, swelling, and pain. As this is neuropathic in origin, conventional approaches to pain management are unsuccessful, but early administration of amitriptyline in a single 25–50 mg dose a couple of hours before sleep normally brings relief. Dosage can be increased to 100 mg or greater if necessary, but patients must be cautioned about drowsiness, and must not drive, operate machinery, etc. Severe cases may develop blistering, sloughing of skin, and gangrene, which should be managed as for severe frostbite once slow rewarming has completed.

Sequelae

Long-term sequelae are more common following non-freezing cold injury, and include chronic pain and sensitization to the cold. Specialist advice is important, and interference with sympathetic innervation, even brief trial blocks, must be avoided, as it worsens the prognosis.

Snow blindness (photokeratitis)

Snow blindness is sunburn of the corneal and conjunctival epithelium covering the front of the eye. Like sunburn, there is a delay between exposure and development of symptoms, usually some 6–12 h. The eye becomes red, swollen, gritty, and very painful. In serious cases victims are incapacitated, as spasm of the eyelids means that they are unable to open their eyes and they develop a severe headache.

Pathophysiology

UV light is a component of sunlight. Because light is reflected off snow, levels of UV radiation in polar areas can be several times greater than in temperate or tropical areas; additionally, in spring, thinning of the ozone layer allows increased amounts of these wavelengths to penetrate the atmosphere. The radiation causes an inflammatory response, with oedema and multiple dry areas over the superficial cornea. The whole surface epithelium of the eye may come away, a process associated with considerable lacrimation. Healing then occurs and subsequent long-term problems are very rare. The retina of the eye is unaffected.

Prevention

UV rays can penetrate cloud so good quality sunglasses should be used in both clear and brightly overcast conditions. Both the front and the side of the eye should be shielded, either by suitable side flaps or by wrap-around spectacles. Some experienced polar travellers find that they rarely experience eye problems; their disregard for eye protection should not encourage novices to emulate them. Should proper sunglasses have been lost, damaged, or rendered useless by recurrent condensation, an effective emergency solution is to recreate Eskimo eye protection by cutting two thin eye slits in a piece of wood, paper, plastic, or fabric, use elastic or string to hold it to the head and use this as a shield for the eyes (Fig. 20.5).

Treatment in the field

- Ensure that the patient has no history of foreign bodies entering the eye. Contact lenses should be removed if still in place.
- Rest in a darkened room or tent.
- Give simple painkillers, such as paracetamol 1 g 4-hrly or ibuprofen 400 mg 8-hrly to relieve pain and headache. In severe cases, a more powerful painkiller such as codeine or tramadol may also be needed.
- Flushing the eye with clean water or saline solutions may relieve discomfort.
- Eye drops that relax ciliary muscle spasm of the pupil (e.g. tropicamide 0.5%) can help in moderate to severe cases, but should not be used if the patient suffers from glaucoma.
- If available, one dose of local anaesthetic eye drops such as tetracaine 0.5% (amethocaine) relieves the initial discomfort, but repeated doses of local anaesthetic drugs are no longer recommended as they may delay healing and increase risk of accidental abrasion.

- Chloramphenicol eye ointment 0.5% three to four times daily is soothing and may prevent infection, although there is some evidence that the regular use of eye ointments may actually slow the healing process.
- The eyes can be double-padded (see Fig. 10.6) to provide relief from photophobia and blinking.

Sequelae

Most cases of snow blindness will recover within 72 h. Seek help and follow up if:

- Infection develops.
- There is evidence of visual loss persisting after eye drops have been discontinued.

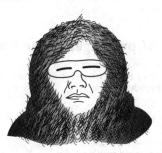

Fig. 20.5 Traditional polar sunshades.

Skin problems

Solar energy is intense in polar areas with strong reflections off the snow, and the radiation intensity may exceed that in equatorial regions. High latitude (owing to thinning of the ozone layer) and altitude increase the risk of sunburn, and a high factor (SP30+) sun cream should be applied liberally. Sunburn is particularly uncomfortable when rays reflected upwards off the snow burn the eyelids and underside of the chin and nostrils.

When persistently exposed to the cold, lips are particularly vulnerable to severe and painful chapping. They may crack and bleed. It is not certain whether this injury is due to sunburn, cold injury caused by the persistent evaporation of moisture from their surface, or the activation of herpetic cold sores. There is no guaranteed protection, but regular application of a moisturizing sunblock may reduce symptoms. The benefits of antiviral cold sore creams are unknown.

Problems of prolonged polar travel

These often occur during exploration, and more recently as a result of the rise in polar racing and challenge trips where individuals or groups are exposed to long periods on the ice.

Health

- Respiratory problems are common—cold dry air.
- Feet—blisters.
- Hands and lips—cracking of skin.
- Psychological factors and team dynamics:
  - Depression.
  - Poor self-care.
  - Team breakdown.
  - Inability to feel positive.
  - Snow blindness.

Technical issues

- Losing tent, tent fire.
- Fueling injury, stoves not lighting.
- Poor navigation.
- Not knowing how to repair kit.
- Running out of food or fuel.
- Communication failures.
- Inability to charge batteries.
- Unpredictability of weather.
- Inability to evacuate unless medical emergency and well insured.
- Nutrition and scurvy.

Resource

For Antarctic news and information see: ℘ http://www.antarctica.ac.uk/about_antarctica

Mountains and high altitude

Section editors
Chris Imray and Chris Johnson

Contributors
Jon Dallimore
Annabel H. Nickol
Andrew J. Pollard
Barry Roberts
George W. Rodway
Jeremy Windsor
Charles Clarke (1st edition)
Christopher Moxon (1st edition)

The high-altitude environment 638
Avalanches 642
Preparing to travel to altitude 648
Humans at altitude 650
High-altitude physiology 654
High-altitude illness 656
Children at altitude 670
Chronic mountain sickness 672

The high-altitude environment

Physical characteristics

High altitude is defined as any altitude >2500 m and is found on all the world's continents. See Table 21.1. Whilst the world's highest peaks are only accessible to well-equipped mountaineers, substantial areas of the American Rockies, the Andes, and the Tibetan plateau are accessible by road. About 140 million people permanently reside above 2500 m, whilst similar numbers travel to altitude for work or recreation each year. The number of trekkers in Nepal rose by 330% from 1982 to 1994, and by 450% from 1994 to 2000. A similar increase has been seen above 6000 m: in the 40 years between 1950 and 1990, 19,810 climbers attempted the highest peaks in Nepal compared to 30,141 between 1990 and 2006.

Mountains do not have to be high to be dangerous—each year the Scottish Highlands claim a number of lives. Anyone venturing onto the hills should have adequate knowledge of their environment and appropriate equipment to manage any difficulties they encounter.

Table 21.1 Altitude and associated physiological changes

Zone	Height (m)	Arterial saturation	Physiological changes
Intermediate	1500–2500	>90%	Physiological changes detectable. Altitude sickness rare but possible with rapid ascent, exercise, and susceptible individual
High	2500–3500	>85–90%	Altitude sickness common when individuals ascend rapidly
Very high	3500–5800	>80%	Altitude sickness common. Marked hypoxaemia during exercise. 5800 m is altitude of highest permanent habitation
Extreme	>5800	<75%	Marked hypoxaemia at rest. Progressive deterioration despite maximal acclimatization. Permanent survival not thought to be possible
'Death zone'	>8000	~55%	Prolonged acclimatization (>6 weeks) essential. Most mountaineers require supplementary oxygen to climb safely. Rapid deterioration inevitable and time spent above this altitude is strictly limited

Adapted from *The High Altitude Medicine Handbook*. Acute altitude illnesses. Imray C, Booth A, Wright A, Bradwell A. *BMJ*. 2011 Aug 15;343:d4943. doi: 10.1136/bmj.d4943

Weather

Weather conditions can be extreme in the mountainous and high-altitude regions of the world. High winds and severe cold may be encountered, though alternatively intense heat and strong UV can also be problematic. (➔ Solar skin damage, p. 266).

Travel and navigation in the mountains

The terrain will dictate the safest and most expeditious means of travel, both to and from base camp as well as on the mountain. High-altitude terrain often requires ropes for safe passage and crevasses, ice falls, or avalanches may be encountered. Crampons, snow shoes, or skis can aid progress while in snowy areas supplies may be brought in using sledges or pulks. GPS and satellite mapping can aid navigation, but must not be relied upon in steep terrain; often a map, compass, and direct vision are the only realistic ways of navigating through difficult mountainous terrain.

Risk assessment

Comprehensive risk assessment is vital for safe travel within these challenging environments and should reflect both the objectives of the expedition together with the skill base and experience of the individuals concerned. (See ➔ Factors influencing risk in the mountains, p. 640).

Environmental impact of humans

Mountain environments are particularly susceptible to the effects of global warming; glacial retreat is now visible in most mountain regions. The delicate ecosystems can be adversely affected by the increased numbers visiting these regions with demands of tourism resulting in deforestation to provide fuel (e.g. Nepal), and pressure on water supplies (e.g. Atacama desert). The impact on local communities can vary: tourism can bring money and improved standards of living, but traditional lifestyles may be irrevocably disrupted. Expeditions must plan to minimize their impact on the environment and this may, for instance, include the need to removal all human and other waste (e.g. Alaska, Antarctica).

Animal, bird, and insect life

Whilst very few predatory animals live at high altitude and particularly above the snow line, precautions against aggressive animals including domestic animals, and diseases with insect vectors (see Chapter 17) need to be taken when travelling to and from high-altitude areas.

Risks of mountaineering

Specific risks in the mountains include:
- Avalanche (see ➔ Avalanches, p. 642).
- Ice or rock fall.
- Adverse weather.
- Reduced atmospheric pressure and oxygen availability.
- Steep and slippery surfaces.
- Navigation.
- Equipment failure.
- Human factors.
- Difficulties accessing food, fuel, water, shelter, and medical help.

Climbing and mountaineering have always been high-risk activities associated with significant death and injury rates, especially when expeditions ascend above 7000 m. Dedicated and experienced climbers accept these risks, but increasingly adventure travellers are buying guided ascents of the great peaks, which may expose them to hazards beyond their skill and understanding.

Mortality rates vary according to a number of factors including the altitude, the technical challenges encountered, and the ability of individuals to acclimatize. They range from 0.031% on Mount Rainier, 0.308% on Denali, to 1.3% on Everest. The death rate on Everest via standard routes is higher for climbers than for Sherpas (2.7% vs 0.4%).[1]

Factors influencing risk in the mountains

- *Choice of area, mountain, and route:* popular, non-technical peaks are likely to be considerably safer than new technical routes in remote areas. A survey of 83 expeditions to unclimbed technical objectives found a mortality rate of 4.3% amongst climbers.
- *Activity:* downhill skiing in resorts is safer than off-piste skiing. Deaths from technical mountaineering in New Zealand are more than 1000 times more common than during treks in Nepal.
- *Access to definitive treatment:* life-threatening injuries at altitude require urgent treatment. Helicopters can rarely rescue stranded mountaineers above 6000 m and require good visibility. At lower altitudes weather conditions may delay evacuation for several days and victims may need to be carried long distances or managed on the mountain.
- *Resources, experience, and expertise of the party:* without a comprehensive medical kit and the expertise to use it, lives can be quickly lost. To prevent life-threatening injuries and illness inexperienced members need close supervision from their guides. The recent trend for commercial organizations to market very challenging objectives as 'adventure holidays' or 'charity treks' to the general public places inexperienced travellers at risk and demands excellent risk management, which is not always apparent.
- *Search and rescue (SAR):* the terrain, remoteness, likely weather, available communications, and local SAR resources all need to be factored when planning an expedition to mountainous regions. Facilities vary enormously between, for instance, the European Alps and the Antarctic Plateau (➔ Search and rescue, p. 139).

1 Firth PG, Zheng H, Windsor JS, Sutherland AI, Imray CH, Moore GW, *et al.* (2008). Mortality on Mount Everest, 1921–2006: descriptive study. *BMJ*, 337, a2654.

Causes of death in the mountains
(Also see ➜ Risk of death, p. 6.)

- *Trauma:* traumatic injuries resulting from falls and collisions are the commonest cause of death in the mountain environment.
- *Cold injury and hypothermia:* since ambient temperature falls by approximately 5.5°C for every 1000 m of height gain, hypothermia and cold injury increase significantly with gains in altitude and can quickly complicate injuries and illnesses.
- *Sudden cardiac death:* the commonest cause of non-traumatic deaths in the mountain environment. Accounts for 52% of deaths during downhill skiing and 30% of mountain hiking fatalities. Extensive coronary artery disease is usually found at postmortem.
- *High-altitude illness:* covered extensively in subsequent sections on high-altitude headache (HAH), acute mountain sickness (AMS), high-altitude pulmonary oedema (HAPE), and high-altitude cerebral oedema (HACE). However, it should be noted that some adventure holiday organizations and charity treks are encouraging people to climb mountains faster than is desirable: this is a particular problem with Kilimanjaro and some Andean mountains where access treks are short.

Avalanches

An avalanche is typically a falling mass of snow, which may contain rocks, ice, or other debris. Avalanches are released by either an increase in stress (fresh snow or weight of a climber/skier) or a decrease in strength of the snow pack caused by the heat of the sun. In developed countries, around 150 people die annually in avalanches;[2] estimates suggest that 90% of victims have triggered the avalanche themselves. Death rates in the high mountain ranges are unknown.

In high mountains snow can fall at any time of year, and wilderness travellers will have to evaluate the risks of terrain and snow pack for themselves. Knowledge of avalanche assessment, prudent group management strategies, and the skills and equipment to effect the rescue of avalanche victims are prerequisites to back-country mountainous snow travel both in summer and winter.

Avalanche deaths result from:
- Burial and suffocation: 65% of deaths.
- Collision with obstacles: 25% of deaths.
- Hypothermia and shock: 10% of deaths.

Overall, only 50% of victims fully buried by an avalanche survive; shallow burial and rapid retrieval significantly improve survival rates.

At up to 15 min buried, survival rates are 90%, but by 35 min the chance of survival is reduced to 30% (Fig. 21.1). Burial depth is related to survivability (Fig. 21.2). This data emphasizes the importance of groups being trained in search and rescue techniques as the 'golden 15–30 minutes' are likely to have passed before the arrival any external search and rescue team.

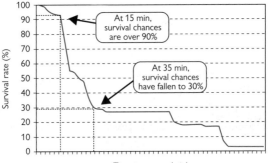

At 15 min, survival chances are over 90%

At 35 min, survival chances have fallen to 30%

Time to rescue (min)

Fig. 21.1 Full burial survival rates.

2 ℘ http://www.avalanche.ca/cac/library/avalanche-accidents

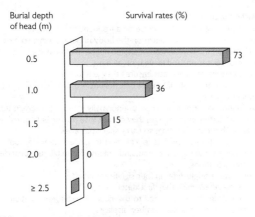

Fig. 21.2 Survival rates by burial depth.

Travel in avalanche-prone areas

- Plan your route to follow safe terrain.
- Are you starting early enough and moving fast enough to avoid sun-exposed slopes later in the day?
- Avoid terrain traps where deep burial is more likely.
- Avoid areas where there is clear evidence of past avalanche activity—including uprooted vegetation, rocks, soil, and snow and ice debris.
- Beware gaps in the vegetation (past avalanche paths?).

Crossing high-risk terrain

- Ensure that avalanche transceivers are set to send.
- Remove ski pole straps, undo all buckles (ski safety straps, rucksack).
- Zip up clothes, put on hat and gloves, cover mouth with a scarf.
- Move gently, one at a time, on a predetermined 'safe' line.
- Don't stop or regroup until you reach an 'island of safety': a ridge, rock outcrop, hill top, forest, or other area out of all potential avalanche paths.
- Use signals to indicate when it is safe for the next person to cross.

Search and rescue

If caught in an avalanche:
- Shout to attract attention.
- Jettison poles, rucksacks, and skis—they will drag you down.
- Try to get to the edge of the avalanche and out of its path.
- Fight to stay on the surface using a swimming motion, particularly just before the avalanche settles.
- Cover your mouth as the avalanche settles and fight to create an air pocket around your face.

Avalanche transceivers
- All modern transceivers operate on a frequency of 457 kHz.
- The transceiver must be worn on the body under clothing, so it cannot be ripped off in an avalanche. It should *not* be in a rucksack or pocket.
- Turn it on, put it on, and leave it on all day.
- Test transceivers daily—this ensures they are turned on.
- Transceivers are in SEND mode unless switched to RECEIVE mode to conduct a search.
- Use lithium batteries which operate normally in very low temperatures. As lithium batteries discharge, they do not lose power but they suddenly go flat without any warning, so carry spare batteries.
- Each type of transceiver has specific performance advantages, but all of them require training, education, and practise for maximum proficiency in search situations.
- Transceiver models differ in four significant ways:
  - The range at which they first detect a signal.
  - How distance and direction to the victim is displayed—audible signals, lights, or digital number displays.
  - How the unit deals with more than one buried victim—a multiple burial scenario.
  - Some models incorporate the 'on button' into the harness strap so it is impossible to wear the device without turning it on. Other models can be worn in the 'off' mode and require the user to activate a switch, which introduces scope for human error.

For these reasons it is important for groups to practise transceiver searching together to appreciate the differences between transceiver models and the search patterns recommended by the manufacturer.

Probe
For detailed searching—or searching for a victim with no transceiver—a proper avalanche probe is necessary. A probe is a thin, sectional aluminium pole, like a tent pole, which assembles into a 2–3 m length that can penetrate even dense snow. You cannot probe effectively with ski poles or ice axes.

Shovel
Effective digging requires a proper shovel since skis, hands, trekking poles, ice axes, and skis are slow and ineffective. Strong, light, collapsible shovels are readily purchased in equipment stores.

Other technologies

With 65% of deaths occurring as a result of suffocation and burial shortly after the avalanche, new approaches have been developed:

- The RECCO® system.[3] Some outdoor clothing, boots, helmets, and other equipment is equipped with a RECCO® reflector which 'enables rapid directional pinpointing of a victim's precise location using harmonic radar'. The two-part system consists of a RECCO® detector used by professional rescue groups and RECCO® reflectors. 'The RECCO system is not intended for self-rescue and is not an alternative to transceiver use in the back-country.'
- *Snorkel:* the Avalung® provides the user with the potential to breathe fresh air directly from the snowpack, rather like a snorkel. In addition, by diverting exhaled air away from the fresh air intake zone it is said to reduce the risk of rebreathing carbon dioxide and so suffocation.
- *Airbags:* another technique (a number of models are available including Airbag Safety Systems, Mammut, and Back Country Access) uses a deployable air bag system stored in a rucksack. Once in an avalanche the carrier pulls an activation handle that rapidly inflates from a re-usable gas cartridge a large (about 200 L) air bag, so reducing the risk of burial and creating an air pocket. Initial reports are very encouraging.

If a party member is caught in an avalanche

- Stop, think, and assess further risk to rescuers before going to help.
- Watch the victim carefully to estimate where they are buried.
- Look for clues as to the path they were swept down—clothing and equipment on the surface—note the last spot seen.
- Count survivors so you know how many victims you are searching for. Multiple burials complicate the transceiver search.
- Make a visual search for any sign of the victim sticking clear of the snow before starting a more complex transceiver search.
- Start a transceiver search; turn rescuers' transceivers to receive.
- Probe search once you have narrowed down the transceiver search.
- Dig the victim out—see ➜ Extrication priorities, p. 645.
- Turn the victim's transceiver off in case of multiple burials.
- Administer medical attention (see ➜ Triage, p. 182).
- Once all victims have been rescued, switch *all* transceivers back to send.

Extrication priorities

(See Fig 21.3.)

- Burial <35 min: extricate as fast as possible. Clear the airway. If the victim is in a critical condition, suspect acute asphyxia or mechanical trauma. Treat accordingly.
- Burial >35 min: assume hypothermia and extricate as gently as possible. Check carefully for an air pocket around the victim's face and for a clear airway; both are paramount to a favourable outcome.
- Following a complete burial (head and trunk), the victim should be monitored for 24 h to observe for pulmonary complications (aspiration and pulmonary oedema) in a hospital with intensive care facilities.

3 🕾 http://www.recco.com

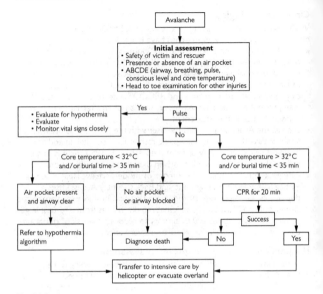

Fig. 21.3 Management of avalanche casualties.

Conclusion

Assessing the snow, developing a sense of which route to take, and generally getting a feel for the level of risk in a snowy mountain environment is not a science and is hard to learn from a book. Even 1 day spent in the mountains with a knowledgeable friend or mountain guide practising the techniques outlined and applying the 'science' will substantially raise your understanding of the hazards associated with snow travel and make you a safer, more respectful mountain traveller. Make sure that everyone in the party is properly equipped and trained to respond effectively in an avalanche emergency. There is no point in being the only 'expert' if you are the one buried in an avalanche.

Resource

🕭 http://www.ultimate-ski.com/features/off-piste-safety.aspx

Preparing to travel to altitude

Preparations

- Physical and mental endurance are essential on multi-day trips. Middle-aged participants in 'adventure' holidays that involve long mountain days must have prepared properly.
- Some experienced high altitude mountaineers will deliberately gain weight in order to offset later losses; however, this should not be due to lack of exercise!
- Make sure that boots are a good fit and well 'broken-in' before starting out.
- Appropriate insurance is essential; it remains difficult, dangerous, and very expensive to evacuate casualties from remote mountain areas.

Having appropriate equipment is not enough; familiarity with when and how to use it is just as important. The 'weekend warrior' or the affluent but inexperienced mountaineer is a potential danger to both himself and his companions.

Clothing

Clothing for travel to high altitude needs to be appropriate for the conditions expected and there is much overlap in the clothing advice for travel to cold (➲ Clothing, p. 618). The relative advantages (insulation below freezing) and disadvantages (poor insulation when wet, weight, and cost) of natural fibres such as down over manmade fibres need to be fully understood.

Medical kits for altitude

A medical kit appropriate for remote travel (see Chapter 28) needs additional drugs such those suitable for HAH, AMS, HAPE, and HACE including acetazolamide, dexamethasone, nifedipine, and sildenafil. Consider emergency medical oxygen if travelling above 6000 m particularly if travelling across a plateau such as in Tibet, as descent is impractical. A Gamow bag or portable hyperbaric chamber is a practical alternative. It is worth considering giving each mountaineer climbing above 6000 m their own mini-medical kit with injectable drugs for HACE and HAPE. These need to be stored on the climber close to the body to prevent freezing.

Pre-departure medical preparations

- Medical checks should identify and treat conditions such as acid reflux, diarrhoea, and constipation.
- Dental check-up as problems may be exacerbated by the cold and pressure changes at altitude.
- If you wear spectacles, take a spare pair and have prescription sun glasses made. Make sure ski goggles are the type that fit easily over glasses.
- Many GPs can advise on the risks of travelling to altitude with common medical conditions.
- Specialist advice is suggested for those patients with significant pulmonary or cardiac valvular disease. Stable coronary artery disease is less problematic.

- Diabetics can travel to altitude but with the proviso that they are stable at low altitude, have a good understanding of their condition, and manage their condition appropriately. Useful advice is available at the Diabetes UK website.[4]
- More esoteric conditions may require the advice of the relevant specialist who also has an interest in altitude. Advice can often be sought from Faculty members of the Diploma in Mountain Medicine.[5]
- Any individual on regular medication needs an adequate supply of drugs, stored appropriately to minimize the effects of heat and cold, readily available in a day sack, with a backup supply in their main kit bag, and a reserve supply stored with the expedition medic.

4 ℘ http://www.diabetes.org.uk/MyLife-YoungAdults/Sport-and-physical-activity/Hiking-at-altitude

5 ℘ http://medex.org.uk/diploma/diploma_holders.php

Humans at altitude

While altitude sickness tends to dominate consideration of the risks of high altitude, more mundane problems can cause hazard and accidents. These include:
- Exhaustion and dehydration (Box 25.1; ➔ Hydration, p. 651).
- Hypothermia and cold injury (➔ Hypothermia, p. 622; ➔ Freezing cold injuries, p. 626).
- UV keratitis (snow blindness) (➔ Snow blindness (photokeratitis), p. 634).
- Poor visibility: whiteout or problems with masks and spectacles (see ➔ Whiteout, p. 613).
- Communication difficulties in strong winds.
- Unstable and slippery terrain.
- Onset of darkness before descent complete.
- Poor decision-making.

Campcraft

High mountain environments are similar to polar regions (see Chapter 20). Tents, skis, and other equipment must be appropriate to the area visited and capable of surviving extreme conditions. Clean and plentiful fresh water supplies (or clean snow) and appropriate and separate siting of latrines are important.

Cooking and eating equipment

Lightweight liquid gas stoves are essential to the success of any expedition, together with plenty of fuel particularly if fresh water is to be obtained by melting snow. Check what is available locally, e.g. white gas (liquid) fuel tends to be the norm in Alaska. At high altitude, propane fuels burn at a lower temperature than butane and a 20/80 propane/butane mix is the best compromise in most situations (➔ Accommodation, heat, light, and fuel, p. 615). Failure of a stove can be a disaster and each stove set must include spares, cleaning tools, windshield, stove stand, and matches in a waterproof container. The equipment should be designed for high-altitude use and will need to be thoroughly tested before departure. At high altitude, all team members should carry a minimum of a cooking pot, lightweight plastic bowl (keeps food warmer than metal), and a metal spoon (doesn't break easily), together with a small scrubber and sterilizing 'wipes' for cleaning.

Sanitation

This is covered in detail in ➔ Humans in polar areas, p. 614.

Nutrition at altitude

'In mountaineering, as in war, it seldom pays to defer a meal if an opportunity for eating offers; at the best the next opportunity may be long in coming, at the worst it may never come again.'

(H. Tilman 1938)

A 5–20% fall in body weight is typical after time spent at high/extreme altitude. Although fat reserves tend to be metabolized first during an expedition, loss of significant amounts of muscle protein also occurs, leading to dramatic effects upon performance. Weight loss at altitude is due to:
- A rise in basal metabolic rate of 10–30%.
- An increase in energy expenditure (up to 20 000 kJ/5000 kcal per day).

- Symptoms of AMS (lethargy, nausea, vomiting, and anorexia).
- Limited availability of food, water, and fuel.
- Possible changes in the absorption of fat, carbohydrate, and protein.
- Alteration in bowel flora and GI infection causing diarrhoea, abdominal pain, and anorexia.

As in all other environments, meticulous attention to kitchen and culinary hygiene as well as personal hygiene will reduce the incidence of GI upsets.

Any expedition venturing above 3500 m will need a period of acclimatization to ensure appetite and physical performance are optimized. Little, however, is gained from spending long periods of time above 5000–6000 m, where appetites falter, cooking is difficult, and weight loss soon becomes apparent.

Where possible, the responsibility of choosing menus and purchasing food should be given to an experienced member of the team. Ideally, local cooks and kitchen staff should be employed. If this is impossible, the quartermaster should be responsible for providing:
- A wide variety of safely prepared meals, snacks, and 'packed lunches', together with an abundant supply of clean, cold water.
- A warm, well-lit mess tent large enough to accommodate the entire expedition comfortably.
- Adequate cooking utensils and crockery, together with appropriate cooking and storage facilities.

Hydration

Climbers need to drink 3–4 L of fluids each day. Dehydration develops quickly at high altitude; a water deficit of as little as 2% has been shown to reduce performance. Water at high altitude is obtained from melting snow, which should be gathered from fresh, uncontaminated sources and added slowly to warm water. Melting large bowls of snow is inefficient and tends to lead to the formation of condensation on outside of pans, which can extinguish the stove's flame. Ideally, water should be boiled, and left to sterilize before drinking (➜ Water purification, p. 102); however, this can often prove impractical.

Diet

In recent years carbohydrate-rich diets have been widely used on high-altitude expeditions. Theoretically, these not only raise the respiratory exchange ratio (R) and improve the partial pressure of oxygen in the alveoli, but they also reflect the preference tissues have for glucose over free fatty acids at altitude. This results in:
- An increased work tolerance and capacity to produce anaerobic energy.
- Improved mental acuity.
- An increased tolerance to altitude and reduction in symptoms of AMS.

A combination of simple and complex carbohydrates should be used to provide a sustained source of energy.

Snacks

During expeditions, small snacks eaten every 2–4 h provide invaluable sources of energy. A good mixture of carbohydrates can be found in power gels, muesli bars, nuts, dried fruit, flapjacks, and biscuits. In addition, modest quantities of simple carbohydrate 'treats', such as boiled sweets and chocolate bars, provide a useful boost to morale.

Meals

Noodles, potatoes, rice, pasta, polenta, and couscous provide ideal sources of carbohydrate. These can be combined with small amounts of meat, fish, eggs, pulses and vegetables, and flavoured with chillies, garlic, pepper, pickles, powdered cheese, butter, or olive oil. Breakfasts are essential for both rehydration and calorie consumption, and should include cereals (porridge or muesli) and breads (chapattis, rotis, etc.) supplemented with spreads (chocolate, peanut butter, etc.) or preserves. At high altitude, foods should be pre-prepared and should only need the addition of hot water (noodles, 'instant' potato). It is vital to sample foods first before taking them to high camps. This provides information on preparation (cooking time, amount of water required) and, most importantly, palatability.

Supplements

In general, additional vitamins and minerals are not necessary during high-altitude expeditions. However, those with iron or folate deficiencies may benefit from supplements, as red cell production is an essential feature of acclimatization.

Sleep at altitude

(See also Chapter 21.)

At high altitude, cold and harsh living conditions can disrupt sleep, while hypoxia directly disturbs sleep by causing a cyclical variation of respiration, known as periodic breathing.

Pathophysiology of sleep disordered breathing at altitude

Reduced oxygen tension (hypoxia) stimulates breathing at high altitude. The hyperventilation lowers carbon dioxide below the critical level required to stimulate breathing, known as the apnoeic threshold. During wakefulness, cortical drives to breathe are maintained; however, during sleep the relative importance of chemical drives to breathe increase, and an apnoea, or pause in breathing, may ensue. Central apnoeas are frequently followed by arousals consisting of increases in heart rate, respiratory rate, and awakening or lightening of sleep, which lower carbon dioxide again, thereby helping to sustain periodic breathing. A brisk hypoxic ventilatory response (HVR) produces a greater overshoot in ventilation, so leading the cycle to repeat itself. Periodic breathing results. Recurrent awakenings or lightening of sleep impair sleep quality, and if the sleep duration period cannot be extended may lead to fatigue the next day.

Prevalence
Periodic breathing and central apnoeas are nearly universal in native low-landers at high altitude. This is in contrast to Sherpa natives who are long-standing high-altitude dwellers, and is attributed to their blunted HVR. With increasing altitudes, the proportion of the night spent in periodic breathing increases, and periodic breathing hyperpnoea/hypopnoea cycle time decreases.

Implications of sleep-disordered breathing at altitude
It is likely that poor sleep and sleep disruption reported by climbers act synergistically with hypoxaemia to impair judgement, vigilance, and safety at extreme altitude. Sleep disturbance at altitude is a feature of AMS and HAPE (⮕ Acute mountain sickness, p. 656; ⮕ High-altitude pulmonary oedema, p. 661) and group members should be able to recognize and take rapid action if someone develops either of these conditions.

Periodic breathing is increased by a brisk HVR. It may be argued that this is a 'good' thing (the brisker HVR is associated with reduced oxygen desaturations during exercise at altitude), or a 'bad' thing (at extreme altitudes ventilation is greater during exercise, and therefore the trekker has less ventilatory reserve between their actual ventilation and maximum voluntary ventilation).

Treatment of periodic breathing
Periodic breathing and nocturnal hypoxaemia diminish with acclimatization. Graduated, slow ascent, allowing time for acclimatization (⮕ Prevention of AMS, p. 659), will improve sleep quality. When severe, descent should be considered.

- Increased sleep duration may compensate in part for reduced sleep quality. This is often impractical during climbing expeditions!
- At extreme altitudes, oxygen supplementation during sleep improves sleep quality.
- Acetazolamide significantly reduces periodic breathing at altitude. It also helps to prevent and treat altitude-related illness (⮕ Drugs in altitude illness, p. 667).
- Temazepam has been shown to reduce periodic breathing at altitude without any impairment of next day vigilance, reaction time, or cognition.

Further reading

Tilman HW (2004). *The Seven Mountain-Travel Books*. Seattle, WA: Mountaineers' Books. (Collection of seven books covering the period 1919–1952.)

High-altitude physiology

Hypoxia and reduced atmospheric pressure

On an ascent to altitude, although the percentage of oxygen is constant (21%), the barometric pressure (PB), and with it the partial pressure of oxygen (PO_2), falls (Table 21.2 and Fig. 21.4). Above 2500 m, this begins to impact upon the arterial oxygen saturation (SaO_2) and the overall content of oxygen in the arterial circulation (CaO_2):

$$CaO_2 \text{ (mL/L)} = 10 \times [Hb] \times (SaO_2 / 100) \times 1.34$$

where [Hb] is the haemoglobin concentration (g/dL).

By 5500 m, atmospheric pressure has dropped to half that at sea level and an unacclimatized human will be distressed. Significant hypoxia develops—oxygen saturations <75% are common in travellers among the great ranges (6000 m): they will be breathless and exercise capacity will be significantly reduced and oxygen saturations will drop further with exercise.[6]

Acclimatization

The fall in CaO2 can be offset by two physiological processes:
- An increase in [Hb]—within a few days of ascending to altitude the [Hb] increases as a fluid shifts from the circulation and into the tissues. Later, this is supplemented by an increase in bone marrow activity and an increase in red cell production.
- An increase in SaO_2—over the course of several hours, the depth and frequency of breathing increases. This not only increases the partial pressure of oxygen in the lungs but also alters the affinity of oxygen to the haemoglobin molecules.

These processes are called acclimatization and have the effect of increasing the convective oxygen delivery to the tissues. Most altitude-related illnesses occur when there has been insufficient time to acclimatize at altitudes >3000 m.

Full acclimatization takes several weeks, and most humans are unable to tolerate ascent rates of more than 400–600 m a day but there is a significant variation in the degree and speed to which individuals are able to acclimatize. A very few climbers have been able to reach the summit of Everest without supplementary oxygen, but such feats are at the extreme limits of human physiology.

Humans spending prolonged periods at high altitude develop long-term physiological responses to the environment (➔ Chronic mountain sickness, p. 672).

6 Major SA, Hogan RJ, Yeates E, Imray CH (2012). Peripheral arterial desaturation is further exacerbated by exercise in adolescents with acute mountain sickness. *Wilderness Environ Med*, 23(1), 15–23.

Table 21.2 Atmospheric characteristics at high altitude

Altitude (m)	Pressure (mmHg)	Temperature (°C)	Inspired oxygen tension (mm Hg)
Sea level	760	0	160
2500	570	−13.75	120
5000	420	−27.5	88
7500	303	−41.25	64

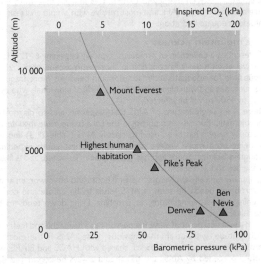

Fig. 21.4 Barometric pressure at altitude.

High-altitude illness

Acclimatization is a slow but necessary process. If ascent is too rapid then high-altitude illnesses such as high altitude headache (HAH), acute mountain sickness (AMS), high-altitude pulmonary oedema (HAPE), and high altitude cerebral oedema (HACE) can occur. Of the latter three, AMS is by far the commonest. Overlap between all four conditions can occur.

High-altitude headache

HAH is a headache that develops within 24 h of ascent >2500 m and resolves within 8 h of descent. HAH often is worse during the night and with exertion. Unlike a common migraine, it resolves after 10–15 min of supplementary oxygen therapy (2 L/min). It is thought that up to 80% of people are affected by HAH, and most resolve with simple analgesic treatment and adequate hydration.

Acute mountain sickness

AMS describes a collection of symptoms typically beginning 6–12 h following arrival at altitude. It is common in those who ascend above 2500 m without time for adequate acclimatization and becomes more frequent at higher altitudes and with higher ascent rates. 59% of individuals who ascend rapidly to 4500 m will be affected.[7]

There is no single feature of AMS that is specific, and so diagnosis can be problematic. For research purposes the *Lake Louise acute mountain sickness scoring system* has been used to classify AMS (Table 21.3) and this is now being used more widely, particularly amongst youth expeditions.[8] A Mountain Sickness Score app has recently been launched, and is likely to increase use and accessibility.[9]

Symptoms typically evolve over several hours and often worsen at night. The throbbing headache seen in AMS tends to be diffuse and constant, worsening with straining, lifting, or coughing. Lying down tends to bring some relief.

From a practical point of view, if a person has a headache and feels unwell at high altitude, without another obvious cause, AMS is the most likely diagnosis. Many features of AMS are shared with HACE and HAPE, which are often preceded by AMS, and this should always be considered during assessment and treatment.[10]

7 Maggiorini M, Buhler B, Walter M, Oelz O (1990). Prevalence of acute mountain sickness in the Swiss Alps. *BMJ*, 301, 853–5.

8 Slingo ME, Lowe FSJ, Pieri ARP, Imray CHE, The British Schools Exploring Society (2012). Visual analogue self-assessment of acute mountain sickness in adolescents: experience from two Himalayan expeditions. *High Alt Med Biol*, 13(3), 185–92.

9 ☏ http://mobogenie.com/download-mountain-sickness-scorer-354024.html

10 ☏ http://www.altitude.org/home.php

Table 21.3 Lake Louise score

Lake Louise acute mountain sickness scoring system

Self-report questionnaire		Clinical assessment	
1. Headache		**6. Change in mental status**	
0	No headache	0	No change in mental status
1	Mild headache	1	Lethargy/lassitude
2	Moderate headache	2	Disorientated/confused
3	Severe headache, incapacitating	3	Stupor/semi-consciousness
2. Gastrointestinal symptoms		4	Coma
0	No gastrointestinal symptoms	**7. Ataxia (heal-to-toe walking)**	
1	Poor appetite or nausea	0	No ataxia
2	Moderate nausea or vomiting	1	Manoeuvres to maintain balance
3	Severe nausea and vomiting, incapacitating	2	Steps off line
3. Fatigue or weakness		3	Falls down
0	Not tired or weak	4	Can't stand
1	Mild fatigue/weakness	**8. Peripheral oedema**	
2	Moderate fatigue/weakness	0	No peripheral oedema
3	Severe fatigue/weakness, incapacitating	1	Peripheral oedema at one location
		2	Peripheral oedema at two or more locations
4. Dizziness/lightheadedness			
0	Not dizzy		
1	Mild dizziness		
2	Moderate dizziness		
3	Severe dizziness, incapacitating		
5. Difficulty sleeping			
0	Slept as well as usual		
1	Did not sleep as well as usual		
2	Woke many times, poor night's sleep		
3	Could not sleep at all		

Developed at Lake Louise in Canada as a tool to standardize diagnostic criteria for AMS during research, the scoring system consists of a self-reported questionnaire and a, less often used, clinical assesment section. In the context of a recent gain in altitude, a score of 3 or more in the questionnaire alone, or 5 when using a combined score, is deemed to indicate AMS. It is sensitive not specific, as many other illness will result in a score greater than 3.

Aetiology

The pathogenesis of AMS is poorly understood. One hypothesis is that AMS represents an early form of HACE, caused by brain swelling and intracerebral pressure symptoms in individuals with insufficient CSF buffer capacity ('tight fit hypothesis'; see ➲ High-altitude cerebral oedema, p. 664).

However, brain swelling has not been demonstrated as early as 6–10 h after ascent, when symptoms of AMS tend to begin. In addition, mild brain swelling is seen equally in those with and without AMS symptoms. Other possible causes are altered fluid balance, free radical-mediated damage, or derangement in cerebral blood flow autoregulation.

In addition, emerging data supports the possibility that resistance to AMS may involve the ability to mount an adequate 'defensive' anti-permeability response during hypoxic exposure. Further investigation is required to confirm the mechanism of development of AMS symptoms. Perhaps most intriguing, however, is accumulating genetic data that are consistent with altitude illness being a polygenic condition with a strong environmental component.

Risk factors
- Rapid ascent 2500 m.
- Altitude above 4500 m.
- Previous history of high-altitude illnesses.
- Long-term residence at low altitude.
- Physical exertion at altitude.
- Pre-existing lung diseases.
- Young age.
- Limited awareness of high-altitude illnesses.

Symptoms
- Headache.
- Anorexia.
- Nausea and vomiting.
- Fatigue.
- Dizziness.
- Sleep disturbance.

Symptoms typically evolve gradually and are worse at night. There are no distinct characteristics, but a headache, typically throbbing in nature, and aggravated either by bending down and/or by Valsalva's manoeuvre, is usually present.

Signs

No specific signs. Some common findings are:
- Peripheral oedema.
- Tachycardia.
- Scattered crackles on auscultation.
- Slightly raised basal temperature.
- Lower oxygen saturations than healthy companions have been observed.
- Elevated diastolic pressure

Management

- *Stop*: do not ascend further if symptoms are present.
- *Rest*: try lying flat on a comfortable surface.
- *Treat*: simple analgesia (the combination of paracetamol 1 g and ibuprofen 400 mg every 6 h is highly effective) and an antiemetic (metoclopramide 10–20 mg every 6 h) if required. Encourage sufferer to drink slowly: 500–1000 mL of water, tea or soup) over the course of 1 h. Avoid alcoholic drinks. (See Fig. 21.5.)
- *Descend* : in cases that do not improve overnight it is advisable to descend 500 m or further, to an altitude where the individual was well. To aid descent consider using:
  - Acetazolamide: 125–250 mg PO twice a day.
  - Dexamethasone: 4 mg PO, IM, or IV four times a day.
  - Supplemental oxygen: (1–5 L/min. Aim for SaO_2 >95%)
  - Hyperbaric chamber: 1–2 h spent in a portable hyperbaric chamber often improves symptoms. Although these effects may only last for a few hours, the use of a chamber may allow those with AMS to descend quicker and more safely.

Prevention of AMS

- Adequate acclimatization.
- Above an altitude of 3000m, sleeping elevation should not increase by >500m a day, resting every 3–4 days.
- Though usually impractical, preacclimatization (daily exposure to simulated altitude for 4 h) is probably beneficial.
- Avoid hard physical exertion for 2–3 days after arrival at altitude (anecdotal evidence).
- Acetazolamide (Diamox®) 250 mg twice a day from 1 day before ascent. Lower doses (125 mg twice a day) may be equally effective.
- Although dexamethasone 4mg twice a day (some doctors recommend 2mg four times a day) has been used and may offer some protection, the use of steroids prophylactically is questionable. Courses should be limited to 7–10 days.

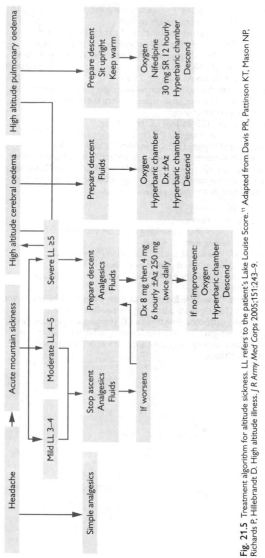

Fig. 21.5 Treatment algorithm for altitude sickness. LL refers to the patient's Lake Louise Score.[11] Adapted from Davis PR, Pattinson KT, Mason NP, Richards P, Hillebrandt D. High altitude illness. *J R Army Med Corps* 2005;151:243–9.

11 Imray C, Booth A, Wright A, Bradwell A (2011). Acute altitude illnesses. *BMJ*, 343, d4943. ℜ http://jysmedicscorner.com/Medicine_files/Acute%20altitude%20illnesses.pdf

High-altitude pulmonary oedema

HAPE is a potentially fatal high-altitude illness in which there is movement of fluid from the capillaries into the alveoli of the lungs. The accumulation of oedema creates a mechanical barrier which impairs gas exchange. The commonest symptoms are tiredness, cough, and shortness of breath. Breathlessness is first seen during exercise but rapidly develops at rest. HAPE resolves quickly on descent.

HAPE typically occurs within 2 to 4 days of arriving at altitude (>2500 m). AMS is frequently but not always associated. There is a strong correlation with altitude attained—6% at 4500 m and 15% at 5500 m. HAPE may be commoner in those who undertake heavy physical exercise. Porters from lowland areas may be at particular risk.

Aetiology

The condition is incompletely understood. However the formation of oedema is likely to be due to an imbalance between fluid entering and exiting the alveolus:

An increase in the build-up of alveolar fluid—this results from the breakdown of the membrane separating the alveoli and capillaries. When blood vessels in the lungs are exposed to hypoxia they respond by contracting (hypoxic pulmonary vasoconstriction (HPVR)). In HAPE this response is patchy, with some blood vessels contracting more than others. There is a resulting breakdown of the alveolar-capillary membrane or stress failure and a leak of fluid and cells into the alveoli. In those with a pre-existing inflammatory condition (i.e. upper respiratory tract infection) the risk of developing HAPE is believed to be significantly greater.

A decrease in the reabsorption of alveolar fluid—even at low altitude small quantities of fluid accumulate in the alveoli. This is normally removed by the lymphatic system and relies upon Na^+/K^+-ATPase pump activity in alveolar epithelial cells. In those susceptible to HAPE, drugs such as salmeterol can increase Na^+/K^+-ATPase activity and prevent the condition from developing.

Risk factors and susceptibility

In addition to those risk factors that predispose to AMS, HAPE is also associated with:

- A history of recent AMS or HACE.
- Male sex.
- Cold.
- Fast ascent (including fast re-ascent in a pre-acclimatized individual).
- Recent respiratory or systemic infection.
- A previous episode of HAPE.
- Blunted hypoxic ventilatory response.
- Small lung volumes.
- Diseases that predispose individuals to pulmonary hypertension (including structural cardiac defects such as absent right pulmonary artery and respiratory disorders such as COPD).

- Genes responsible for transcribing substances responsible for changes in pulmonary artery pressure (endothelin, angiotensin II, and nitric oxide) and alveolar fluid removal (surfactant, Na^+/K^+-ATPase) have been found in those with HAPE. However their contribution to the development of this condition is not yet clear.[12]

Symptoms
- Fatigue.
- Shortness of breath.
- Cough, initially dry, becoming wet.
- Haemoptysis.
- Chest pain.
- Symptoms of AMS and HACE can also commonly occur.

Signs
- *Grade 1: mild*. Minor symptoms with heavy exertion. Mild tachycardia and increased respiratory rate at rest. No limitations to normal activities.
- *Grade 2: moderate*. Patient is ambulatory, but normal activities are reduced. Tachycardia and tachypnoea are present. Weakness, dyspnoea, and cough are evident to others. Rales may be present.
- *Grade 3: serious*. Symptoms are present at rest. The patient may be unable to walk and prefer to rest. Simple tasks may be impossible. Senses may be dulled. Confusion and disorientation may be present. Tachycardia and tachypnoea are present. Rales are easily heard.
- *Grade 4: severe*. Patient is severely obtunded or comatose and cannot respond logically to questions or commands. Patient is unable to sit or stand. Exhibits noisy breathing with sounds of fluid in the airways. There is marked tachycardia and tachypnoea.

Differential diagnosis
- Dry persistent cough is common at altitude, independent of HAPE.
- Respiratory tract infection or pneumonia.
- Asthma.
- Carbon monoxide poisoning.
- Congestive cardiac failure.
- Myocardial infarction.
- Panic attack.
- Pulmonary embolism.

Investigations (when available)
- Pulse oximetry: a low arterial oxygen saturation compared to healthy, well-acclimatized individuals who have shared the same ascent profile.
- Radiology: changes can be highly variable. However, HAPE sufferers eventually develop asymmetric areas of 'cotton wool' infiltrates in the mid and lower zones of the lung field. These often begin in the right mid zone and eventually spread across to the left. The apices and costophrenic angles are usually spared. Signs of cardiogenic pulmonary oedema are usually absent. X-ray and CT changes resolve quickly following recovery.

12 Scherrer U, Rexhaj E, Jayet PY, Allemann Y, Sartori C (2010). New insights in the pathogenesis of high-altitude pulmonary edema. *Prog Cardiovasc Dis*, 52(6), 485–92.

- Electrocardiography : typically shows a sinus tachycardia and changes compatible with acute pulmonary hypertension including right axis deviation and bundle branch block; peaked P waves in leads II, III, and aVF; and an increase in the depth of precordial S waves. Cardiac catheter studies have shown elevated pulmonary artery pressure.
- Chest ultrasound: the presence of pulmonary oedema can result in the formation of 'comet-tail artefacts' on ultrasound scanning. These can provide an objective assessment of pulmonary oedema, and can be used to monitor the course of the disease.
- Blood tests: the majority of laboratory investigations are normal in HAPE however a mild neutrophil leucocytosis is sometimes seen.

Management

Descent is the 'gold standard' treatment for HAPE. A descent of just a few hundred metres can often prove beneficial. In severe cases the subject should not be self-ambulatory and should ideally be carried by pack animal, porter or mechanized transport. When descent is not possible (weather, terrain nightfall, etc.) other treatments may help prevent further deterioration:

- Sit patient up.
- Supplemental oxygen by face mask (titrate to SaO_2 >95%—up to 10 L/min) and/or hyperbaric chamber.
- Nifedipine 30 mg PO twice a day or 20 mg PO three times a day slow-release preparation.
- Dexamethasone 8 mg initially then 4 mg PO/IM/IV four times a day if HACE is suspected.

Prevention

- Slow ascent: above 3000 m, ascend at a rate of 500 m/day and include a rest day every 3–4 days. Avoid strenuous exertion while acclimatizing.
- Manage AMS: in the event of AMS symptoms developing follow the 'Stop, Rest, Treat and Descend' approach.
- Modify behaviour: avoid heavy physical exertion for 2–3 days after arriving at a new altitude and descend quickly if HAPE symptoms arise.

In those with a prior history of HAPE the following have been shown to reduce the incidence and severity of a relapse:

- Nifedipine 30 mg PO twice a day or 20 mg PO three times a day Slow-release preparation—'gold standard' prophylactic treatment for those with a previous history of HAPE.
- Salmeterol 125 microgram inhaler twice a day. Of limited clinical use and is thought to act by improving lung water clearance, it may not be as effective as nifedipine; many experts recommend its use only in combination with nifedipine.
- Tadalafil 10 mg twice a day—limited clinical use. Along with other phosphodiesterase inhibitors, tadalafil reduces pulmonary artery pressure in those with a history of HAPE. It is unclear what effect tadalafil and nifedipine have when used in combination.

High-altitude cerebral oedema

HACE is a rare but potentially fatal condition that can occur at altitudes above 2500 m. Approximately 1–3% of those travelling above 5000 m will develop the condition. Up to 20% of those who present with HAPE will also have signs of HACE, whilst up to 50% of those who die from HAPE also have evidence of HACE on autopsy. A low threshold to treat both conditions is needed.

In most cases those who develop HACE will first have symptoms of AMS. However, at very high altitudes (above 6000 m) HACE can occasionally develop without symptoms of AMS.

Aetiology

The exact pathophysiology of HACE remains to be determined. Cerebral blood flow increases both at altitude and in AMS, and there appears to be a generalized capillary leakage. There also appears to be evidence of impaired cerebral autoregulation on acute exposure to altitude.

The symptoms of AMS and of raised intracranial pressure appear similar, with headaches, nausea, and photophobia being features of both conditions. In both severe AMS and HACE, CSF pressures were found to be elevated compared with that after recovery, and subjects dying from AMS have evidence of cerebral oedema on autopsy. Computerized axial tomography demonstrates diffuse low-density areas consistent with oedema in subjects with HACE.

Disruption of the blood–brain barrier (BBB) may be important and is likely to occur in HACE. This results in:
1. The activation of platelets resulting in the formation of thrombi.
2. The release of neutrophils triggering an inflammatory response.

Since all those who ascend to altitude experience an increase in cerebral blood flow, it may be differences in this response to the exposed BBB that may explain why only a small proportion of those who ascend to altitude develop HACE. Two main hypotheses have been proposed: vasogenic (increased cerebral blood flow) and cytotoxic (local cellular response). A number of different molecules have been implicated in weakening the BBB during hypoxia. These include bradykinin, histamine, arachidonic acid, oxygen and hydroxyl free-radicals, nitric oxide, noradrenaline, and vascular endothelium growth factor (VEGF). VEGF has been shown to increase in rats exposed to hypoxic conditions and also in humans after exercise.

Relief of HAH with dexamethasone provides indirect evidence of the importance of cerebral oedema and vascular permeability in HAH since dexamethasone suppresses lipid peroxidation, blocks VEGF, and reduces endothelial permeability.

Risk factors

These are similar to AMS and HAPE. Gradual acclimatization and correct treatment of AMS reduces the risk of brain oedema during the early stages of ascent to high altitudes. Little can be done to prevent sudden brain oedema at extreme altitudes—it is vital to recognize the condition promptly and act swiftly.

No pre-ascent evaluation is helpful, a difference from HAPE.

Symptoms

HACE sufferers are often unaware of any changes to their condition. Colleagues may report recent symptoms of other high altitude illnesses such as AMS and HAPE.

- Headache.
- Nausea.
- Hallucination.
- Disorientation.
- Confusion.

Signs

HACE is distinguished from AMS by the presence of neurological signs. In those with AMS, the appearance of new neurological signs should necessitate urgent evacuation and treatment for HACE.

- *Ataxia*: commonest sign identified in those with HACE. Identified by observing a short distance of heel to toe walking interrupted by a 180° turn. A positive sharpened Rhomberg test is often seen. In severe cases victims may be unable to stand. Differences in tone, power, and reflexes can also occur.
- *Plantar reflexes* are abnormal in 34% of HACE sufferers.
- *Cranial nerve palsies*: although rare, palsies to the III, IV, VI, and XII are seen.
- *Behavioural changes*: victims may appear unusually tired, irritable, confused, forgetful, elated, or prone to bouts of irrational behaviour. Memory and orientation is often impaired. Hallucinations are occasionally seen.
- *Urinary signs*: in 48% of those with HACE urinary incontinence or retention is reported.
- *Visual* : retinal haemorrhages and papilledema are seen on fundoscopy.

Investigations

HACE is a clinical diagnosis. Anyone exhibiting these signs and symptoms following a recent ascent to altitude should be assumed to have HACE and evacuated as soon as possible.

In hospital the following tests are useful:

- *CT scan*: an increase in ICP reveals compression of the ventricles and changes to the gyri and sulci on the surface of the cerebral hemispheres.
- *MRI scan*: shows formation of oedema in the white matter. This is often concentrated in the splenium of the corpus callosum. Grey matter is largely unaffected by HACE.

Changes seen on CT and MRI may take weeks or even months to resolve after clinical recovery.

Management

Like HAPE, descent is the 'gold standard' treatment for HACE. When this is prevented by significant compromise or poor conditions, other treatments may help prevent further deterioration:

- Supplemental oxygen by mask (aim for SaO_2 >95%).
- Dexamethasone 8 mg (IV or IM) initially, followed by 4 mg every 4 h.
- Nifedipine 30 mg PO twice daily or 20 mg PO three times daily slow-release preparation if coexistent HAPE is suspected.
- Use of a hyperbaric recompression bag.

Prevention

- Adequate acclimatization.
- Above an altitude of 3000m, sleeping elevation should not increase by >500m a day, resting every 3–4 days.

- Avoid hard physical exertion for 2–3 days after arrival at altitude (anecdotal evidence).
- Early descent on any appearance of symptoms (rapidly reversed in early stages).
- Prevention of AMS/HAPE may reduce the risk of HACE.
- Acetazolamide (Diamox®) 125–250 mg twice a day from 1 day before ascent.
- Dexamethasone 4 mg four times a day may offer some protection.

Portable hyperbaric chambers
(See Fig. 21.6 and ♫ http://www.high-altitude-medicine.com/hyperbaric.html)

Now carried by many larger high-altitude expeditions, these are capsules constructed from lightweight airtight materials into which a person can be zipped. The capsule is then inflated with a foot or hand pump. This results in a rapid increase in barometric pressure within the chamber and a simulated descent. Manual pumping, with hand or foot pump, must continue intermittently, even after inflation, to allow CO_2 clearance.

Single-man portable devices weigh 4.8–6.5 kg and cost between US$1400 and US$2400. Hyperbaric chambers have been shown to treat all forms of altitude illness effectively; however, the effect does not persist long after removal from the chamber and should not replace descent as the primary treatment. Such bags must be used with care:

- Prior to setting out on an expedition the chamber needs to be checked that it is complete (including piping and foot pump) and airtight and the supervisor is familiar with its operation.
- Ensure the subject can clear their ears (to avoid barotrauma).
- Ensure a constant clean air supply to casualty.
- Position bag so that casualty lies in head-up position.
- Position the chamber in a flat, sheltered area that is set away from any potential dangers.
- Monitor casualty's condition continuously to ensure that they remain breathing and do not vomit (it is dangerous to put a patient who cannot protect their airway into the bag).

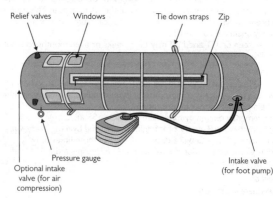

Relief valves Windows Tie down straps Zip

Pressure gauge
Optional intake valve (for air compression)

Intake valve (for foot pump)

Fig. 21.6 Gamow bag.

High-altitude retinal haemorrhages

(See Plate 24 and ➲ High-altitude retinopathy, p. 332.)

Retinal haemorrhages (in the nerve fibre layer) are common above 5000 m and are not necessarily related to AMS. They do not predispose to cerebral oedema and rarely interfere with vision unless found over the macula. No treatment is usually necessary but if vision becomes blurred or fails, descent is advisable. Permanent visual loss is exceptional. Haemorrhages not affecting vision are not known to have any clinical significance and do not warrant descent. Haemorrhages have been induced by strenuous exercise, which increases BP and decreases the arterial oxygen saturation levels.

Drugs in altitude illness

Acetazolamide (Diamox®)

Acetazolamide is a carbonic anhydrase inhibitor which affects renal bicarbonate excretion to produce a metabolic acidosis and therefore increased respiratory drive. This can be used for:

- *Prophylaxis*: drug of choice in at-risk individuals. Recommended dose: 125–250 mg twice a day, or 500 mg once a day of slow-release preparation, beginning 1 day before ascent to altitude; child 2.5 mg/kg twice a day. The dose of 250 mg twice a day is supported by several trials and a different meta-analysis. A single 125 mg dose can reduce abnormal breathing patterns and therefore improve sleep at altitude.
- *Treatment of AMS*: 250 mg three times a day; child 2.5 mg/kg three times a day (max 250 mg/dose).

Common side effects

Nausea and vomiting, anorexia, dizziness, tingling in hands, and an odd taste in the mouth. While most people tolerate acetazolamide well, others experience significant side effects and it is recommended that people try it before using it as prophylaxis at altitude. It has been argued that since the risk of AMS depends upon the ascent rate, the absolute altitude attained, and the individual's susceptibility, the exact dose prescribed should take these factors into account.

Dexamethasone

A glucocorticoid steroid that can be used for:

- *Prevention and treatment of AMS* (in individuals intolerant to acetazolamide): unknown action. Unlike acetazolamide, dexamethasone does not aid acclimatization. If stopped suddenly, AMS can quickly develop.
- *Prophylaxis*: 8 mg/day in divided doses (e.g. 4 mg twice a day).
- *Treatment of AMS*: 4 mg four times a day; child 0.15 mg/kg/dose four times a day (maximum 4 mg/dose).
- *Treatment of HACE*: 8 mg initially PO, IM or IV then 4 mg four times a day; child 0.15 mg/kg/dose four times a day.
- *Treatment of AMS*: 4 mg four times a day PO or IV; child 0.15 mg/kg/dose PO four times a day (maximum 4 mg/dose). Relieves symptoms but not physiological abnormalities. May be used in conjunction with acetazolamide.

Common side effects

Usually none with short courses; steroid psychosis occurs rarely. However, if used for more than a few days side effects can quickly multiply. An 'Addisonian crisis' has been reported on Mount Everest, complicated by GI bleeding and a number of other side effects related to dexamethasone use.

Nifedipine

A calcium channel blocker that inhibits hypoxic pulmonary vasoconstriction at altitude and therefore causes pulmonary artery pressure to fall. It can be used for:

- *Prevention of HAPE* in susceptible individuals: has been shown to reduce the incidence significantly in people of known susceptibility. 20 mg PO slow-release preparation three times a day.
- *Treatment of HAPE*: drug treatment is secondary to descent and/or supplementary oxygen which address the primary cause. 20 mg PO slow-release preparation four times a day. Child 0.5 mg/kg/dose PO three times a day— ideally slow-release preparation (maximum 20 mg/dose).

Some authors recommend a 10 mg sublingual tablet taken initially but this has been known to cause significant hypotension that may prevent descent for several hours.

Common side effects

Headache, dizziness, and postural hypotension. The latter, which is serious as it may hamper descent, is less likely with a slow-release preparation.

Sildenafil

Sildenafil (Viagra®) is a phosphodiesterase inhibitor widely used for the treatment of erectile dysfunction. It is also effective in the treatment of HAPE by increasing pulmonary nitric oxide (NO) levels resulting in smooth muscle relaxation and a lowering of pulmonary artery pressures.

- *Prevention of HAPE*: in susceptible individuals, sildenafil has been shown to reduce the incidence of HAPE. Dosage: 20 mg orally three times daily or 30–60 mg sustained-release for prevention of HAPE. The drug should be started on the day of ascent and continued for 72 h at higher altitudes. Tadalafil (Cialis®) 10 mg orally twice a day has also been described in the prevention of HAPE.
- *Treatment of HAPE*: drug treatment is secondary to descent and/or supplementary oxygen which address the primary cause. 10 mg orally once then 20 mg sustained-release four times daily.
- *Common side effects*: postural hypotension and reflex tachycardia. Dizziness and nausea can also be problematic

Salmeterol

Salmeterol is normally in the treatment of asthma but since it upregulates pulmonary sodium transport across alveolar membranes increasing clearance of alveolar fluid it has been described in the prevention of HAPE.

- *Dose*: 50 micrograms (2 puffs) inhaled twice daily starting the day prior to ascent and continued for 2 days at maximum altitude.
- *Common side effects*: mild tachycardia.

Children at altitude

Improved access and the growth of adventure tourism mean that increasing numbers of lowland children are travelling to high altitude. Here they are exposed to the same risks as those described for adults, including environmental and meteorological hazards, and altitude illness, for which the parent, guardian, school, or guide must recognize responsibility. While a carefully planned adventure in high-altitude areas with older children can be beneficial, taking young children to high altitude in remote regions may not be in their best interests.

Altitude illness in lowland children ascending to height

- Although there are few studies that have considered altitude illness in children, available data indicate that AMS and HAPE probably occur at about the same rate as in adults, though one study found higher rates.
- Intercurrent illness may increase the risk of altitude illness in children.
- Symptoms of altitude illness are especially difficult to recognize in preverbal children and the classic symptoms of AMS are not reported by children <5 years of age.
- In preschool children, irritability, fussiness, food refusal, lethargy, decreased playfulness, difficulty sleeping, and excessive crying may be the symptoms noted, but these are difficult to distinguish from symptoms related to other causes including intercurrent illness and even just a change of normal routine.
- A Children's Lake Louise Score or 'fussiness' score has been developed for study of AMS in children. See Table 21.4.
- The risk of late recognition of altitude illness in children can be reduced by vigilance and an assumption that any non-specific symptoms may indicate the onset of AMS or early HAPE/HACE.
- AMS, HAPE, and HACE in children should be managed in the same way as described earlier for adults (paediatric doses of drugs for prophylaxis and treatment are given in ➜ Drugs in altitude illness, p. 667.
- As with adults, AMS may be prevented by slow graded ascent: above an altitude of 3000m, sleeping elevation should not increase by >500m a day, resting every 3-4 days.
- Where a rapid ascent with a child is unavoidable, the use of drug therapy for prophylaxis is reasonable as for adults.

Infants residing at altitude

There is evidence that infants (<1 year of age) who are exposed to high-altitude environments for prolonged periods may develop symptomatic complications as a result of maladaptation:

- Newborns at altitude have low oxygen saturations at birth which may interfere with normal adaptation of the circulation to *ex utero* life. Persistence of a patent ductus arteriosus is more common at altitude and all infants should receive supplementary oxygen after delivery to encourage ductal closure.

- Both infants born at altitude and infants travelling to altitude during the first year of life may develop symptomatic high-altitude pulmonary hypertension (SHAPH) in response to altitude hypoxia.
- The length of exposure necessary for SHAPH is unknown and it is recommended that infants residing at high altitude are monitored by a cardiologist.
- SHAPH is associated with muscularization of peripheral pulmonary arterioles and right ventricular hypertrophy, which may lead to heart failure.
- Treatment of SHAPH includes oxygen therapy and descent.

Cold, snow, and sun

As a result of their high surface area to volume ratio, children are especially susceptible to the cold (including wind chill), particularly if they are being carried and are therefore not generating heat through exercise.

- Minimize risk of hypothermia and cold injury by paying attention to thermal balance.
- Ensure they wear adequate windproof, waterproof, insulating clothing, even if there are complaints about its comfort and fashion standards.
- Children being carried in packs or slings are at risk of hypothermia and/or frostbite of the extremities.
- Goggles should be worn to avoid snow blindness.
- Sun protection should be provided using clothing and sunblock creams.

Table 21.4 The Children's Lake Louise Score (CLLS) is used in children aged 4 or younger. A diagnosis of AMS can be made if there has been a recent gain in altitude and the CLLS is greater than, or equal, to 7

	0	1	2	3	4, 5, 6
Amount of unexplained fussiness	Range from 0 (no fussiness) to 6 (constant fussiness when awake)				
Intensity of fussiness	Range from 0 (no fussiness) to 6 (severe fussiness when awake)				
Appetite	Normal	Slightly less than normal	Much less than normal	Vomiting or not eating	
Playfulness	Normal	Playing slightly less	Playing much less than normal	Not playing	
Ability to Sleep	Normal	Slightly less or more than normal	Much less or more than normal	Not able to sleep	

Chronic mountain sickness

In South America, high-altitude miners working for prolonged periods above 3000 m develop pathologically high haemoglobin concentrations (>22 g/dL) that may result in pulmonary hypertension and cardiac failure (chronic mountain sickness (CMS)—Monge's disease). Ethnic Tibetans seem better able to cope at high altitude, with only a small proportion of those living at up to 4000 m affected, but Chinese immigrants living on the Tibetan plateau may experience significant complications and infant mortality is high.

Definition

A clinical syndrome that occurs in natives or lifelong residents above 2500 m. CMS is characterized by:
- A high haemoglobin concentration (females >19 g/dL; males >21 g/dL).
- Severe hypoxaemia.
- Pulmonary hypertension which may evolve into cor pulmonale and congestive cardiac failure.

Typically, the clinical features of CMS gradually disappear with descent and return following re-ascent.

Prevalence

- Occurs in ~5% of permanent high-altitude residents.
- In La Paz (3600 m), 6–8% of male population and 28% of hospital inpatients have CMS.
- CMS is commoner in men, elderly, smokers, those exposed to environmental pollution and individuals with respiratory diseases. Conditions associated with hypoventilation (i.e. kyphoscoliosis and obesity) are also associated with CMS.
- CMS is rarer in those populations who have resided at altitude for many generations. On the Tibetan plateau, CMS prevalence is 5.6% in Han Chinese and just 1.2% in Tibetan natives.

Pathophysiology

Hyperventilation is a common feature of healthy high-altitude residents. CMS occurs in those who under ventilate, resulting in relative hypoxaemia, an exaggerated polycythaemic response, and a greater degree of pulmonary hypertension.

Clinical picture

- *Symptoms:* decreased exercise tolerance, disturbed sleep, headaches, dizziness, tinnitus and paraesthesia.
- *Signs:* clubbing. Dark, erythematous facial features. Cyanosis in nail beds, ears and lips. Pronounced pulmonary second sound and occasionally a soft mid-systolic ejection murmur on auscultation. Evidence of congestive cardiac failure.
- *Investigations:* chest X-ray shows cardiac enlargement and prominent pulmonary vasculature. ECG reveals right axis deviation, negative T waves in V1 and elevated P waves in II, III, and aVF. Lung function tests are normal in CMS unless primary lung diseases are present.

Treatment

- *Acute:* rapid descent. Supplemental oxygen (aim for SaO₂ >95%).
- *Chronic:* the 'gold standard' long-term treatment for CMS is permanent residence at low altitude. Polycythaemia settles within weeks of descent, however cardiovascular changes may take months or even years to resolve. In those who choose to remain at altitude medical therapies are available. Acetazolamide 250 mg once daily or medroxyprogesterone have both been used with some success.

Further reading

Bärtsch P, Mairbäurl H, Maggiorini M, Swenson E (2005). Physiological aspects of high-altitude pulmonary edema. *J Appl Physiol*, 98, 1101–10.

Imray C, Booth A, Wright A, Bradwell A (2011). Acute altitude illnesses. *BMJ*, 343, d4943.

Imray CHE (2012). Acetazolamide for the prophylaxis of acute mountain sickness. *BMJ*, 345, e7077.

Luks AM, McIntosh SE, Grissom CK, Auerbach PS, Rodway G, Schoene RB, *et al.* (2010). Wilderness Medical Society consensus guidelines for the prevention and treatment of acute altitude illness. *Wilderness Environ Med*, 21, 146–55.

Pollard AJ, Murdoch DR (2003). *The High Altitude Medicine Handbook,* 3rd edn, pp. 7–34. Oxford: Radcliffe.

Wilson MH, Newman S, Imray CH (2009). The cerebral effects of ascent to high altitudes. *Lancet Neurol*, 8(2), 175–91.

Chapter 22

Inland and coastal waters

Section editor
Chris Johnson

Contributors
Paddy Morgan
Andy Watt

Aquatic environments *676*
Rescue *682*
Humans in aquatic environments *686*
Immersion and drowning *688*
Canoeing and kayaking *692*
White-water rafting *695*
Medical problems in small craft *696*

Aquatic environments

Drowning is the third leading cause of accidental death worldwide (after road traffic injuries and falls) and results in about 450,000 deaths a year,[1,2] >70% of which involve alcohol. Serious medical problems such as seizures, ischaemic heart disease, and strokes may cause a person to collapse into water and then drown as a secondary event. In 2013, the RNLI in Britain and Ireland rescued 8384 people at sea, with a further 21,938 aided by beach lifeguards—but sophisticated rescue services are not universally available.

Aquatic environments, whether oceans, rivers, or lakes, are very complex, being affected by the flows of water, their interaction with surrounding land, and the interplay with other physical forces such as the wind. Expeditions using rivers or lakes as routes of communication also have to contend with the nature of the surrounding terrain and the local weather conditions.

All expedition risk assessments should consider aquatic hazards.

Water's edge

Most deaths from drowning occur close to shore. Effective risk assessment requires an understanding of the nature of the coastal terrain or river hydrology.

Gradient

- *Vertical or steep edges:* increase risk of slip into water of unknown depth, the edges may be unstable (e.g. decaying canal banks), and make it difficult to rescue a casualty.
- *Steeply sloping beaches:* create dumping waves, and are prone to fast run-offs that can knock people off their feet.
- *Shallow beaches:* often have long tidal ranges with rapid flows that can strand people on sandbanks.
- *Rapids:* form as gradients increase, encouraging white-water activities, but fast currents increase risk for anyone in the water.

Construction

- *Shale/coral:* painful to walk on, sharp pieces can penetrate the skin and cause infections. Formal surgical exploration may be required to remove the infective focus.
- *Sand:* difficult to see animals such as rays that may be trodden on. May produce inshore holes, sandbanks, and rip currents.
- *Rock type:* softer limestone and sandstone riverbeds erode into 'holes' that can trap or damage feet and equipment.
- *Boat launching areas:* should avoid coral, urchins, dangerous currents, and other water users.

---

1 Peden MM, McGee K (2003). The epidemiology of drowning worldwide. *Inj Control Saf Promot*, 10, 195–9.

2 Idris AH, Berg RA, Bierens J, Bossaert L, Branche CM, Gabrielli A, et al. (2003). Recommended guidelines for uniform reporting of data from drowning: the 'Utstein style'. *Resuscitation*, 59, 45–57.

Landscape
- Sandbanks: may falsely reassure about water depth; an incoming tide may produce a deep inshore zone between bather and the shore.
- *Inshore holes:* troughs that run parallel to the shore that can be several feet deep, up to 50 m wide, and several hundred metres long. Rip currents develop as waves break over a sandbar and then run out to sea via the inshore hole.
- *Piers, outcrops:* can also create rip currents. May be surrounded by sharp barnacles, submerged objects and waste.
- *Waste:* glass, oil, and other discarded objects.
- *Flora:* falling coconuts can cause severe head injuries. The Manchineel tree (*Hippomane mancinella*), found in countries bordering the Caribbean, has caustic sap and highly toxic fruits and leaves; don't shelter under these trees. In some countries they are marked by a red cross or band on their trunk, elsewhere you need to be wary.
- On small rivers in wooded areas, fallen trees lying across the river are very hazardous to small craft which may become jammed underneath.
- Coastal landscape may prevent landing by sea kayak and small boats, cliffs may generate strong downdrafts and erratic wave patterns.

Water

Offshore
- Tides, currents, and weather can vary unpredictably; seek local knowledge, although this can be hard to obtain in remote locations.
- Self-rescue is difficult offshore from exposed and inaccessible coastlines.
- Incoming tides can isolate people on sandbanks, and at the midpoint of 'flooding' can raise the level of the sea very dramatically in a short period of time. Outgoing tides can pull people and boats offshore. Both flows can be exacerbated by strong winds or storms.
- *Inshore drift:* a current lateral to shore. Can displace water users into more dangerous areas.
- *Rip current:* a body of water moving in a direction other than the general flow. If it is trapped behind a sandbank as the tide retreats water will flow quickly through deep channels. The flow is strongest when the waves breaking over a sand bar are at their maximum; and minimal over the rip channel. Rip currents can vary from a couple of metres wide to over 50 m, and on rare occasions flow hundreds of metres offshore. The flow will vary with the tides. Identifying features include:
  - Discoloration of the water from disturbance of silt or sand.
  - Darker water surrounding the main current flow.
  - Floating debris or foam on the surface.
  - Surface changes such as rippled water while the surrounding area is calm.
  - Waves breaking on either side of the rip.

If caught in a rip current: float, attract attention, and wait. Some rip currents will re-circulate you to the shore, sandbank or out to sea. If you are a competent swimmer you can consider swimming out of the rip aiming parallel to the shore and towards the breaking waves.

Rivers

- Risks vary markedly according to the gradient, depth, and flow rate of water. Drop a stick in the river—if it moves faster than walking pace, the energy of the system is enough to knock you off your feet.
- Fast-flowing rivers are likely to have stony bottoms, with sudden variations in depth; slow-flowing rivers have muddy bottoms, often with weeds. The outer side of a river bend will have the faster flow.
- Flash floods are a serious risk in mountain regions. In glacial areas the water level will rise rapidly with melt water towards the afternoon. Identify any upstream dams or hydroelectric stations that may suddenly release massive volumes of water.
- Rapids may change from year to year, affected by alterations to the riverbed and the volume of water flowing. Define the extent and complexity of portage if craft need to be transported around waterfalls and rapids.
- Rivers may run through gorges from which escape is difficult; in flat areas, marshes and mud may make access and egress difficult.
- On managed rivers, the unbroken stoppers of artificial weirs are a hazard; river confluences produce eddy currents.
- Narrow, muddy, or wet rock riverside paths increase risk that a slip will cause injury or fall into water, especially during portages.

Waves

- *Dumping waves* occur if the bottom is steep. They peak rapidly and drop the entire force of the wave into the floor, commonly pulling people off their feet and increasing the chance of spinal injury.
- *Spilling waves* have a gradual slope; white water 'spills' down the front of the wave. The point of breaking is dependent on the wind direction.
- *Surging waves* never break, lose speed, or gain height. They 'surge' into the beach and retreat as quickly, possibly dragging people into deep water.
- *Tidal river bores* are predictable phenomena that sweep up estuarine rivers. Surfing them is increasingly popular, but significant skill is required and the rivers can be unpredictable.
- *Standing* waves, seen on rivers, maintain their position relative to the current. They can trap craft and people wearing buoyancy aids.
- *'Stoppers'* are the big hazard on rivers. They re-circulate vertically upstream, creating a wave that can trap boats in a pounding maelstrom that has a high risk of retention and capsize.

Sea

- Coastal navigation is affected by tides, currents, and visibility.
- Compass and maps or charts vital in case any electronic methods fail; in any case, preserving your map reading skills is also important. Both maps + electronic methods should be carried by other paddlers as backup. GPS systems can use a lot of batteries, but can plot mileage, and are useful for positive fix and emergency positioning.
- For longer sea trips, estimate 10–15 miles a day (includes bad weather holdups).

- Rock hopping, i.e. dodging around rocky shores is good fun and raises skills, but runs the risk of damage to both gear and, if capsized, to body.
- *Coasteering*—navigation along the inter-tidal shoreline using a combination of walking, rock climbing, and swimming is increasing in popularity. Safety demands appropriate equipment, knowledge of ledges above and below water and tidal flows especially when youngsters are participating.

Tsunami, jökulhlaup, and flash floods

Although rare, these natural phenomena can be catastrophic, devastating everything in their path, and leaving infra-structure wrecked. Many coastal countries have tsunami warning systems; expeditions must be aware of local alarms, the escape routes to higher ground, and designated muster points. In mountainous areas the overflow or breaching of glacial outflow lakes occasionally leads to catastrophic flooding. Many landscapes in Iceland have been formed as a result of flooding secondary to volcanic activity under the ice-caps; jökulhlaup.

- If you have time: exit buildings and head to high ground on foot.
- If the water level is already rising, or high ground is too far away, go to the top of a well-constructed building near an exit and wait for initial surge to pass.
- If time allows put passport, communications (EPIRB, satellite phone) into a waterproof bag and fix firmly to yourself.
- If buoyancy aids are available, put them on as soon as possible.
- If on a boat, head offshore as the wave height will be less.
- Post disaster: identify all party members and contact the local embassy or consulate to inform them of your predicament.
- Secondary floods, landslides, and building collapse are common.
- Water will be contaminated; purification of drinking water is essential.
- You may feel morally obliged to assist with disaster relief. Balance your involvement with the risk to yourself and your group of exposure to pathogens, depletion of expedition equipment, and the inevitable difficulties in finding clean food and safe water.

Other issues

- *Depth:* compared to shallow areas, deep water will usually appear darker and be associated with less surface disturbance.
- *Submerged objects:* rocks, tree roots, sunken vehicles, and outlet pipes are difficult to recognize. In calm areas look for unexpected waves breaking over the obstruction. Obstructions can form 'strainers' in a river system, trapping swimmers against them.
- *Plants, reeds, seaweed:* can easily entrap swimmers or waders; use small gentle strokes to escape. Dense vegetation may hide snakes, crocodiles, etc. Floating debris is common after storm weather.
- *Quality:* rivers and coastlines may be polluted by industrial, agricultural, or bacteriological effluent. Determine local dumping areas and sewage outlets. Smell or coloured algae foam can be an indication of hazardous zones. Problems commonest soon after heavy rain that overwhelms sewage systems.

Weather

- *Wind* affects wave strength and formation, cools the skin, masks sunburn, and increases the risk of hypothermia. Down drafts near cliffs can be fierce.
- *Rain* reduces visibility, increases the risk of hypothermia, and steep catchment areas can result in rapid change in river level.
- *Ultraviolet light* from the sun reflects off the surface of the water, increasing exposure to radiation. Tropical climates encourage scanty clothing. Splash water washes off protective sun block creams. Minimize hazards by appropriate behaviour, clothing, and UV protection. UV exposure is greater at altitude. Reflected glare may affect underside of chin, nose, eyebrows, and eyes (the use of good quality sunglasses will reduce risk of long-term damage; ➔ Solar skin damage, p. 266). On the plus side, UV light reduces the pathogen load of natural bodies of water; minimum load is in the 2–3 h post midday.
- *Weather reports* are important; if there are no reports available you may have to rely on your own personal observations and barometric analysis. In the USA/Canada, weather reports are transmitted continuously; several organizations provide satellite text weather messaging services, and phone apps are available.
- For kayakers and canoeists, cold and wet weather leads to shorter days paddling and consequent pressure on schedules.

Travel on water

- Getting craft and stores safely to and from a river can be challenging. River bridges, harbours and quays provide good landing points and escape routes, but away from such fixed locations, carefully planning is required.
- Itineraries must consider the unpredictable stresses of multi-day journeys, which considerably exceed those of shorter leisure trips.
- Escape routes and rescue plans must be considered especially in areas where access to the water is difficult.
- Maps may not accurately highlight the physical characteristics of shorelines and riverbanks.
- Portage routes must be planned and appropriate loads taken.

Navigation

- On the water, most navigating is done from the boat ('read and run') as stopping to inspect rapids ('scouting') is a lot slower.
- Need to be able to recognize white-water dangers—mainly 'stoppers' and small whirlpools below big water rapids, but also sumps, undercuts, ledge drops, waterfalls, and the risks of broaching and pinning.
- Need to understand river flows as expressed by European metric cubic metres per second (cumecs) or American cubic feet per second (cfs). 1 cumecs = 35.3 cfs.
- Coastal navigation is affected by tides, currents, and visibility.
- Navigation through swamps, reed beds, and tunda shield terrain where there are numerous lakes and low hills can be exceptionally challenging. GPS may provide a position, but maps may be hard to interpret.

Environmental impact of humans
- Away from centres of population and tourist destinations, communities at the water's edge are often small, remote and poor, possibly with only tenuous road access to the outside world.
- Sewage and garbage are diffuse and everywhere, especially after heavy rains.
- Fish traps are occasionally placed in small channels at water's edge or shallow seas.

Rescue

However stressful the situation, never add to the death toll; maintain your own and others' safety. Have a realistic view of your own abilities and, unless highly skilled, avoid direct contact with a panicking casualty. Local rescue services may be primitive or non-existent.

Preventing accidents

Risk management

All expeditions working on or near water must consider the possibility of immersion and plan rescue procedures.

- Drowning often occurs very quickly and unexpectedly.
- A personal flotation device dramatically improves the chance of surviving an immersion—but only if it is worn. You may not have enough time to put it on if you are not already wearing it.
- Accidents often happen out of reach of other party members. Use a buddy system to keep in touch with other team members.
- Many incidents could be avoided with good risk assessment.

Rivers

- Shouted commands are unreliable above the roar of moving water; if possible, discuss among rescuers before starting the rescue, personal radios if available may assist.
- At river rapids: identify hazards, agree run, and decide running order.
- In difficult areas, 'set safety' by distributing team members with appropriate rescue equipment in advance of the boats in case rescue is required.
- Remember 'reach, throw, wade, tow'; recognizing the hazards with each technique. Learn and practise proper use of throwbags.
- Wading risks foot entrapment, and is best done with a paddle for support; or better as a pair or threesome, linking arms and with safety set downstream.
- Ropes and karabiners may assist during rescues, but add to the hazard if people are not properly trained in their use.

Around coasts

- There are many options for communication around coasts. Mobile or satellite phones and VHF radios enable surface-to-shore communications. Equipment should ideally allow communication with both rescue centres and rescue craft on a variety of frequencies.
- GPS-PLB (personal locator beacons) are cheaper and smaller than EPIRB and have good battery life. They have world cover—in the UK, if the device is registered, the signal goes through Falmouth to local coastguards; and keeps transmitting for 10 h. A SPOT satellite GPS messenger sends pre-programmed text messages and also has buttons for routine plots of progress.[3]
- Other vessels may be involved in rescue, so read relevant textbooks on managing such a rescue and also understand actions to take during helicopter rescue (see ➲ Helicopter evacuation, p. 722).

3 ☞ www.international.findmespot.com

Rescue techniques

See Table 22.1.

Table 22.1 Rescue techniques

Choice	Intervention	Suitability and risk
1st	Signal and shout	Effective for disorientated, weak, or injured swimmer. Low risk to rescuer
2nd	Reach	Casualties that are within physical reach, or in reach with pole/stick, etc. Potential to be pulled in
3rd	Throw	Floatable aids or rope effective for weak/injured swimmers. Rope throwing requires practise
4th	Boat or dingy	Limited by availability, operator skill, time to set up, and water conditions
5th	Swim with an aid	Swimming with floatable aid, can allow a small distance to be kept from casualty or assist tow.
6th	Swim and tow	High risk owing to physical contact with panicking casualty. Energy sapping procedure. Avoid obstructing victim's airway with towing technique

Unconscious casualty

Approach swiftly; turn the casualty into a supine position. Prompt expired air ventilation (EAV) increases survival if the casualty is not breathing properly. Balance difficulties of administering rescue breaths against the time taken to exit the water, and rescuer's capability to perform the skill. If there is only a short distance to safety—exit and then resuscitate; if a longer swim is involved, and you have the skill and strength, attempt in-water EAV. Casualties often vomit—be prepared.

Post-immersion collapse syndrome

Prolonged immersion creates dehydration, with BP supported by hydrostatic pressure of water on limbs. Rescue in horizontal position if practical. Vertical extraction carries the risk of cardiovascular collapse and death.

Injuries

Certain aquatic accidents predispose to life-threatening injuries. These include fractures and head injuries from high-velocity impacts such as fast watercraft, cliff diving, or anybody in heavy surf. Surfers and those diving into shallow water are at high risk of cervical spine injuries, which are otherwise relatively uncommon.

Mass rescue

If more than one casualty is present, rescue must be prioritized. (See Table 22.2.)

Table 22.2 Priority of rescue

1st	Non-swimmer	Head going under water and unable to maintain a direction
2nd	Weak swimmer	Able to hold position and direction of sight but not move
3rd	Injured swimmer	Holds position, swims slowly, communicates injury
4th	Unconscious	Usually face down. If the casualty is seen to go unconscious they are first priority to minimize period of hypoxaemia. But if period of hypoxia is unknown, victim may be dead and extraction of body from water will prevent rescue of other casualties

Immersion

There are four phases following immersion into water below the thermon-eutral temperature of 30°C (see Fig. 22.1):

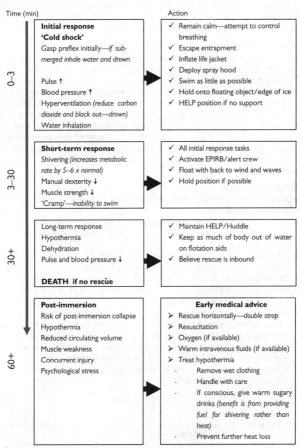

Time (min)

0–3

Initial response
'Cold shock'
Gasp preflex initially—*if submerged inhale water and drown*

Pulse ↑
Blood pressure ↑
Hyperventilation *(reduce carbon dioxide and black out—drown)*
Water inhalation

Action
- ✓ Remain calm—attempt to control breathing
- ✓ Escape entrapment
- ✓ Inflate life jacket
- ✓ Deploy spray hood
- ✓ Swim as little as possible
- ✓ Hold onto floating object/edge of ice
- ✓ HELP position if no support

3–30

Short-term response
Shivering *(increases metabolic rate by 5–6 x normal)*
Manual dexterity ↓
Muscle strength ↓
'Cramp'—*inability to swim*

- ✓ All initial response tasks
- ✓ Activate EPIRB/alert crew
- ✓ Float with back to wind and waves
- ✓ Hold position if possible

30+

Long-term response
Hypothermia
Dehydration
Pulse and blood pressure ↓

DEATH if no rescue

- ✓ Maintain HELP/Huddle
- ✓ Keep as much of body out of water on flotation aids
- ✓ Believe rescue is inbound

60+

Post-immersion
Risk of post-immersion collapse
Hypothermia
Reduced circulating volume
Muscle weakness
Concurrent injury
Psychological stress

Early medical advice
- ➤ Rescue horizontally—*double strop*
- ➤ Resuscitation
- ➤ Oxygen (if available)
- ➤ Warm intravenous fluids (if available)
- ➤ Treat hypothermia
  - – Remove wet clothing
  - – Handle with care
  - – If conscious, give warm sugary drinks *(benefit is from providing fuel for shivering rather than heat)*
  - – Prevent further heat loss

†Time to death depends on various factors (weight/water temperature/clothing/wind, etc.)

HELP: Heat Escape Lessening Position.

EPIRB: Emergency Positioning Indicating Rescue Beacon—a satellite rescue beacon.

Fig. 22.1 Responses to immersion.

- Initial response.
- Short-term response.
- Long-term response.
- Post-immersion response.

The colder the water the more dramatic the response. Consider whether a sudden illness such as epileptic seizure or myocardial infarction may have caused the casualty to fall into the water.

Basic resuscitation

Follow international guidelines[5] but, as the likely cause is primary respiratory failure, complete five initial breaths and 1 min of CPR before going for help. Approximately 2/3 of drowning victims will vomit—try to keep the airway clear by turning the head to face downhill. This will allow any fluid or vomit to drain away. Overall, only 0.5% of drowning victims will have associated spinal injuries so care of the spinal cord is of secondary importance unless there is a high index of suspicion: head injury or mechanism, e.g. dive into shallow water. If suspected, and enough rescuers are present, extract the casualty horizontally from the water with cervical spine control and log-roll to clear the airway if required. Hypothermia and shock are common, even in tropical climates.

Advanced techniques

- An automatic external defibrillator may reveal electrical heart activity if pulses are impalpable.
- All post-drowning victims are hypothermic until proven otherwise. Shivering is a good prognostic sign. Warm appropriately (➔ Field management, p. 624).
- Administer high-flow oxygen (if available) during resuscitation and recovery, ideally titrated to pulse oximetry (if available).
- Dehydration and acidosis can develop from hypoxia and physiological effects of prolonged immersion. Consider warm IV fluids if available, monitor urine output and respiratory rate.
- Acute respiratory distress syndrome (ARDS) can develop up to 72 h post-immersion. It presents as a non-cardiogenic pulmonary oedema caused by the irritation of water in the lungs, and requires hospitalization and ventilatory support.[6] If there is likely to be a delay in getting the patient to hospital and the casualty develops wheeze, consider regular hydrocortisone together with salbutamol inhalers/ nebulizers, and furosemide.[7]

5 Soar J, Perkins GD, Abbas G Alfonzo A, Barelli A, Bierens JJ, et al. (2010) European Resuscitation Council Guidelines for Resuscitation 2010 Section 8. Cardiac arrest in special circumstances: Electrolyte abnormalities, poisoning, drowning, accidental hypothermia, hyperthermia, asthma, anaphylaxis, cardiac surgery, trauma, pregnancy, electrocution. *Resuscitation*, 81, 1400–33.

6 Tipton MJ, Golden FS (2011). A proposed decision-making guide for the search, rescue and resuscitation of submersion (head under) victims based on expert opinion. *Resuscitation*, 82(7), 819–24.

7 Van Berkel M, Bierens J, Lie R, de Rooy TP, Kool LJ, van de Velde EA, et al. (1996). Pulmonary oedema, pneumonia and mortality in submersion victims; a retrospective study in 125 patients. *Intensive Care Med*, 22(2), 101–7.

Aspiration pneumonia can develop later. Antibiotics are usually not required, but prophylactic antibiotics may be appropriate in remote areas, or if the casualty shows signs of fever or sepsis. Consider other fungal or parasitic pathogens if aspirated water was potentially dirty, e.g. ditches, sewers or frequented by rodents (see ➡ Leptospirosis p. 471).

All survivors of an immersion incident who may have inhaled water should be triaged to ascertain whether they require admission to a hospital capable of offering advanced respiratory support.

A cough post immersion is not a criterion for admission.

Immediate, (as is practicable), admission is required if a cough is present *plus* one of: productive sputum or 'foam', fever, respiratory distress, or cardiac compromise.

Discontinuing resuscitation and rescue attempts

Good quality survival following prolonged immersion can occur, particularly if water is very cold. Attempt basic resuscitation wherever practical and, if possible, evacuate to a hospital capable of advanced re-warming techniques such as cardiopulmonary bypass. After prolonged hypothermia or cardiac arrest, the core temperature should be re-stabilized at 33°C for 72 h before returning to normothermia.

Survival is extremely unlikely if the victim has been submerged (head under) for >30 min in water warmer than 6°C, and >90 min in water <6°C. Expeditions in remote areas should attempt to resuscitate and re-warm a casualty, but will have to adopt a pragmatic approach to ceasing resuscitation attempts (see also ➡ Hypothermia, p. 622).

Resources

Surf Life Saving GB: ℅ http://www.surflifesaving.org.uk

Transport Canada. *Marine Safety*: ℅ http://www.tc.gc.ca/MarineSafety

Canoeing and kayaking

Canoes are open boats manoeuvred by sitting or kneeling using single-blade paddles, but the term is often used generically to include kayaks, which are enclosed craft, paddled sitting using a double-blade paddle. Kayaks are more manoeuvrable and manage waves and white water better. Sea kayaks can carry reasonable loads and manage longer trips; river kayaks have limited space for gear and food. Canoes are more suitable for lakes or slow rivers and can carry heavy loads. These craft may be used to explore remote areas, for other recreations such as fishing, or for the challenge of white water trips.

Preparation

- Fitness appropriate to the challenge is vital, especially for multiday trips, which are far more exhausting than day excursions. Any fitness training is worthwhile, but most important preparation is 'time in boat'.
- Good paddling and rafting technique reduces the risk of shoulder and back injuries.
- Learn to lift weights and loaded boats safely and efficiently.
- Team working is vital for a successful expedition. Disputes about goals are a major factor in expedition 'failures'. Before you go, it is important to establish what you are all in it for—a challenging paddle, a holiday, or something in between?
- Consider immunizations against waterborne hepatitis A and polio, also rabies for remote areas and oral cholera (Dukoral®) for some urban centres.
- Consider if other treatments such as antimalarial drugs are required.
- Get treatment for dental problems, back pain, and piles before departure—if these conditions worsen on the trip, they may force you to abandon the trip or may spoil the journey for your mates.

Accommodation and campcraft

- Commonest site for accidents, especially if alcohol is involved.
- Acceptable sites can be infrequent and may have limited space for camping. Keep gear, especially boats, above high-water mark.
- Lightweight tents are used but with limited space in boats for gear, if weather is warm and biting insects not an issue, save weight by using a lightweight tarpaulin for the group, propped up with paddles and throwlines, and/or bivi bags. Down sleeping bags pack small, but are unreliable if damp. Double bag them, or choose the bulkier artificial fibre bags that retain insulation even if damp.

Heat, light, and fuel

- Carry fuel, driftwood makes good fires but may not be available.
- Gas canisters are light, but always check local availability as they cannot be taken on aircraft.
- Kerosene or petrol will probably be available locally, but quality may vary and soot may clog stove nozzles: take several prickers. Fuel bottles must have perfect seals to prevent smelly contamination and damage of other gear and food.

Water supplies

(See also ➲ Water purification, p. 102.)

- Sea, rivers, and lakes are recipients of sewage and, in urban areas, street run-off with oils and animal and human faeces.
- At sea on coastal trips, it is vital to know the next source of fresh water. If location unknown prior to departure, take adequate water. Water bladders with pipe to mouth are useful for daytime paddling. Consider a flask of boiled water, useful for a brew in the first half of the day, and as a source of clean water for cuts etc.
- In river kayaks, a filter can be bulky and may develop unseen breakages and leaks. Canoes, rafts, and sea kayaks, have more space to carry filters. An alternative to a filter is to use chlorine dioxide or iodine, easy to carry as an emergency supply. Take sufficient dropper bottles with you to fill up with iodine.
- Lakes and coastal seas may develop harmful algae blooms (HABs), containing toxic or otherwise harmful phytoplankton such as dinoflagellates of the genus *Alexandrium* and *Karenia*, or diatoms of the genus *Pseudo-nitzschia*. Such blooms often take on a red or brown hue and are known colloquially as 'red tides'.
- Biting insects and snails may be vectors for parasites.

Nutrition

Ensure adequate food and water supplies available during day to counter-act fatigue. In remote locations it may be difficult to buy food; expedition rations may then be restricted to less palatable freeze-dried or tinned alter-natives. Keep food and water cool by storing low in the boat's hull, with heavy items central to maintain balance.

Sanitation

At sea, some carry a marked pee bottle, but its use can be difficult in rough water, and groups may need to raft up. More difficult for women, although some use a 'slipper' type bottle.

Faecal matter degrades slowly in toilet pits on beaches. Small or popular beaches can get overloaded unless a management plan is in place. In many North American National Parks you are required to carry out your toilet waste.

Clothing

Wind and water combine to chill the body, so effective protective gear is necessary, but overheating can also be an issue with hard exercise and impermeable fabrics.

Wetsuits tend not to be used in kayaking expeditions—if you're expect-ing to get wet, then a drycag is better at keeping you dry and warm, although damaged and leaking drycags are hard to repair effectively. If you are only expecting exposure to spray, then wear a comfortable paddling top cuffed at neck and wrists over a synthetic or merino wool vest. Dry suits can cause overheating, chafing, become punctured, and may be uncomfortable. Following coastal trips wash all kit in fresh water each evening to minimize damage and chafing. Effective UV protection is necessary in sunny places.

Footwear should cope with slippery, rough ground and bearing the weight of boats while the sole must be flexible enough to fit in cramped cockpits.

Spectacles should be tied firmly with thin yachting cord; proprietary cords with quick-fit rubber ends don't hold them well in turbulent water.

Safety

- Get used to wearing buoyancy aids whenever close to water.
- Wherever possible in difficult water, ensure there are backup or rescue craft.
- Use a buddy system; in bigger groups appoint front and rear paddlers. Split large groups into smaller units.
- Work as a team and know where everyone is. Communication within the group is vital; even small, experienced groups make a point at the beginning and end of each day of having a briefing on the day past and the day to come. All sea kayakers carry waterproof VHF radios for both inter-group and outside contact.
- Agree hand signals and methods of communication that will work despite wind or water noise.
- When scouting rapids, agree routes and running order with safety crafts or throw lines positioned below rapids.
- Helmets, paddles, and cagoules should be brightly coloured, perhaps even using fluorescent tape on dark-coloured gear.
- If travelling with a guiding company using their equipment, check the experience, qualifications, and first-aid training of the guides together with the age and serviceability of the vessels.
- Self-rescue is important; kayakers should be able to self-right after a roll even in heavy water, and practise other rescue techniques such as towing.

White-water rafting

White-water rafting is an exhilarating active sport usually led by professional guides, who can safely guide novices through reasonably hard rapids. Multiday trips are true river journeys, offering unique access to wilderness areas.

Although white-water rafting may appear dangerous, accident rates are low if basic safety rules are followed. A survey in the USA (West Virginia, 200 injuries) showed that most injuries occur in the raft: 1/3 to the face, 1/3 cuts—especially to the hands, and 1/6 fractures.

Evaluating the raft company

Good companies should run well-organized trips, but local competition can reduce prices to the detriment of safety. Check:

- The experience of the guides and their qualifications.
- How often they have run the river.
- Age and serviceability of the rafts.
- Buoyancy aids and helmets provided.
- Appropriateness of safety briefing.
- Whether another craft (raft or kayak) will accompany your raft.

Preparations

- You need to be reasonably fit.
- Safer if you can swim, you should certainly not be scared of water.
- In developing countries consider hepatitis A vaccination.
- Clothing should include a peaked sun cap and good river sandals with either buckles or Velcro® fastening.
- Take a small medical kit, including paracetamol, plasters, and sun screen, and iodine for grazes, cuts and emergency water sterilization.

On the water

- Use sun-protection.
- Drink plenty of clean water to prevent dehydration.
- Wear your buoyancy aid whenever you are close to flowing water.

At camps

- Sterilize water effectively.
- Follow local sanitation rules.
- Careful hand hygiene using soap and water or alcohol gel.
- Beware of twists and sprains on rocks especially at night.
- Beware of the campfire.

Medical problems in small craft

Serious medical issues

Immersion and drowning

(See also ⮕ Immersion and drowning, p. 688.)

Sudden immersion in very cold water, especially in those less habituated to it, activates the cold shock response: 'gasp and hyperventilation', which reduces the time available to attempt a roll and can increase risk of drowning. Above rapids, experienced paddlers often douse their faces in cold water as this may reduce the reflex.

Non-freezing cold injury

(See also ⮕ Non-freezing cold injury, p. 632.)

Also known as trench foot or pernio, cold injury is possible in very cold waters if feet are immersed in cold water for prolonged periods. May occur during spring rafting especially in high latitudes. Recognized by pain and discoloration of the foot; it can cause prolonged disability.

Hypothermia

(See also ⮕ Hypothermia, p. 622.)

Clearly a risk with prolonged exposure to water and spray, not necessarily very cold. More likely at end of the day, if people are less experienced, have rolled, or have inadequate clothing. Look out for non-specific, poorer functioning, often in a less experienced team mate, who likely won't recognize it, and thus you will have to take decisions on their behalf. Cut the day short, camp, rewarm, and feed.

Shoulder dislocation

(For relocation see ⮕ Shoulder and upper arm injuries, p. 422.)

A particular risk for less experienced paddlers unfamiliar with the power of, and the reaction times needed, on big water. Once injured the risk of a recurrent dislocation is high (up to 50% in first time dislocations), while a weakened vulnerable shoulder will reduce future capability to deal with difficult waters. Older paddlers with a dislocation tend to injure the rotator cuff muscles surrounding the shoulder joint. Dislocation is common when the paddle arm is lifted high and forcibly abducted: as when bracing against a wave, or during an imminent capsize. Proper paddling technique involves keeping the hands low and not reaching too far to the side.

Head and neck injuries

(See also ⮕ Airway, p. 186; ⮕ Head injury, p. 312.)

May occur as a result of:
- Collisions with paddles or other crew members.
- Collision with overhanging vegetation.
- Colliding with a rock in the water after fall from craft; if swimming, point your feet downstream or towards any rocks.

Common medical problems

Seasickness

(See also ➲ Seasickness, p. 718.)

May be debilitating and hazardous during rough water paddling. Risk factors include fatigue, cold, fear, and watching compass regularly. Sea-sickness is exhausting; sufferers may require rest, food, fluids, and understanding from other expedition members.

Dehydration

An easily overlooked problem particularly common when rafting in the heat, but risk is high even in the Arctic where humidity can be very low. Early signs are vague symptoms such as headache, light headiness, and lethargy and are difficult to recognize unless you are on the lookout for them. Some people avoid drinking much during the day to reduce toilet trips, but then rehydrate during the evening; a risky strategy unless you are very aware of your fluid status.

Back, neck, and muscle problems

Stiff and knotted muscles, especially in neck and between shoulder blades, are common on multi-day trips, and after moving heavy craft. Stretching exercises before and after paddling are worthwhile; together with firm massages of 'knots' at end of the day. If non-specific pain affects your paddling, try keeping the elbow low during the paddle action.

Sea paddlers can get leg strain through constant sitting in the same position. Take the weight off the leg muscles especially in the groin by placing a filled drybag under the knees.

Low back trouble is common in kayakers, especially as the kayaking posture flexes the lower lumbar spine against its natural lordosis. If you suffer from back problems:

- Review your flexibility exercises before departure.
- Use proper lifting techniques.
- Consider lifting aids such as straps or portable trolleys.
- Fit a good backrest with effective lumbar or pelvic support.
- Back, pelvis, and thigh strains are a risk in contemporary tightly strapped play boats. On the flatter river sections, you should be able to release your legs easily.

Tenosynovitis

Tenosynovitis of wrist tendon is a repetitive strain injury (RSI) due to flexion and extension of the wrist while using a feathered paddle. Pain can be severe and crepitus dramatic. Point tenderness distinguishes this from a non-specific sprain.

Treatment requires complete rest, but on a long journey the paddler may be unable or unwilling to comply. Prescribe an NSAID painkiller such as ibuprofen or diclofenac, or simple analgesic if contraindications to NSAID (➲ Painkillers, p. 348). A wrist splint or neoprene support may help. Icing (if practical) and elevation in sling may assist recovery.

Alterations to paddling technique may help:

- A common cause is gripping paddle too tightly ('overgrip'), try a looser grip especially when injured wrist is on upper part of stroke.
- Use a larger diameter paddle shaft, possibly with cranked shaft.
- Change from right to left paddle feather, or vice versa.
- Alter feather angle, although this may not help much once pain has started.

Blisters
(See also ➲ Blisters, p. 276.)

Water softens the skin. Blisters are fairly common on multi-day trips, even amongst experienced paddlers. Strap tape or moleskin over 'hot spots' or early blisters, and change the way you grip the paddle. If blisters burst, treat as a simple cut.

Burns
(See also ➲ Burns, p. 280.)

Common when wood fires used. Immediate action to cool the flesh is vital, usually immersing affected area in the water for a period is best. If the burn is severe enough to require a burns dressing, then the challenge on the water is keeping that dressing dry: try duct tape and plastic bags.

Piles
(See also ➲ Haemorrhoids (piles), p. 397.)

Common in kayakers, they may be precipitated by both diarrhoea, or by constipation associated with dehydrated foods. Sufferers should consider treatment before departure—they will only get worse.

Ear problems
A common complaint of kayakers is a sensation of 'water in the ear' with deafness. This can be caused either by a blocked Eustachian tube (possibly secondary to an upper respiratory tract infection) or by extensive wet wax in ear canal, causing a blockage external to the tympanic membrane. These can be hard to treat. Try to unblock the Eustachian tube:
• By inhaling steam.
• Using a decongestant such as Actifed®.
• Swallowing hard.
• Using a Valsalva manoeuvre—but avoid this technique in the case of active nasal infection with green snot as it can make things worse.

You are unlikely to persuade an enthusiastic kayaker to avoid rolling, so it is likely the symptom won't clear up until after the trip ends. Flying, especially during descent, can be painful if Eustachian tubes are blocked and occasionally leads to tympanic rupture.

Bony exostoses of the ear canal ('surfer's ear') are associated with frequent cold-water impact during years of kayak rolling. When ear canal obstruction exceeds 50%, the risk of infection increases and hearing is impaired. Some experienced kayakers have >80% obstruction. Operations to excise the exostoses don't always give symptom-free recovery. Prevent by using custom earplugs and a neoprene hood—although these do reduce hearing and therefore safety. Prevention is especially important for athletic youngsters in playboats, who are, at an increasingly younger age, being exposed to frequent immersion in cold water.

Otitis external is an infection of the external ear canal that may be itchy or painful. Common in tropical humid zones, treatment requires good aural toilet, helped by acetic acid (or vinegar) and alcohol. Use an ear plug of cotton wool with an astringent such as Vaseline® or aluminium sulphate. Persistent or severe infections may require antibiotic drops to deal with an acute infection, or steroids if chronic eczema develops.

Cuts, grazes, and skin problems
(See also ➔ Wound types and management, p. 272.)

Cuts and grazes should be cleaned with filtered or sterilized water to eliminate risk of contaminating wound with sand or pathogens. Keep a bottle of clean water handy available for such minor emergencies. Cuts on the water have a significant risk of infection. Clean and close as soon as possible with sutures or glue, although glue often wears off after a couple of days. Adhesive skin closure strips are useless in the wet. Uninfected wounds become waterproof after 24 h, but until initial healing has taken place try to keep dry.

Fungal skin infections are common in hot climates, while sun and wind can lead to chapped lips.

Jellyfish stings
(See also ➔ Venomous marine animals, p. 566.)
• Avoid rubbing skin as pressure increases discharge from sting.
• Scrape skin with stiff plastic like an old credit card.
• Rinse area well with sea water (fresh water is hypotonic to stinging cells and they will explode in its presence—exacerbating the irritation).
• Ice and elevate affected area.
• Use an antihistamine (e.g. diphenhydramine) cream or spray.
• Don't pee on the sting—it's an old wife's tale.

Burn out and stress
Rushed itineraries lead to chronic mild exhaustion. On challenging sea trips, safe landings can be hours away, but all team members have to be able to the face consequent fatigue and fear. Don't push weaker members into challenging coastlines or attempting rapids above their skill level. On week-long trips, the nadir of physical fatigue and emotions can come around day 4, then improves. Recognition of variation in moods is important to prevent over-reaction to apparent 'difficult behaviour'.

Limited medical kit items for small craft
(See also Chapter 28.)

Often lack of space restricts choice of supplies. Pack in zipper plastic storage bags or waterproof container/dry bags, leaving lots of air within the bag or barrel so it floats if displaced in a capsize.
• Plastic dropper bottle for iodine solution (one per paddler).
• One large bandage (cut to size required).
• Suitable painkillers (see Table 28.1).
• Multitool with knife and/or scissors (probably in main repair kit).
• Antibiotic ear drops (e.g. Betnesol-N®), cotton wool, and petroleum gel.
• Hand cream, lip salve.
• Seasickness tablets.
• Tape—duct tape sticks best, but doesn't stretch.
• Sub-tropical trips—cotton wool, and petroleum gel and consider calamine lotion for sunburn.

Resources
Brown G (2006). *Sea Kayak*. Bangor: Pesda Press.
ℰ http://www.seakayakwithgordonbrown.com

DVDs on skills, rescue, and technological/helicopter/lifeboat rescue:
ℰ http://www.pesdapress.com

Ferrero F. (2006). *Whitewater Safety and Rescue*, 2nd ed. Bangor: Pesda Press.

Safety Code of American Whitewater:
ℰ http://www.americanwhitewater.org/content/Wiki/safety:start

Chapter 23

Offshore

Section editor
Chris Johnson

Contributors
Spike Briggs
Campbell MacKenzie

The environment 702
Risk assessment 704
Environmental impact of sailors 706
Preparations for voyage 712
Offshore medical kits 716
Offshore medical problems 718
Emergency procedures 722

The environment

> 'They who go down to the sea in ships and
> take their leisure in deep waters.'
>
> (Psalm 107, verse 23)

Physical characteristics

- *Isolation* from assistance is a major factor when assessing the fitness of crew, planning medical kits, and arranging medical shore support.
- *Extreme weather conditions*—high winds, wave impact, motion, salt water, humidity, heat, cold, and frequent immersion—should be expected, and prepared for.
- *Trauma, illness, and physical danger* are medical and mental challenges, and are common; pre-existing medical conditions may relapse.
- *Seasickness* is a frequent and often disabling condition. It can usually be treated effectively, but vomiting may prevent absorption of other oral medications or contraceptives.
- *Living conditions* are enclosed, cramped, and often difficult to keep clean, leading to the risk of community infection. Well-planned watch-keeping schedules are essential to minimize fatigue.
- *Nutrition and hydration* are essential factors in maintaining team health and performance.
- *Team dynamics* are central to every facet of boat performance; a happy and healthy boat performs well.

Weather

Weather forecasts are increasingly accurate and can be accessed anywhere. GRIB (GRIdded Binary) files are readily available from a variety of websites via satellite phone or single side band radio (SSB), giving high definition of weather conditions local to a yacht's position, but a forecast is only helpful if accessed in good time and interpreted correctly. Think ahead, get information, and plan accordingly.

Be prepared for anything. Bad weather takes a toll on crew and boat; both must be in the best condition possible, and both require regular maintenance. Hot, humid tropical weather in the tropics can lead to exhaustion, dehydration, infections, and sunburn. Prolonged cold conditions make it hard to dry anything and can lead to insidious development of hypothermia (→ Hypothermia, p. 622).

Trauma and deterioration of medical conditions are most likely during poor weather. Plan accordingly: where is the best place for the medical kit to be accessed when the boat is falling off 10 m waves, and where is the best place to put a casualty so they do not come to further harm, and can be examined and treated?

Navigation

You should always know where you are and where you are heading. Keep in contact with a shore-based facility; if disaster strikes rescuers need to know where to look for you.

- *Global Positioning System*: over the past 25 years, universal access to GPS has made navigation far more accurate and less dependent upon weather conditions. Always have a least one backup system, and another system that gives latitude and longitude that can be plotted on a paper chart.
- *Electricity*: all technical systems require electricity, which also requires multiple backups. Solar panels or a wind turbine can provide an alternative power source to the ship's generator. Electrical power for several days must be available in a life raft as well.
- *Paper charts* (Standard Nautical Charts) and Pilots (Sailing Directions) covering all sail areas and ports of call are still essential items and board.
- *Astronavigation* is the ultimate backup plan but requires detailed training and frequent practice to be reasonably accurate.

Risk assessment

Both yacht racing and cruising involve significant risk:[1]
- One death per 200,000 miles or 60 man-years of sailing.
- One major incident per 10,000 miles.
- One minor incident per 2750 miles.

Specific risk factors
- Crew composition and fitness.
- Proposed route:
  - Distance from land (in/out of helicopter range of 200 miles).
  - Distance from frequented shipping routes.
  - Special obstacles, e.g. ice, fog, other shipping.
  - Piracy is a risk in some regions. See: ℘ https://www.gov.uk/
    sea-river-and-piracy-safety
- Length of time at sea.
- On-board medical skill.
- Shore support.
- Medical kit contents.
- Communication availability.

Search and rescue

Ocean sailing can put a yacht crew >2 weeks from useful medical help.
Crews might have to cope with serious medical problems during this time,
and must have a realistic expectation of what is possible if someone is seri-
ously injured or falls ill. Communication must be reliable, and may be via:
- Marine radio (VHF and SSB) when within range of shore.
- Satellite telephones (email or voice).
- Inmarsat Standard C.

Telemedicine is increasingly common but requires video or image transmission and reception, together with the medical expertise to interpret those
images. Shore support for medical emergencies is possible via international
maritime rescue coordination centres such as MRCC Falmouth (a Maritime
and Coastguard Agency service). There are various other organizations that
provide support for expeditions to remote places, such as Medical Support
Offshore Ltd, based in Southampton, UK, and the British Antarctic Survey
Medical Unit (BASMU), based at Derriford Hospital, Plymouth, UK. Larger
expeditions may organize their own shore medical support team that can
then be tailored to the crew's specific requirements.

    Helicopters can fly ~200 nautical miles from the nearest base, and expedi-
tions beyond this range should be planned more rigorously.

1 Osborne T (1990). First aid, illness and accidents on board: a Cruising Committee survey. *Cruising Summer Ed*. Cruising Association, pp. 12–15.

Environmental impact of sailors

- Sailing takes place in some of the most pristine environments on the planet. Respect this.
- Plastic and other non-perishable detritus already despoil every ocean—do not add to this, take all rubbish to land.
- Do not release oil or other hydrocarbons at sea—oil slicks can have a profound impact on sea life and birds.
- Do not release sewage if it could make landfall within 24 h.
- Consider where you drop the anchor and the effect of the chain when the boat swings on its mooring.
- Do not closely pursue marine animals such as cetaceans and sharks, and do not stray close to seabird nesting colonies.
- Make full use of solar and wind generators, and minimize use of the ship's engines.
- Think about the type of anti-foulant used—this can have serious detrimental effects on local wildlife in crowded moorings.
- Music can add to the atmosphere on board, but not in a quiet anchorage. It will annoy local wildlife and those anchored nearby.

Humans on long voyages

Sailing in remote areas is no longer the preserve of the young and fit.

Journeys. Rigorous, remoter, longer, colder or tropical routes require fitter crew and better medical training for skipper and medic.

Crew should be physically fit prior to the expedition, with particular attention paid to cardiopulmonary fitness and lower limb strength, which will decline when confined on board a yacht for several weeks. Short-handed crew work harder, become more exhausted, and consequently incur more injuries and illnesses.

Personal space is limited, but will be ameliorated by having ownership of at least some space, no matter how small.

Weather whether cold, hot or rough can be exhausting. With no escape crew have to cope whatever the weather. Storms don't blow forever, although at the time they may feel as if they do.

Eating at sea is a communal activity. Personal choice is reduced with less opportunity for 'grazing' or indulgences. Food supplies must take into account personal dietary restrictions. Occasional treats may prevent mutiny.

Patience and tolerance are essential if the crew are to remain happy and efficient. When in close proximity, noises and smells must be tolerated by the observer, and minimized by the emitter.

Boredom may sometimes beset crew; youngsters are particularly at risk. Usually they can be distracted by a never-ending list of maintenance tasks, but reading, schooling, a structure for the day and pastimes such as musical instruments may alleviate occasional tedium.

Fear and danger are real concerns offshore. Rough weather, accidents, other emergencies, and even possibly the catastrophic experience of having to take to a life raft after a vessel sinks, bring out both the worst and the best in crew. They may react by becoming aggressive or withdrawn and depressed. Mutual watchfulness and support, with honesty about one's own emotions, will result in a strong team more likely to remain cohesive, and survive.

Accommodation

Typically about half of all injuries happen below decks. Think what below decks would be like should the boat turn on its side, or even upside down. Consider how you would escape if the boat remained upside down (a problem with yachts if they lose their keel), and how you would do this in the dark.

Formal standards for accommodation at sea only apply to commercial vessels. Other vessels come in all shapes and sizes, accommodation varies from air-conditioned state rooms with en-suite facilities on super yachts, to hot-bunking cots on racing boats.

Racing boats are stripped out, with no soft coatings on surfaces, which are unforgiving as a result. Crew sleep in sleeping bags on 'cots': fabric slung between two longitudinal poles with a 'lee cloth' to prevent unscheduled exits in rough weather. Commonly members of the off-watch climb into the bunk just vacated by the on-watch, a process known as 'hot-bunking'. Sleeping weight is kept on the windward side, or towards the stern when sailing downwind.

Cruising boats tend to be heavier, but better equipped than racing boats. They may have recognizable bunks, but still with lee cloths to prevent falls.

Dampness due to the saltwater environment and humidity is ever-present. Take any opportunity when it rains to wash clothing in fresh water coming off the boom, (let the rain wash the salt off the mainsail first). Damp bedding has reduced insulation and is less pleasant to sleep in, so take any opportunity to dry it out.

Heat, light, and fuel

Fuel is invariably diesel—used to run the main boat engine, power a generator for recharging the boat's batteries and possibly a desalinator for producing freshwater from seawater.

Heat can be supplied by solid fuel stoves, gas heaters, or diesel drip-feed heaters, either on a demand basis or as a 'central heating' system. Each type of system has advantages and disadvantages in terms of cost, responsiveness, ease of use, and service requirements.

Electricity is usually supplied from a 12V or 24V DC system battery bank, with inverters to create a 240V AC supply. The battery bank can be charged by a diesel generator, possibly supplemented by solar panels, wind turbine or water turbines. A boat without fuel or electricity will have no outside communication (apart from emergency systems), no meteorological information or external navigational aids, and perhaps only a limited supply of water. During pre-voyage planning it is essential to anticipate fuel usage and add a generous safety margin. Fuel consumption should be monitored regularly to ensure the lights and computers stay on.

Water supplies

Fresh water consumption on boats varies enormously, but generally ranges from 5 to 30 L/day per person on a well-run cruising yacht.

Fresh water tanks

Boats are usually equipped with several fresh water tanks, to ensure that the entire fresh water supply is not lost if one tank is breached or contaminated. These tanks are situated low in the boat to keep the centre of gravity low, and also distributed symmetrically to minimize effect on boat trim. When re-filling tanks from a shore supply, test for taste and clarity. Discovery of contaminated water in the tanks when at sea may terminate a voyage prematurely.

Desalinators

At sea a desalinator is commonly used to replenish supplies. Water is pumped under pressure through a fine filter, removing sodium chloride, other electrolytes, larger particles, and bacteria by a process known as 'reverse osmosis'. Desalinators may be powered by electricity, or can be manually powered—a process very tiring for the crew. Apart from collecting rain water, manual desalination the only available means of producing fresh water in a life raft.

Rainwater

Rainwater can provide sporadic supplies of fresh water, but collection systems must initially be thoroughly flushed to prevent salt contamination of existing supplies.

Nutrition

Energy expenditure varies enormously offshore but may reach 6000 calories/day, depending on weather conditions, ambient temperature, and body size. Plan accordingly for the number of crew and anticipated length of voyage, then add a generous safety margin.

- Think about where you may be able to re-provision—local ports and local foods.
- It is common sense not to run out of provisions but it does happen on racing boats when weight is pared to a bare minimum with little margin for error.
- Arranging provisions by day and week is a sensible way to make sure food is used at a sustainable rate.
- Airtight containers are mandatory for dry provisions.
- Tins, jars, and other pre-prepared meals are heavy so food in bags is more efficient in terms of weight and storage space. It's a good idea to remove paper labels from tins and jars, and write the contents on the tin with an indelible marker pen.
- Dried provisions are often used, including freeze-dried food. It is critically important that this is re-hydrated properly prior to eating, as partially hydrated food may cause catastrophic constipation.

- Frozen foods require a freezer and perishable foods require a fridge, both run by electricity or gas. Make a plan in case fridge or freezer fails, and don't depend on the foodstuffs kept in them.
- Fresh foods are a boon, but after a week at sea, there won't be much left. Plan a balanced diet once the fresh food has run out.
- Convenience foods and the occasional treat will keep the crew going during an extended period of rough weather, and may prevent discord.

Cleanliness

It is mandatory to keep the boat and crew clean at all times. This has to be built in to the ethos of the crew, and a rota for cleaning below decks helps. Personal cleanliness is personal, but excessive body odour affects others, and does nothing for team dynamics. Main routes of infection are faecal–oral, skin to skin, and skin to infected surfaces to skin. Skin infections such as impetigo can run through a crew in a very short period of time, as can gut infections.

Develop a culture in which hand washing is mandatory:

- After using the toilet.
- Before any form of food handling or preparation.
- Antiseptic wipes or alcohol gel dispensers are convenient and effective on any sort of boat.

Waste water

(See ♪ http://www.rya.org.uk for additional advice.)

Toilets

Toilets on boats may range from one that looks like the one in your home, to a bucket for chucking. In between, most boat toilets (or 'heads') have small-diameter outlet drain pipes and a hand-operated pump, using sea-water to flush the toilet. They block easily and are difficult to unblock, so it is forbidden to put sanitary products or other items down them. Toilet paper is usually acceptable. Provide a bin with plastic bag liner for waste that cannot be put down the toilet. This will need to be stored until disposed of ashore.

Sewage

- Empty holding tanks >3 miles offshore, in the open sea, where waste will be quickly diluted and dispersed by wave actions and currents. Preferably where sewage will take more than 24 h to reach land.
- In marinas, use shore facilities and brief your crew to do likewise. Use holding tanks or a portable toilet if you regularly sail in areas of poor flushing such as estuaries, inland waterways, and inlets, and when visiting crowded anchorages.
- Chemical toilets use toxic substances and must be emptied ashore into the regular sewage system. Plan ahead as they can be difficult to carry and few pump out (sanitation) facilities will accept chemical toilet waste.
- When visiting new sites, give consideration to the environmental sensitivity of the area before using your sea toilet.

Grey water

- Choose environmentally sensitive products—avoiding chlorine and bleach that can be toxic to flora and fauna, and phosphates that encourage algal growth.
- Keep oils and other food waste onboard and dispose of with non-recyclable rubbish.
- Minimize use of soaps and detergents in onboard sinks, showers, and washing machines. The sink on your boat needs to be treated differently to those in your home—it will block more easily.
- If using a washing machine on board, switch to a detergent-free washball, or use less ecologically damaging washing powders—a must in inland waterways.
- Consider re-plumbing your wastewater system so that all sewage, grey and black water, including that from dishwashers and washing machines, is diverted to a holding tank, especially if you keep your boat in enclosed waters such as inland waterways and marinas.

Preparations for voyage

Numerous tasks demand attention prior to departure, such as:
- Fitting out.
- Planning for safety.
- Victualling.
- Examining charts, pilot books, and weather information.

Thought must be given to the crew's health and welfare, an area at worst neglected, at best given low priority in the work schedule. Such time is well spent and may dictate the success or failure of the trip.

Crew selection

Sailing in remote areas is no longer the preserve of the young and fit.
- Crew should be generally physically fit prior to the expedition, with particular attention paid to cardiopulmonary fitness and lower limb strength, both of which will decline when confined on board a yacht for periods of weeks.
- There is greater risk taking crew who are dependent on oral medication for life-threatening conditions, such as organ transplant, epilepsy, or severe heart disease. Seasickness may prevent absorption of the medication. Conditions such as type 1 diabetes mellitus and severe asthma also carry greater risk offshore.
- More stringent exclusion criteria should be applied to expeditions beyond helicopter range, possibly excluding sailors with those conditions mentioned here.
- The Maritime and Coastguard Agency (MCA) guidelines[2] provide a structure for assessing potential crew with pre-existing medical conditions.

Medical screening

- Mostly, there is little choice in who makes up the crew, and often their medical problems will be well known. However, it is worth taking a step back and formally assessing the risk.
- Medical screening may take the form of a self-declaration questionnaire, with or without confirmation by the family doctor who is aware of the medical history, or it may be formal physical examination and testing.
- Such screening will appear onerous but will avoid potentially serious complications that may endanger the whole boat.
- All crew should have a dental check-up and appropriate treatment before departure.
- Crew should have current immunizations for tetanus, diphtheria, meningitis A and C, hepatitis A and B, and typhoid. Other immunizations (eg for yellow fever) and chemoprophylaxis (eg for malaria) may be required depending on the ports-of-call.

2 Maritime and Coastguard Agency (2010). *Seafarer Medical Examination System and Medical and Eyesight Standards: Application of the Merchant Shipping (Maritime Labour Convention) (Medical Certification) Regulations 2010.* Merchant Shipping Notice 1822(M). Southampton: MCA.

Crew medic

Crew will understandably expect that, should they be struck down, treatment on board will be the best available in the circumstances. Ideally, a suitable crew member, preferably with some form of medical or para-medical background such as paramedic, nurse, fire-fighter, or police officer, should be designated to provide medical care on-board. In the absence of someone with professional qualifications, the most important factors are motivation and knowledge. Whether or not medics have a qualification, appropriate training for working in remote and difficult conditions, together with early involvement gives ownership of the process and will improve outcome. Both the medic and the skipper should receive appropriate training. There should be clear mechanisms of support including medical manuals on board, and guidance on how to seek shore advice and help.

Medical support

In all medical emergencies, the universal advice is to seek medical advice early. This requires some form of communication system that works reliably in all locations, and the sources of advice must be known beforehand. Medical support may be arranged with a specific provider or, in an emergency, shore support is possible through the system of Maritime Rescue Coordination centres.

Ports of call

It is worthwhile investigating facilities at all ports of call, both scheduled and ones identified for use in an emergency. Local rescue facilities and hospital services may be limited, so prior knowledge may affect planning a suitable response in an emergency.

Restocking medical supplies may be a problem in areas where the local language is not English. However, most drugs are available in most places, although names and packaging will vary. Ensure the local port customs office knows you have a medical kit on board, so it is properly cleared in and out of port. This may save time and red faces if the kit comes to light as part of a search of the vessel.

Insurance

Medical insurance is advisable for all crew. It should provide cover for:
- Rescue from remote locations.
- Emergency treatment in local hospitals.
- Repatriation.
- Cost of medicines.

The medic and skipper may require additional insurance to cover them to treat fellow crew members in territorial waters or in ports-of-call. Insurance companies may require medical details of all crew. Adequate insurance is particularly important if a crew member might be landed in the USA and associated territories, as medical costs there can be extremely high.

Clothing

Clothing is the barrier between the crew and the elements. It has to be right for each crew, and no one solution is suitable for all. A triple layer system is most commonly used:

- *Base layer*—close fitting, usually made from merino wool, silk, or other synthetic material, but always a material with good wicking properties that can be worn for extended periods of weeks or more. Long arms and long legs are usual.
- *Mid-layer*—reasonably close fitting, made from a fleece-type material, its main function being thermal insulation. The mid-layer may range from a relatively thin, micro-fleece one-piece suit, to a waterproof, breathable jacket and salopettes combination. The shell layer may have a degree of water and wind resistance.
- *Outer-layer* is the main barrier against the elements, and typically comprises a jacket or smock top, with trousers that reach up to chest level. The jacket will usually have a high collar, incorporating a hood that can be zipped up to protect the majority of the face. The outer-layer invariably has reflective patches on the shoulders to aid locating crew in the event of a man-overboard at night. A safety harness may sometimes be built into the structure of the jacket.
- *Seaboots* must be properly fitted before departure. Loose boots are hazardous and may cause a trip and fall, whereas excessively tight boots may restrict blood supply to the feet, causing uncomfortably cold feet, and possibly other complications such as 'cockpit foot'—a non-freezing cold injury (see ⮕ Non-freezing cold injury, p. 632). Boots should allow adequate space for a pair of reasonably thick socks.
- *Gloves and hats*—essential in cold climes. Take spares. Sun hats are also essential in virtually all areas of the oceans.
- *Sunglasses*—although strictly not clothing, these are essential due to the increased glare from the water (similar to the effect on snow) and may cause photokeratitis after a relatively short period of exposure. Wrap-around glasses are the most effective type.

Offshore medical kits

(Also see Chapter 28.)

Contents and quantities

The contents and quantities of the medical kit are similar for any expedition to a remote location, and must take into account:

- Duration of expedition.
- Number of crew.
- Type of voyage—racing is inherently more dangerous than cruising.
- Proposed route and distance from definitive help.
- Medical expertise on-board.
- Medical history of the crew members.
- Opportunities for re-supply in ports of call: generally English-speaking countries are easier for replenishment—drug availability, dosages, and names vary widely in other countries.

The MCA have formulated a recommended kit list[3] for various classes of commercial vessel, with proposed quantities of medications.

Other kit lists have been proposed for non-commercial vessels, such as different types of yacht,[4] taking in to account the specific requirements of boats that are racing, or those venturing to isolated and stormy areas of the world's oceans, and for smaller yachts with less storage space.

Organization

Kits need to be clearly planned and organized:

- By body system in to separate transparent bags or boxes.
- Additional separate bags should contain:
  - Emergency/resuscitation drugs.
  - Hardware.
  - IV/IM drugs, needles, syringes.
  - IV fluid (if carried).
- Controlled drugs (e.g. morphine) must be kept secure and usage fully documented.
- First aid books, medical reference manuals, and the *British National Formulary* (or similar pharmacopoeia) should be included.
- Oxygen cylinders and concentrators, and marine defibrillators are also possible additions to the medical kit, but involve regular update training, servicing, and are only one link in a chain of survival.

---

3 Maritime and Coastguard Agency (2003). *Ships' Medical Stores*. Merchant Shipping Notice 1768 (M&F). Southampton: MCA.

4 Briggs S, Mackenzie C (2008). *Skipper's Medical Emergency Handbook*, pp. 205–7. London: Adlard Coles Nautical.

Grab bag

A specific medical kit to be taken to the life raft if abandoning ship that may also double as emergency treatment bag should contain:

- Emergency analgesics (oral and IM).
- Seasickness medications (a large stock and including drugs that can be absorbed by routes other than oral).
- Antibiotics.
- Rehydration salts.
- Suturing kit.
- Immobilization splints, strapping, bandages.

Always restock from the main kit if an item is used.

Offshore medical problems

Seasickness

- The three stages of mal de mer:
  - 'I feel sick.'
  - 'I think I'm going to die.'
  - 'I'm worried I'm not going to die.'
- A common and disabling condition; untreatable in <10%.
- Symptoms include nausea, sweating, vomiting, fatigue, loss of appetite, reduction in bowel action, dry mouth.
- Prevention is better than a cure; commencing medication 24 h before leaving port is likely to be most effective.
- Behavioural adaptations may lessen the effects of motion: staying on deck, focusing on the horizon, helming, avoiding chart work down below, avoiding unpleasant smells, eating small meals regularly.
- Drug therapy may be effective in >90% of sufferers; however, each individual varies in their response and it is worth finding the best drug or combination of drugs for each person.
- There is a wealth of evidence for and against most common remedies which include cinnarizine (Stugeron®), hyoscine hydrobromide (Scopoderm®), domperidone, prochlorperazine (Stemetil®), and ondansetron.
- Drug delivery may be cutaneous, buccal, oral, rectal, IM, or IV.
- Some remedies have side effects such as dry mouth, blurred vision, drowsiness, and urinary hesitancy.
- Dehydration and hypothermia may occur more readily in severe seasickness, requiring active treatment.
- Seasickness susceptibility in females is linked to the menstrual cycle. At these times, they may be more susceptible, and perhaps suffer more.
- Sickness usually improves after 48 h but may return if rough weather follows a period of relative calm.
- Remember that if a sufferer is dependent on oral medication (anti-epileptics, treatments for heart conditions, oral contraceptive pill, etc.) they may well not absorb the medication, and be at considerable risk of untoward medical deterioration. In these circumstances there should be increased emphasis on treating seasickness. Pre-planning is essential.
- Being sick over the side carries the real risk of following the vomit. Use a bucket.

Trauma

All types of sport and impact injuries may be encountered. Half of all injuries occur below decks.[5] The susceptibility to injury does not seem to be related to age of crew, but may be affected by work pattern on-board.

---

5 Price CJS, Spalding TJW, McKenzie C (2002). Patterns of illness and injury encountered in amateur ocean yacht racing: an analysis of the British Telecom Round the World Yacht Race 1996–1997. *Br J Sports Med*, 36, 457–62.

Injuries may be life-threatening and include:
- Head injuries (➔ Head injury, p. 312).
- Long bone fractures (➔ Fractures, p. 418).
- Blunt chest and abdominal trauma (see Chapter 7).
- Pelvic fractures (➔ Pelvic fractures, p. 436).
- Therapeutic manoeuvres that may be required include:
  - Chest drains.
  - Limb splints and cervical spine immobilizers.
  - Reduction of fractures and dislocations.
  - Simple local anaesthetic nerve blocks.
  - IV access and fluid resuscitation.
  - Nasogastric tubes and urinary catheters.
  - Skin suturing or stapling (Steri-Strips™ and tissue glue are of limited use in the marine environment).

Skin

Sun, salt water, heat, cold, damp, and friction have a deleterious effect on the skin. Common complaints include:
- Salt water boils (➔ Other infective skin lesions, p. 293).
- Gunwhale bum.
- Prickly heat.
- Cockpit foot (non-freezing cold injury; ➔ Non-freezing cold injury, p. 632).
- Rope burns.
- Sunburn.

Skin infections (such as impetigo and fungal infections of groin and foot) in the close yacht environment are also common. Personal hygiene is essential, and regular below-decks cleaning should occur. Skin and wound infections should be treated with antibiotics which include activity against the bacterium *Staphylococcus aureus*. Hypertrophy of the skin leads to the development of 'sausage fingers' and a dangerous reduction in dexterity. Barrier cream, moisturizers, and protective clothing such as gloves may reduce this process. Skin and lips must be protected against the sun.

Dehydration

A serious and potentially life-threatening condition, which can have many causes, including:
- Seasickness.
- Hot weather.
- Hard physical work in heavy clothing.
- Inadequately rehydrated freeze-dried food.
- Distraction from the process of regular rehydration.
- Unwillingness to undress to pass water regularly, so intentional limitation of fluid intake.

Rehydration may be undertaken orally (with Dioralyte®, for instance), rectally, or intravenously, which requires special medical training.

Proper personal hydration has to be part of the team ethos.

Immersion and drowning

(See also ➲ Immersion and drowning, p. 688.)

- Prevention is better than cure.
- The man-overboard drill should be clearly understood and practised by all on board, to facilitate rapid recovery.
- The routine use of harnesses, life jackets with spray hoods, immersion-activated lights, and personal EPIRBs (emergency radio beacons) should be part of the ethos of the boat.
- Concurrent injury is common in the process of being swept over the side.
- Immersion in cold water causes uncontrolled rapid breathing and tachycardia.
- Initial action in the water should be to stay still, trying to minimize seawater aspiration during initial gasps, then limit physical exertion, and heat loss by facing away from the weather. Adopt HELP position if practicable (Fig. 23.1 and Fig. 23.2). In calm waters these positions help to conserve heat, but they are less effective and safe in rough seas, where individuals could be thrown against each other, risking injury.
- Recovery should be in the horizontal position as far as possible to prevent circulatory collapse.
- Victims may require full resuscitation, rewarming, and supportive therapy for a prolonged period following recovery.

See ➲ Field management, p. 624 for more details.

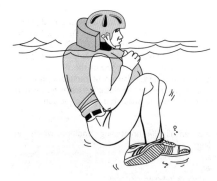

Fig. 23.1 HELP survival position. If alone in the water assume this position to minimize heat loss from head, neck, sides of body, and groin region.

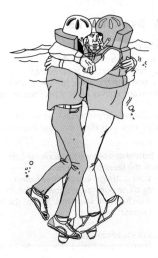

Fig. 23.2 HELP survival position. If two or more people are in water together, form a huddle so that sides of body are close together.

Emergency procedures

Helicopter evacuation

- A very costly resource to be used wisely. Not without risk to boat and helicopter crew. Training exercises are invaluable.
- Good communication with shore and helicopter crew is essential to ensure coordination and convey medical information regarding the victim.
- The normal range for helicopter rescue is within 200 nautical miles, occasionally using a fixed wing plane to locate the boat initially.

Method

- Brief your crew beforehand—it will be too noisy later.
- Communicate with the helicopter on VHF.
- The boat should steer a straight course close hauled on port, with the helicopter hovering off to port (avoids downdraft hitting yacht).
- Rescue will take place from the starboard door of the helicopter and the port side of the boat.
- Be prepared:
  - Clear the deck of loose objects.
  - Do as the helicopter crew tell you; they are the experts!
  - Use gloves.
  - The victim should be dressed and ready, with medical record attached.
  - All crew should be clipped to the boat.
- Initially, a weighted 'hi-line' is dropped from the helicopter. Do not touch until it has earthed in water or on the boat.
- Do not attach the line to the boat and avoid it getting snagged. For safety, coil it into a bucket.
- A diver descends on the main lifting wire; pull him in to the boat.
- Follow his directions.
- A single or double strop or stretcher may be used.
- In rough weather, recovery may be from a life raft trailed astern, or directly from the water.

Life raft evacuation

(Always ensure regular life raft servicing.)

- Only abandon a boat if it is sinking under your feet.
- Anticipate the possibility and be prepared. Each crewman should have a pre-assigned abandonment task.
- All crew get very seasick in a life raft; take medications beforehand.
- Take the grab bag (see ➲ Grab bag, p. 717).
- Other essential items (see ISAF recommended list[6]).
- Water (as much as possible) and portable water maker if carried.
- Weatherproof clothing and life jackets (put on before entering raft).

---

6 International Sailing Federation (2012). *Offshore Special Regulations Appendix A Part 1 and 2.*
🔖 http://www.sailing.org/tools/documents/OSR2012AppAP109122011-[11750].pdf
🔖 http://www.sailing.org/tools/documents/OSR2012AppAP209122011Book-[11751].pdf

- VHF radio.
- Satellite/mobile phones (the latter if inshore).
- Flares.
- EPIRB(s).
- Polythene or waterproof bags for vomit, faeces, urine.
- Toilet paper.
- Torches.
- Handheld GPS.
- Food.
- Crew get very sick, dehydrated, may be injured, and mentally traumatized by losing their boat.

Man overboard (MOB)

- A frightening experience for all on-board, particularly for the one in the water.
- Staying on board is obviously the best plan. Do this by adopting the following strategies:
  - Use safe techniques on deck and avoid overt risk-taking behaviour.
  - One hand for the boat and one for yourself.
  - Embed the use of harnesses, lifelines, jackstays, and life jackets in the ethos of the boat.
  - Consider all crew carrying personal EPIRB, mini-flares, waterproof torch, proximity- or water-activated alarm.
- Practise regularly, particularly recovery from the water. Decide the best route for recovery—over the sides, from the stern, etc. Plan practices thoroughly, so they don't themselves become an emergency.
- Specific actions in the event of MOB:
  - A loud shout to alert all on-deck.
  - One crew keeps pointing and tracking the crew in the water.
  - Press the MOB button on the boat GPS to record position of event.
  - Deploy all MOB equipment—Dan buoy, horseshoe buoy.
  - Adopt a sailing pattern to return to the crew in the water (e.g. crash stop, reach-turn-reach).
  - If using the engine, approach alongside the crew in the water in neutral or engine stopped.
  - Recover in the horizontal position if the crew has been in the water for an extended period. If this isn't possible, do not delay recovery, but place in horizontal position when on deck, and reassess.
  - It may be necessary, in the event the crew in the water is unconscious, to put a suitably clothed crew in to the water on a line, to assist with recovery.
  - Remember—the crew may have sustained injury before, or on the way over the side, so once recovered from the water, perform a full assessment using the ABCDE approach (see Chapter 7).
  - If the MOB is not recovered immediately, consider making a MAYDAY call for assistance.

Resources

Adventure Medical Kits: ℛ http://adventuremedicalkits.com

Cruising Association: M http://www.cruising.org.uk

Medical Support Offshore: ℛ http://msos.org.uk

Royal Ocean Racing Club (RORC): ℛ http://www.rorc.org

The Maritime and Coastguard Agency (2014). *Ships Captain's Medical Guide.* 22nd edn, HMSO. ℛ https://www.gov.uk/government/publications/the-ship-captains-medical-guide

The Maritime and Coastguard Agency: ℛ http://www.mcga.gov.uk

The Royal Yachting Association: ℛ http://www.rya.org.uk

Maritime medical training courses
Medical Care at Sea: The Maritime and Coastguard Agency.

Elementary First Aid: The Maritime and Coastguard Agency.

Medical First Aid at Sea: The Maritime and Coastguard Agency.

Sea Survival Course, Elementary First Aid: The Royal Yachting Association.

Further reading

Briggs S, Mackenzie C (2008). *Skipper's Medical Emergency Handbook.* London: Adlard Coles Nautical.
Cold Water Casualty Video (1990). British Defence Library A3788. Institute of Naval Medicine.
Golden F, Tipton M (2002). *Essentials of Sea Survival.* Leeds: Human Kinetics.
Howarth F, Howarth M (2002). *The Grab Bag—Your Ultimate Guide to Liferaft Survival.* London: Adlard Coles Nautical.
(1997). World Health Organization.
Weiss EA, Jacobs M. *A Comprehensive Guide to Marine Medicine.* Adventure Medical Kits, Oakland, USA.
World Health Organization (1997). *International Medical Guide for Ships,* 2nd edn. Geneva:

Chapter 24

Underwater

Section editor
Chris Johnson

Contributors
Robert Conway
Lesley F. Thomson
Andy Pitkin (1st edition)

Reviewer
Rose Drew

The underwater environment 726
Preparations before travel 730
Diving medicine 732
Effects of high-pressure gases 734
Decompression sickness 736
Barotrauma 740
Other problems 742

The underwater environment

'Il faut aller voir.'

(Jacques Cousteau)

Increased ease of travel and the rise in adventure tourism has enabled many more people to explore the underwater world. A variety of specialist breathing equipment has been developed to extend the duration and range of underwater exploration. However, prolonged immersion under pressure can lead to a variety of medical problems.

Medical personnel on diving expeditions should not only understand the medical problems associated with underwater work but also broader medical conditions common to all expeditions. Appropriate medical equipment and casualty evacuation plans should be in place prior to the start of the expedition. Underwater activities on expeditions include:

• Marine biology and conservation work.
• Underwater archaeology including wreck diving.
• Cave diving.
• Marine salvage.
• Fishing—shellfish collection or spear gun.

Commercial activities within the oil or mining industries, governed by stringent commercial diving regulations and medical examinations, are not covered in this chapter.

Contrary to popular belief, shark attacks and the bends are rare on diving expeditions. Common medical problems include:

• GI upsets.
• Minor trauma.
• Ear problems secondary to repetitive diving.
• Soft tissue injuries.
• Secondary infections.

Decompression illness (encompassing decompression sickness and barotrauma) is rare, but may be life threatening and require immediate intervention in a specialist centre for recompression and hyperbaric oxygen treatment.

Physical characteristics of the underwater environment

Environmental conditions expose divers to risks of seasickness, hypothermia, drowning, and marine envenomation. Waves and swell may lead to trauma during water entry or exit from boat or shore; strong currents, tides or poor visibility may cause a diver to become separated and lost. Intensely hot or cold climates expose equipment and divers to physical and physiological stresses.

Weather

Climatic conditions at depth may be both different and more constant than those on the surface, but atmospheric conditions govern the ease with which the transition between land and water is made. Both currents and squalls may make it difficult to return to boat or beach.

Travel

Diving equipment is bulky and transport may be logistically difficult. Several airlines allow extra weight for this equipment if booked in advance (either free or at a discounted rate). Cabin pressures in commercial airliners are equivalent to a journey to altitude (about 2500 m/8000 ft) and may precipitate decompression sickness. There are recommendations for the limits to diving for a time period before flying, and these should be strictly imposed for safety. Divers should not fly within 12 h of a single, non-decompression dive or within 24 h after repetitive, multiple day, or decompression diving.

Types of underwater activity

The simplest methods to explore underwater include snorkelling or breath-hold diving (free-diving). Most expeditions use scuba (self-contained underwater breathing apparatus), using cylinders filled with compressed air. Nitrox (higher oxygen concentration than air) can be used to reduce the risks of decompression sickness or to increase the duration of safe diving. Technical divers often use rebreathing apparatus and gas mixtures of oxygen, nitrogen, and helium to prolong the length and durations of a dive.

Snorkelling and breath-hold ('free') diving

A snorkel enables a diver to breathe at the surface whilst still visualizing objects beneath. Many swimmers use snorkels for short breath-hold dives without training in free-diving.

Free-diving is both a recreational activity and a competitive sport where breath is held throughout a period underwater. The term may include activities such as underwater hockey or synchronized swimming, but at the more extreme end, competitive free-diving involves apnoea during swims for maximum distance or depth, or static breath-hold duration. Athletes train to endure high carbon dioxide (CO_2) levels, low oxygen (O_2) levels, and lactic acidosis. Movement in swimming is relaxed and energy efficient. Competitors winning depth records often have unique morphology and an unusual amount of blood fills the space left in the chest by compressed lung tissue as depth increases. Specific risks include aspiration, drowning, otitis externa, ear barotrauma during descent or ascent, lung squeeze causing pulmonary haemorrhage and haemoptysis, and shallow or deep water blackout.

Self-contained underwater breathing apparatus

Scuba divers breathe compressed air or nitrox from cylinders. Dive depth and duration is calculated from decompression tables or dive computers. These utilize mathematical algorithms to guide dive time according to the maximum depth reached during the dive. The dive should be planned with maximum depth established prior to diving, and calculations to ensure the cylinders contain sufficient gas for the whole dive including any safety or decompression stops. Divers usually dive in buddy pairs for safety and enjoyment. This chapter mainly concentrates on the medical problems associated with scuba diving.

Technical (saturation) diving

A breathing mixture of oxygen, nitrogen, and helium can be used with specific equipment to expand the depth and duration of diving (e.g. cave or wreck penetration). The use of gas mixtures is uncommon on remote expeditions due to expense, logistics, and the difficulties of equipment maintenance. Dives are usually significantly longer and deeper than recreational scuba diving, with lengthy decompression schedules of several hours, restricting when the diver can surface. Technical diving requires advanced training and use of either open (produces bubbles like scuba) or closed rebreathing circuits.[1] Treatment of decompression sickness is the same for scuba, however if injury occurs during the dive it may prove fatal, with mortality quoted up to 1:100 divers.[2]

Risk assessment for diving expeditions

General risk assessments should be made as for all expeditions (see ⊃ Risk management, p. 68). Diving practice and safety can often be improved by running introductory talks on diving-related illness and treatment including first aid, not least because the non-diving expedition members will form the main team helping to treat a sick diver.

Be careful storing oxygen cylinders; keep them cool and away from sources of fire. Check where they can be refilled locally and if the expedition is due to run for longer periods, where they can be serviced. Keep the generator for refilling air cylinders away from vehicle fumes or personnel smoking; this can cause carbon monoxide (CO) to enter the breathing gas, which is dangerous at pressure.

Be aware of specific points of danger—the entry and exit from water to shore or boat; managing boat handling during pick-up. Have and practise a search protocol to use if a diver is lost underwater or on the surface. Surface marker buoys help to locate divers on surfacing, and there are several electronic diver-locating systems on the market (e.g. ENOS, Sea Marshall).

Search and rescue

Dive profiles should be planned using tables or dive computer algorithms. Divers should have adequate equipment to signal boats if surfacing out of eyesight or in rough sea conditions. These include whistles, surface marker buoys, and torches or strobes at night. If a boat crew loses a dive team then they should begin the search at the point of last contact, taking into account prevailing currents. Searching should take the form of a systematic approach using linear, sweeping or circular search patterns. If after initial searching dive teams are still missing, emergency services should be contacted, if available, in order to broaden search patterns.

---

1 Mitchell SJ, Doolette DJ (2013). Recreational technical diving part 1: an introduction to diving and technical diving methods and activities. *Diving Hyperb Med*, 43(2), 86–93.

2 Fock AW (2013). Analysis of recreational closed-circuit rebreather deaths 1998–2010. *Diving Hyperb Med*, 43(2), 78–85.

Environmental impact

Look but do not touch. Training, good buoyancy control, and diving within one's limits are key to protecting the marine environment. Never remove or disturb the underwater environment. In particular be aware of damaging fragile coral structures with fins and only collect marine animals if warranted and correct permissions have been sought prior to diving. Respect wreck diving policies on war graves and do not disturb remains.

Preparations before travel

Clothing

Be familiar with diving equipment. Buoyancy is greater in new wet or dry suits leading to unexpected rapid ascent. Over-weighted divers may sink. Longer and repetitive exposure may lead to the necessity for a thicker wetsuit in any given water temperature so consider extra thickness. Seek expert advice if unsure.

Specific equipment

Many diving accidents involve the use of new, unfamiliar, or faulty equipment. Induced panic is common. Appropriate experience is more important than paper qualifications. Train and practise in a safe environment. Medics should work closely with expedition leaders to ensure divers are familiar with their equipment and safety procedures, and that initial 'check' dives are in shallow water with good visibility.

Pre-departure medical preparations

A medic with scuba diving qualifications is often better placed to understand and influence the diving practice on an expedition and its implications on potential illness or injury. Familiarization with practical issues, equipment, safe use of decompression tables, and dive computers is vital. Diving medicine courses are widely available and a diving expedition doctor should possess appropriate knowledge.

Medical kits

Diving expeditions should consider including the following additional items to their general medical kit (see Chapter 28 and ➲ Diving expeditions, p. 808):

- O_2 supplies with an appropriate delivery system. The filling system in the host country will need to be compatible with the equipment taken, and appropriate volumes for evacuation must be calculated. Rebreathing systems are available; by using lower gas flows these provide longer duration of supply.
- IV fluids and cannulas.
- Seasickness prophylaxis.
- Urinary catheter for neurological bends.
- Antibiotic ± steroid eardrops.
- Liquid decongestant.
- Alcohol ear drops.
- Auroscope and tendon hammer.
- Chest drain/underwater sealed drain or Heimlich valve.

Fitness to dive

Fitness to dive requirements vary between international training organizations. Ultimately, some general standards apply, modified according to the remoteness of the expedition and physical diving activity. Decisions regarding fitness to dive should be made prior to the expedition departure; if necessary seek advice from experienced diving physicians. The basic principle is that any condition that may unexpectedly impair a diver's ability to exert themselves physically or that may cause a sudden alteration in conscious level will usually mean that the candidate is unfit to dive. (See Table 24.1.)

Table 24.1 Potential medical conditions

System	Condition	Acceptability for diving
Cardiac	Hypertension	Normally compatible
	Dysrhythmias	Normally absolute contraindication
	Ischaemia	Strict criteria must be met to dive
	Septal defect/patent foramen ovale	Shunt dependent, closure currently often advised. Obtain cardiology input
Respiratory	Obstructive airway disease	COPD/emphysema, asthma. Asthma is absolute contraindication in Australasia but relative in Europe/USA
	Acute upper respiratory tract infection	No diving until fully resolved
Neurological	Epilepsy	Contraindicated unless convulsion-free and off medication for 5 years
	Severe head injury	May return to diving after review by diving physician
Metabolic	Type 1 diabetes	Allowed if no hypoglycaemic unawareness or end-organ damage and review by diving physician
ENT	Tympanic membrane barotrauma	Perforation 4 weeks, otherwise 24–48 h
	Sinusitis	Acutely is a contraindication; avoid decongestants
Psychiatric	Depression/anxiety	Requiring medication requires discussion with diving physician
Other	Lack of physical fitness	BMI >35 kg/m²
	Decompression illness	Review by diving physician
	Poor dental work	May result in dental pain, review dental work pre-departure (Chapter 11)
	Pregnancy	No research on effects on fetus, therefore diving should be avoided

Diving medicine

See Table 24.2 for medical concerns.

Table 24.2 Medical concerns on diving expeditions

Environment	Trauma	Heat illness/hypothermia
	Sunburn	Marine envenomation
	Dehydration	Near drowning
	Motion sickness	Waterborne disease
Diving	Barotrauma	Decompression sickness
Breathing gas	Nitrogen narcosis	CO poisoning
	Hypercapnia	Oxygen toxicity (e.g. nitrox)
Other	Local diseases, e.g. tropical	Otitis externa
	GI upset	Psychological problems/panic

Safe practice when diving

Dive conservatively and well within limits, guided by tables or computer algorithms. Minimize the number of dives each day (preferable a maximum of two or three depending on depth) with rest days (no diving) every 3–4 days. Safety stops at 3–6 m for 3–5 min significantly reduce intravascular bubbles. Beware of psychological pressure to push diving limits if project is behind schedule.

Casualty evacuation (medevac) plan

Introduce yourself to the local recompression chamber at the start of the expedition. This can help to establish the facilities available and make the chamber facility aware of the diving expedition. Local staff will have knowledge of diving conditions or venomous marine life. It may be useful to visit the local hospital(s) to ascertain appropriateness of other medical facilities.

A medevac plan should include:-

- Recompression chamber—emergency phone number, staff contact numbers.
- Transport—type (e.g. boat, road vehicle, aircraft); how many patients fit into vehicle (buddy may also need treatment).
- Distance/time to and from recompression facility.
- Aeronautical transfer (pressurized or fly close to sea level).
- Calculation of O_2 requirement for two people (plus contingency). Is O_2 supplied on transport?
- Are medical personnel available with the transport. Should the expedition medic go with them (and if so, how will they return)?

Always remember to take passport, insurance details, patient family contact details, credit card and mobile phone.

Medevac letter

A medical letter accompanying an affected diver should include:

- Diver—name, date of birth.
- Maximum depth, duration, and any decompression stops of dive. Include the diver's computer if possible.
- Details of precipitating factor, e.g. rapid ascent.
- Time of surfacing.
- Time of onset of symptoms.
- Description of symptoms.
- Symptom progression (improving/worsening).
- Treatment given—any improvement?
- Previous dives (maximum depth, duration, surface intervals) including preceding days.
- Past medical history, including previous decompression sickness.
- Prescription medicines/use of recreational drugs or alcohol.
- Any allergies.

Diving physics

Most diving expeditions will use scuba with cylinders containing breathing gas, typically compressed air at 200 bar (atmospheres). A regulator valve reduces this high pressure so the diver breathes at a pressure equal to that of the surrounding water. For every 10 m/33 ft depth, water pressure increases by 1 atmosphere. The density of breathed air increases with depth; at 10 m it is twice the density of surface air, so more nitrogen molecules are inhaled and absorbed with each breath. The nitrogen dissolves in blood and tissues and can result in decompression sickness during or after ascent.

Air may be enriched with oxygen to make 'nitrox'. Reducing the inhaled nitrogen concentration enables longer dive durations and reduces the risk of decompression sickness. However, it increases the risk of acute oxygen toxicity and the permitted maximum diving depth must take this into account. (See Table 24.3.)

Table 24.3 Diving physics

Depth (metres)	Relative volume of balloon	Density	Partial pressure of oxygen (PO_2)	Partial pressure of nitrogen (PN_2)
Surface	1	× 1	0.21	0.79
10	½	× 2	0.42	1.58
20	⅓	× 3	0.63	2.37
30	¼	× 4	0.84	3.16
40	⅕	× 5	1.05	3.95

The risk of DCS and circulatory microbubbles following a single dive has been well researched; tables and computer algorithms give consistent analysis of the risks. However, multiple dives, particularly on consecutive days may lead to accumulation of nitrogen in the tissues and very few repetitive dive profiles have been fully researched. Any mathematical error in the tables or physiological variation between divers could increase the risk of decompression sickness.

Effects of high-pressure gases

Nitrogen narcosis

High partial pressures of nitrogen cause anaesthetic-like effects. Jacques Cousteau lost friends to this condition and described it as 'rapture of the deep'. Euphoric effects develop between 10 m and 30 m, below 50 m the effects can be life-threatening. Individual susceptibility varies; divers are usually unaware of being affected and, without appropriate training, oblivious to its danger. They may react inappropriately and put themselves at risk.

Typical symptoms (with increasing depth):
- Tunnel vision, euphoria, apprehension.
- Inability to manage complex tasks.
- Tinnitus.
- Drowsiness.
- Loss of consciousness.

The condition may be exacerbated by hypercapnia, exertion, cold water, and darkness. Symptoms resolve rapidly on ascent. Buddy divers need to take charge of an affected diver.

Hypercapnia (carbon dioxide retention)

The increased density of gas at depth affects resistance to breathing, and so with increased depth the compressed air 'feels thicker'. Alongside this a normal regulator has some in-built resistance to breathing. Exertion, such as swimming against a current, will magnify these effects leading to build up of CO_2 and 'air hunger'.

Risk factors include:
- Resistance to breathing in regulator.
- Excessive exertion, over-weighted diver.
- High gas density (excessive depth for gas mixture used).
- Exhaustion of CO_2 scrubber in divers using re-breathing system.
- Poor dive practice, e.g. some divers may exhibit 'skip-breathing', deliberately hypo-ventilating in order to conserve air!

Symptoms include:
- Headache.
- Strong feelings of panic.
- Flushing.
- Palpitations.
- Breathlessness.
- Eventual loss of consciousness.

Once recognized, try to rest and reassure the affected diver. Ascend at normal rate to minimize risk of barotrauma or decompression sickness. Assistance may be required if diver is over-weighted or panicking.

Carbon monoxide poisoning

CO is colourless, odourless, and hazardous as it binds to haemoglobin to prevent O_2 transport in the bloodstream. Scuba cylinder supplies may be contaminated if the breathing gas compressor intake is sited downwind of a source of combustion. Even a small amount of CO may cause symptoms as the partial pressure of CO will increase with depth, increasing the likelihood/severity of symptoms, which include:

- Headache.
- General malaise.
- Nausea.
- Poor coordination.
- Weakness.
- Unconsciousness leading to death.

Management
- 100% O_2 reduces the half-life ($t_{1/2}$) of CO from around 4 h to 1 h.
- In severe cases hyperbaric O_2 therapy (at 3 atm—if available) can reduce the $t_{1/2}$ to <30 min.
- Check compressor, servicing schedules, tanks, semi-closed circuits.

Acute (CNS) oxygen toxicity

Oxygen breathed at partial pressures greater than PO_2 >1.6 bar (160 kPa) can be harmful. The risk of toxicity increases with PO_2, duration of exposure, degree of exertion, and associated hypercapnia.

Symptoms include:
- Facial (especially lip), diaphragmatic, and other muscle twitching.
- Visual disturbances (e.g. central and peripheral visual field defects).
- Nausea, vertigo, tinnitus.
- Dysphoria ('sensation of impending doom').
- Convulsions (may be the first manifestation).

Management
Reduce PO_2 immediately (e.g. ascend, switch gas mix).
  Convulsions occurring under water are potentially fatal:
- Maintain diver's depth during initial tonic phase of the seizure, to prevent barotraumas caused by uncontrolled ascent.
- Attempt to keep mouthpiece in casualty's mouth if possible.
- Recover to the surface and treat any secondary illness, e.g. barotrauma.

The seizure will resolve immediately once PO_2 is reduced and will not require further treatment or restriction of diving. O_2 toxicity is a risk in recompression chambers when breathing 100% O_2, although higher PO_2 are tolerated, thought to be due to inactivity.

Decompression sickness

Decompression sickness (DCS), or 'the bends', is caused by gas that has dissolved within body tissues under pressure during a dive, re-emerging as bubbles when pressure reduces during or after ascent. The bubbles (usually nitrogen) may be intravascular, extravascular, or both, depending on gas load, and cause clinical syndromes depending on their location. Small bubbles merge into larger ones leading to bubble growth. Intravascular bubbles cause emboli leading to hypoxic damage. Secondary clotting and inflammatory cascades are activated at bubble/blood interfaces. Rapid recompression and O_2 administration compress gases back into solution, provide a concentration gradient for nitrogen elimination and supply O_2 to hypoxic tissues. (See Table 24.4.)

Table 24.4 Symptoms of decompression sickness

System	Symptoms
Musculoskeletal	Limb pain
Neurological	Paraesthesia (often with limb pain)
	Epigastric/girdle/back pain
	Limb weakness (most commonly legs)
	Loss of balance/coordination
	General malaise or fatigue
	Cognitive dysfunction
	Urinary retention
	Visual disturbance (often 'wavy lines')
Temporary	Petechial rash (may indicate high inert gas load)
	Marbled rash (rare)
	Lymphatic obstruction (rare)
Cardiorespiratory	Cough, frothy bloodstained sputum—'the chokes'
	Dyspnoea
	Chest pain
	Collapse

Onset of symptoms varies from several minutes to hours after a dive. DCS may be precipitated by ascent to altitude even days after diving or occur following a single dive within decompression limits.

There is an increased risk of DCS following:
• Rapid ascent.
• Missed decompression stops.
• Repetitive diving over several days.
• Physical exercise soon after diving.
• Ascent to altitude (flights, mountain passes).
• Coincidental illness (particularly if dehydrated: fever or hungover).
• Obesity.

Field treatment

DCS is often hard to recognize. Concealment and denial are common amongst divers because of the perceived stigma attached to decompression illness, as well as possible cognitive dysfunction and lethargy in the patient. Encouragement and awareness should be addressed prior to expedition departure.

Initial management

- Resuscitation: ABC.
- Administer 100% O_2 via rebreather mask or demand regulator.
- Lie flat if there is any concern for cerebral gas embolism.
- Give fluids: oral if the diver is alert, otherwise IV.
- Early neurological examination, repeated regularly.
- Seek expert advice (via available communications system).
- Do not forget the buddy.
- Consider early evacuation to recompression facility.

NB Symptoms may resolve during treatment with O_2, but (especially with neurological presentations) relapse is common without hyperbaric therapy. Do not stop transfer to medical facility even if symptoms appear resolved.

Evacuation

- Recompression becomes less effective as each hour passes. Most benefit is obtained within 6 h of onset, but some cases respond even after several days.
- First aid (O_2, fluids) should continue during transport.
- Keep dive computers/record of previous dives with the casualty.
- Unpressurized aircraft should be flown at the lowest safe altitude.
- Recompression treatment (and evacuation) is very expensive and divers should be appropriately insured.

Recompression treatment

Recompression protocols typically start with compression to 2.8 atm (18 m/60 ft) on 100% O_2, with subsequent treatment based on clinical response. Most cases are treatable using US Navy Table 6 (RN Table 62)[3] with extensions if necessary. In remote areas, hyperbaric facilities may be limited and unable to sustain a treatment longer than this, even if it is required. Further hyperbaric O_2 sessions may then be given to improve any residual manifestations.

In-water recompression

A controversial technique. It has been used when a casualty is in an extremely remote location with no means of evacuation to dedicated facility or awaiting retrieval. If conscious level is reduced use a full face mask and have an attendant in the water. Hypothermia, seizures, and aspiration are potential risks. No high-level evidence currently supports its use.[4]

---

3 ⟳ http://www.londondivingchamber.co.uk/index.php?id=theory&page=2

4 Lipmann J, Mitchell S (2005). *Deeper into Diving*, 2nd ed. Victoria: JL Publications.

Patent foramen ovale

A patent foramen ovale (PFO) is an opening in the heart between the left and right atria, which normally closes after birth. PFOs that are around 0.5–1 cm in size can cause bubbles to pass directly from venous to arterial circulation, bypassing the usual filtering of bubbles by the lungs, leading to emboli which cause damage to tissues.

Rapid onset of neurological, cardiovascular, and skin DCS (occurring within 30 min of surfacing) has been linked with the presence of a large PFO. The risk of DCS increases with the size of the shunt, and divers are often advised to be screened for a PFO using bubble contrast echocardiography after developing DCS. Current guidance suggests PFO closure using a transcatheter technique.

Barotrauma

Barotrauma is tissue damage due to a change in pressure altering the volume within gas-filled spaces such as sinuses, middle ear, facemask, teeth, gut, and lungs. Pressure must be equalized to avoid 'squeeze' during descent or 'overpressure' during ascent from a dive. The volume of an enclosed gas-filled space varies inversely with pressure (Boyle's law). Gas volume changes are greatest closest to the surface and most problems occur within 10 m (33 ft) of the surface.

Middle ear (tympanic membrane) barotrauma

- Common.
- Pressure/pain on ascent or descent.
- 'Muffled' hearing post-dive owing to middle ear effusion.
- Caloric vertigo under water with sudden relief of pain suggests perforation.
- Tympanic membrane may appear inflamed and retracted.
- Return to diving: 24–48 h if no perforation has occurred. If perforation is present, diving should be avoided for at least 28 days and full otolaryngological review should be sought.

Inner ear barotrauma

- Rare.
- Rupture of the round window caused by pressure differential between inner and middle ear, usually because of excessive Valsalva manoeuvres.
- Severe persistent vertigo, distinguishable from transient vertigo on ascent and caloric vertigo from tympanic membrane perforation. Associated with a sensorineural hearing loss.
- Difficult to differentiate from decompression illness affecting the inner ear which may also cause severe vertigo; diagnosis may rest on the response to hyperbaric O_2 therapy.

Pulmonary barotrauma

Rapid expansion of alveolar gas during a fast ascent must be vented through the transmitting airways. If this cannot occur, due to the diver forgetting to exhale, a closed glottis, or obstruction, it may rupture into surrounding structures or pulmonary blood vessels. *Always* consider life-threatening cerebral arterial gas embolism (see ➲ Cerebral arterial gas embolism, p. 741) following rapid ascent. Air expansion may cause the following:

Pneumothorax
- Air escapes into the pleural cavity.
- Symptoms include chest pain, breathlessness, and cardiovascular collapse.
- ABC approach, standard needle decompression using large-bore cannula plus chest drain.

Pneumomediastinum
- Air enters the mediastinum.
- Symptoms include central chest pain, voice change, neck swelling, subcutaneous emphysema, and cardiovascular collapse.
- ABC, O_2 (may be required for several hours) and evacuation to a specialist centre.

Cerebral arterial gas embolism
- Air enters pulmonary capillaries.
- Difficult to distinguish from DCS, but rapid time of onset (often within minutes of surfacing) may influence your likely diagnosis.
- Symptoms include loss of consciousness, convulsions, and/or neurological deficits such as hemiparesis, weakness, or dysphasia.
- Treat as for DCS. ABC, 100% O_2, and hyperbaric recompression.
- Examine for other signs of barotrauma.

Other problems

Otitis externa

A common problem associated with repetitive diving. Exposure to water and subsequent shifts in pH cause bacterial growth in the external ear canal leading to skin inflammation. Symptoms include:

- Painful ears.
- Inability to equalize.
- Hearing loss if severe.

Treatment

- Meticulous attention to hygiene, ensure ears are dried thoroughly after immersion.
- Some divers recommend alcohol drops to dry out outer ear after diving.
- Steroid plus antibiotic eardrops may help in severe cases.
- Breaks in diving schedule may be required.
- Condition increases incidence of tympanic membrane perforation.

Hypoxia

Altered consciousness as a result of reduced inspired O_2 concentrations is rare, but should be excluded as a cause if a diver using a semi- or closed-circuit rebreathing apparatus develops an impaired cognitive state during a dive.

Other conditions

- Trauma—see Chapter 7.
- Sunburn—see ➔ Solar skin damage, p. 266.
- Dehydration—see ➔ Fluids and electrolytes, p. 760.
- Motion sickness—see ➔ Seasickness, p. 718.
- Heat-related illness—see ➔ Heat-related illnesses (HRIs), p. 748.
- Hypothermia—see ➔ Hypothermia, p. 622.
- Marine envenomation including coral cuts—see ➔ Venomous marine animals, p. 566.
- Water aspiration and drowning—see ➔ Immersion and drowning, p. 688.
- Water-borne disease—see ➔ Water-borne infections, p. 687.

Expert advice

Relevant bodies include:

- UK water: at sea call the Marine Coastguard Agency on VHF Channel 16, DSC Channel 70, or call 999 and ask for the Coastguard.
- British Hyperbaric Associations National Diving Helpline (England and Northern Ireland): +44 7831 151523.
- Scotland: +44 845 408 6008 (Aberdeen).
- Europe: +39 6 4211 8685 (Divers Alert Network).
- Africa: +27 828 106010 or 0800-020111 in South Africa (Divers Alert Network).
- Asia: +10 4500 9113 (Korea) +81 3 3812 4999 (Japan)
- Australasia and the Pacific: +61 8 8212 9242 (Australia) or +64 9 445 8454 (New Zealand).
- In the USA/Caribbean: +1 919 684 8111 (Divers Alert Network).

Resources

Divers Alert Network: ◈ http://www.diversalertnetwork.org

London Diving Chamber. *Royal Navy Treatment Table 62*: ◈ http://www.londondivingchamber.co.uk/index.php?id=theory&page=2

The Rubicon Foundation: ◈ http://www.rubicon-foundation.org

UK Sports Diving Committee: ◈ http://uksdmc.co.uk

Further reading

British Thoracic Society Fitness to Dive Group, Subgroup of the British Thoracic Society Standards of Care Committee (2003). British Thoracic Society guidelines on respiratory aspects of fitness for diving. *Thorax*, 58, 3–13.

Edmonds C, Lowry C, Pennefather I, Walker R (2005). *Diving and Subaquatic Medicine*, 4th ed. London: Hodder Arnold.

Brubakk AO (2000).On-site recompression treatment is acceptable for DCI. *Journal of the South Pacific Underwater Medicine Society* 30, pp.166–73.

Chapter 25

Hot, dry environments: deserts

Section editor
Chris Johnson

Contributors
Jon Dallimore
Sundeep Dhillon
Shane Winser

Reviewer
Harvey Pynn

The environment 746
Heat-related illnesses (HRIs) 748
Pathophysiology of HRIs 750
Acclimatization to heat 754
Prevention of HRIs 756
Fluids and electrolytes 760
Treatment of HRIs 764
Other heat-related problems 766

The environment

Two of the most popular expedition destinations, deserts and tropical forests, seem very different. Deserts appear barren, arid, and have a very limited range of highly adapted plants and animals, while in contrast the hot and humid tropical forests (Chapter 26) offer the world's richest land ecosystem.

Both environments require humans to live and work in high temperatures, but the high humidity in forests places additional stresses on body physiology. Those living in temperate climates such as Northern Europe rarely experience heat waves, and may be physically and mentally unprepared for heat stress. Heat-related illness is a cause of death amongst travellers including previously fit young adults. Endurance athletes and the military are especially at risk as they deliberately push their bodies even when conditions are hazardous. An occasional short spell of heat in an otherwise temperate zone is especially hazardous to endurance competitors as they will have little physiological acclimatization to the conditions.

Deserts

A desert is a region with little vegetation and much exposed bare soil, where average annual rainfall is <20% of the amount needed to support optimum plant growth, and where plants and animals show clear adaptations for survival during long droughts. Covering almost 20% of the Earth's landmass, deserts are mainly found between 25° and 35° north and south of the equator, and are home to around 1 billion people.

Some deserts consist of the sand dunes of popular imagination, but others are rocky wastelands or semi-arid grasslands. Diurnal and seasonal temperature ranges can be considerable, with the landscape sculpted by freeze/thaw cycles and by powerful winds driving sand, soil or snow.[1]

Clothing and footwear

Wear light, loose-fitting clothes made of natural materials that allow air to circulate and sweat to evaporate. Protect the head with a hat, scarf, or keffiyeh (shemagh). Shorts and T-shirts are also convenient and usually perfectly adequate, but be conscious that such dress—particularly if worn by women—may cause offence in some countries. Where possible check the ultraviolet protection factor (UVF) offered by clothing—some materials are more effective at preventing sunburn than others. Exposed skin must be properly protected by sunblock while both sunglasses and goggles are essential.

Footwear needs to be light, comfortable, and tough; boots, shoes, and trainers all have disadvantages. Enclosed feet become sweaty, smelly, soft, and prone to fungal infections. On the other hand, bare feet or light shoes expose the feet to heat from the ground, injury by rock or thorns, and bites from snakes or scorpions. In sand and gravel deserts, walking sandals, trainers, or desert boots suffice; heavier footwear is required in stony and volcanic areas.

1 ℘ http://www.unep.org/geo/gdoutlook/016.asp

Bases and campsites

It is possible to travel for months in deserts without the need for formal shelter. A camp bed off the ground is protection against snakes and scorpions (but remember to shake your shoes out in the morning). A tent or impregnated mosquito net will protect against insects. Guard the area against human or large animal invasion. Beware of making camps in dry riverbeds or wadis, which can be susceptible to flash flooding from rainfall miles away.

Travel

Most desert expeditions use vehicles. These must be well maintained and have adequate tyres, tool kits, and spares to cope with the stresses of travel. Fuel consumption will be high. Ensure the party knows how to extricate a bogged vehicle, and do not lose the vehicle keys.

Travellers relying on more traditional travel methods require suitable skills in animal husbandry to keep pack animals healthy, content, and tethered at night.

Navigation

Journey times are often very long. Maps may be unreliable and roads little more than parallel tracks on the ground, invisible if the wind is blowing. GPS devices are invaluable, but ensure suitable backup.

Risk management

Difficult travel

Considerable reserves of water, fuel, and food are essential to ensure safety in the event of bad weather, mechanical failure, or navigational problems.

Dust storms

Dust storms can develop with little warning in any arid or semi-arid environment. These take the form of an advancing wall of dust and debris that may be miles long and several thousand feet high; they can appear from any direction though generally follow the prevailing winds. Most storms pass within an hour, but some persist for several hours. High winds can destroy tents and strip campsites bare. Health risks include suffocation and silicosis from dust inhalation, and extremely low visibility both on roads and in the air leading to disorientation and the possibility of serious accident.

Flora and fauna

Snakes and scorpions (see Chapter 17) live in deserts and may enter discarded footwear or containers. Plants in arid areas can have thorns, tough spiny surfaces, or serrated leaves.

Survival strategies in a dust storm

- Don't panic!
- Avoid travelling in dust storms if at all possible.
- If caught in a dust storm while driving, get off the road. Turn off driving lights and turn on emergency flashers.
- If out in the open with a dust storm coming your way, sit down with your back to the wind, and cover your head with your clothes to keep dust out of your eyes, nose, mouth, and ears (a dry shemagh or bandana is ideal—wet clothing will quickly become clogged up).

Heat-related illnesses (HRIs)

In hot weather a major environmental risk is that of developing some form of HRI. Humans originated in tropical regions and most people can adapt well to heat, but only after a period of acclimatization. Individuals vary considerably in their tolerance to heat stress, and the underlying mechanisms are not fully understood. Many people successfully complete endurance races such as the Marathon des Sables and Amazon Marathon in hot environments without incident, yet others tragically die whilst exercising on a hot day in temperate latitudes. Ultimately, if the duration and intensity is sufficiently challenging, everyone is vulnerable. Prolonged heat adds to the physiological stress and the risk of serious HRI is greatest following several days of exposure to hot and humid conditions.

Epidemiology

Classical heatstroke affects humans trapped in hot, unventilated environments, e.g. workers in mines, prisoners, stowaways in freight containers, or children left in cars during heat waves. Individuals with impaired thermoregulation such as infants, the elderly, people with underlying medical conditions, or those taking drugs known to interfere with thermoregulation are at greater risk (see Box 25.3). Increasing summer temperatures in normally temperate areas (exacerbated by urban environments where buildings can store heat and so raise night-time temperatures by 5°C) are producing urban heat waves and deaths amongst the frail and elderly. The 2003 European heat wave is thought to have been responsible for an extra 70,000 deaths, mainly in France. In the UK, the annual average mortality from classical heatstroke is thought to be about 40 cases per year.

The constant heat of jungles and urban environments constitutes a greater physiological stress than that found in deserts, where the nights are often cool.

Exertional heat stroke (EHS) occurs as a result of physical exercise, and cases may develop even in otherwise temperate conditions if someone becomes dehydrated or overexerts themselves, sometimes in inappropriate clothing. It typically occurs during military training or during endurance sporting events. EHS is much more likely on expeditions than classical heatstroke.

Hyperthermia is also associated with stimulant recreational drugs such as cocaine, ecstasy, and amphetamines (Box 25.3).

Heat exhaustion

Heat exhaustion is the most commonly encountered form of HRI. It occurs when the cardiac output is insufficient to meet the demands of increased blood flow to the skin, working muscles, and vital organs. The effects are compounded by a decreased effective plasma volume (redistribution of blood), dehydration, and salt loss due to sweating. Heat exhaustion does not result in any organ damage and some individuals may be fit to resume normal activities after 24–48 h.

Exertional heat stroke

EHS is defined as a core body temperature of >40°C caused by strenuous exercise and/or environmental heat exposure which is associated with central nervous system dysfunction and multiple-system organ failure (usually cardiovascular collapse). Heat shock proteins and cytokines contribute to a systemic inflammatory response syndrome (SIRS) similar to that seen in other critical illnesses.

EHS is most often associated with pale, sweaty skin, as opposed to the hot, dry, flushed skin of classical heat stroke. As tissue temperatures rise, cell membranes and enzyme-dependent energy systems are disrupted leading to variable cell and organ dysfunction and death. The extent of injury relates both to the duration of exposure and the severity of the rise in core temperature, but the seriousness of the condition cannot be predicted from these two parameters alone, and requires laboratory confirmation.

Unfortunately the symptoms of EHS are non-specific. Anyone looking unwell, or behaving abnormally in a hot and/or humid environment, or during vigorous exercise in a temperate environment, should be managed as a victim of HRI until proven otherwise. Typically sufferers from EHS will have more than 2/3 of the symptoms (see Box 25.1), while someone who has a febrile illness instead of a HRI will show 1/3 or fewer. The box may be used as a prompt and all symptoms and signs should be sought.

> ### Box 25.1 Heat exhaustion and heatstroke present with the following features:
>
> - Weakness.
> - Lethargy.
> - Headache.
> - Dizziness.
> - Nausea.
> - Vomiting.
> - Diarrhoea.
> - Fatigue.
> - Hysteria.
> - Anxiety.
> - Confusion.
> - Staggering.
> - Impaired judgement.
> - Hyperventilation.
> - Collapse.
> - Convulsions.
> - Loss of consciousness.
> - Muscle cramps.
> - Irrational behaviour.
> - Coma.

Incidence

EHS is not always recognized and may be diagnosed as exercise-associated collapse. The incidence is unknown, but appears to be on the rise as more people take up long-distance and endurance sporting events. In the US military, the incidence rose eightfold between 1981 and 2001 to 14.5 cases per 100,000 soldiers. In Singapore's hot, humid climate the incidence in the military may be as high as 350 cases per 100,000 soldiers.

Differential diagnosis of EHS in a previously fit person

- Hypoglycaemia—especially if diabetic.
- Hyponatraemia—excess rehydration with plain water.
- Drug toxicity—including alcohol.
- Ischaemic heart disease.
- Cerebrovascular event.
- Epilepsy.
- Head injury.
- Acute onset of fever, especially malaria.

Inability to reduce core temperature below 39°C with evaporative cooling suggests that a febrile co-morbid condition may be present.

Pathophysiology of HRIs

Core temperature is the temperature of the vital organs such as brain, heart, liver, and kidneys. Normally it should remain relatively constant regardless of environmental conditions and at rest should be between 35.5°C and 37°C, with a measurement above 37.5°C being abnormal. However, during vigorous and prolonged exercise, such as long-distance running on a hot day, core temperature rises and measurements up to 41°C have been recorded without apparent harm to the subject. Temperatures above 41°C are almost always abnormal and harmful.

Surrounding the body core is a shell of tissues at a lower temperature, the size of which depends upon the balance between heat generation and heat loss. In hot conditions, metabolic heat generated in the core has to be transferred to the skin, a process that involves substantial increases in skin blood flow.

The most critical factor in predicting the severity of injury is the duration of heat exposure following collapse. An elevated core temperature of 42–43°C can be tolerated for short periods (5–10 min) with little damage. For example, exertional heat stroke during military training usually involves short exposures and rapid treatment; there may be large numbers of casualties, but the mortality rate is relatively low. During the papal visit to Denver, Colorado in 1993, there were 18,000 symptomatic victims among the crowd but no deaths, as the organizers ensured that immediate help was available. If body temperature remains persistently elevated, body metabolism becomes deranged and enzymes denature. The destructive processes are listed in Box 25.2.

Box 25.2 Pathophysiology of heat stroke

- Cellular oxidative phosphorylation becomes uncoupled at temperatures >42°C.
- Cellular damage is directly proportional to the temperature and exposure time.
- Compensatory mechanisms for heat dissipation fail.
- Dehydration increases the sodium/potassium pump activity and increases metabolic rate.
- Complications may arise in multiple organ systems:
  - *CNS*: oedema and petechial haemorrhages cause focal and generalized damage.
  - *Muscle*: skeletal muscles show widespread degeneration of fibres. Rhabdomyolysis releases myoglobin, potassium, creatinine phosphokinase, and purines (which are metabolized into uric acid) into the circulation.
  - *Lungs*: non-cardiogenic pulmonary oedema.
  - *Kidneys*: oliguric acute renal failure due to renal ischaemia, muscle breakdown products, DIC, hyperuricaemia and hypovolaemia. Renal failure occurs in up to 35%.
  - *Blood*: DIC (poor prognosis), thrombocytopaenia, leucocytosis. Thermal injury to endothelium releases thromboplastins which result in intravascular thrombosis and secondary fibrinolysis.
  - *Metabolic*: metabolic acidosis, respiratory alkalosis, hypoglycaemia, hyper- or hypokalaemia.

Physics of heat transfer

Heat transfer and hence changes in body temperature take place as a result of radiation, conduction, convection, and evaporation.

- *Radiation*: the direct transfer of heat between the body surface and all other sources of radiant energy. The main source of radiant energy in hot climates is the sun. Under clear daytime desert skies the sun can cause great heat stress, but at night heat radiates away from warm bodies.
- *Conduction*: the direct transfer of heat between the body and any solid in contact with it, particularly the ground. Conduction ceases when the two solids in contact reach thermal equilibrium.
- *Convection*: the removal of heat through the flow of one substance over another. Convection augments conductive heat transfer and prevents thermal equilibrium developing by constantly replacing one of the materials so heat transfer can continue.

The rate of heat transfer by conduction, convection, and radiation is dependent on the difference in temperature between the body surface and the materials or radiating surfaces in the environment. If the body surface is warmer than the environment, the body will lose energy to the environment. However, very warm air or surfaces will transfer heat to the body by conduction/convection, and sunlit surfaces or sky will transfer heat to the body by radiation.

- *Evaporation*: heat can be lost indirectly by evaporation of sweat. Each litre of sweat evaporated from the body surface at 30°C removes approximately 580 kcal (140 kJ) of heat energy. If sweat drips off the body, it has not been allowed to evaporate, and therefore no heat is lost. Sweating (and therefore evaporative heat loss) occurs when internal heat production exceeds the capacity of direct routes of heat transfer to dissipate it. Importantly, when the environment is sufficiently hot to cause heat gain by the direct transfer routes, evaporative cooling is the only thermoregulatory mechanism available to control body temperature.

Biology of heat transfer

80% of metabolic energy is produced as heat in muscles—by normal metabolism, during exercise, and through shivering—and is conducted to the skin, where it is lost to the environment. The circulation of the blood augments and regulates this heat transfer by varying superficial blood flow. Clothing further modifies heat loss by acting either as a conductor or an insulator. At rest at 20°C, conduction and convection account for only about 10% of our heat loss, the majority occurring by radiation.

Once environmental temperature rises above 35°C it is impossible to lose heat through conduction, convection, or radiation. Our ability to survive and function in higher temperatures depends upon the ability to sweat.

Sweating allows the body to lose heat at any environmental temperature through evaporation, but evaporative heat loss can only occur if the air is not saturated with water vapour. So, sweating is most efficient in hot dry deserts and is less effective in hot humid rain forests. Humidity has a greater effect on the ability to lose heat than the absolute temperature.[2] (See Table 25.1.)

2 Morimoto T (1998). Heat loss mechanisms. In CM Blatteis (ed.) *Physiology and Pathophysiology of Temperature Regulation*. Singapore, p. 80–90. Singapore: World Scientific Publishing.

Table 25.1 Heat transfer

Mode of heat transfer	Contribution		
	25°C	30°C	35°C
Radiation	67%	41%	4%
Conduction and convection	10%	33%	6%
Evaporation	23%	26%	90%

The body's response to thermal stress

Changes in temperature are detected by both sensory nerve endings in the skin and by direct sensing of blood temperature in the hypothalamus of the brain. At rest, the skin receives around 9% of the total circulating blood flow. A rise in core temperature of as little as 0.1°C will increase skin blood flow to dissipate the heat, and under high heat stress skin blood flow can increase fourfold. Heat energy is then lost directly to the environment by a combination of radiation, conduction, convection, and by evaporation of sweat. High environmental temperatures also lead to behavioural changes such as reduced activity, seeking shade, and drinking more.

During physical work blood flow is directed to the working muscles and away from the intestines. This limits the ability of the gut to absorb water to around 1200 mL/h. If the rate of fluid lost in sweat exceeds this amount, then dehydration will occur. Anyone working in these conditions must be allowed adequate rest periods with fluid replacement. If blood flow is further distributed to the skin to allow evaporative heat loss, then the effective circulating volume is further decreased. An adequate blood volume is therefore required to ensure that thermoregulatory blood flow can occur.

Measurement of core temperature

(See also Chapter 3.)

Measuring body temperature accurately is difficult and medics need to be aware of the limitations of the various techniques. In hospital the best ways to measure core temperature are by the use of central venous or oesophageal sensors but neither is practical on most expeditions.

Rectal temperature can be measured using simple portable equipment, but there may be poor correlation between the rectal temperature and the severity of symptoms; fatalities have been reported with rectal temperatures of 39.5°C, while victims have survived core temperatures of 47°C. During active cooling, there may be rapid changes in temperature of the blood as demonstrated by the sudden onset of shivering, but there is a significant lag before the body temperature change is seen rectally.[3]

---

3 Greenes DS, Fleisher GR (2004). When body temperature changes, does rectal temperature lag?. *J Pediatr*, 144(6), 824–6.

A systemic review of febrile critically ill patients concluded that rectal temperatures were overestimated and inaccurate, but oral and tympanic temperatures more accurately reflected core (pulmonary artery catheter) temperature.[4]

Oral temperature measurement requires a conscious, cooperative patient and accurate placement of the bulb underneath the tongue for sufficient time to ensure thermal equilibrium. The patient should not breathe through the mouth during temperature measurement.

The tympanic membrane shares its blood supply with the hypothalamus (the body's thermostat) and changes in body temperature are measureable sooner at the tympanic membrane than at other external sites. Ear temperature probably offers the best compromise between the lag associated with rectal temperature measurement and the impracticalities and inaccuracies of oral temperature measurement, particularly in a semi-conscious patient.

However, for ease of use, most infrared ear thermometers are calibrated to read the mid-canal temperature, rather than the temperature of the tympanic membrane and this region is more susceptible to error. Some thermometers (e.g. Braun Thermoscan® models) correct for the site of measurement, but false readings may occur for a variety of reasons. Proper technique is important—a clean probe cover should be used each time, the ear must be free of wax and water, and the ear canal should be straightened (pull the ear up and back). If in doubt, treat the clinical signs rather than be reassured by a single measurement of temperature.

4 Jefferies SS, Weatherall MM, Young PP, Beasley RR (2011). A systematic review of the accuracy of peripheral thermometry in estimating core temperatures among febrile critically ill patients. *Crit Care Resusc*, 13(3), 194–9.

Acclimatization to heat

Full acclimatization to heat develops at different rates in different individuals; typically 10–14 days are required for all the physiological changes to develop. The rate of acclimatization depends upon factors, including body shape, the severity of the heat stress, and pre-existing physical fitness.

> **Benefits of acclimatization**
> * Reduced resting heart rate.
> * Increased blood volume.
> * Reduced core and skin temperature.
> * Decreased salt loss in sweat (may drop from 60 mmol/L to 5 mmol/L).
> * Increased sweat production (at lower core temperatures).
> * Increased blood flow to skin.
> * Improved renal sodium and water retention (aldosterone mediated).
> * Increased plasma proteins maintain extracellular fluid volume and reduce tachycardias.
> * Decreased glycogen consumption.
> * Improved ability to exercise (Fig. 25.1).

Physiological acclimatization enhances evaporative heat loss while reducing cardiovascular strain. Exercise becomes easier and exercise syncope, common on day 1, rapidly declines to zero by day 5. The increased sweat rate (0.5 L/h to 2 L/h), coupled with the increased blood flow, can increase heat loss by a factor of 20, but requires a significant increase in water consumption before, during, and after activity.

Some degree of acclimatization can be obtained in temperate climates before departure. Hot baths twice a day, saunas, and exercising while wearing more clothing than normal may be effective. In a hot dry climate, rapid acclimatization requires about 2 h of exercise per day sufficient to raise heart rate to around two-thirds of maximum, which should be conducted during the cooler hours of the morning or evening. Acclimatization may be delayed if substantial portions of the day are spent in air-conditioned environments. In comparison to dry heat, acclimatizing to hot humid climates, especially if the heat is unremitting, is much harder, and initial exercise tolerance will be substantially lower.

Sweating can only remove heat if there is sufficient fluid to spare. Sweat production rates can reach 2 L an hour for short periods and can be up to 15 L a day. In low-humidity environments such as deserts where evaporation is rapid, the daily cooling capacity of the sweating mechanism is adequate to maintain body temperature even during vigorous work, but in humid environments such as tropical forest, evaporation is ineffective and slow, so exercise must be limited to avoid overheating.

Sweat is a hypotonic (dilute) solution of sodium chloride. The concentration of sodium chloride in sweat depends on the sweat rate and the degree of acclimatization. Higher sweating rates reduce the opportunity to conserve salt, and the sweat salt concentration rises, but acclimatized sweat glands conserve salt more effectively by producing more hypotonic sweat. In addition to conserving salt in sweat, humans acclimatized to heat start sweating at lower body temperatures and their kidneys conserve salt more effectively. As a consequence, an acclimatized person in a hot environment requires no more salt than an unacclimatized individual in temperate conditions, and can maintain lower body temperatures for any degree of heat stress.

Jungle acclimatization readily transfers to desert climates (hot and dry) but the reverse journey requires further acclimatization to humidity. The benefits of acclimatization are lost over 20–40 days after returning to a temperate environment.

Prevention of HRIs

Heat stress is the product of the interaction between:
- The individual.
- The environment: temperature, wind, sun, and humidity.
- The workload of the task being undertaken.

Prevention of HRI

- Identify individuals at risk.
- Monitor environmental heat stress (ideally the wet bulb globe temperature (WBGT), see ➜ Evaluating environmental heat stress, p. 757).
- Adjust the daily aims of the expedition accordingly.
- Educate everyone about the nature of HRI: prevention, early recognition, and treatment.
- Provide adequate clean drinking water, shade, and latrines (inadequate toilet facilities may discourage drinking).
- Ensure that a robust medical evacuation system is in place.

Assessment of risk must consider each of these factors.

The individual

An individual is best able to cope with heat stress when:
- Fully hydrated.
- Physically fit.
- Acclimatized.
- Well nourished.
- Well rested.

Dehydration reduces both blood flow and sweating, so that a dehydrated person has reduced ability to maintain a constant body temperature in the heat. Acclimatization and physical fitness enable high temperatures to be tolerated better, but do not reduce water requirements; indeed, a fit acclimatized person will usually drink more than a new arrival to a hot environment.

Thermoregulation can be impaired by:
- Lack of sleep.
- Missed meals.
- Fever or recent pyrexial illness.
- Sunburn.
- Recent air travel.
- Use of therapeutic medications (see Box 25.3).
- Other causes of relative dehydration such as diarrhoea and menstruation.

People with any of these conditions should be watched closely for signs of heat distress and should avoid excessive exertion. If one member of a party develops symptoms of heat stress, then leaders and medics should assume that everyone else in that group who has been exposed to similar heat stress is a potential heat casualty.

A few individuals appear to have a genetic predisposition to developing a HRI. Previous HRI should alert one to a recurrence. However the data is variable and victims of previous exertional heat stroke may cope perfectly well with subsequent heat stress.

Box 25.3 Medications that increase risk of HRI

- Alcohol.
- Amphetamines.
- Antihistamines.
- Beta blockers.
- Desmopressin.
- Laxatives.
- Phenothiazines.
- Theophylline.

- ACE inhibitors.
- Anticholinergics.
- Calcium channel blockers.
- Cocaine.
- Diuretics.
- Major tranquillizers.
- SSRI antidepressants.
- Tricyclic antidepressants.

Evaluating environmental heat stress

Four environmental characteristics influence perceived heat stress:
- Air temperature.
- Solar (or radiant heat) load.
- Absolute humidity.
- Wind speed.

Environmental heat stress can vary greatly and unpredictably over short periods of time and space. On a calm, sunny day an open field may present a greater heat stress than an adjacent forest, but on a windy, cloudy day the forest may present the greater heat stress.

Three of these four factors are combined into an internationally accepted measure of heat stress, the WBGT index, developed by the US military in the 1950s.
- Dry bulb (Tamb)—measures ambient air temperature in the shade.
- Black globe (Tg)—measures solar load.
- Wet bulb (Tw)—measures absolute humidity.

$$WBGT = 0.7Tw + 0.2Tg + 0.1Tamb$$

Several manufacturers now produce relatively cheap devices capable of measuring and calculating WGBT; suppliers can be readily accessed on-line. In some states in the USA, measurement of WGBT is mandatory before sports are played in hot weather, with risk management procedures dependent upon the heat stress. Elsewhere organizers of sporting events and expedition leaders should consider planning activities around the value of WGBT. Further details of this and other temperature indices, including use of ambient temperature are available at: ℘ http://www.bom.gov.au/info/thermal_stress

If you do not have access to equipment for measuring WBGT, consider evaluating heat stress using the workload calculations (see Table 25.2 and ➔ Workload calculations, p. 758).

The wet bulb temperature is the most important component of the WBGT index, which reflects the thermoregulatory importance of evaporation in hot (especially humid) environments, but the index does not include wind speed, another important environmental modifier, within its calculation. Air movement increases convective heat transfer and will assist evaporation; cool winds reduce heat stress, but hot winds increase it. The American College of Sports Medicine provides guidelines for exercise in hot environments and recommends cancelling sporting events if the WBGT is >28°C.

Table 25.2 Recommended maximum workloads in various conditions

	Workload			Work-rest cycle (per hour)
	Light	Medium	Heavy	
WGBT	30.0	26.7	25.0	Continuous work
	30.6	28.0	25.9	45 min work/15 min rest
	31.4	29.4	27.9	30 min work/30 min rest
	32.2	31.1	30.0	15 min work/45 min rest

Workload calculations

For expeditions lacking meteorological facilities, an alternative method of judging a safe workload pattern has been suggested:

- Each individual should work out their maximum heart rate (220 minus their age in years) (e.g. a 40-year-old will have a maximum heart rate of 220–40 = 180 beats/min).
- The group should all work to the lowest figure obtained.
- Multiply the age-adjusted maximum heart rate by 0.75 (e.g. 75% age-adjusted maximum = 180 × 0.75=135 beats/min).
- The group should undertake the proposed activity for one work period (e.g. 30 min) under close supervision.
- Immediately after this initial work period all should recheck their heart rates.
- If anyone's heart rate exceeds the 75% age-adjusted maximum, the next working period should be reduced by 1/3 (e.g. to 20 min with 40 min rest).
- The group should rest in the shade and rehydrate for the remainder of the hour.
- Repeat the process until the 75% age-adjusted maximum is not exceeded.
- Unless they are lean, athletic, and very fit, women tend to tolerate heat less well than men, and their exercise rates should be adjusted accordingly.
- Fig. 25.1 indicates the rapid improvements in exercise tolerance that develop with acclimatization.

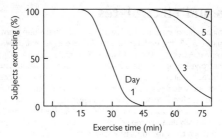

Fig. 25.1 Improved exercise duration with acclimatization during a standard exercise regime in hot conditions. Reproduced from Piantadosi CA (2003). *The Biology of Human Survival*, with permission from Oxford University Press.

Fluids and electrolytes

Maintaining an appropriate fluid balance during the transition from a cool to a hot climate, or during endurance sporting events is difficult. Inadequate fluid intake, excessive ingestion of water, and inadequate or inappropriate use of electrolyte supplements can all lead to serious health issues. Fluid and electrolyte requirements will change as the body becomes acclimatized to heat. Each individual will have different needs at different times and this makes it hard to offer firm advice on requirements.

A reduction in total body water (TBW) of 1% affects thermoregulation and losses of 2% significantly impair physical and mental performance. Thirst is a poor stimulus to drink and TBW losses of 5–10% have been tolerated in experiments. Fluid must be consumed before, during and after physical activity to maintain normal (eu-) hydration. This is most easily assessed by measuring the specific gravity of the first urine of the day (a specific gravity of ≤1.020 can be considered as euhydrated), along with changes in daily body weight performed at the same time (and before and after activity). Weight loss is common on expeditions and caused not only by dehydration, but also by increased work-load, GI upset, and decreased appetite due to heat and unfamiliar food.

Even when a person is significantly dehydrated, urine is still produced and the volume of fluid required to return to full hydration must be at least 1.5 times that lost in sweat (assuming the individual was fully hydrated before the onset of activity). Women have a lower proportion of water in their bodies and may be at greater risk of dehydration than men.

Dehydration

If an individual drinks only enough to satisfy their thirst they may become chronically dehydrated, particularly if they drink substantial amounts of caffeine-containing drinks, which act as diuretics. It is essential that personnel working hard in any environment are made aware of the need to drink water despite not feeling thirsty. Expedition leaders must enforce work/rest cycles, and provide adequate shade. If toilet facilities are unpleasant or lack privacy, travellers may seek to avoid visits by drinking less. Clean and screened facilities will encourage proper drinking habits—especially if the party consists of easily embarrassed youngsters.

Thirsty = dehydrated. Dehydrated *does not* = thirsty

Hydration can be monitored by the colour and quantity of urine along with how often one needs to pass urine. Dark yellow urine is a sure indicator that the individual is dehydrated, as is the need to urinate less than twice a day. Medical officers should check lying and standing BP; a difference of >15 mmHg in the systolic pressure suggests dehydration.

Diabetics need to maintain good glucose control as blood glucose >10 mmol/L will result in glucose in the urine and consequent osmotic diuresis producing lighter urine. This could be mistaken as indicating adequate hydration whereas in reality it would be masking, and at the same time, worsening dehydration.

Water supplies

In hot environments, water losses can reach 15 L per day per person. Complete replacement requires realistic estimates of potable water requirements, adequate water logistics, and individuals who understand and act on their water requirement. Water for hygiene will be needed in addition to water for drinking.

Where water supplies are unsafe, expedition leaders must ensure that adequate provision exists to purify sufficient water for the group's requirements. This may be flavoured to increase palatability. If chlorine or iodine is used, there should be a method of removing the taste at the point of use (see → Water purification, p. 102). Bottled water supplies purchased in local markets may be contaminated, discarded bottles having been recycled by being refilled from the nearest water source. Carbonated water may be preferable as it is harder to tamper with. Carbonated water and soft drinks will fill the stomach with carbon dioxide before sufficient water has been ingested to combat dehydration, and should not be relied upon as the only source of fluid.

Choice of replacement fluid

New arrivals in a hot climate will lose more salt in their sweat than normal and should supplement their salt intake until they become acclimatized. Salt tablets are best avoided as they contain an unknown amount of sodium and may irritate the stomach. Table salt should be readily available at meal times. Salt can be added to fluids in sensible amounts. Soups are an excellent source of both fluid and electrolytes.

The oral rehydration solution recommended by the WHO has a sodium content of 60–90 mmol/L, but the high sodium content of this significantly reduces palatability, resulting in reduced consumption. Whilst life-saving for diarrhoeal illnesses, its use cannot be recommended for fluid replacement in healthy people operating in the heat.

Sports drinks manufacturers have heavily promoted their products as the ideal way for active adults to replace the water and salt lost in sweat. Their value is controversial, with some athletes believing that they increase endurance and reduce the risk of heat cramps, whilst others doubt their value. Some sports drinks are sold as powders. Dissolving excessive amounts of powder in the hope of increasing absorbed energy produces hypertonic fluids that do not quench thirst and enhance the effects of dehydration. Always mix such powders according to instructions.

A 2012 *BMJ* review concluded that water remains the best replacement fluid, but that over-hydration is a bigger risk than dehydration during running events up to marathon length.[5] However this advice may not apply when prolonged heat exposure leads to substantial additional salt losses.

5 Cohen DD (2012). The truth about sports drinks. *BMJ*, 345, e4737–7.

Fluid-induced hyponatraemia

In the absence of serious HRI or renal failure, dehydration by itself does not cause unconsciousness. Competitors participating in endurance races can develop symptomatic hyponatraemia if they drink excessive amounts of plain water or hypotonic fluids. Stomach bloating, weakness, and collapse may be followed by unconsciousness.

- Hospitalization is necessary.
- Cerebral oedema can develop.
- Avoid giving further water.
- The bladder should be catheterized and urine output monitored.
- Avoid oral fluids. Salt-containing foods may be given during recovery.
- Hypertonic saline (3%) can be infused slowly IV.

The use of desmopressin (DDAVP®) for the treatment of nocturnal enuresis has been linked to the death of a young traveller on an expedition (see ➜ Nocturnal enuresis, p. 525).

Without laboratory facilities it will probably be impossible to distinguish between collapse from symptomatic hyponatraemia and collapse as a result of a heat related illness. Both are life-threatening conditions and require urgent medical support.

Treatment of HRIs

Treatment should focus on returning the victim's body temperature to the normal range as rapidly as possible in the prevailing situation (see Table 25.3).

Remove the casualty from the source of heat and place them in the shade. Lying down maximizes heat loss, but only if the ground or mattress is no warmer than the surrounding environment. A string hammock is ideal for encouraging heat loss as it enables air to circulate over the whole body.

The most rapid cooling (with lowest morbidity and mortality) is achieved by immersing a casualty in a bath or pool of iced-water. A children's paddling pool may be a suitable piece of first-aid equipment for expeditions or event organizers to consider. Aggressive cooling using ice-water soaked towels in combination with ice packs to the head, neck, axillae and groin also achieves reasonable cooling. Evaporative cooling using wet towels and fanning is less effective, especially in humid conditions, but is probably the mainstay of treatment on expeditions. The casualty should be continuously sprayed with cold water and fanned to encourage evaporation. A wet sheet may be wrapped around the casualty instead and kept constantly moist.

In some countries a simple solution to heat exhaustion is to lie the victim in a tepid running stream, but beware that they could become unconscious, that the stream could be polluted, or that aggressive animals may be encountered.

Oral or IV fluids may be given, the latter being more effective in serious cases. At the Hajj pilgrimage, cold IV infusions of up to 1 L of normal saline or dextrose saline at 5°C for heatstroke and 12°C for heat exhaustion have been used successfully. Frequently casualties also suffer from hypoglycaemia, and glucose should be administered orally or IV to all casualties. No more than 2 L of IV fluids are normally required.

A heat-injured casualty who has not been cooled and yet is shivering is seriously ill. They may complain bitterly of feeling cold. They will not feel hot or thirsty. They will look pale and have cold skin. They will want to be wrapped in warm clothing, which only increases their core temperature further, as does shivering. They must have their core temperature measured to exclude HRI or a febrile illness such as malaria.

During cooling, the return to a normal temperature is often associated with shivering. It is important to continue to monitor core temperature, as the casualty's thermoregulatory capacity has been damaged and these individuals are at continued risk of either hyperthermia or hypothermia.

Some of the effects of heatstroke, e.g. renal or hepatic failure, only develop after 24–72 h. As it is impossible to distinguish accurately between heat exhaustion and heatstroke, all casualties should be evacuated to a hospital with intensive care facilities.

Advanced medical care

- Airway—unconscious patients require support and may need intubation and ventilation.
- Cardiorespiratory collapse—IV fluids and BP monitoring required.
- Fitting—may require IV lorazepam or rectal diazepam.
- Renal failure—may require catheterization to monitor urine output and dialysis.
- Liver failure—may develop several days after initial episode.
- Body temperature characteristically remains unstable for several days following a severe acute episode.
- Dantrolene—used in the treatment of malignant hyperpyrexia does *not* appear to help.
- Antipyretics—including anti-inflammatories such as NSAIDs and paracetamol (acetaminophen) are valueless and might exacerbate renal and hepatic failure.
- In serious cases of heat stroke, the value of a period of controlled induced hypothermia, similar to that employed following cardiac arrest, should be considered.

Table 25.3 The seven Rs of managing HRI

Recognize signs and symptoms	If in doubt—treat as heat injury.
Rest casualty in shade	Get rest of group under cover and drinking water.
Remove all clothing	Strip to underwear.
Resuscitate	Maintain ABC.
Reduce temperature ASAP	Evaporative cooling and iv fluids.
Rehydrate	Oral or intravenous fluids.
Rush to hospital	Evacuate all heat casualties.

Other heat-related problems

Heat syncope

Fainting on standing in the heat is thought to occur because of blood pooling in the legs and increased blood flow to the skin. When standing, the blood supply to the brain is temporarily interrupted, causing loss of consciousness. Although most cases of heat syncope are harmless, the potential for HRI should be considered, especially following physical work in the heat, or after the acclimatization period. Treat with rest in the cool and oral fluids.

Heat oedema

Mild swelling of the limbs may be experienced during the first few days of exposure to heat, during the time when the plasma volume increases to allow for the increased blood flow to the skin. Cutaneous vasodilatation and pooling of increased interstitial fluid in dependent extremities results in swelling of the hands and feet. It is self-limiting, resolving in a few days.

Exercise associated muscle (heat) cramps

Heat cramps are painful skeletal muscle spasms following prolonged exercise, often in the heat. They usually occur in the arms, legs, or abdomen from prolonged exercise and are thought to be due to dilutional hyponatremia, but also occur in cool conditions, e.g. swimming. Treatment is rest, prolonged stretches of affected muscle groups, and oral sodium replacement. If the individual is otherwise well, there is no association with HRI, but a raised core temperature should be treated promptly.

Miliaria rubra ('prickly heat')

Miliaria rubra is an inflammatory skin eruption, which appears in actively sweating skin in humid conditions (or skin covered by clothing in dry environments). Each lesion represents a blocked sweat gland, which cannot function efficiently. The risk of HRI is increased in proportion to the amount of skin surface involved. Sleeplessness due to itching and secondary infection of occluded glands may further affect thermoregulation. Miliaria is treated by cooling and drying affected skin, avoiding sweating, controlling infection, and relieving itching. Sweat gland function recovers with replacement of the damaged skin, which takes 7–10 days.

Prevent if practicable by wearing loose, airy cotton clothing and taking regular cool showers. Treatment consists of frequent bathing in cool water, gently dabbing dry to prevent further damage, and application of talcum powder or calamine lotion. Air conditioning can help if available. Sedative antihistamines such as chlorphenamine (Piriton®) may help to relieve symptoms and promote sleep at night, but sedative drugs should be avoided during the daytime as they may increase risk of accidents with machetes, etc.

NB Many general travellers who claim to have had 'prickly heat' may actually be describing polymorphic light eruption.

Sunburn

Sunburn reduces the thermoregulatory capacity of skin and also affects central thermoregulation; prevent by insisting on the use of adequate sun protection. Sunburnt individuals should be protected from significant heat stress until the burn has healed (see also ➔ Solar skin damage, p. 266).

Skin infections

Wound and skin infections are common in hot conditions and are covered in Chapter 9.

Resources

Singapore Army evidence-based guidelines for the management of heat illness: ℘ http://www.guideline.gov/content.aspx?id=39341

American College of Sports Medicine Position Stands—*Exertional Heat Illness during Training and Competition*: ℘ http://journals.lww.com/acsm-msse/Fulltext/2007/03000/Exertional_Heat_Illness_during_Training_and.20.aspx

Exercise and fluid replacement: ℘ http://journals.lww.com/acsm-msse/Fulltext/2007/02000/Exercise_and_Fluid_Replacement.22.aspx

Further reading

O'Brien KK, Leon LR, Kenefick RQ (2011). Clinical management of heat-related illnesses. In P Auerbach (ed) *Wilderness Medicine*, 6th edn, pp. Mosby.
Walden J (2001). *Jungle Travel and Survival*. Guilford, CT: The Lyons Press.

Chapter 26

Hot, humid environments: tropical forest

Section editors
James Moore, Chris Johnson, and Shane Winser

Contributors
James Moore
Jon Dallimore
Paul Richards
Shane Winser

Reviewer
Harvey Pynn

The tropical forest environment 770
Risk assessment for tropical forest travel 774
Travel in tropical forests 776
Accommodation and campcraft in tropical forests 778
Water and sanitation in tropical forests 781
Humans in the tropics 782
Tropical-related illness 786

NB This chapter should be read in conjunction with Chapter 25, particularly the sections on heat illness.

The tropical forest environment

Tropical forests cover a dwindling 5% of the Earth's landmass, and are defined by their location (between the tropic of Cancer and the tropic of Capricorn). They can be broadly separated into five types:
- *Lowland equatorial evergreen forests*: archetypical tropical forest such as the Amazon and Congo Basins.
- *Moist deciduous forests*: Central American, Caribbean, Indian, and Indochina.
- *Montane rain forests*: cloud forests found between 1500 and 3000 m, e.g. Bolivian Yungas or Malaysian Cameron Highlands.
- Flooded forests.
- Freshwater swamps.

Expedition preparations should be tailored to the particular biome visited. Primary (un-logged) rain forest, where the high tree canopy suppresses ground growth, is more open and easier to travel through than logged forest. Logging removes the tall canopy trees allowing more light to reach the forest floor and creating greater secondary plant growth. Travel becomes restricted to pre-cut trails.

Weather

During the day, tropical forests are hot and humid, often with little breeze to give respite, but at night they become much cooler, and travellers in montane forests will require a blanket or lightweight sleeping bag. The forest floor, especially in flooded forests, may be under water for much of the year.

Rainfall levels vary between biomes, they can exceed 2 m annually. Seasonal variations in weather patterns (such as dryer seasons or monsoons) can be expected, depending on the forest type and location. Typically, cumulonimbus storm clouds develop during the day, leading to intense rainfall mid to late afternoon.

Humidity

The combination of high temperatures and high rainfall ensure the humidity remains high for much of the year in most tropical forests, affecting not only the health of individuals, but also the operation of equipment. Everything gets damp, and it is very difficult to dry things out. Silica gel sachets may help to reduce moisture in medical kits, bags, and containers holding sensitive and electronic equipment.

Biting insects

Insects are the most prolific of all creatures in the tropical forest environment and will rapidly invade every part of camp life. Insects can bite, irritate, and infest; they may transmit serious illnesses such as malaria (➜ Malaria, p. 480) and dengue fever (➜ Dengue fever ('break bone' fever), p. 465). They may be attracted by:
- Carbon dioxide from respiration or stoves.
- Scented deodorants or antiperspirants.
- Smelly feet and boots.
- Food.
- Poor personal hygiene.

- During the day wear appropriate clothing that should include good ankle and leg protection. Diethyl-toluamide (DEET)-impregnated wrist and ankle bands may help repel insects.
- The hazardous malaria-carrying mosquitoes emerge at dusk and usually bite during the night. During daylight clothing needs to be appropriate to the task in hand. Once dusk falls it is sensible to spend as much time as possible wearing appropriately protective clothing and remaining inside screened accommodation. At night sleep under permethrin impregnated mosquito nets.

Insect protection and repellents
(See also Box 15.3)
The annoyance and hazard of insects may be reduced by use of:
- *DEET*: which can help in the prevention of mass insect invasion. A few squirts on tassels wound around the strings of a hammock, or on the guy ropes of a tent will divert insects elsewhere. Note: DEET in high concentrations will dissolve man-made fibres and plastics. 50% DEET is adequate for most uses.
- *20% picaridin*: a modern repellent of comparable efficacy to DEET that does not degrade man-made fibres.
- *P-menthane-3,8-diol (PMD)* is an isolate of the lemon eucalyptus plant and has been shown to have similar efficacy to DEET although much shorter duration of action. It must not be used on children under the age of 3 and can cause irritation to the eyes.
- Smoke from a campfire.
- Insecticides such as permethrin.
- Insect repellent coils can help in enclosed spaces.
- Reducing the amount of artificial light used after sunset.

Other repellents such as citronella oil or candles, or 'Skin-so-soft®' have not been shown to be as efficacious and should be avoided. Remember that the half-life of most repellents applied to skin is reduced in hot, humid conditions, as sweat will remove the agent.

See also ➲ Arthropods, p. 560.

Other animals
Tropical forests are home to several species of animals large enough to cause harm to humans (see Chapter 17). To minimize the risk of a dangerous encounter:
- Obtain good local knowledge about dangerous animals.
- When siting camp, avoid animal tracks—especially if they lead to a waterhole. Be particularly wary of wild boar, peccaries, hippo, crocodile, and elephant.
- Store food in appropriate containers, away from sleeping and communal areas.
- Be cautious around rivers and lakes. Large reptiles and animals will attack whilst humans and animals are near the water's edge.

Birds

Generally birds do not pose a physical threat to humans although large birds such as the cassowary have been known to cause serious injuries if provoked. They may, however, be vectors for transmittable diseases such as salmonella and bird flu.

See also: ➔ Ectoparasitic infestations, p. 286.

Plant hazards

(See also Chapter 18.)

Approximately 2/3 of all plant species grow within tropical forests. Consuming any part of an unidentified plant is hazardous, as is remaining below a rotten tree whose branches could break, or any species liable to drop nuts or fruit. Many plants and grasses can cause irritation and or injury.

Plants are a natural source of food for insects and animals and so have developed defence mechanisms. Many contain poisons in their fruit, sap, flesh or foliage; e.g. *Solanum americanum* (American nightshade) that contains the neurotoxin solanidine, or the highly poisonous *Strychnos nux-vomica*, also known as the strychnine tree. If human skin comes into contact with these plants it should be irrigated as rapidly as possible; itching and discomfort can be relieved using topical steroids. In more serious cases parental corticosteroids and hydrocortisone cream may be required, and very occasionally these plants may cause an anaphylactic reaction (see Fig. 8.8).

Identification of the toxic plant will be difficult without extensive subject knowledge, but useful for appropriate treatment guidelines. Where possible the use of telemedicine and remote-photographic identification should be considered. Individuals should be made aware of the dangers of eating unidentified plants and fruit found in the tropical forest, or drinking water collected from vines or leaves.

Other plants protect themselves by spines, barbs and needles, e.g. *Acacia cuspidifolia* (Wait-a-while), or many of the 600 species of *Calameae*—commonly known as rattan. Foreign bodies left in the skin after contact with spine-bearing plants should be removed rapidly, observed for infection, and treated accordingly.

Finally, some plants use a combination of needles and poisons, such as *Dendrocnide moroides*, or the 'stinging bush' native to northeastern Australia and Indonesia. This species is clothed in hollow silica hairs filled with a potent neurotoxin. On contact, silica hairs penetrate the skin and remain stuck, releasing toxin and causing pain and discomfort for several weeks. The irritant hairs can be removed using adhesive tape or hair-removal waxing strips.

Risk assessment for tropical forest travel

Before embarking on a tropical forest expedition, consider how the environment is likely to affect the participants' safety. Important risk factors include:

Topography

- Falls due to steep-sided ravines and cliffs.
- Rivers prone to flash flooding.
- Thick vegetation hindering communications and navigation.

Climate

- High rainfall.
- High humidity.
- High temperatures.

Forest living and travel

- Deadfall—dead trees and branches supported by the canopy but which can fall down in even light winds.
- Falling branches and debris in recently logged forest.
- Trip hazards—muddy, slippery paths, roots, rattan.
- Lack of ambient light—particularly at dusk when sunset occurs in a matter of minutes.
- Contact with poisonous and spine-bearing plants is likely. The dappled light found under the canopy makes it impractical to wear sunglasses, leaving eyes unprotected.
- Risk of sunburn especially when travelling by river.
- Camp design and layout.
- Hazards around the camp.
- A requirement for lost-person search procedures (see ➲ Search and rescue, p. 776).

Health and well-being

- Heat—new arrivals must acclimatize to the environment, heat. and humidity. Physical exertion must be limited until full acclimatization has occurred. Death from heat stroke may occur. Visitors should be aware of the hazards of both dehydration and hyponatraemia (Chapter 25).
- Water supplies must take account of high fluid requirements—especially amongst poorly acclimatized newcomers.
- Biting insects (see ➲ Biting insects, p. 770) and hazardous plants (Chapter 18).
- Transmittable diseases, especially dengue (see ➲ Dengue fever ('break bone' fever), p. 465) and malaria (➲ Malaria, p. 480).
- Cuts and grazes will become infected much more quickly in tropical climates if not given prompt and careful wound management and untreated can lead to tropical ulcers (➲ Tropical ulcers, p. 292).
- Tropical immersion foot and other fungal infections (➲ Tropical immersion foot, p. 787).
- Jungle psychology (➲ Psychological stress, p. 786).

Travel

- Journey times must take account of difficulty of terrain.
- Exercise duration and loads carried must be limited until the team has acclimatized to the environment.
- Consider how a non-ambulant casualty could be evacuated.

Risk assessments should be kept short, and clearly identify what actions need to be taken by individuals to prevent serious foreseeable incidents occurring. See also Risk Management, p. 68.

Travel in tropical forests

Traditionally travel through forests has been by foot or waterway, but in recent years roads have been cut through many tropical forests in an attempt to obtain natural resources. Planning should consider not only normal movement through the forest, but also how supplies can be brought in or a casualty evacuated.

For most non-natives the forest micro-topography, high temperatures and humidity means that travel by foot will be slow and physically demanding. Waterways provide easier and faster passage, and can provide access to remote areas by canoe, powerboat, float plane, or helicopter, although they have their own hazards including fast currents, waterfalls and cataracts, submerged obstacles and debris, and reptiles, hippopotamuses and other large animals.

Forest roads may be poorly maintained and hazardous with large vehicles travelling at speed. Avoid driving at night. In the event of a traffic accident warning signals should be placed by or in the road several hundred metres either side of the accident and it is essential to carefully search the surrounding jungle for casualties thrown clear but hidden by dense foliage.

Navigation

The absence of visible references, such as the sun or landmarks, makes navigation in tropical forests difficult. Without visual references, winding paths and difficult terrain can be very disorientating. Any available maps are likely to be large scale, making accurate navigation and pacing difficult although large navigable waterways are often well charted.

Steep valleys and high tree canopies restrict the use of satellite navigation and communication equipment. Electronic navigation equipment should not be relied on in tropical regions—as with anything electronic, they are prone to failure.

The most accurate and safest method of navigation in tropical regions is by using reliable local guides and a good compass.

Search and rescue

(See also ➲ Missing persons, p. 140.)

Locating lost or injured casualties is very difficult in tropical forests. Shouts and cries do not carry far, while visibility is very restricted both on the ground and from above, limiting the use of aids such as heliographs, smoke or flares. Electronic emergency aids, such as emergency position indicating radio beacons (EPIRBs) can warn rescue agencies of a problem but amid dense vegetation on steep hillsides it can still be very difficult to locate a party. Even if a helicopter is available, topography, weather conditions, and tall trees can make it impossible to land or winch a casualty, who may have to be transported some distance to a clearing and then nursed for an extended period until medevac becomes possible.

Rescue times can be significantly reduced through meticulous planning. Ensure external agencies have:

- Daily estimated location/route.
- Potential deviations from travel plans.
- Pre-arranged situation-reports ('sit-reps').
- Pre-arranged rescue plan, including use of local guides/agencies.
- Expedition members should be briefed on 'lost and found' procedures. If separated from a group and disorientated, individuals should be briefed to remain where they are, provided that the location is safe. Tropical forests are notoriously confusing and following 'hunches' or unconfirmed paths in an attempt to relocate is likely to get the individual even more lost. No member should leave camp without a personal survival kit (\bigodot Useful equipment, p. 784).

Accommodation and campcraft in tropical forests

Living comfortably in the jungle requires knowledge and sound fieldcraft, which should if possible be learned and practised before arrival. Managed successfully, tropical forests can be an immensely satisfying environment in which to live and work.

Campsite management

- Evaluate planned campsites. Look up: site shelters away from rotting trees or branches that could crash down (so-called deadfall).
- Consider the animals and insects likely to be affected by setting up camp. Minimize interference with animal's natural food supplies and carefully assess areas for the presence of insect colonies such as hornet nests.
- Low river banks are access points to and from the water for wild animals. Check potential campsite for animal spoor and droppings.
- Ensure all paths around the camp are well marked and clear from obstacles.
- Protect group areas from rain using tarpaulins or other forms of shelter.
- Sleep off the ground to avoid snakes, scorpions, etc. A hammock, mosquito net and basha combination is the best form of accommodation in the jungle. Hammocks are now available with an integrated mosquito net, which reduces complicated sleeping set-ups and the number of guy-ropes needed to tie to trees.
- Expedition medics will benefit from an 'over-sized' basha or tarpaulin, allowing more space should they need to assess and treat patients.
- Clearing enough ground for tents can take a lot of energy and it can be difficult to remove stumps effectively. If used, tents should have a midge mesh, sewn-in bucket-type groundsheet and zips that seal the entrance. They can be stiflingly hot and heavy when wet.
- Leaf litter can hide snakes and scorpions, so this is best cleared from the ground beneath hammocks and around tent entrances.
- Abandoned native shelters may be structurally unsound and can harbour spiders, ants, rodents, and snakes which feed off them. Even when the fauna have left, they are potential sources of infections such as histoplasmosis (see ➜ Histoplasmosis, p. 794) and Chagas' disease (see ➜ American trypanosomiasis (Chagas' disease), p. 493).

Campfires

Sitting around a campfire is one of the most enjoyable aspects of being in the wilderness. Campfires provide:

- Warmth.
- A place to cook.
- A means to purify water.
- A way to dispose of rubbish.
- Security against animals.
- A great camp atmosphere.

However, they can cause:
- Burn injuries (**⊃** Burns, p. 280), through carelessness or horseplay.
- Damage to the camp.
- Damage to the wider environment.

Positioning a campfire
- Designate a specific area for the fire at least 3 m from scrub, grass, or other potential combustibles.
- Beware of overhanging foliage. Animals living in a forest canopy, for instance, will soon descend when gassed by noxious fumes from a campfire.
- If possible, create a fire surround with non-porous rocks. Porous rocks can explode when heated.
- Make sure there is a sensible distance between the fire and any tents/ hammocks or supplies.
- Consider the wind direction and speed. If sparks are likely to fly, reconsider the appropriateness of an open fire.
- Keep the fuel stores well away from the fire and prevailing winds.
- Have a supply of water ready to extinguish the fire if required.
- Fires that have been left to burn out or extinguished with sand have been shown to hold temperatures of 100°C 8 h later. In contrast, a fire extinguished with water has a temperature of 50°C only 10 min later.
- Campfires can consume significant amounts of fuel in relatively short periods of time. Be careful not to exhaust wood supplies needed by local communities.
- *Finally. . .* never leave a fire unattended.

Fuel
- Fuel is one of the most important components of living and surviving in the tropical forest. Fuel is required for heating, cooking, sterilizing water, and generating light. The most common source of fuel used in the tropical forest is wood and one should not underestimate quantities required for even modest use. Wood should be collected and stored with care as snakes and scorpions will often use woodpiles as homes or shelters. Keep it well away from the kitchen and living areas.
- Those responsible for collecting and using wood fuel should learn to use it efficiently, reducing the environmental impact.
- Petroleum and diesel should be stored in a well-marked place away from any fires or cooking areas. When siting the fuel dump ensure there is no possibility of accidental spillage reaching water-sources.
- Ideally there should be a method of extinguishing any fire around fuel storage areas, such as buckets of water/sand or extinguishers.

Light
- Tropical sunsets are considerably shorter than those in the northern and southern latitudes and it is important that individuals have a torch with them at all times. The jungle canopy dims sunlight during the day and causes an almost complete 'blackout' at night.
- Key areas of camp should be well lit or easily identified at night:
  - The communal area.
  - The latrines.
  - The kitchen.
  - The medic's basha.

- Even with a generator it may be impractical to keep a camp lit at all times for the duration of the expedition. Battery-powered lights work well but will eventually require new cells. Teams must learn to conserve light source energy and always have a backup in case of emergency.
- Glow-sticks are a useful source of emergency light. However, they have a limited light duration and emit sufficient light to be seen but not to use as a torch.
- Lanterns are commonly used for light on expeditions. These are generally run on liquid fuels (sometimes under pressure) or gas. Not only are these are an obvious fire hazard, but they also emit fumes which are poisonous in enclosed spaces.
- Single-cell LED lights are very useful as an emergency light. They are low cost and often have intermittent or flashing settings. Placing one inside a balloon will create a large, glowing sphere.

Water and sanitation in tropical forests

(See also ➔ Water purification, p. 102; ➔ Sanitation and latrines, p. 108.)

Water

In the tropics. daily drinking fluid requirements may rise from the 3 L per day typically required in temperate zones to as much as 8 L per day. By their very nature, tropical forests have an abundance of water; however, it is not always easily accessible.

Water can be collected from streams, wells, rivers, and lakes but must be treated appropriately before use. If a ground water-source is unavailable, consider the use of tarpaulins or bashas to collect and funnel rainwater. It is wise to filter and treat rainwater to remove particles collected from the canopy.

Each member of the team should carry at least 2 L of water with them at all times.

Sanitation

Careful disposal of human waste in the jungle is important as it can quickly find its way into water sources or the animal food chain.

Jungle latrines

In tropical forests the top 15 cm is where most bacterial activity takes place, so only a shallow scrape or latrine trench is required. Latrines should be sited downstream of any local water source but away from water to mini-mize risk of contamination.

'Longdrop latrines' are not appropriate in most jungle environments. Unless professionally designed and sited, they do not allow for the natural decomposition process to occur.

Toilet paper and sanitary items

If storing toilet paper and sanitary items at the latrine, make sure they are kept in a container suitable for the conditions present, preferably animal- and waterproof.

Toilet paper and sanitary items should be burnt. This can be on an indi-vidual basis, or stored and collected as part of the latrine rota, then burnt at the end of the day with other rubbish.

Latrine rota

Where possible, a latrine rota should be established. Tasks include:
• Digging new trenches.
• Re-siting urinals.
• The marking of new/old latrines.
• Ensuring an adequate supply of toilet paper is available.
• Ensuring that there is sufficient alcohol gel for hand cleaning.
• Ensuring there is soap/detergent by the water.
• Burning toilet paper and sanitary items.

See also ➔ Sanitation and latrines, p. 108.

Humans in the tropics

Humans in heat and high humidity

In hot climates, the human body becomes increasingly dependent upon sweating to maintain normal body temperature. But in tropical forests, high humidity and lack of breeze limit evaporation rates. At around 80% relative humidity perspiration fails to evaporate, drastically reducing its cooling effect. Perspiration is only an effective cooling mechanism if the moisture evaporates on or close to the skin surface, but in hot, humid conditions sweat frequently runs off ineffectively, continuing to dehydrate the individual. Until acclimatized, this fluid loss will be associated with salt depletion.

Expedition leaders must be very aware of the debilitating and potentially hazardous combination of heat and humidity experienced by new arrivals in the tropics. Heat illness is discussed in Chapter 25 (see ➔ Heat related illnesses (HRIs), p. 748).

- Evaluate environmental heat stress using the WGBT index (➔ Evaluating environmental heat stress, p. 757). Weather conditions in the tropics are usually consistent which should permit analysis of likely heat stresses before departure. However, heat waves or unusually high humidity on arrival may require plans for activity to be further modified.
- The American College of Sports Medicine recommends cancelling sporting events if the WBGT is above 28°C. Pressures of an expedition may make it hard to limit exercise in certain circumstances, but youngsters in particular should not be required to trek long distances in heat and humidity.
- Until team members have acclimatized, maximum work intensity and duration must be adjusted according to the ambient heat and humidity levels (Table 25.2).
- It is important to get both fluid balance and salt intake correct. Both dehydration and excessive intake of water can be hazardous. Fluid loss through sweat alone in humid environments can exceed 2 L per hour, therefore fluid and electrolyte replacement is vital. Ensure adequate fluid, salt, and carbohydrate intake throughout the day. Add salt to food rather than relying on salt tablets. Oral rehydration sachets are useful for electrolyte replacement but ideally should only be used in the presence of illness. Excessive fluid intake can lead to hyponatraemia (➔ Fluid-induced hyponatraemia, p. 762).

Clothing and equipment

The tropical forest environment is unforgiving in its treatment of clothing and equipment. Without proper care both will degrade rapidly, as a result of environmental conditions and effects from flora and fauna. Clothing should be manufactured from tough, snag-proof, man-made fibres. Natural fibres rapidly become waterlogged through sweat and rain. Clothing should cover arms and legs to prevent scratches and reduce the effect of insect, animal and reptile bites. In some areas of the tropics, locals will wear 'snake-gaiters' or 'leech protectors'– canvas or cloth over socks to the knees.

- Waterproof clothing will keep rainwater out, but increase the wearer's body temperature, thus leading to counterproductive sweating inside the clothing.

- Accept daytime wetness. Rinse kit in camp and re-wear wet next day. Keep a dry set of clothing in a plastic bag for evening and bedtime use to preserve comfort and skin.
- Never go barefoot or wear sandals; you risk cuts, insect or snake bites, larva migrans, jiggers, etc.
- Use boots with good treads that dry quickly. De-roofed blisters could develop into ulcers, so ensure that boots are properly worn-in before entering the jungle.
- Waterproof socks, such as Sealskinz™ are useful should one need to get up at night and keep feet dry.
- Cover up—long sleeves and trousers protect you from irritant plants and insect bites.
- Lycra shorts will help to prevent leeches and other insects from reaching the more intimate body parts.
- Gloves protect against sawgrass cuts, especially when using a machete.
- Hats with a brim protect against sun, rain, and barbed leaves.

Personal skills

- In camp, personal sleeping space should be kept clean and tidy. When not in use, kit should be kept packed away and bags fastened shut to prevent infestation by insects, snakes, or other small animals. Mosquito nets should be tied up and off the ground.
- At night, ensure boots are kept off the ground, upside-down on sticks, or with the boot-neck fastened shut or blocked. Open boots can attract scorpions, snakes, and spiders. Check every time you put your boots back on!
- Minimize risk of insect bites (➡ Biting insects, p. 770; Box 15.3).
- Be wary of snakes and scorpions (➡ Venomous land animals, p. 550).
- Avoid trauma. Learn correct use of machete—sheathed when carried and not in use.
- Practise crossing rivers safely, but avoid where possible.
- On log bridges, balance is aided by fixing eyes ahead and use of a walking pole.
- Drink only sterilized water and maintain appropriate personal and food hygiene. Beware water contamination with heavy metals such as mercury from gold mining in the Amazon. This will not be removed by boiling, but filters using activated carbon should reduce the risk (➡ Water purification, p. 102).
- Learn to navigate using map and compass. GPS is useful but may require wide clearings as the canopy impedes the signal. Use trails, walk in file keeping team members in sight, use guides, and place a designated person at the back of the group as tail marker.
- Rise at dawn, eat and drink, and make a camp an hour before nightfall, as it will take at least an hour to put up bashas or hammocks, and get a fire lit before the sudden arrival of the tropical night.
- Respect local customs, including those of dress (➡ Cultural clashes, p. 113).
- Theft—many expeditions are supplied with food, equipment, and clothing costing more than the local village's annual income. Overt displays of wealth should be avoided.
- Avoid ingesting hallucinogenic plants, or other native drugs (➡ Dangers of living off the land, p. 578).

Useful equipment

- *Machete:* a key piece of tropical forest kit is the machete or parang. It should be made of a tool-grade steel or similar and come with a file or sharpening steel to maintain a sharp edge. Before using a machete ensure the area is safe and free from others. Only the first person in the column should have an open machete. A wrist loop is useful. Cut using small movements and stand leading with the dominant leg and hand, i.e. if you hold the machete in your right hand, have your right leg forward. Ensure inexperienced group members are given sufficient training in the use of machetes.
- *Dry bags:* are very helpful to keep your kit dry in camp, during rain or while crossing rivers.
- *Slings and karabiners* are useful for keeping kit off the ground.
- *Paracord and 'gaffa' tape* will fix most things in the jungle.
- *An umbrella*—ideal for walking around camp in a downpour.
- Personal survival kit: many seasoned tropical forest veterans will recommend keeping an army-style 'belt kit'. This holds, within a few belt pouches, enough equipment to survive a night or two in the jungle alone. Amongst other things it would contain:
  - A sturdy pocket knife.
  - A whistle.
  - A compass.
  - A torch.
  - A fire-lighting kit.
    —Lighter.
    —Tinder/accelerant.
    —Flint and steel.
  - Water purification tablets.
  - Paracord.
  - An energy bar or other snack.

The most important part about any piece of equipment is to know how to use it before it is required. This is especially true in the tropics.

Tropical-related illness

Heat illnesses—see ➲ Heat related illnesses (HRIs), p. 748.
Acclimatization to heat—see ➲ Acclimatization to heat, p. 754.
Treatment of heat illnesses—see ➲ Treatment of HRIs, p. 764.

Psychological stress

Unfamiliar sounds, smells, fear of animals, disease, the intense darkness of night, or the isolation of sleeping exposed in a hammock in a strange place may contribute to anxiety. Encourage team members to learn about the environment, listen to the local guides, and become informed. Fear arises from unfamiliarity and uncertainty; knowledge helps you to find the forest accommodating rather than intimidating.

Prolonged exposure to wet discomfort saps morale, so regular return to a comfortable environment such as a well-constructed base camp is important. 'Social time', particularly for sharing the evening meal and general relaxed chat, is important for team integrity and morale.

All expedition members should be briefed on:
- Bite prevention and malaria chemoprophylaxis.
- Safety, lost person, and search and rescue plan.
- Hammocks/machete/clothing.
- Dangers of the heat and humidity.
- Ensuring an appropriate water intake.
- Deadfall (dead timber in the canopy that may fall in high winds).
- Animal hazards.
- First-aid treatment of snake and other bites/stings.
- Water hazards.

Stress that some diseases such as malaria will not manifest themselves until after return, and that in the event of an illness doctors must be informed of the recent overseas trip. GPs in a temperate country may be unfamiliar with the signs and symptoms of tropical illness and it may be appropriate to seek referral to a specialist infectious or tropical disease unit.

Finally it is important that team members are sufficiently fit for jungle life. Poor physical fitness makes it harder to cope with the cardiovascular effects of heat stress and acclimatization takes longer. Overweight individuals are at increased risk from heat related illness, both because excess body fat acts as insulation and because they have to use extra energy to move around arduous and demanding terrain.

Tropical ulcers

See ➲ Tropical ulcers, p. 292.

Tropical immersion foot

Tropical immersion foot is a dermatological condition resulting from the skin being in contact with warm water for over 48 h. The skin becomes hyperhydrated, ulcerates, and breaks down. Although difficult, prevention is far better than cure:

- Allow time every night for foot care.
- In the evenings, ensure feet are clean and dry.
- Use a light dusting of medicated foot powder.
- When possible and where appropriate, use flip-flops or sandals around camp to give feet 'air-time'.

Other fungal infections

(See Chapter 9.)

Tropical infections

(See Chapter 15.)

- *Yellow fever* (→ Yellow fever, p. 464) occurs in South America and Africa, with 90% of cases reported from Africa.
- *African trypanosomiasis (sleeping sickness)* occurs in a number of smallish areas scattered throughout West, Central, East, and southern Africa (→ African trypanosomiasis (sleeping sickness), p. 492 and → American trypanosomiasis (Chagas' disease), p. 493).
- *Lassa fever* (West Africa) and Bolivian, Argentine, and Venezuelan haemorrhagic fevers (→ Arenaviruses: Lassa fever (West Africa) and Bolivian, Argentine, and Venezuelan haemorrhagic fevers, p. 466).

Leishmaniasis

- *Marburg* and *Ebola viruses* which have caused epidemics of highly fatal haemorrhagic fever in Equatorial Africa, Congo DR, Sierra Leone, and Uganda (→ Filoviruses: Marburg and Ebola viruses, p. 467).
- Elephantiasis (lymphatic filariasis) (→ Elephantiasis (lymphatic filariasis), p. 494).
- *Melioidosis*, a dangerous infection caused by soil-dwelling bacteria in South East Asia, Northern Australia, and the tropical Americas (→ Melioidosis, p. 472).

Tropical medical kits

Medical kits for tropical forest expeditions should be robust and designed to keep water out. The rugged and humid nature of the jungle will quickly cause medicine labels to degrade, metal components to rust, and kit bags to fail.

The medical kit should be kept in a dry, well-ventilated area and be sealed sufficiently to prevent insect invasion. Consider the use of silica gel to keep the contents dry.

For discussion of contents, see Chapter 28.

Chapter 27

Caving

Section editor
Chris Johnson

Contributor
Paul Cooper

The underground environment 790
Humans underground 791
Risk management underground 792
Specific medical problems for cavers 794

The underground environment

Deep, tight caves are found both near to civilization and in very remote areas, the latter adding to the logistic difficulties. In some parts of the world, especially south-east Asia, accessing caves may be hazardous because landmines and other munitions from past conflicts may be strewn around outside, or abandoned inside. When searching for entrances in heavy undergrowth, beware of snakes and other venomous animals.

Caves are dangerous places. Lighting can depend upon torches, ceilings and floors are often uneven and may be slippery. Flooding is a possibility. Communications with the surface may be very limited. You are unlikely to survive a significant accident, and therefore *take care*, as rescue is likely to be limited to helping out the 'walking wounded'. However, caves are amongst the last unexplored areas on Earth and there are some great places to find!

Colonies of bats and birds, as well as ground creatures like to live in caves. They can spread disease to humans, while humans may be vectors aiding the spread of animal diseases.

Caves usually have a fairly constant low temperature of 5–8°C. Hypothermia (❷ Hypothermia, p. 622) is a significant risk especially where running or falling water creates high humidity, spray, and cave draughts, all of which intensify the chilling effect. It is a particular risk if you have to wait around for some time, or if you have to make an unanticipated bivouac; a space blanket kept in your pocket or helmet could be a life-saver.

Cave exploration often involves diving (see ❷ Cave diving, p. 793 and Chapter 24).

Types of caving expedition

Caving expeditions may be:

- Large expeditions, based at one site, often for several weeks. These are usually exploring a large cave system, will have many members, and will often have a specified medical officer. Deep cave exploration requires major logistic support.
- Smaller lightweight expeditions, with fewer members, often reconnaissance, the caving may be less challenging, but may be more remote.

Humans underground

Clothing

Typical cave clothing is impermeable and traps perspiration, so a prolonged wait at a pitch head after a vigorous climb can be very cold; the combination of a wet shell garment with damp undergarments leads to rapid heat loss. Up to half the heat loss from an otherwise well-insulated person is from the head, so keep a silk or fleece balaclava in your pocket and put it on when stationary. Cold injury, either hypothermia (➲ Hypothermia, p. 622) or non-freezing peripheral cold injury (trench foot ➲ Non-freezing cold injury, p. 632), is a risk during prolonged trips, especially in wet caves. Modern materials offer significant improvements; ensure that expedition members unfamiliar with the subterranean environment—e.g. scientists accompanying the trip—receive appropriate advice on gear.

Hygiene

Strict food handling and sanitation arrangements are essential underground. Latrine arrangements vary depending on the nature of the cave; many modern underground camping expeditions will bring out solid matter in plastic bags. Alcohol gel hand lotion should be available at the camp, but may not protect against viral gastroenteritis. When washing is impractical, baby wipes are useful for personal hygiene.

Minor injuries

(See ➲ Wounds, p. 268; ➲ Wound types and management, p. 272.)

'Crutch rot', split fingers, and minor foot injuries, blisters, and the like are common. Experienced cavers have their own views on how to deal with what are usually just minor irritations. Tissue superglue, used to repair skin splits on fingers and feet, is a useful addition to the underground first-aid kit.

Risk management underground

Rescue

Caving has a fatal accident rate twice that of climbing accidents in the UK (although the risk is still much lower than climbing in the Greater Ranges), but a relatively low non-fatal accident rate.[1] Some accidents, e.g. those caused by rock falls, may be unavoidable, but others are preventable. Be careful 'pushing the cave' when tired or cold. The low non-fatal accident rate indicates that there is a low margin for error and that death is common if something goes wrong. A relatively minor injury is likely to be fatal if the victim is unable to assist during the extraction. Small independent expeditions are usually incapable of mounting a major rescue without outside help.

An excellent cave rescue ropework manual, currently in the second edition, is available at ✆ http://www.lifeonaline.com. If planning to explore vertical caves, purchase and download the manual, and practise the techniques before departure.

Harness hang (also known as suspension trauma)

If someone is immobile upright in a harness for some time, the usual muscle pump in the legs ceases and venous return to the heart is impeded. This can lead to syncope with loss of consciousness. Usually when someone faints, they fall to the ground, venous return is restored, and cerebral perfusion resumes. However, in a harness this correction cannot occur, and the resultant loss of cerebral blood flow may be rapidly fatal. Cavers are particularly at risk when they are immobile in a harness on a rope, especially if unconscious. The first priority if you have an unconscious companion hanging on a rope, maybe knocked out from a falling rock, is to swing them horizontal, so that their legs, heart, and head are all at the same level. This will probably mean moving the point of suspension down to their waist, obviously taking suitable precautions to ensure that they don't come off the rope. You may only have a few minutes, so act quickly, but get them either horizontal, or ideally off the rope as soon as possible.

Bad air

Bad air is an issue in some caves, although you should usually be aware of the risks beforehand. The gases in question result from decaying organic matter, including guano, in caves with poor ventilation. Carbon monoxide monitors and supplementary oxygen may be required. Important gases are:
- Methane:
  - Odourless, lighter than air, disperses.
  - Formed from organic matter, common in coalmines.
  - Potential asphyxiation hazard.
  - Highly explosive, so avoid any naked flames, such as carbide lights, candles, or cooking stoves.

1 Mohr PD (2000). Gauging risk. *Descent*, 153, 20–4.

- Hydrogen sulphide:
  - Smells of rotten eggs; any such smell should prompt a rapid exit from the cave.
  - Early symptoms include headache, dizziness, numbness, and tingling.
  - May inactivate the olfactory nerves, rapidly reducing ability to sense scent, hence a false perception that it has gone.
  - Heavier than air, accumulates in caves with poor ventilation.
  - Present in volcanic areas.
  - Highly toxic, combining with haemoglobin and with cytochromes in a manner similar to cyanide to block cellular metabolism rapidly.

Biosecurity

Since 2006, bats in the northeastern USA and Canada have been dying in vast numbers as a result of white nose syndrome (WNS), a condition associated with fungal growth *(Geomyces destructans)* around the muzzles and wings of hibernating bats. European bats carry the fungus, but appear resistant to its effects. Direct bat-to-bat contact appears necessary for transmission, but the role of humans in its spread is debated, and Europeans caving in North America should ensure all their clothing and equipment has been carefully cleaned.

Cave diving

(See also Chapter 24.)

Scuba diving in caves is notoriously dangerous, with a significant number of fatalities amongst both inexperienced divers and those pushing the limits of exploration. The clarity of water in cave sumps can distort depth perception, subterranean currents may drag divers, while silt can suddenly reduce visibility. Safety can be enhanced by:

- Adequate prior experience and training in safer environments.
- Use of a continuous guide line to open water.
- Strict operation of depth rules.
- Breathing mixture management—no more than 1/3 of the supply used during access phase.
- Use of three independent sources of light.
- Additional information on aspects of diving medicine can be found in Chapter 24.

Specific medical problems for cavers

Cavers are at risk of catching some specific infectious diseases. If you consider that any of these pose a risk in the area that you plan to visit, seek expert advice before you go. Consult the Cave-Associated Disease Database, which is maintained by Dr Charles F. Cicciarella, Department of Kinesiology, Louisiana Tech University: ℘ http://www.latech.edu/education/faculty/cicciarella/cavedis/cave-disease-table2_1.html

American trypanosomiasis

(Chagas disease; see ➋ American trypanosomiasis (Chagas' disease), p. 493.)

Protozoan infection transmitted by faeces of tritomine bugs; widespread in South America. Infection develops through contamination of skin.

Histoplasmosis

A fungal infection inhaled from infected bats' droppings. It results in chronic malaise and, as it is usually diagnosed following chest X-ray (which may resemble sarcoid), it is not readily diagnosed in the field. Symptoms of severe pneumonia which are unresponsive to antibiotics would merit evacuation for a chest X-ray and investigation (treatment is with IV amphotericin). Although it may resolve spontaneously, specialist treatment with antifungals is likely to be required.

Leishmaniasis

(See ➋ Leishmaniasis, p. 490.)

Transmitted by sand flies, especially in China.

Leptospirosis

(See ➋ Leptospirosis, p. 471.)

Transmitted by exposure to water contaminated by rodent urine. It presents with an acute generalized febrile illness, usually with jaundice, and specialist investigation may be needed to distinguish it from other febrile illnesses in the tropics.

Rabies

(See ➋ Rabies, p. 461.)

Transmitted by cave bats. If visiting caves in areas where it is prevalent, ensure the party has been immunized pre-departure. European bats carry bat lyssaviruses 2, a rabies-like infection. The only case of UK-acquired rabies since 1902 was in a licensed bat handler bitten by an infected bat. There have only been four documented cases of humans being infected by a European bat lyssavirus in the past 25 years.

Relapsing fever

(See ⊃ Ticks, p. 288.)

Caused by a *Borrelia* spirochaete and transmitted by tick or louse. Tick-borne relapsing fever is prevalent on the west coast of North America and is common in caves, with an intermediate animal host. It results in a relapsing fever (!), together with headaches, abdominal pains, and myalgia. Treatment is with tetracycline, but this can result in a Jarisch–Herxheimer reaction (a severe allergic reaction due to the antibiotic killing large numbers of the organism).

St Louis encephalitis

Occurs in epidemics in the southern USA, and may be of particular risk to cavers as the intermediate host includes bats.

Skin problems

Siopel® silicone cream is recommended for macerated skin produced by prolonged contact with wetsuits.

Chapter 28

Medical kits

Section editor
Chris Johnson

Contributors
Jon Dallimore
Robert Conway
Penelope B. Granger
Burjor K. Langdana
Campbell MacKenzie
Daniel S. Morris

Medical kits and supplies 798
Personal medical kit 800
Team medical kit 802
Extra drugs and equipment for special environments 808
Extra materials for those with special skills 810

NB This chapter suggests the type of drug supplies and equipment that would be suitable for a medium-sized climbing expedition spending 6 weeks in a remote area. The kit is compatible with the advice given within individual chapters of this book.

However, this list should not be regarded as definitive, nor do we endorse any individual manufacturer's products. Factors such as the nature of the expedition, the skills of the medics, and the ease of access to high-quality medical facilities, together with cost and weight will all affect the extent of medical kit.

Medical kits and supplies

It is never possible to deal with every possible accident or illness—even with a large amount of medical equipment. Items from medical kits are used most frequently for blisters, headaches, minor cuts and sprains, sunburn, diarrhoea, and insect bites. Similar illnesses and accidents occur on all expeditions, but clearly extra drugs and equipment may be needed to deal with problems in particular environments.

It is often difficult to judge how much medical equipment to take and this will depend on:

- The size of the party, the duration of the trip, and its remoteness.
- The number of outlying camps.
- The likelihood of having to treat local staff and villagers (➲ Treating local people, not part of the expedition, p. 120).
- Local medical facilities.
- The medical knowledge of the team members/medic.
- Communications with other camps and remote medical help.

Obtaining supplies

Buying medical supplies from a retailer can be costly, and acquiring, packing, and labelling a medical kit can be time-consuming. Local pharmacists and NHS hospital trusts may be able to help by providing drugs at cost. Technically, GPs should not give NHS prescriptions for illnesses which may be acquired outside the UK, but many do.

In some parts of the world, prescription drugs are available over the counter but they may be counterfeit and the quality cannot be guaranteed.

Drug export

Expeditions carrying reasonable quantities of drugs are unlikely to encounter problems at customs when entering a country. However, it may be useful to have a doctor's letter stating that the drugs are for the personal use of the expedition team members and are not the subject of any commercial transaction.

Controlled drugs

Wherever possible, avoid taking 'controlled' drugs. A Home Office licence is required and must be returned within 28 days of return to the UK. For more details see ℘ http://www.gov.uk/controlled-drugs-licences-fees-and-returns. Any controlled drugs dispensed should be recorded in a controlled drugs register.

Be aware that drugs that are freely available in one country may be controlled or proscribed in another.

Storage and transport

- Where possible, avoid liquid medicines.
- Obtain tablets in blister packs—loose-packed tablets can disintegrate during the rigours of an expedition.
- Avoid splitting the medical kit between several team members—a vital piece of equipment may be 2 h walk away!

- Wrap the whole kit in waterproof/dustproof packaging (e.g. re-sealable polythene bags or in plastic boxes).
- Try to pack items which are used together in the same box, e.g. cotton buds, fluorescein strips, tetracaine, and chloramphenicol ointment for eye problems.
- Label each box with a laminated, waterproof list of its contents on the lid. If the kit is marked with a large red cross it may attract attention and be a target for thieves—medical supplies are very valuable in many parts of the world.
- Full instructions should be provided with each medical kit.
- A small personal medical kit should be carried by each expedition member at all times.

Personal medical kit

Each team member should carry a small supply of first-aid equipment for their own personal use. This should be kept in a compact waterproof and re-sealable container or bag.

- Paracetamol or preferred painkiller.
- Adhesive plasters.
- Antiseptic wipes.
- Blister kit.
- Piriton® or similar antihistamine.
- Insect repellent.
- Sunblock cream.
- Biox® for water purification.
- Rehydration sachets (e.g. Dioralyte®).

In addition, team members should carry sufficient personal medication for the duration of the trip, including antimalarials.

Team medical kit

The list in Table 28.1 indicates the types of drugs and equipment that a group of 20 people on a 6-week, high-altitude mountaineering expedition might wish to assemble. However, this list should only be regarded as indicative of the sort of kit required which may vary according to the exact nature of the work, the logistics available, and the skills of the medics.

In this text our treatment recommendations have been restricted to a relatively limited range of drugs and equipment that we feel most medics could use with reasonable safety. It is likely that a specialist in a particular area of medicine would want to take additional materials (➔ Extra drugs and equipment for special environments, p. 808; ➔ Extra materials for those with special skills, p. 810) and more specialist kit.

Table 28.1 Drugs and equipment list

Antimicrobials	Amounts
Azithromycin 500 mg	20 tablets
Ceftriaxone for injection 2 g	5 ampoules
Chloramphenicol (eye) ointment 1%	3 × 4 g
Ciprofloxacin 500 mg	50 tablets
Clarithromycin 250 mg	40 tablets
Co-amoxiclav 250/125	84 tablets
Doxycycline 100 mg	56 capsules
Fluconazole 150 mg	4 tablets
Gentisone® HC (ear drops)	10 mL × 4
Mebendazole 100 mg	20 tablets
Metronidazole 400 mg	100 tablets
Metronidazole suppositories 1 g	10
Rabies vaccine 1 mL (lyophilized)	2
Riamet® malaria treatment pack	2
Valaciclovir 500 mg	10 tablets
Painkillers, local anaesthetics/sedatives	
Aspirin 300 mg	32 tablets
Bupivacaine 0.5% injection	10 mL × 5
Co-codamol 30/500	80 tablets
Diclofenac 50 mg	100 tablets
Diclofenac 75 mg suppositories	5
Ibuprofen 400 mg	80 tablets
GTN spray	1
Ketamine for injection (50 mg/mL)	2 vials

(continued)

Table 28.1 (*Cont.*)

Lidocaine 1% for injection	5 mL × 10
Lidocaine gel	2 tubes
Lorazepam for injection 2 mg	5 ampoules
Midazolam for injection (10 mg/5 mL)	5 ampoules
Paracetamol 500 mg	100 tablets
Tetracaine (amethocaine) eye drops	6 single dose units
Zopiclone 7.5 mg	20 tablets
Gastrointestinal	
Antacid tablets	100 tablets
Bisacodyl	20 tablets
Buccastem 3 mg buccal tablets	10 tablets
Oral rehydration solution sachets	40 sachets
GlucoGel®	2 ampoules
Loperamide 2 mg	50 capsules
Omeprazole 20 mg	56 tablets
Ondansetron 4 mg	10 tablets
Prochlorperazine 5 mg	56 tablets
Prochlorperazine injection 12.5 mg	5 ampoules
Prochlorperazine suppositories 25 mg	10
Cardiovascular	
Atropine for injection 600 micrograms	5 ampoules
Bisoprolol 5 mg	20 tablets
Furosemide 40 mg	10 tablets
Respiratory/allergy	
Adrenaline 1:1000	5 × 1 mL
Beclometasone inhaler 100 micrograms	2
Chlorphenamine 4 mg	40 tablets
Chlorphenamine injection 10 mg	5 ampoules
Adrenaline auto-injector	2
Hydrocortisone injection 100 mg	10 ampoules
Otrivine-Antistin® (eye drops) 10 mL	2
Prednisolone EC 5 mg	112 tablets
Salbutamol inhaler	2
Spacer device	1

(continued)

Table 28.1 (*Cont.*)

Altitude	
Acetazolamide 250 mg	100 tablets
Dexamethasone 2 mg	40 tablets
Dexamethasone for injection 4 mg/mL, 1 mL ampoules	5
Nifedipine MR caps 10 mg	20 capsules
EmOx®	1 set
Portable altitude chamber	1
Creams and ointments	
Aciclovir cream (Zovirax®)	2 g × 6
Aqueous cream	50 g tube
Clotrimazole cream	20 g × 6
Haemorrhoidal cream	1
Hydrocortisone cream 1%	30 g × 4
Mupirocin cream	15 g × 6
Silver nitrate cautery sticks	5
Terbinafine 1% cream	30 g × 4
Topical steroid/antibiotic ear drops	10 mL × 4
Tropicamide 1%	5 single dose units
Airway care—supplies for appropriately trained individuals	
Bag-valve mask apparatus	1
ETT 6 mm for tracheostomy	1
ETTs 7, 8 mm	2 of each
LMA sizes 3, 4, 5	2 of each
Catheter mounts for above	2
Insertion bougie for ETTs	1
Handheld suction unit	1
Laryngoscope	1
Nasopharyngeal airway Size 5, 6	2
Oro-pharyngeal airways Size 2, 3, 4	2 of each
Oxygen cylinder	1
Oxygen tubing	1
Pulse oximeter	1
Major trauma	
Bladder syringe 50 mL	2
Blizzard blanket®	1
Catheter bag and tubing	2

(*continued*)

Table 28.1 (*Cont.*)

Cervical collar (adjustable)	2
Chest drain 32 F	2
Combat application tourniquet	1
Disposable scalpels	2
Gloves sterile (medium)	10 pairs
Heimlich valve	2
Kendrick traction device	1
Clinical gloves (non-sterile)	100
Nasogastric tube 12 FG	2
Needle holder	1
QuikClot® 1st Response Advanced Clotting Sponge 25 g	Pack of 5
Safety pins	12
Sam splint	2
Scissors	1
Skin staples and remover	1
Sutures:	4
2/0 silk straight	5
4/0 non-absorbable suture	5
5/0 non-absorbable suture	
Tissue glue	1
Toothed forceps	1
Tranexamic acid 100 mg/mL, 5 mL ampoules	5
Tuff Cut® scissors	1
Urinary catheter 14 FG	2
Examination/other	
Blood glucose monitoring equipment	1
Dental first-aid kit	1
Fluorescein eye test strips	10
Head torch, pen torch	1
Malaria ICT	1
Stethoscope	1
Thermometer (digital)	1
Thermometer (low reading)	1
Tick remover	2
Urine pregnancy kit	2

(continued)

Table 28.1 (*Cont.*)

Dressings	
Adhesive plasters	50 assorted
Alcohol swabs	100 × 2
Crepe bandages 5 cm	5
Dressing No. 15	2
Eye dressing No. 16	4
Gauze swabs 5 × 5 cm²	100
Hypoallergenic tape 2.5 cm	2 rolls
Non-adherent dressing 5 cm²	5
Non-adherent dressing 10 cm²	5
Steri-Strips™, assorted	4 packets
Triangular bandages	8
Tubigrip (knee/ankle)	10 m of each
Vaseline gauze 10 cm²	10
Cling wrap	1 roll
Zinc oxide tape	2 rolls
Injection equipment and intravenous fluids	
2 mL, 5 mL, 10 mL syringes	20 of each
1 mL insulin syringes (rabies intradermal)	5
Blue, green, orange needles	20 of each
Glucose 5%	500 mL × 4
Ringers Lactate (Hartmanns) 1 L	1000 mL × 3
Giving sets	5
IV cannulae 14 G, 18 G	10 of each
Normal saline 1 L	1000 mL × 3
Sharps box	1

Reference texts

This book is available in a digital as well as a printed version. An up-to-date *BNF* or other pharmacopoeia should be carried at all times - to check drug doses, side effects and contraindications. Digital drug guides such as the *BNF* app or *Epocrates* app can reduce the need for a relatively heavy book—although rely upon a charged and functioning phone or tablet. Also see: ℘ http://www.medicines.org.uk

Specialist equipment

The use of these items requires special training and so will depend on the medical skills in the group:

- Stethoscope.
- Anaeroid sphygmomanometer.
- Auriscope/ophthalmoscope.
- Oropharyngeal/nasopharyngeal airways.
- Nasogastric tube.
- Urinary catheter.
- Chest drains and Heimlich valves, or Thoraquik, for pneumothorax.
- Suturing equipment.
- Dental forceps, if skilled.
- Snake (or other) anti-venom.

Extra drugs and equipment for special environments

Malaria medication

(See ❯ Chemoprophylactic drugs and combinations, p. 485.)

Take spare prophylactic antimalarials if the expedition is going to a region where malaria is endemic—someone always loses their tablets! Also take a different and appropriate drug for standby (prospective) treatment of a fever that could be malaria (e.g. Riamet® (co-artemether or malarone (atovaquone-proguanil))). Rapid diagnostic tests for malaria can be very useful (❯ Diagnosis, p. 482). Mosquito nets should be re-treated with permethrin every 3–6 months (depending on the amount of rain and UV exposure); always carry spare permethrin together with protective gloves.

Sailing, boating, or canoeing

(See Chapter 22 and Chapter 23.)

Participants develop chapped hands, salt water boils, and sunburn. Lanolin-based hand cream is useful and cinnarizine is recommended for seasickness.

Grab bag

A specific medical kit to be taken to the life raft if abandoning ship that may also double as an emergency treatment bag should contain:
• Emergency analgesics (oral and IM).
• Seasickness medications (a large stock and including drugs that can be absorbed by routes other than oral).
• Antibiotics.
• Rehydration salts.
• Suturing kit.
• Immobilization splints, strapping, bandages.

Tropical areas

(See Chapter 26.)

Wound infections are common, and small individual iodine tincture bottles are recommended to clean wounds plus additional topical antibiotics. Anti-venoms for snakes, scorpions, etc. may be considered for high-risk areas and occupations plus several long 10 cm-wide crepe bandages for pressure immobilization (❯ Treatment of snake-bite, p. 553).

Diving expeditions

(See Chapter 24.)

Otitis externa (diver's ear) is common; take extra antibacterial eardrops (e.g. Gentisone® HC) and consider aluminium acetate or distilled water after each dive. Oxygen, chest drains, and ventilation equipment may be needed. Find out where decompression facilities exist before you need them! Consider additional antibiotics for marine wound infections.

Mountain expeditions

(See Chapter 21.)

Oxygen is bulky and heavy but is essential for any trip above 6000 m. EmOx® is used by some groups – chemical oxygen from the reaction of percarbonate, manganese and water. Acetazolamide, nifedipine, and dexamethasone should certainly be carried. Consider the excellent Kendrick traction device for thigh fractures as these can be life-saving in remote areas—they are lightweight (around 500 g) and are very popular with mountain rescue teams.

Desert environments

(See Chapter 25.)

Dehydration and heat-related illnesses are of major concern. Strongly consider IV fluids and plenty of cannulae and giving sets. Total block sun cream and goggles to keep sand out of eyes are recommended.

Extra materials for those with special skills

Ocular first-aid kit
The first-aid kit listed here is lightweight and will fit into a small pouch.

Equipment
- Pentorch 9 blue filter.
- Pocket ophthalmoscope.
- Magnifying loupe.
- Eye pads.
- Eye shield.
- Surgical tape.
- pH paper.
- Minor operations kit.
- Single-use drops ('Minims'®):
  - Tetracaine (amethocaine)/oxybuprocaine (topical anaesthetic).
  - Fluorescein 1% (use only after topical anaesthetic for corneal staining).
  - Cyclopentolate 1% (pupil dilation and pain relief).
  - Artificial tears (dry eyes and snow blindness).
  - Tropicamide 1% (for pupil dilation).
  - Pilocarpine 2% (for reversal of pupil dilation by tropicamide).

Other topical medication:
- Antibiotic ointment and drops (e.g. chloramphenicol) (conjunctivitis, any minor infection, or snow blindness).
- Ofloxacin (reserve for more serious corneal infection and all contact lens-related infection).
- Sodium cromoglicate (allergic conjunctivitis).
- Fluorometholone (mild steroid; use cautiously in snow blindness).
- These drops are given four times daily except ofloxacin, which can be given hourly for serious corneal infection.
- Remember oral analgesia is required for a painful eye.

Useful equipment and drugs for ENT problems
- Head torch.
- Forceps.
- Nasal tampons.
- Gentisone® HC ointment.
- Amoxicillin.
- Silver nitrate sticks.

Remote dentistry kit list
Suppliers: The Dental Directory, 6 Perry Way, Witham, Essex, CM8 3SX, UK. Tel: 01376 391 100, ℘ http://www.dental-directory.co.uk

Some items may well be duplicated within your standard medical kit.

Instruments (sterile disposable kits available which come with their own tray):

- Two dental mirrors (size 3).
- One flat-plastic (a stainless steel instrument for placing dental filling material onto tooth).
- College tweezers.
- Spoon excavator (medium)—for scraping out soft caries (tooth decay).
- Spencer Wells suturing forceps.
- Fine curved surgical scissors.
- One double ended stainless steel cement mixing spatula.
- One glazed mixing paper pad for mixing and moulding temporary filling materials.
- Disposable scalpel (number 15 blade).
- Cold sterilization tablets.

Medicaments

- Temporary filling materials—glass ionomer powder + liquid or intermediate restorative material (IRM), Cavit™.
- Chlorhexidine 0.2% mouthwash (Corsodyl®).
- Duraphat® (high fluoride varnish).
- Ledermix® paste.
- Antibiotics—co-amoxiclav 500/125 mg, metronidazole 200 mg, and clindamycin 150 mg.
- Painkillers—ibuprofen, paracetamol, codeine-phosphate.
- Dental local anaesthetic cartridges—2% lidocaine with 1:80,000 adrenaline and 3% prilocaine with felypressin. Allow 4 cartridges per person.
- Toothpaste for sensitive teeth.
- Eugenol (oil of cloves) topical analgesic.

Others

- Sterile gloves.
- Cotton wool rolls.
- 3/0 black silk or Vicryl® suture on fine semilunar needle.
- Rapid IMF (wire-free, easy to remove intermaxillary fixation).
- Stainless steel wire for eyelet wiring (24 G for eyelets, 26 G for ligatures) or electrical cord for harvesting copper wire.
- Safety-plus disposable syringes—27 G long (can be used in upper and lower jaw).
- 5 mL syringe with blunt needles (for irrigation and flushing out debris below operculum).

Practicals

- Two head torches + batteries.
- Gas aerosol suitable for camera cleaning—ideal for drying teeth and cavities.

Optional equipment (if you have gained experience in their use)

- Upper single root extraction forceps.
- Upper molar extraction forceps left and right.
- Lower molar extraction forceps.
- Lower single root extraction forceps.
- Fine Luxator or Elevator-Couplands Chisel Size 2.

Index

A

Abbreviated Mental Test
  Score 253
abdominal examination 172
abdominal pain 65–6,
  384–95, 412–13
abrasions 276
abscesses 278
Acanthamoeba 294
acclimatization 654, 754–5
accommodation, see
  campsites
acetaminophen 93–4, 95
acetazolamide 667
Achilles tendon 444
achlorous algae 294
Acinetobacter baumannii 503
Acinetobacter spp. 294
ackee 580–1
acromio-clavicular joint 422
acute abdomen 384–5, 386
acute chest infection 376–8
acute confusional
  states 523–4
acute mountain
  sickness 656–61
acute oxygen toxicity 735
acute respiratory distress
  syndrome 690–1
acute urinary
  retention 387, 406–7
adrenaline
  auto-injectors 54, 560–1
Aeromonas
  hydrophila 294, 295
African tick fever 478–9
African trypanosomiasis 492
ageing 58
airbags 645
air evacuation 153–4
airway
  anatomy 300, 301
  assessment and manage-
    ment 186–8, 214
  medical kit supplies 804
  obstruction 224, 225
alcohol abuse/
  misuse 519, 539
alcohol withdrawal 539
allergic dermatitis 579
allergies 54, 803
alligators 545–6
altitude, see high altitude
  headings
alum 103

amatoxin poisoning 583
American trypanosomiasis
  493, 794
amoeba 294
amoebic dysentery 401
AMPLE history 204
amputations 277, 433
anaesthesia 585–605
  dental 358–61
  hand 435
  ketamine 600–1
  local infiltra-
    tion 590–3, 802–3
  peripheral nerve
    blocks 594–5
  spinal 596–8
anal fissure 397
analgesics 93–4, 95, 802–3
Anapen™ 560–1
anaphylactic shock 236–7,
  238
anaphylaxis 54, 236–7, 238
Anaplasma
  phagocytophilum 503
Ancylostoma 496
Ancylostoma braziliense 290
Ancylostoma caninum 290
animal hazards 82–3,
  541–76, 610–11, 639,
  687, 771
ankle injuries 445
ankle strapping 453
annelids 570
anorexia nervosa 524
anterior draw test 440–2
antibiotic-resistant
  bacteria 502–3
antihypertensives 52
antimalarials 62, 485–6, 487
antimicrobials 802
antivenom 550–65
ant stings 560–1
anxiety disorders 519, 522
appendicitis 65–6,
  386, 390–2
application forms 518
Aqua Pure Traveller™ 106
Aquatab™ tablets 104
Arcanobacterium
  haemolyticum 503
arenaviruses 466
argasid ticks 288
Argentine haemorrhagic
  fever 466
arm
  forearm injuries 426–7

  supports and
    slings 420, 421
  upper arm injuries 422–4
arthropods 560–1
Ascaris lumbricoides 496
Asperger's syndrome 525
aspiration 688
aspiration pneumonia 691
asthma 50, 380–2
athlete's foot 298
atmospheric
  pressure 756, 758
atovaquone–proguanil 486
attention deficit hyperactivity disorders 525
atypical mycobacteria 477
Auchmeromyia luteola 289–90
Australian bat lyssavirus
  502
autism spectrum
  conditions 525
automated external
  defibrillators 217
autonomic conflict 688
autonomy 112
avalanche probes 644
avalanches 642–7
avalanche
  transceivers 142, 644
Avalung® 645
avian influenza
  H5N1 501
  H7N9 502
aviophobia 522
Avloclor® 486
AVPU scale 202, 215
axillary nerve block 595

B

Bacillus cereus 400
back pain 450–1, 697
bacterial infections 470–9,
  502–3
bacterial meningitis 319,
  473, 474
bacterial vaginosis 509
bad air 792–3
bad news 528, 532
Balamuthia
  mandrillaris 294, 504
bandages 270
barometric pressure 655
barotrauma 334, 740–1
bases, see campsites
basic life support 220–2

bats
  lyssavirus 502, 794
  white nose syndrome 793
Battle's sign 313
BCG 37, 476
beacons 142, 163–4,
  613, 682
bears 542–3, 611
bed bugs 287
bed nets 484–5
bed-wetting 525
beefworm 289–90
bee stings 560–1, 561
Behçet's disease 511
bends 736–8
beneficence 112
benzodiazepines 602
bereavement 528
berne 289–90
biceps, long head
  rupture 424
big cats 543
bilharzia 498, 499
biliary colic 386, 389
binge eating disorder 524
Biox Aqua™ 104
birds 611
bites and stings 63, 276,
  284–5, 544, 550–72,
  699, 770–1
blackouts 316–19, 319
blanket (and poles)
  stretcher 152
blast injuries 207
bleeding 269; see also
  haemorrhage
blister beetles 562, 563
blisters 276–7, 698
Blood Care Foundation
  137
blood pressure 174–5
blood supplies 137
blow-out fractures 308–10
'blue bottle' 568–9
boats, see sailing
body lice (Pediculus
  humanus) 286
body temperature 174,
  622–5, 623, 686–7,
  750–3, 752–3
boiling water 104
Bolivian haemorrhagic
  fever 466
bot fly 289–90
boxing glove dressing 431
box jellyfish 568–9
break bone fever 465–6
breaking bad news 532
breath-hold diving 727
breathing
  children 66
  emergencies 190–3, 214

normal rate 66, 175
shortness of breath 246–7
bristle worms 570
British Standard: BS8848 19
broad arm sling 420, 421
brucellosis 470
bruises 276
buccal/labial intraligamentary injection 362
bullimia nervosa 524
bunyaviruses 467–9
buoyancy aids 686–7
bupivacaine 590
burn out 699
burns 280–3, 698
bursitis
  olecranon 426
  patella 440
  subacromial 423
Buruli ulcer 477

C

calcaneal fractures 446
calf pain 444
Callitroga
  hominivorax 289–90
calorific requirements 98
Camelbak 106
camels 544
campfires 778–9
campsites 22, 82–3,
  107, 615, 650, 692,
  747, 778–80
Campylobacter 401
candidiasis 509
canoeing 692–4, 808
capillary refill time 175, 417
carbohydrates 100
carbon dioxide retention 734
carbon monoxide
  poisoning 615–16, 735
cardiogenic shock 235
cardiopulmonary resuscitation
  (CPR) 220–2
cardiovascular disease 53
cardiovascular drugs 803
carotid pulse 174
casualty evacuation, see
  medical evacuation
catering personnel 96
caterpillar stings 562
catfish 547
causation 77–8
caving 789–95
celebrities 128
cellulitis 278
  orbital 330–1
  preseptal 331
centipedes 565
cerebral arterial gas
  embolism 741

cerebral perfusion
  pressure 314
cervical collars 200
cervical
  spine 199–200, 200–1
cestodes 499
Chagas' disease 493, 794
chain of survival 216
chair carry 151
chancroid 511
charity organizations 17
chemical eye injury 328
chest
  drains 192
  examination 171–2
  flail chest 193, 372–3
  infections 376–8
  pain 242–4, 370
  sucking wound 193
chiggers 287
chigoe flea 290
chikungunya fever 468–9
children
  in cold weather 614–15
  consent issues 23
  health issues 62–7
  at high altitude 670–1
chlamydia 507, 508, 509
chloramine T 104
chlorine 104
chlorine dioxide 104
chloroquine 486
choking 224, 225
cholangitis 389
cholecystitis 386, 389
cholera 401, 402
cholera vaccine 33
Chromobacterium
  violaceum 294
chronic fatigue syndrome 56
chronic mountain
  sickness 672–3
Chrysomyia bessania 289–90
ciguatera poisoning 574
Cimex 287
circulation 194–5, 214–15
clavicle fractures 422
clinical competence 116–17
clinical
  measurements 174–5
Clostridium perfringens 400
clothing 63, 285, 485,
  618–19, 648, 686–7,
  693–4, 714, 746,
  782–4, 791
cnidarian sting 568–9
coagulation–flocculation
  103
  with disinfection 105
coastal waters 675–00
Cochliomyia
  hominivorax 289–90

codeine 93–4, 95
coelenterate sting 568–9
cold climates 607–36
cold injury 626–32
collapse 212
collar and cuff sling 420, 421
Colles' fracture 428
coma 248–9
commercial
  expeditions 17, 78
common cold 336
communication 144–5,
  160–4, 682, 704
compartment
  syndrome 443
conduct disorders 525
condylar fractures 306
cone shells 570, 571
confidentiality 23
confusion 252, 523–4
Congo floor
  maggots 289–90
conjunctivitis 326–7
consciousness 175, 249
consent 23
constipation 404
consultations 22
contact dermatitis 579
contact lenses 325, 619
continuing care 206
contraception 410–11
controlled drugs 42, 798
contusions 276
convulsions 254–5
convulsive syncope 317
cooking, see food storage
  and preparation
cooking gas 615, 650, 692
coprine poisoning 582
coral 568–9
Cordylobia
  anthropophaga 289–90
core temperature 622–5,
  750–3
cornea 327–8
coryza 336
COSPAS-SARSAT 163–4
costs 16–18
cougars 543
cowbane 580–1
crab 287
creams 804
creeping eruption 290
crew selection 712
cricothyroidotomy 188
Crimean–Congo haemor-
  rhagic fever 467
crisis management 133–67
critical incident
  debriefing 527
crocodiles 545–6
Crohn's disease 54–5

cruciate ligaments 442
crush injury 234, 277
Cryptosporidium spp.
  103, 400
cubomedusoids 568–9
cultural adjustment 517
cultural clashes 113–15
currents 677
cutaneous larva migrans 290
cutaneous leishmaniasis 490
cuts 272–3, 699
Cyclospora cayetanensis 504
cyclosporiasis 504
cytomegalovirus 458–9

D

Daintree ulcer 477
deadfall 774
death 6–8, 166–7, 641
deathcap mushroom 582–3
debriefing 527, 530–1
decision-making 116–17
decompression
  sickness 736–8
DEET 771
dehydration 65, 240, 616,
  651, 697, 719, 760
delirium 252, 253
dengue fever 465–6
Depo-Provera® 410
depression 522–4
Dermatobia hominis 289–90
dermatophytosis 296
desalinators 708
deserts 745–67, 809
desmopressin 525
dexamethasone 667–8
diabetes 50–2, 256–8
diabetic ketoacidosis 258
Diamox® 667
diarrhoea 65, 398–403
diazepam 602
diclofenac 93–4, 95
diet 98–100, 651
digital nerve block 592
diphtheria 470–1
disability 202, 215
disabled travellers 55–6
disaster medicine 130–1
dislocations 420
  elbow 426
  fingers 431
  foot 446–7
  hand 431
  hip 437
  jaw (TMJ) 309–10
  knee 441
  patellar 441
  shoulder 422–3, 696

thumb 431
toe 446
diverticulitis 387, 391–2
diving 725–43, 793, 808
documentation 89–90, 155
dogs 544
doxycyline 486
dressings 270, 806
drinking bottle filters 106
drowning 676–81, 688–91,
  696, 720
drowsiness 64
drugs
  abuse/misuse 519, 538–9
  controlled drugs 42, 798
  exporting 42, 798
  list of supplies for team
    medical kit 802
  obtaining supplies 42, 798
  prescribing and
    administration 92–4
  storage 86, 798–9
dry eyes 327
Dukoral™ 33
dumping waves 678
dust storms 747
duty of care 76, 118
dysentery 398–401
dyspnoea 246–7

E

eardrum rupture 334
ear problems 334, 698,
  740, 742
ear temperature 753
eating disorders 519, 524
Ebola virus 467
echinoderms 570
ectoparasites 286–91
ectopic
  pregnancy 387, 394–5
EHIC form 74–5
Ehrlichia chaffeensis 503
Ehrlichia ewingii 503
elbow injuries 426–7
electrolytes 760–2
elephantiasis 494, 495
elephants 544
el torsalo 289–90
email 162
emergency response
  plan 136–9
emerging infections 500–4
empowerment 113
endotracheal tubes 187
energy
  requirements 98, 616
entamoeba 401
ENT equipment and
  drugs 810
enteric fevers 477–8

Enterobius vermicularis 497
Enterococcus faecium 503
enterotoxigenic *Escherichia coli* (ETEC) 33
environmental control 203, 215
environmental impact 82–3, 124–5, 613, 639, 681, 686–7, 729
epicondylitis 426
Epidermophyton 296
epididymitis 408
epilepsy 53, 318–19
EpiPen® 54, 560–1
epistaxis 335
ergotism 583
erucism 562
erysipeloid 294, 295
Erysipelothrix rhusiopathiae 294, 295
erythema migrans 472
Escherichia coli 33, 400, 503
escorpión 560
ETHANE report 144–5
ethics 112–15
evacuation 12–13, 24, 146, 153–6, 366–7, 722–3, 732–3
examination 170–3
exercised-induced muscle cramps 766
exertional heat stroke 748, 749
expedition medical officer
essential skills 45
role 20–5
expedition medicine 2–3
scope 4–5
specialist courses 45
types of medical problems 10–11
expeditions 2–3
assessing 18
costs 16–18
destinations 4–5
information sources 18
interaction with other expeditions 124
joining 16–18
post-expedition issues 25, 60, 540
team selection 26
types 16–17
expired air ventilation 683
explosions 207
exposure 203, 215
extensor tendon injuries 432
extreme challenges 17
eyelid laceration 328–9

eyes 324–32, 559, 619, 634–5

F

face
bone fractures 306–10
examination 171
injuries 302–3
lacerations 304
faecal waste 108–9
fainting 317, 319
falciparum malaria 480–9
fascia iliaca block 594, 595
fats 100
favism 581
favus 581
feet, see foot
felon 297
femoral
fractures 194–5, 437–8
femoral pulse 174
fever 64, 262–3
filarial worms 494
film projects 17, 126–8
finger injuries 431, 433
finger nails 297, 298, 434
fire ants 560–1
fireman's carry 150–1
first-aid training 44–5
fish
bites and stings 546–7, 566–9
poisonous 574–6
fitness to dive 730, 731
flail chest 193, 372–3
flash floods 679
Flavobacterium spp. 294
fleas 286, 289–91
flexor tendon injuries 432
floods 679
fluid-induced hyponatraemia 762
fluid intake 651, 760–2
flukes 498–9
flumazenil 602
flush drowning 688
flying
divers 727
phobia 522
fly larvae 289–91
focal seizures 318
folliculitis 511, 512
food storage and preparation 96–7, 616, 650–1, 693, 708–9
foot
injuries 446–7
non-freezing cold injury 632
skin conditions 296–8

tropical immersion foot 787
footwear 619, 632, 714, 746
forearm injuries 426–7
foreign body
cornea 327–8
ear canal 334
nasal 335
throat 336
under nails 434
fractures 418
ankle 445
blow-out 308–10
calcaneal 446
clavicle 424
Colles' 430
condylar 306
distal radius 428
elbow 426
facial bones 306–10
femoral 194–5, 437–8
foot 446–7
forearm 427
hand 431
hip 437
humerus 424
knee 440–1
mandibular 306, 307
maxillary 307
metatarsal 446
nasal 308
orbital 308–10
patella 440, 442
pelvic 195, 436–7
radial head 427
ramus 306
rib 372–3
scaphoid 428
shoulder 424
stress 446
tibial 443
tibial tuberosity 442
toe 446
zygomatic 307–8
free diving 727
freezing cold injury 626–31
frostbite 628–31
frostnip 626–8, 628
fuel 615, 650, 692, 707, 779
'fugu' 574
fungal infections 296, 298
fungi 577–84

G

gallstone disease 388–9
gamekeeper's thumb 431
Gamow bag 666

gar fish 547
gastrointestinal bleed-
    ing 260, 261, 396–7
gastrointestinal drugs 803
gastrointestinal
    obstruction 392
gastro-oesophageal reflux
    disease 388
generalized seizures 318–19
genital herpes 510–11
genital lumps 511
genital sores and
    ulcers 510–11
genital warts 511, 512
giardiasis (Giardia lamblia)
    102, 400
Gila monster 560
gingivitis 350
Glasgow Coma
    Scale 203, 312–13
golfer's elbow 426
gonorrhoea 507, 508, 509
good practice 118
'Good Samaritan' cover 78
grab bag 717, 808
green whistle 602
grief 528
group A streptococci 503
group meetings 114
Guedel airway 187
gynaecology 410–13
gyromitrin poisoning 583

H

haemarthrosis 440
haematoma block 593
haemorrhage 194–5, 196,
    214–15, 269
haemorrhoids 397, 698
haemothorax 193
Haglund's spur
    deformity 444
hallucinogenics 539
hand
    examination 171, 430
    hygiene 109
    injuries 430–2
    local anaesthesia 435
    skin conditions 296–8
hantavirus haemor-
    rhagic fever with renal
    syndrome 468
hantavirus pulmonary
    syndrome 468
harness hang 792
harvest mites 287
head
    anatomy 300, 301
    injuries 304–5,
        312–15, 696

headache 250, 251, 656
head lice (Pediculus
    capitis) 286
healers 122
health clinics 84–6
health questionnaire 47
heart attack 371
heat cramps 766
heat exhaustion 748, 749
heat oedema 766
heat-related
    illness 240, 748–53
heat stress 757–8
heatstroke 748, 749, 750
heat syncope 766
Heimlich valve 191
helicopter evacuation 153,
    154, 722
helminths 496–7
HELP survival position 720
hepatitis, viral 458–9
hepatitis A vaccine 33
hepatitis B vaccine 34
hernias 387, 393
herpetic whitlow 297
HF radios 164
high altitude 325, 332,
    637–73, 804
high-altitude cerebral
    oedema (HACE) 664–6
high-altitude headache 656
high-altitude pulmonary
    oedema (HAPE) 661–6
high-altitude
    retinopathy 332, 667
high-arm sling 420, 421
high-pressure gases 734–5
hip injuries 436–8
hippopotamuses 545
histamine-like
    syndrome 574
histoplasmosis 794
history-taking 170, 215
HIV 56, 512–14
honey bees 561
hook worm 496
hornets 560–1
horses 544
hostage-taking 534–6
hot environments
    deserts 745–67, 809
    tropical
        forest 769–87, 808
human bocavirus 502
human bot fly 289–90
human immunodeficiency
    virus 56, 512–14
human waste
    disposal 108–9
humerus fracture 424
humidity 770, 782

'hunting response' 614–17
hydration, see dehydration
hydrogen sulphide 793
hyenas 545
hygiene 22, 88–90.3; see
    also personal hygiene
Hymenoptera stings 560–1
hyperbaric chambers 666
hypercapnia 734
hypertension 52
hyperthermia 240, 748
hypnotics 539
hypobaric hypoxia 154
hypoglycaemia 256
hyponatraemia 762
hypothermia 622–5, 688,
    696, 790
hypovolaemic shock 234
hypoxia 654, 742

I

ibotenic poisoning 582
ibuprofen 93–4, 95
illness assessment
    form 176–7
iloprost 629
immersion 688–91,
    696, 720
immersion foot 632
immunizations 28–40, 62
immunosuppression 56
incident reports 24
indigestion 388
infectious
    diseases 455–14, 620
inferior dental block 358
infestations 286–91
inflammatory bowel
    disease 54–5
influenza
    avian (H5N1) 501
    avian (H7N9) 502
    pandemic swine flu
        (H1N1) 502
influenza vaccine 34
informed consent 23
ingrowing toenails 296,
    297
injection equipment 806
inland waters 675–95
insect bites and stings 63,
    284–5, 560–5, 770–1
insecticide-treated nets 484
insect repellents 484–5, 771
inshore drift 677
institutional expeditions 16
insulin 52
insurance 74–5, 79, 713
intellectual disorders 524–5
Internet 162

interpersonal disharmony 114–15
interviews 518
intestinal obstruction 386
intestinal worms 496–7
intra-oral lacerations 304
intravenous fluids 195, 806
in-water recompression 737
iodine 104
Irukandji syndrome 569
ISOBAR 144–5
Ixiaro® 35
ixodid ticks 288

J

jaguars 543
Jamaican vomiting sickness 580–1
Japanese encephalitis 460
Japanese encephalitis vaccine 35
Jarisch–Herxheimer reaction 795
jaw
  dislocation 309–10
  fracture 306, 307
jellyfish 568—569, 699
jet lag 322–3
Jext® 54
jigger flea 290
jumper ants 560–1
justice 113

K

kala-azar 490
Katadyne silver 104
Katayama fever 498
kayaking 686–7, 692–4, 698
ketamine 600–1, 602
kidnapping 534–6
killer bees 561
kitchens 96–7
kite surfing 686–7
Klebsiella pneumoniae 503
knee injuries 440–2
Komodo dragon 560
konzo 581
Korean haemorrhagic fever 468

L

lacerations 272–3, 304, 328–9, 447
Lachman test 442
Lake Louise score 656–9, 671
Lariam® 62, 485–6
larva currens 496
laryngeal mask airways 187

LASEK/LASIK 325
Lassa fever 466
lateral collateral ligament 441
lathyrism 581
latrines 108, 781, 791
leadership 114–15
learning disorders 524–5
ledermix paste 348, 349
leeches 290–1
legal issues 76–9
leishmaniasis 490, 787, 794
leopards 543
lepidopterism 562
leprosy 477
leptospirosis 471, 794
Lewis 'hunting response' 614–17
lice 286–7
lidocaine 590
life rafts 722–3
ligament injuries
  ankle 445
  hand 431
  knee 441–2
lightning 208–9
limb injuries 173, 416–17
lions 543
lip laceration 304
liver flukes 499
living off the land 578
lizard bites 560
local anaesthesia 590–3, 802–3
  dental 358–61
  hand 435
local people 24, 118, 120–2
log roll 148, 149
long head of biceps rupture 424
loss of consciousness 175, 249
lost persons 140–2
low back pain 450–1, 697
lower gastrointestinal bleeding 396–7
lower leg injuries 443
Ludwig's angina 366–7
Lyme disease 472
lymphatic filariasis 494, 495

M

machete 784
McMurray's test 440–2
maggots 289–90
malaria 480–9, 808
Malarivon® 486
Malarone® 62, 486
Malassezia furfur 296
mallet finger 433

mandibular fractures 306, 307
man overboard 723
Mantoux test 476
Marburg virus 467
marine animals 566–76
marine wound infections 294–5
mastoiditis 334
mauve stinger 569
maxillary fractures 307
maxillofacial examination 302–3
medial collateral ligament 441
media projects 17, 126–8
medical assistance companies 158
medical crisis management 133–67
medical evacuation (medevac) 12–13, 24, 146, 153–6, 366–7, 722–3, 732–3
medical insurance 74–5
medical kits and supplies 42–3, 66–7, 86, 604–5, 648, 699, 716–17, 730, 787, 797–811
medical screening 21, 46–8, 712
medical training 44–5
medicines, seedrugs
Mediterranean boutonneuse fever 478–9
mefloquine 485–6
melatonin 323
melioidosis 472–3
meningitis 473
meningococcal meningitis 473
meningococcal meningitis vaccine 32
meniscal injuries 442
menstruation 410–11
mental illness 519
MERS-CoV 501
metatarsal fractures 446
methane 792
methoxyflurane 602
Mexican bearded lizard 560
Micropure™ tablets 104
microsporidiasis 504
Microsporum 296
midazolam 602
Middle East respiratory syndrome coronavirus 501
migraine 320–1
miliaria rubra (prickly heat) 63, 766
Millbank bags 103
millipedes 565

missing persons 140–2
mites 287
Mittelschmerz pain 394
MMR vaccine 28, 30
mobile phones 142, 613
molluscs 570
molluscum
    contagiosum 511, 512
Monge's disease 672–3
monitoring 175
monitor lizards 560
monkey pox virus 502
Mooncup® 411
moose 611
morphine 93–4, 95, 373
mosquito nets and
    repellents 484–5
moth stings 562
mountain lions 543
mountains 637–73, 809
mouth lacerations 304
mouthwashes 350
moving casualties 148–52
mucocutaneous
    leishmaniasis 490
muscarinic poisoning 582
muscle cramps 766
muscle knots 697
mushroom poisoning 582–3
Mycobacterium avium 477
Mycobacterium chelonae 477
Mycobacterium fortuitum
    477
Mycobacterium
    intracellulare 477
Mycobacterium leprae 477
Mycobacterium marinum 294,
    295, 477
Mycobacterium
    tuberculosis 475–6
Mycobacterium ulcerans 477
myiasis 289–91
myocardial infarction 371

N

Naegleria 294
nails 296, 297, 298, 434
Nairobi eye 562, 563
nasal foreign bodies 335
nasal fractures 308
nasal injuries 304
nasopharyngeal airway 187
navigation 612, 639, 678–9,
    680, 703, 747, 776
Necator 496
neck injuries 171, 198–201,
    304–5, 696, 697
needle fish 547
negligence 76–8
nematodes 496
nervous system 173

neurocysticercosis 319
neurogenic shock 235–6
neurotoxic shellfish
    poisoning 574–5
Nexplanon® 410
NEXUS guidelines 199–200
nifedipine 668
Nipah virus 502
nitrogen narcosis 734
nitrox 733
Nivaquine® 486
nocturnal enuresis 525
non-freezing cold injury 627,
    632, 696
non-maleficence 112
non-specific
    urethritis 507, 508
non-steroidal
    anti-inflammatory
    drugs 93–4, 95
norovirus 400
Norwegian scabies 287
nose
    bleeds 335
    foreign bodies 335
    fractures 308
    injuries 304
nursing care 88–90, 156
nutrition 650–3, 693, 708–9

O

obesity 56
observations 89–90
observations chart 232
obstructive jaundice 389
obstructive sleep apnoea
    syndrome 323
ocean voyages 701–24
octopus 570, 571
ocular first-aid kit 810
offshore 701–24
ointments 804
older travellers 58–60
olecranon bursitis 426
onchocerciasis 494, 495
onychomycosis 298
open fractures 195
operational debriefing 527
opioids 93–4, 538
optic nerve function 326
oral rehydration
    solution 65, 761–2
orbital cellulitis 330–1
orbital compartment
    syndrome 331
orbital fracture 308–10
orellanine poisoning 583
orf 297
oriental sore 490
Orientia
    tsutsugamushi 478–9, 503

oropharyngeal airway 187
otitis externa 334, 698, 742
otitis media 334
ovarian conditions 394
oxygen toxicity 735

P

Package Travel Regulations
    (1992) 17
paddy foot 632
pain control 93–4,
    95, 802–3
Paludrine® 486
pancreatitis 386, 389
panda eyes 313
panic disorder 522
paracetamol 93–4, 95
paralytic shellfish
    poisoning 574–6
paramyxoviruses 502
paratyphoid 477–8
paronychia 297
partial seizures 318
patella
    bursitis 440
    dislocation 441
    fracture 440, 442
    tendon rupture 442
patent foramen ovale 738
peccaries 545
Pediculus capitis 286
Pediculus humanus 286
pelvic fractures 195, 436–7
pelvic inflammatory
    disease 395
penetrating eye injuries
    329
penicillin allergy 236–7,
    265
penthrox 602
peptic ulcer 386, 388
perianal abscess 404–5
perianal haematoma 404
pericoronitis 350
periodic breathing 652–3
periods 410–11
peripheral nerve
    block 594–5
peritonsillar abscess 336
permissive hypotension
    195
personal accident
    insurance 75
personal clashes 114–15
personal flotation
    devices 686–7
personal hygiene 22, 88–9,
    109, 616, 709, 791
personal liability
    insurance 75
personal medical kit 800

personal survival kit 784
phagedenic ulcers 292
pharyngitis 336
photokeratitis (snow blindness) 327, 634–5
photorefractive keratectomy 325
physiotherapy 452–4
picaridin 771
pigs 545
piles 397, 698
pilonidal abscess 405
pin worms 497
piranhas 547
pityriasis 296
Pityrosporum orbiculare 296
plague 474
plantar fasciitis 447
plants 577–84, 772
Plesiomonas shigelloides 294
P-methane-3, 8-diol (PMD) 771
pneumococcal meningitis 474
pneumomediastinum 741
pneumothorax 190—192, 374, 740
poisoning
    carbon monoxide 615–16, 735
    fish and shellfish 574–6
    hydrogen sulphide 793
    plants and fungi 580–4
polar bears 543, 611
polar expeditions 607–36
poliomyelitis 459, 460
Portuguese man o'war 568–9
post-expedition issues 25, 60, 540
post-expedition medical 25
post-expedition medical questionnaire 21
post-immersion collapse syndrome 683
post-traumatic amnesia 312–13
post-traumatic stress disorder 530–1
pre-existing medical conditions 50–6
pregnancy
    diving 731
    malaria 488
preseptal cellulitis 331
pressure-immobilization 554–5
pressure-pad 554–5, 555
prickly heat 63, 766
prilocaine 590
primary assessment 214–15
private expeditions 17

professional clashes 114–15
professional indemnity insurance 75, 79
proguanil 486
Project Renala 122
prostatitis 408–9
protein 99
Prototheca spp. 294
protozoal infections 401
prowords 161
Pseudomonas aeruginosa 294, 297
psilocybin poisoning 582
psychiatric problems 55, 515–40
psychogenic blackouts 319
psychological debriefing 530–1
psychological first aid 527
psychological health screening 518–392
psychological issues 88, 515–40, 786
psychosis 523–4
pubic lice (*Pthirus pubis*) 286
public health 121
public liability insurance 75
puffer fish 574
Pulex irritans 286
pulmonary barotrauma 740–1
pulmonary embolus 235
pulse 174
puma 543
puncture wounds 276
PUR™ 105
putsi fly 289–90
pyelonephritis 406
pyogenic *Streptococcus* 294

Q

quadriceps tendon rupture 442
quinsy 336

R

rabies 458–69, 794
rabies vaccine 36
racing boats 707
radial keratotomy 325
radial pulse 174
radio communication 144–5, 162, 164
radius fractures 427, 428
rafting 695
ramus fracture 306
rapid primary assessment 214–15
RECCO® system 645

recovery position 226, 227
recreational drugs 538–9
rectal bleeding 396–7
rectal temperature 752–3
'red tide' 574–5, 693
refractive surgery 325
rehydration
    solutions 65, 761–2
relapsing fever 795
remote areas 2–3
renal colic 387, 407
repatriation 146, 158, 167
rescue, see search and rescue
respiratory drugs 803
respiratory problems, see breathing
respiratory rate 66, 175
resuscitation 216–18
retinal haemorrhages 332, 667
reverse drag 148, 149
reverse osmosis filters 105
Rhodoccus equi 503
rib fractures 372–3
Rickettsia spp. 478–9
Rift valley fever 468
ringworm 296
rip current 677
risk assessment and management 24, 68–73, 610, 639–40, 704, 728, 747, 774–5, 792–3
river blindness 494, 495
rivers 678
road traffic collisions 144–5
Rocky Mountain spotted fever 478–9
Romaña's sign 493
rope sling 151
rotator cuff injuries 423
rotavirus 400
round worm 496
Royal Geographical Society 18
rule of nines 280–1

S

sailing
    coastal waters 675–00
    offshore 701–24
St Anthony's fire 583
St Louis encephalitis 795
salmeterol 668
Salmonella 401
Salmonella paratyphi 477–8
Salmonella typhi 477–8, 503
salpingitis 387
salt 761–2
sanatorium 85

sanitary towels/
tampons 109, 411
sanitation 108–9, 617, 693,
709–10, 781, 791
Sarcoptes scabei 287
SARS 500
satellite beacons 142,
163–4, 613, 682
satellite phones 162–4
saturation diving 728
scabies mites 287
scalp lacerations 304
scaphoid fractures 428
scene management 144–5
schistosomiasis 319, 498,
499
scombroid poisoning 574
scorpion stings 564
screw worm flies 289–90
scrotal pain 408–9
scrub typhus 478–9, 503
scuba diving 727, 733, 793
sea anemones 568–9
sea expeditions
coastal waters 675–00
offshore 701–24
seal finger 294, 295
seals 611
sea nettle 568–9
search and rescue (SAR) 75,
139, 613, 643—644,
682–4, 704, 728,
776–7, 792
seasickness 697–9, 718
sea snakes 566, 567
sea urchin 570
sea wasp 568–9
secondary
survey 204—205, 215
sedation 602, 802–3
seizures 318–19
self-contained underwater
breathing apparatus
(scuba) 727, 733, 793
self-harm 519
septal haematoma 308
septic shock 234
settling tanks 103
severe acute respiratory syndrome (SARS) 500
sexual assault 165
sexually transmitted
infection 506–14
sharks 546
shellfish poisoning 574–6
shelter limb 632
Shigella 401
shock 228–40
shortness of breath 246–7
shoulder injuries 422–4, 696
sick bay 85
Siedel's test 329

sildenafil 668
silver compounds 104
Simmond's test 444
skier's thumb 431
skin 265–98, 579, 636, 699,
719, 795
ski pulks 614–15
sleep distur-
bances 322–3, 652–3
sleeping sickness 492
sling carry 151
slings 420, 421
snake bites 549, 550–9
snorkelling 727
snow blindness 327, 634–5
snow holes 615
sodium thiosulphate 104
solar skin
damage 266–7, 680
sore throat 336
Spanish fly 562, 563
Spaso method 422–3
spectacles 619
sphygmomanometer 174
spider bites 562
spilling waves 678
spinal anaesthesia 596–8
spinal injuries 198–201,
448—449
spitting cobra 559
splinters 277
splints 416, 417
sports drinks 761–2
standard of care 77
standby emergency
treatment 488
standing waves 678
Staphylococcus aureus
294, 400
antibiotic-resistant 503
PVL-positive strains 503
staples 273
starfish 570
*Stenotrophomonas
maltophilia* 503
Steripen™ 105
Steri-Strips™ 272
Stimson's method 423
stimulants 538
stinging bush 772
stingrays 568
stings and bites 63, 276,
284–5, 544, 550–72,
699, 770–1
'stoppers' 678
strangulated hernia 387, 393
strapping 452–4
Streptococcus pyogenes 503
stress 517, 520, 699, 786
stress fractures 446
stretchers 152
strongyloidiasis 496

subacromial bursitis 423
submersion 688
subungual haematoma 434
sucking chest wound 193
suicide attempts 519
sunblocks 63
sunburn 63, 266–7, 767
sun protection factor
(SPF) 267
sunscreens 63, 267
supraspinatus tendinitis 423
surfing 686–7
surgical airway 188
surging waves 678
suspension trauma 792
sutures 273, 274
sweating 751, 754–5, 782
swim failure 688
swimmer's itch 498
swimming 686–7
swine flu 502
Swiss field staging
system 622
symptomatic high-altitude
pulmonary hypertension
(SHAPH) 671
syncope 317, 319, 766
syphilis 510–11

T

Taenia spp. 499
talus fractures 446
tampons 109, 411
tapeworms 499
taping 452–4
team building 26
team medical kit 802–7
team selection 26
technical diving 728
teeth
avulsion 354–6
crowns and bridges
352–3
extractions 364–5
fillings 351
luxation 354
pre-departure
preparations 340–1
toothache 344–50
telemedicine 160–4
telephones 162
television
projects 17, 126–8
temporomandibular joint
dislocation 309–10
tendon injuries
Achilles 444
hand 432
knee 442
tennis elbow 426
tenosynovitis 428, 697

tension
  pneumothorax 190–1
testicular torsion 408
tetanus 475
tetrodotoxin poisoning 574
ThoraQuik® 191
thermometers 622–5, 753
thirst 760–2
throat 336
thrombolysis 629
thrush (candidiasis) 509
thumb dislocations 431
tibial fractures 443
tibial tuberosity
  fractures 442
tick-borne
  encephalitis 460–1
tick-borne encephalitis
  vaccine 37
ticks 288, 565
tidal river bores 678
tides 677
tied hands crawl 150–1
tigers 543
tinea 296
tinea pedis 298
tinea unguium 298
tinea versicolor 296
tissue glue 273
toe fractures and
  dislocations 446
toenails 296, 297
tongue injuries 304
tonsillitis 336
toothache 344–50;
  see also teeth
tourniquets 196
tracheostomy 188
tramadol 93–4, 95
tranexamic acid 195
trauma 179–209, 526–8,
  548, 718–19, 804–5
travel 612, 639, 643, 648–9,
  680, 727, 747, 774,
  775, 776–7
traveller's diarrhoea 400
travel package 17
trench foot 632
triage 182, 183, 184
Trichomonas vaginalis 509
Trichophyton 296
Trichuris 497
trombiculid mites 287
tropical forests 769–87, 808
tropical immersion foot 787
tropical ulcers 292
trypanosomiasis 492,
  493, 794
tsunami 679
tuberculosis 475–6

tuberculosis vaccine 37, 476
Tuffier's line 596
tumbu fly 289–90
Tunga penetrans 290
tungiasis 289–91
tungosis 290
tympanic membrane
  rupture 334
typhoid 402–3, 477–8
typhoid vaccine 38
typhus 478–9

U

UK International Emergency
  Trauma Register
  (UKIETR) 131
ulcerative colitis 54–5
ultraviolet radiation
  skin damage 266, 680
  water treatment 105
'umbles' 622–5
Uncinaria stenocephala 290
underground
  activities 789–95
underwater
  activities 725–43
upper arm injuries 422–4
upper gastrointestinal
  bleeding 396
upper respiratory tract 336
ureteric (renal)
  colic 387, 407
urethral discharge 507–8
urethritis 406
urinary
  retention 387, 406–7
urinary tract
  infection 406, 412
urine disposal 108
urological problems 406–7

V

vaccinations 28–40, 62
vaginal irritation/
  discharge 411, 508–9
Venezuelan haemorrhagic
  fever 466
venomous
  animals 549, 550–72
ver du cayor 289–90
ver macaque 289–90
VHF radios 164
Viagra® 668
Vibramycin® 486
vibrios 294
viral encephalitis 460–1
viral haemorrhagic
  fevers 464–9

viral hepatitis 458–9
viral infections 458–69,
  500–4
visceral leishmaniasis 490
visual loss 326
vomiting 398–403

W

wasp stings 560–1
water-borne disease 102–3,
  294–5, 687
water filters 105
water intake 102–7, 616,
  651, 760–2
'water in the ear' 698
water pumps 105
water purification 102–7
water's edge 676–7
water supplies 102–7, 616,
  651, 693, 708, 761, 781
waves 678
wave splash 688
weather 608, 639, 680, 702,
  726, 770
West Nile fever 461
wet bulb globe
  temperature 757–8
whale finger 294, 295
whip worm 497
white nose syndrome 793
whiteout 613
white-water rafting 695
whitlow 297
wilderness medicine 2–3
wildlife, see animal hazards
windchill index 608–11
windsurfing 686–7
wolves 544
workload 758
work references 518
worm infections 496–7
wounds 268–77
  infection 270, 278, 294–5
wrist injuries 428, 697

X

Xenopsylla spp. 286

Y

yellow fever 464
yellow fever vaccine 28,
  38–9, 464
yellow jackets 560–1

Z

zygomatic fractures 307–8